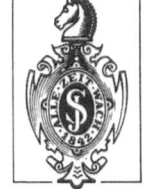

Ian J. Forbes   Anthony S-Y. Leong

Essential Oncology of the Lymphocyte

With 99 Figures

Springer-Verlag
London Berlin Heidelberg New York
Paris Tokyo

Ian J. Forbes, MB, BS, MD (Adel), FRACP, FRCPA
Reader in Medicine, University of Adelaide, and Senior Visiting
Medical Specialist, The Queen Elizabeth Hospital, Woodville, South
Australia.

Anthony S-Y. Leong, MB, BS, MD (Adel), FRCPA, FRCPath, FCAP
Director of Surgical Pathology, Institute of Medical and Veterinary
Science, Adelaide, and Clinical Reader, Department of Pathology,
University of Adelaide, South Australia.

ISBN-13:978-1-4471-1469-7   e-ISBN-13:978-1-4471-1467-3
DOI: 10.1007/978-1-4471-1467-3

British Library Cataloguing in Publication Data
Forbes, I. J.
Essential oncology of the lymphocyte.
1. Leukemia
I. Title   II. Leong, A.S-Y.
616.99'419 RC643
ISBN-13:978-1-4471-1469-7

Library of Congress Cataloging-in-Publication Data
Forbes, I. J. (Ian James), 1930–
Essential oncology of the lymphocyte.
Includes bibliographies and index.
1. Lymphomas. I. Leong, A. S.-Y. (Anthony Siew-Yin), 1945–. II. Title. [DNLM: 1.
Leukemia-pathology. 2. Lymphocytes-pathology. 3. Lymphoma-pathology. QZ 350
F693e] RC280.L9F57   1987   616.99'4   87–12734
ISBN-13:978-1-4471-1469-7 (U.S.)

©Springer-Verlag Berlin Heidelberg 1987
Softcover reprint of the hardcover 1st edition 1987

Filmset by H Charlesworth & Co Ltd, Huddersfield

To Jan and Wendy Guat, our wives.

Preface

This book has been written from two points of view: firstly, from the viewpoint of those who are involved in the diagnosis and treatment of lymphoid malignancies, who must meet the challenge of integrating the new biological insights into their knowledge of these diseases; and secondly, from the viewpoint of those who are involved in basic biological approaches to malignancy and immunology, who wish to know more about the function of the lymphoid tissues and their malignant diseases.

Neoplasia of lymphocytes is a focus for considering many of the most important biological advances impinging on cancer in the past two or three decades, because malignant lymphoproliferative diseases offer unequalled opportunities for studying many aspects of cancer. We probably know more about lymphocytes than other normal cells because of the ease with which they can be obtained. For the same reason we probably know more about malignant lymphocytes. One or other aspect of most of the momentous advances in biology of the past two or three decades has implications for lymphoid malignancies: hybridoma technology and the use of monoclonal antibodies, gene technology, the understanding of oncogenes and growth factors in the control of growth and differentiation, insights into causation of cancer by potent tumour promoters such as the phorbol esters and by viruses, and knowledge of the control of growth function of lymphocytes themselves. Conversely, many of the advances in understanding lymphocytic leukaemias and lymphomas have implications for other cancers.

The way pathologists and clinicians look at chronic lymphocytic leukaemia and malignant lymphomas has been changing rapidly in the past two decades, and greater changes are imminent. Diagnosis of the malignant lymphoproliferative diseases was made on a combination of clinical and histological features until the 1960s, when a new basis for comprehending lymphomas began to develop out of the rapidly expanding investigation of the immune system. Determination of immunological phenotypes in the 1970s showed that lymphoid malignancies represented proliferations of subsets of the lymphocytes and sometimes of the monocyte-macrophage lineage, thus adding to the precision of diagnosis and classification. The next step was to consider the lymphoproliferative malignancies in functional terms. Monoclonal antibodies were quickly used to classify the lymphoproliferative diseases and to characterise maturation stages. Genetic probes, already in widespread use, open up greater possibilities. They may show the presence of viral genomes, demonstrate the cell lineage and reveal the normal and abnormal activity of oncogenes and genes encoding growth factors. These new technologies bring a new dimension to the study of processes occurring within normal and malignant lymphoid follicles, rapidly changing the interpretation of lymphoid tissue pathology. Epstein–Barr virus, in Burkitt's lymphoma, and the two recently discovered human T leukaemia/lymphoma viruses, HTLV-I and HTLV-III (now renamed HIV), associated with adult T cell leukaemia/lymphoma (ATL) and the acquired immunodeficiency syndrome (AIDS), respectively, have presented an unprecedented stimulus to investigation of the viral pathogenesis of cancer in man.

The ultimate aim of prevention and cure will be achieved only by understanding the diseases. While this may seem daunting, the discoveries of recent years give cause for real excitement and optimism.

Acknowledgments

We thank Prof. Dr. H. Kirchner, Prof. Dr. L. Gissmann, Prof. Dr. M. Pawlita and Dr. V. Kinzel of the Deutsches Krebsforschungs- zentrum, Heidelberg; Dr. B. Dörken and Dr. A. Pezzuto of the Universitätspoliklinik, Heidelberg; Dr. Andrea Mastro, Department of Microbiology, Pennsylvania State University; Dr. Judy Layton, Ludwig Institute for Cancer Research, Melbourne; Dr. Judith Ford, Department of Genetics, Dr. Graeme Russ, Renal Unit, and Dr. Prudence Cowled, Department of Medicine, The Queen Elizabeth Hospital, Woodville, for help with sections of the manuscript, Mrs. Lorraine McKenzie for the graphic illustrations and Miss I. Doskatsch, Librarian of the Queen Elizabeth Hospital, for help with references.

Adelaide, 1987   Ian J. Forbes
                                                                               Anthony S-Y. Leong

Contents

Abbreviations

AC   accessory cells
ABC   avidin-biotin peroxidase complex
ACTH   adrenocorticotrophic hormone
ADA   adenosine deaminase
ADCC   antibody-dependent cell-mediated cytotoxicity
AEC   3-amino-9-ethylcarbazole
AEF   allogeneic effector factor
AET   amino-ethylisothiouronium bromide
AEV   avian erythroblastosis virus
AIDS   acquired immunodeficiency syndrome
AIHA   autoimmune haemolytic anaemia
ALL   acute lymphoblastic leukaemia
ALV   avian leukosis virus
AML   acute myeloblastic leukaemia
AMP   adenosine monophosphate
A-MuLV   Abelson murine leukaemia virus
AMV   avian myeloblastosis virus
ANAE   α-naphthyl acetate esterase
ANLL   acute non-lymphocytic leukaemia
APC   antigen-presenting cell
APUD   amine precursor uptake and decarboxylation
AT   ataxia telangiectasia
ATL   adult T cell leukaemia/lymphoma
ATLA   ATL-antigen
ATP   adenine triphosphate
ATPase   adenine triphosphatase
AZT   3'-azido-3'-deoxythymidine
BALB-MSV   BALB mouse sarcoma virus
BCDF   B cell differentiation factor
BCG   Bacille Calmette-Guérin
BCGF   B cell growth factor

BEF   B cell-derived enhancing factor
BFU-E   burst-forming cell (erythrocytic)
BL   Burkitt's lymphoma
BLV   bovine leukaemia virus
BMF   B cell maturation factor
BrUdR   bromodeoxyuridine
BSF   B cell stimulatory factor
C_H constant region of immunoglobulin heavy chain
C_L constant region of immunoglobulin light chain
C3b   component of complement
C3bi   component of complement
CALLA   common acute lymphoblastic leukaemia antigen
cAMP   cyclic adenosine 3',5'-cyclic monophosphate
CCAD   chronic cold agglutinin disease
CD   cluster of differentiation (antigen specificity)
cDNA   complementary DNA
cGMP   cyclic guanosine monophosphate
cIg   cytoplasmic immunoglobulin
CLL   chronic lymphocytic leukaemia
CML   cell-mediated lympholysis
CML   chronic myelogenous leukaemia
CMP   cytidine monophosphate
C_μ cytoplasmic μ immunoglobulin
con A   concanavalin A
CR   complement receptor
CRPV   cottontail rabbit papillomavirus
CSF   colony-stimulating factor
CTCL   cutaneous T cell lymphoma
CTL   cytotoxic T lymphocyte
CVID   common variable immunodeficiency
D   immunoglobulin diversity gene
DAB   3,3-diaminobenzidine tetra-hydrachloride
DAG   diacylglycerol
dCF   deoxycoformycin
DHL   diffuse histiocytic lymphoma
DMBA   dimethylbenzanthracene
dmin   double minute chromosomes
DMSO   dimethyl sulphoxide
DNA   deoxyribonucleic acid
DP, DQ, DR   major histocompatibility gene regions
DRC   dendritic reticulum cell
DTH   delayed type hypersensitivity
E   erythrocyte (usually sheep erythrocyte if unqualified)

EBNA EBV-associated nuclear antigen
EBV Epstein–Barr virus
EGF epidermal growth factor
ER erythrocyte (usually sheep) receptor
F(ab)$_2$ fragment of antibody containing antibody-combining sites
FACS flourescence-activated cell sorter
FBJ-MSV FBJ osteosarcoma virus
Fc fragment of antibody containing constant regions
FcR Fc receptor
FeLV feline leukaemia virus
FeSV feline sarcoma virus
FITC fluorescein isothiocyanate
G$_0$ zero growth phase of the cell cycle
G$_1$ first phase of the cell growth cycle
G-binding protein guanine triphosphate binding proteins
G-CSF granulocyte colony-stimulating factor
GDP guanosine diphosphate
G6PD glucose-6-phosphate dehydrogenase
GM-CSF granulocyte-macrophage colony-stimulating factor
GTP guanosine triphosphate
GVHR graft versus host reaction
H heavy chain of immunoglobulin
H-2 major histocompatibility system in mice
HaSV Harvey murine sarcoma virus
HBsAg hepatitis B surface antigen
HBV hepatitis B virus
HCD heavy chain diseases
HCL hairy cell leukaemia
HD Hodgkin's disease
HIV human immunodeficiency virus (new name for HTLV-III)
HLA human leucocyte A (old name for histocompatibility complex)
HLA-A, HLA-B MHC class I loci
HLA-D, HLA-DR MHC class II loci
HMG high motility group
^{3}H-PDBu tritiated phorbol dibutyrate
HPV human papilloma virus
HSR homogeneously staining regions
HTLV human T cell leukaemia/lymphoma virus
HVT herpesvirus of turkeys
Ia immunity-associated (old term used for MHC class II)
IBL immunoblastic lymphadenopathy
IDRC interdigitating reticulum cell
IFN interferon

Ig   immunoglobulin
IGF-I   insulin-like growth factor I
IGF-II   insulin-like growth factor II
IL-1   interleukin 1
IL-2   interleukin 2
IP$_3$ inositol triphosphate
IPSID   immunoproliferative small intestinal disease
Ir gene   immune response gene
IVS   intervening sequence of DNA between J and C genes
J   joining gene linking D and J genes
J$_L$ light chain joining gene
kD   kilodalton
KiSV   Kirsten murine sarcoma virus
L   light chain of immunoglobulin
LAF   lymphocyte activating factor
LAK   lymphokine-activated killer
LCA   leucocyte common antigen
LFA-1   lymphocyte-function-associated-1
LGL   large granular lymphocyte
LIF   leucocyte inhibitory factor
LL   lymphoblastic lymphoma
LPS   (bacterial) lipopolysaccharide
LSCL   lymphosarcoma cell leukaemia
LTR   long terminal repeat
MAF   macrophage activating factor
MALT   mucosa-associated lymphoid tissue, GALT
M-CSF   monocyte colony-stimulating factor
MDP   muramyl-L-alanyl-D-isoglutamine peptide
2 ME   2-mercaptoethanol
MEM   minimum essential medium
MER   mouse erythrocyte receptor
MESA   myoepithelial sialadenitis
MF   mycosis fungoides
MGUS   monoclonal gammopathy of undetermined significance
MHC   major histocompatibility complex
MIF   migration inhibition factor
MLR   mixed lymphocyte reaction
Mo-MSV   Moloney murine sarcoma virus
Mo-MuLV   Moloney leukaemogenic virus
mRNA   messenger RNA
MSV   murine sarcoma virus
Multi-CSF   multi-colony-stimulating factor
MuLV   murine leukaemia virus

MuSV   murine sarcoma virus
NBTCL   node-based T cell lymphoma
NCI   nuclear contour index
NGF   nerve growth factor
NHL   non-Hodgkin's lymphoma
NK   natural killer
NMU   nitroso-methyl-urea
NPC   nasopharyngeal carcinoma
NSE   non-specific esterase
OAG   oleoylaceylglycerol
PAP   peroxidase-antiperoxidase
PAS   periodic-acid Schiff
PBA   polyclonal B cell activator
PBS   phosphate-buffered saline
PC   phosphatidylcholine
PDBu   phorbol dibutyrate
PDD   phorbol didecanoate
PDGF   platelet-derived growth factor
PE   phosphatidylethanolamine
PHA   phytohaemagglutinin
PI   phosphatidylinositol
PIP$_2$ PI 4, 5-biphophate
PKC   protein kinase C
PLL   prolymphocytic leukaemia
PNA   peanut agglutinin
PS   phosphatidylserine
PWM   pokeweed mitogen
R2   second receptor for mouse erythrocytes
RadLV   radiation leukaemia virus
RaSV   Rasheed sarcoma virus
RES   reticuloendothelial system
RFLP   restriction fragment length polymorphism
RNA   ribonucleic acid
RPA   12-retinoylphorbol-13-acetate
RPMI 1640   Roswell Park Memorial Institute 1640 (culture medium)
RSV   Rous sarcoma virus
SAC   *Staphylococcus aureus* Cowan strain 1
SAF   stem cell activating factor
SB   MHC class II gene region
SCID   severe combined immunodeficiency
sIg   surface immunoglobulin
SIRS   soluble immune response suppressor
SPA   staphylococcal protein A

SS   Sézary syndrome
SSV   simian sarcoma virus
STLV   simian T lymphoma/leukaemia virus
SV40   simian vacuolating virus 40
TAF   T cell activating factor
T-ALL   T acute lymphoblastic leukaemia
TCGF   T cell growth factor
T-CLL   T cell chronic lymphocytic leukaemia
TD   thymus-dependent
TdT   terminal deoxynucleotidyl transferase
ter   telomere
$\mathbf{T_\gamma}$ T cell subset possessing Fc_γ receptors
$\mathbf{TGF_\alpha}$ transforming growth factor alpha
$\mathbf{TGF_\beta}$ transforming growth factor beta
T-HCL   T hairy cell leukaemia
TI   thymus-independent
T-IBS   T immunoblastic sarcoma
T-LL   T lymphoblastic lymphoma
$\mathbf{T_\mu}$ T cell subset possessing Fc_μ receptors
TNF   tumour necrosis factor
TNP   trinitrophenol
TPA   12-*O*-tetradecanoylphorbol-13-acetate
T-PLL   T prolymphocytic leukaemia
TRAP   tartrate-resistant acid phosphatase
TRF   T cell replacing factor
TSeF   T suppressor effector factor
TSiF   T suppressor inducer factor
$\mathbf{V_H}$ variable region of immunoglobulin heavy chain
$\mathbf{V_L}$ variable region of immunoglobulin light chain
WDLL   well-differentiated lymphocytic lymphoma

1 Cancer Biology

Introduction

With the accumulating knowledge about all kinds of cancer, a number of important concepts have evolved. These relate to the manner in which neoplasia commences and to the behaviour of malignant cells (Table 1.1). The concepts apply both to lymphoid as well as non-lymphoid malignancy. Cancers of lymphocytes have been particularly important in confirming and illustrating some of these concepts.

Cancer cells proliferate inappropriately, accumulate locally, invade the surrounding tissues and release cells that generate new collections of proliferating cells in distant sites. All of these properties are possessed by malignant lymphocytes, although there are other subtle differences between solid tumours and leukaemias.

Malignant tumours frequently have benign counterparts, for example an adenomatous polyp is a benign counterpart of carcinoma of the colon. Benign tumours become malignant. There are benign counterparts of some lymphoid

Table 1.1. Some concepts applying generally to cancer

1. A cancer develops from a single cell, and therefore
2. A cancer represents expansion of a monoclonal population
3. New subclones develop constantly throughout the life of a cancer, as a result of mutation and other changes in the genome
4. The fundamental abnormality of malignant cells is abnormal regulation of proliferation and differentiation, resulting from abnormalities of the genome
5. Cancers develop from stem cells which differentiate to some extent, rather than from mature cells which dedifferentiate
6. The ultimate cause of cancer is an abnormality of the genome. Abnormality of gene regulation is an essential part of this abnormality of the genome
7. Arrest of differentiation is an essential component of the biology of cancers
9. The aetiology of cancers is usually mutifactorial
10. The development of most cancers is a multistep process
11. Cancers become progressively more malignant

malignancies, such as benign monoclonal lymphocytosis (versus chronic lympho-cytic leukaemia, CLL) and·benign monoclonal gammopathy (versus multiple myeloma).

Solid tumours generally rely heavily on ingrowth of benign stromal elements. When experimental cancers are passaged in animals, the stromal tissues of the new growths are derived from the hosts and not from the donors. Cancer cells from rapidly proliferating tumours grow only sparsely in vitro, presumably because they lack the support of mesodermal tissues and growth factors derived from the host.

How do leukaemias differ from solid tumours? Leukaemic cells do not require a fixed relationship to the supporting stroma. However, leukaemias probably have a tissue-based malignant stem cell population. This population may require support for growth, either from mesodermal tissues, or in the form of diffusible growth factors secreted by the mesodermal stroma. Circulating leukaemic cells may be rather inert, as, for example, in CLL. This inertia may be due partly to qualities of the malignant cells themselves, but their environment in the blood may also lack stimuli for growth and activation.

It has been suggested that fewer genetic changes may be required for the development of leukaemia as opposed to solid cancers (Temin 1984). A normal lymphocyte is already invasive and metastatic, but differs from a neoplastic cell in that its proliferation is under rigid control by external factors.

Development of Cancers from Single Cells

Cancers are believed to develop from single cells (Klein and Klein 1985). Leukaemias and solid tumours can be transferred in experimental animals by inoculation of a single cell. No two tumours are exactly alike, even if induced by the same agent, in the same type of target cell of the same inbred host (Klein 1984). This uniqueness of each cancer has been a strong argument that each cancer arises in one cell.

It may be thought that if a cancer begins from a single cell, all of the progeny of that cell should be the same. They would all belong to the same clone, or to express it in another way, cancers should be monoclonal. However, there is a possibility of change in some of the the progeny, in the same way as the original cancer cell changed to become malignant. All multicellular organisms derive from a single cell, but during the process of development very distinct subclones develop, giving rise to cells with different appearance (phenotype) and function. A strict definition of monoclonality is that every cell is genetically identical, that is, that each cell in the clone has the same genes (genotype). This cannot be deduced from the phenotype, because different genes are expressed during different phases of the growth and differentiation of cells. Both proliferation and differentiation result from an orderly expression of genes. Cells of a single clone may not be phenotypically identical if they are not in the same phase of the cell cycle, because all cells express some different characteristics at different phases of the cell cycle. Similarly, cells of the same clone may not look the same if cells of the clone undergo differentiation. As an example, both normal and malignant clones of lymphocytes may contain undifferentiated and well-differentiated members.

Several techniques have been used to study whether tumours are monoclonal:

1. *Karyotype assays*, especially G banding.

2. *Estimation of DNA frequency distributions*, by showing a distinct peak in preparations of aneuploid cells.

3. *Demonstration of the identity of gene products*, e.g. isoenzymes of glucose-6-phosphate dehydrogenase (G6PD), and immunoglobulins. Evidence of monoclonality comes from studies of the isoenzymes of G6PD, encoded on the X chromosome. In all female cells either the maternal or the paternal X chromosome is randomly inactivated and remains inactivated throughout subsequent generations. As a result, all progeny of a cell, constituting a clone, have either an active paternal or maternal X chromosome. If the two X chromosomes differ at a given locus, the product of that genetic locus in an individual cell will depend upon which X chromosome is active in that cell. One such gene on the X chromosome encodes the enzyme G6PD. The gene exists in slightly differing forms, alleles A and B, which encode enzymes with slightly differing amino acid sequences, recognisable by differing electrophoretic mobilities. The presence in tumours of either enzyme type A or type B only, when tissues of the host express both, i.e. in heterozygotes, is taken as evidence of clonal origin of the tumour. Theoretically, at least, a tumour could produce two isoenzymes if it arose before X-inactivation.

Benign tumours considered monoclonal on the basis of G6PD typing are uterine fibroids, common warts and thyroid adenomas; malignant tumours considered monoclonal on this basis include melanoma, some diffuse B cell lymphomas, carcinomas of the cervix and thyroid, chronic myelogenous leukaemia, Burkitt's lymphoma and polycythaemia.

4. *Comparison of the properties of clones derived in culture from single cells* (so-called clonogenic assays).

5. *Molecular DNA analysis.* Genetic analysis can now be carried out on cells from females heterozygous at the G6PD locus. If the alleles differ, they may be found on DNA restriction fragments differing in size and having differing degrees of methylation (Wainscoat and Thien 1985).

Monoclonality of lymphoid neoplasms can be determined in several ways. The least satisfactory is determination of surface markers and antigens reacting with monoclonal antibodies. Expression in B lymphomas of the same immunoglobulin light chain, either κ or λ, by all of the neoplastic cells is good, but still presumptive, evidence of monoclonality. The most powerful demonstration uses the techniques of molecular genetic analysis. When a lymphocyte arises from a stem cell, the genes for its specific antigen receptors undergo a rearrangement to form the gene encoding its individual receptor. Each gene formed in this way is unique for the individual lymphocyte. All progeny of a lymphocyte inherit the unique configuration of the receptor gene. A population of lymphocytes can be shown unequivocally to be progeny of a single lymphocyte by demonstrating that they all have the same configuration in the genes encoding their antigen receptors. There is no guarantee, however, that cells bearing this mark of inheritance do not undergo mutation in other genes. To prove monoclonality, in the strictest sense, it would be necessary to show that all of the genes of the population are the same. The ultimate evidence would be DNA base sequence identity of the whole genome of all cells in a tumour.

Some doubt has been expressed as to the monoclonality of neuroendocrine (amine precursor uptake and decarboxylation, APUD) tumours (Pearse 1985). These tumours may secrete several peptides and amines. It is difficult to explain how different tumours in one patient may produce different peptides and amines, if they belong to the same clone. It has been argued that all of the tumours in the one patient possess the same genes, which constitute a large family of related genes (a "multigene family") but express them differently, depending on their site. Put another way, the phenotypic difference may depend on different expression of genes in response to different environmental influences.

It is now believed that tumours are not truly monoclonal (Yarbro 1985). The evolution of a tumour results in the successive appearance of subclones (Fig. 1.1). These subclones will still have most of the properties of the original unique malignant cell from which they are derived. The subclones arise because of a change in some part of the genome, a mutation. Genetic analysis of the non-immunoglobulin genes should show differences in different subclones, but each new, more malignant, subclone developing during the life of a B cell tumour will still bear the trade-mark, as it were, of the unique immunoglobulin rearrangement, showing that it is a close relative of the original clone.

Some tumours are made up of more than one major clone, as in lymphoid tumours developing in immunosuppressed persons. Field changes, reflected by dysplasia and metaplasia, lead to the development of successive primary tumours in the bladder, bronchi, skin and elsewhere. It is possible for many cells to undergo

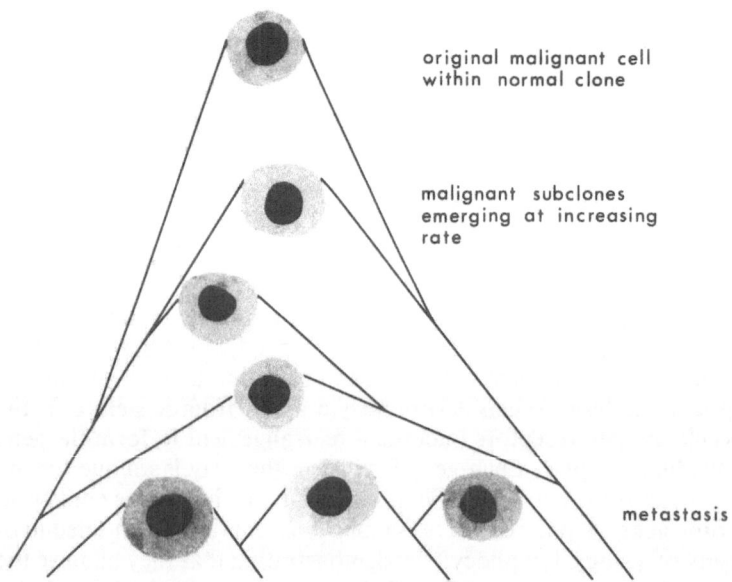

original malignant cell within normal clone

malignant subclones emerging at increasing rate

metastasis

Fig. 1.1. Heterogeneity of a cancer. The progeny of the original malignant cell from which a cancer arises constitute the first clone. Within this clone mutant cells arise from which dominant subclones develop, having a survival advantage, through, for example, faster division or through a longer survival of the individual cells. Some clones may have potential to metastasise. Treatment, such as chemotherapy, selects out clones having a survival advantage in the presence of the drug. This evolutionary process occurs in all cancers, leading to progression of the malignancy.

the initial step towards malignant transformation, but usually the progeny of only one emerges as clinically evident tumour. Biclonal B cell lymphomas have been identified occasionally, with two subpopulations of tumour cells, each producing a different immunoglobulin molecule (Sklar et al. 1984; Wolfe and Borowitz 1984). Two populations of malignant lymphocytes have occasionally been identified in one patient by staining with anti-idiotype antibodies, and the distinctness of the malignant populations has been confirmed by demonstrating distinct, unique immunoglobulin chain gene rearrangements. Rearrangement of immunoglobulin genes can only occur once per allele. Analysis of immunoglobulin chain gene rearrangements has shown that more than one malignant clone may exist in lymphomas arising in severely immunosuppressed recipients of cardiac transplants (Cleary and Sklar 1984).

Diversity of Tumour Cells

Apart from the diversity resulting from supporting, non-malignant cells within a tumour, diversity is a feature of cancers and represents the evolution of progressive cancer (Fig. 1.1). This diversity is the fundamental reason for failure of treatment of advanced cancer. Subclones arise constantly during chemotherapy, with new or differing enzyme patterns enabling them to resist the lethal effects of chemotherapeutic drugs. The resistance of these subclones is based on genetic changes, particularly gene amplification (Goldie and Coldman 1985).

Metastases show this clonal diversity. Metastases which colonise particular organs preferentially can be selected from tumours in experimental animals. Metastatic cells will show distinctive features identifying them as progeny of a single cell, but will differ genetically from the parent cell in some respects.

In summary, new subclones emerge successively which may replace the old, or may colonise new territory. This is a logical extension of the concept of the multistep origin of cancers, discussed in Chapter 4.

Differentiation of Malignant Cells

Cancer cells have long been described as dedifferentiated, as if they started from a fully differentiated cell and became progressively less differentiated as the tumour develops. Actually, when tumour cells arise they are immature and they become mature, i.e. differentiate to some extent. As time passes, tumours often become less differentiated, because of the increasing failure of the progeny of the malignant stem cells to differentiate.

The idea of dedifferentiation presupposes that a cell can go backwards in the differentiation sequence, but this is highly improbable. The rearrangement of receptor genes that occurs when a lymphocyte arises from its stem cell appears to be stable and irreversible. In the case of a B cell the receptor is immunoglobulin and in the case of the T cell it is the newly recognised Ti receptor. Reversion of Ig or Ti receptor genes back to the germline state appears not to occur in lymphoid tumours.

One important problem is to recognise the cells which are the targets for malignant transformation. In epithelial tumours an origin in dysplastic cells can often be assumed with reasonable confidence. Removal of dysplastic epithelium prevents the development of the cancer. One cell within a field of abnormal cells eventually takes the final step to the malignant state. It is surprising that multiple primary tumours are not observed more frequently. Nevertheless, many cancers arise from markedly abnormal epithelia, for example in the mouth, bronchial mucosa and bladder. A second cancer arises within 12 months of treatment of a primary bladder carcinoma in 10% of cases. Studies of the epithelium of the uterine cervix show a pattern of progression from dysplasia, to carcinoma in situ, to invasive carcinoma over a period of 10–20 years.

The target cells for malignant transformation in the lymphocytic malignancies have not been recognised with any certainty (Foon et al. 1982). They must arise at a stage of lymphoid differentiation at which rearrangement of receptor genes has taken place. Otherwise it would not be possible to show that they are tumours of lymphocytes. Cells of the tumour inherit the unique receptor gene rearrangement of its progenitor.

The state of differentiation attained by malignant cells in solid cancers as well as leukaemias is not fixed, either within a population at any one time, or from time to time. In pre-B acute lymphoblastic leukaemia (ALL), variable numbers of cells synthesising cytoplasmic μ immunoglobulin chains ($c\mu+$ cells) are found (Greaves et al. 1980), indicating a variable degree of maturation. The state of differentiation of the population of malignant cells in chronic lymphocytic leukaemia also varies in a given patient from time to time, and the average extent of differentiation may change during the course of the disease. This shift is usually towards a more undifferentiated state, although change to a greater degree of differentiation is also seen in B cell leukaemias.

It has been suggested that a malignant tumour arises from a more primitive cell than does a benign tumour (Pierce 1983). This idea, however, raises difficulties in explaining the development of a malignant tumour from a benign tumour. We cannot be sure that the malignant cell develops from one of the cells of the benign neoplasm, but it seems highly likely. According to Pierce, benign tumours are multiclonal and the less malignant clones initially enjoy a growth advantage. The malignant clone develops later from a minor clone within the benign tumour. All clones have developed originally from a single precursor.

The fundamental point, however, is that the cells from which cancers grow are relatively undifferentiated, having the potential to multiply continuously while retaining some capacity to differentiate. Tumours must contain stem cells that are capable of "self renewal", which means that when they divide, one of the progeny goes on to proliferate and mature, while the other stays in the same undifferentiated state as its precursor. Most cell types have a relatively short life span after they reach full maturity. If there were no stem cell population there would be a relentless drift towards maturity and all clones would eventually die out.

Although the fundamental characteristic of malignant cells is disordered growth, i.e. abnormally regulated proliferation and differentiation, cancers still require support for growth. This support is not merely the supply of nutrients. Growth is a highly coordinated process, resulting from interplay between the environment and the cell. The abnormality in this interplay could lie either in the environment or in the cell. In subsequent chapters we will discuss the concept that the abnormality in established cancers lies in the genome. This abnormality involves particularly the responses of malignant cells to growth factors in the environment. On the other hand, the malignant state usually arises from environmental influences on the genome, often as a result of damage over many cell generations.

References

Cleary ML, Sklar J (1984) Lymphoproliferative disorders in cardiac transplant recipients are multiclonal lymphomas. Lancet II: 489–493

Foon KA, Schroff RW, Gale RP (1982) Surface markers on leukemia and lymphoma cells: recent advances. Blood 60: 1–19

Goldie JH, Coldman AJ (1985) Genetic instability in the development of drug resistance. Semin Oncol 12: 222–230

Greaves M, Verbi W, Volger L (1980) Antigenic and enzymatic phenotypes of the pre-B subclass of acute lymphoblastic leukaemia. Leuk Res 3: 353–362

Klein G (1984) Cooperation of oncogenes in B-cell neoplasia. Introductory remarks. Curr Top Microbiol Immunol 113: 1–5

Klein G, Klein E (1985) Evolution of tumours and the impact of molecular oncology. Nature 315: 190–195

Pearse AGE (1985) Clonality and endocrine peptide (APUD) tumours. In: Polak JM, Bloom SR (eds) Endocrine tumours. Churchill Livingstone, Edinburgh, pp 82–93

Pierce GB (1983) The cancer cell and its control by the embryo. Am J Pathol 113: 117–123

Sklar J, Cleary ML, Thielmans K, Grawlow J, Warnke R, Levy R (1984) Biclonal B cell lymphoma. N Engl J Med 311: 20–27

Temin HM (1984) Do we understand the genetic mechanisms of oncogenesis? Keynote address for Honey Harbor meeting on cellular and molecular biology of neoplasia, 2–6 October, 1983. J Cell Physiol Suppl 3: 1–11

Wainscoat JS, Thien SL (1985) Polymorphism in human DNA: application to cancer studies. Trends Biochem Sci 10: 474–476

Wolfe JA, Borowitz MJ (1984) Composite lymphoma: a unique case with two immunologically distinct B cell neoplasms. Am J Clin Pathol 81: 526–528

Yarbro JW (1985) Introduction. Heterogeneity and new biology. Semin Oncol 12: 201–222 (editorial)

2　Derangement of the Genome as a Cause of Cancer

Introduction

Cancer is the result of malignant transformation of the genome of an individual cell which is passed on to its progeny. The ultimate cause of cancer is an abnormality of the genome. Several kinds of abnormality may be involved: abnormal regulation, i.e. over- or underactivation of genes, failure of expression of genes, or alteration of a gene resulting in a product that vitally affects cell function.

The mechanism by which cancer arises is mutation, in the broadest sense, i.e. damage to individual DNA base sequences of nucleotides, or addition, deletion, translocation or transposition of parts of chromosomes. DNA is constantly exposed to the risk of damage, both from the noxious agents in the environment and from spontaneous degeneration. The outcome of damage to DNA depends on the fidelity and completeness of physiological repair processes. Errors can also occur during replication. Non-lethal damage, followed by repair with a change in nucleotide sequence, constitutes a mutation that will persist in any descendant cells. It is highly likely that most mutations represent errors in DNA introduced during the process of repair after some type of damage by physical or chemical agents (Burnet 1982).

The best studied mutations are those affecting the DNA of structural genes that encode identifiable protein products such as enzymes or fixed structures of the cell. These mutations are manifested as changes in the amino acid sequence of the gene products. However, some three-quarters of the DNA in the mammalian genome does not code for recognisable proteins and is probably involved in controlling the function of the genome, for example in the initiation of synthesis of RNA copies. This regulatory DNA is replicated by the same processes as structural DNA and is presumably subject to the same risks of mutation.

The first step in chemical carcinogenesis, initiation, involves an alteration of a gene or genes. The potent tumour promoter 12-O-tetradecanoylphorbol-13-acetate (TPA), discussed in Chapter 4 (see p. 29), may cause chromosomal aberrations. Further genomic damage may occur during the progression of a tumour. Abnormalities of large segments of the genome seem to be involved in the common cancers (Cairns 1981), rather than mutations of a few base pairs. As an example, asbestos, unequivocally a carcinogen, produces major chromosomal abnormalities, but is not mutagenic in the sense of causing damage to a few base pairs. Nevertheless, a carcinogen may initiate the malignant process by causing a point mutation in an oncogene. Oncogenes, discussed in Chapter 6, are genes that are activated during the growth and development of cells. Burnet (1982) proposed that carcinogenesis is the accumulation of a series of genetic errors over a period of years in successive cell generations of a clonal line of cells.

The Chromosomes

The human karyotype consists of 22 pairs of autosomal chromosomes and a pair of sex chromosomes (XX in females and XY in males). The autosomes are named 1 to 22 in order of decreasing size, with the single exception of 22 and 21 (21 being smaller than 22). The short arm of each chromosome is delineated by the symbol "p" and the long arm by "q" (Fig. 2.1). Chromosomes are conventionally arranged in nominated pairs, with the p arms uppermost, and ordered 1 to 22. Such an arranged karyotype is called a karyogram.

Banding techniques make possible the identification of every chromosome in the human karyotype. Cells of tumours may be harvested directly or cultured for varying periods before being arrested in metaphase by a microtubule inhibitor such as colchicine. Metaphase spreads are prepared by hypotonic rupture of cells, which are then spread on glass slides and treated in various ways to produce a banding pattern. The karyotype of malignant cells can be compared with the

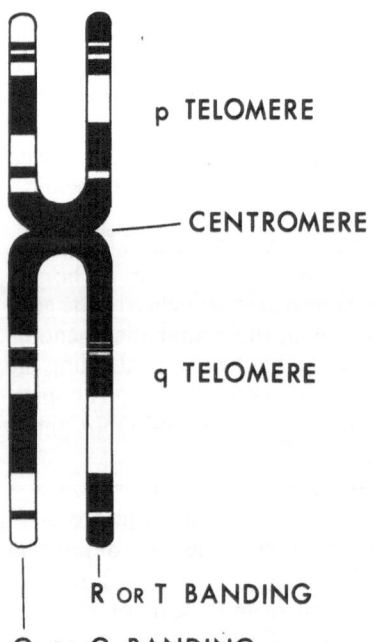

p TELOMERE

CENTROMERE

q TELOMERE

R OR T BANDING

Q OR G BANDING

Fig. 2.1. Nomenclature of the chromosome: *Q*, quinacrine; *G*, Giemsa; *R*, reverse; *T*, terminal; *p*, the short arm; *q*, the long arm. The central, joined portion is known as the *centromere*.

constitutional karyotype of peripheral blood T cells (in which mitosis has been induced by phytohaemagglutinin), fibroblasts or other non-malignant cells.

With the development of these banding techniques in the early 1970s there was a need for a nomenclature which would define both the regions of each chromosome and the types of arrangements which could occur. The details of the nomenclature are outlined in the Report of the 1971 Paris Conference (1972), although further refinements have since been made (Harnden et al. 1981). According to this nomenclature, chromosome bands are numbered from the centromere, as band 1, to the distal telomere (ter). Metaphase band regions seen in the most contracted state of the chromosome can be resolved, when the chromosome is in a less contracted state, into further smaller bands which are also numbered from the centromere. As an example, band 22q11 should be read as the small band, within region 1, closest to the centromere on the long arm of chromosome 22.

Translocations are written with the prefix "t" and the chromosomes involved in the translocation are bracketed in order of size and separated by semicolons. In the most commonly used shorthand nomenclature, a second bracket encloses the breakpoints of the translocations as they apply, in order, to each of the nominated chromosomes. As an example the translocation, discussed on p. 16, which gives rise to the Philadelphia chromosome in chronic myelogenous leukaemia (CML), is written t(9;22)(q34;q11).

In translocations involving two acrocentric chromosomes, i.e. chromosomes having centromeres near the end, it is possible to form either dicentric or monocentric chromosomes. When a chromosome is monocentric it may be difficult to identify the source of the centromere. Such translocations may be written in such a way as to define the observation without overinterpretation, e.g. t(14;22)(14qter-cen-22qter) implies that the long arms of chromosomes 14 and 22 have been involved in a translocation, with retention of a single centromere, the source of which is unknown. Figure 2.2 depicts chromosomal abnormalities of leukaemic lymphocytes from a patient with chronic lymphocytic leukaemia (CLL).

Chromosomal Abnormalities in Cancer

Chromosomal rearrangements in neoplasia may be important because they result in close approximation of DNA sequences that are normally far apart, or cause loss of critically important segments. The result may be abnormal activation of normal genes, including oncogenes, or the creation of new abnormal sequences coding for abnormal proteins, as recently shown in CML. Acquired chromosomal defects, confined to the tumour cells, are present in most neoplasms, and the number increases during the course of most cancers. Mapping of the genes at the sites of deletions, translocations and rearrangements is one of the most exciting advances in the understanding of the mechanisms of the abnormal regulation of the genome in cancer (Table 2.1; see also Table 15.1, p. 202, and Table 18.1, p. 291). The number of chromosomal defects shown to be associated consistently with particular types of human cancer has grown considerably in the past few years (Yunis 1981,1984; Mitelman 1983; Croce and Klein 1985; Human Gene Mapping 8 1985).

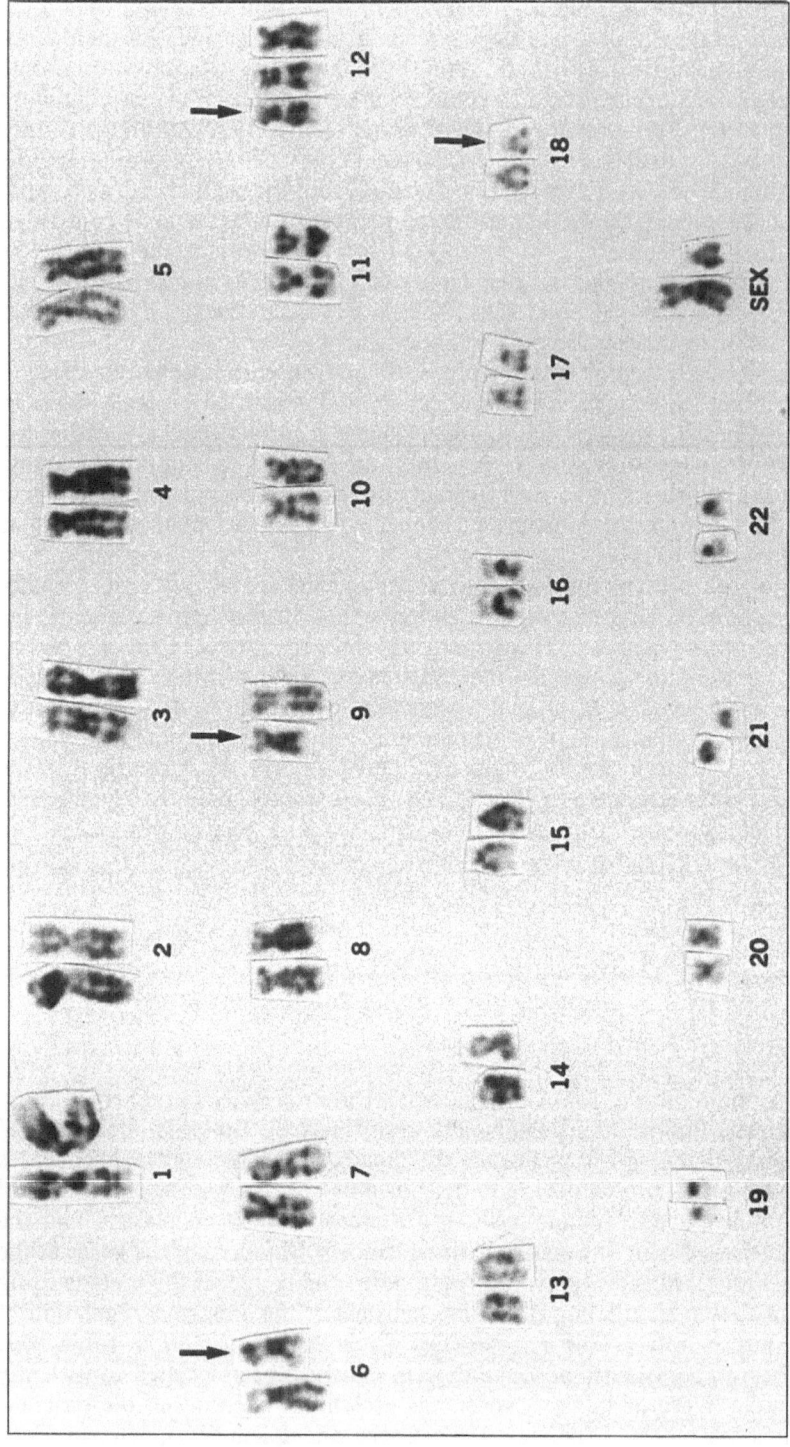

Fig. 2.2. Karyogram from lymphocytes in CLL. This metaphase spread shows trisomy of chromosome 12, unbalanced translocations involving the long arm of chromosome 9 and deletions of chromosomes 6 and 18 (arrowed). The 18 deletion appears to be interstitial, i.e. within the chromosome. The translocation of chromosome 9 could be to 6q, but the reciprocal chromosome is not identified. These abnormalities may be written in shorthand as 47,XY, + 12, del (6)(q15:), t(9;?)(q12:?), del (18)(q11->q21). (Courtesy of Dr. J. Ford, The Queen Elizabeth Hospital, Woodville, South Australia).

Table 2.1. Some important cancer-related loci on human chromosomes

Chromosome 1	
c-N-*ras*	1p22 and/or p12-p11
c-*ski*	1q22-qter
Thyroid stimulating hormone	1p22
c-*src*-2	1p36-p34
NGF β polypeptide	
Chromosome 2	
Ig κ chain	2p12 (2p11)
CD8	2pter-p12
c-N-*myc*	2p24-p23
IFN$_{β3}$	2p23-qter
IL-1	2q13-q21
TGF$_α$	2p13
Fragile site	2q13
Chromosome 3	
c-*raf*-1	3p25-p
transferrin	3q21-q26.1
transferrin receptor	3q26.2-qter
Chromosome 4	
IL-2	4q26-q28
EGF	4q25-q27
OKT10	
CD2	
c-*raf*-2	
Chromosome 5	
c-*fms*	5q34
glucocorticoid receptor	5q11-q13
IFN$_{β2}$	5p
Chromosome 6	
c-Ki-*ras*-1	6p23-q12 (6p11–12)
c-*yes* H	
MHC class I (A,B,C)	6p21.3
MHC class II (DP,DQ,DR)	6p21.3
Complement C2, C3BR	6p21.3
C3DR, C4A, C4B	
c-*myb*	6q15-q24 (6q23)
Fragile site	6p23
Chromosome 7	
Ti γ chain	7p15
c-*erb*-B	7p14–7p12
EGF receptor	7p13–7p11
Fragile site	7p11.2
Ti β chain	7q32–7q35
Chromosome 8	
c-*mos*	8q11
Fragile site	8q22.1
c-*myc*	8q24 (8q24.1)
BL translocation site	8q24

Table 2.1. (*continued*)

Chromosome 9
Fragile site   9p21
IFN$_\alpha$ qter-p13
IFN$_{\beta3}$ 9p24-p13
methylthioadenosine phosphorylase   9p21–22
Fragile site   9q32
c-*abl*   9q34 (9q34.1)

Chromosome 10
IL-2 receptor   10p15-p14
Fragile site   10q23.3
Fragile site   10q25.2
Vimentin

Chromosome 11
c-Ha-*ras*-1   11pter-p15.6 (11p14.1)
c-*ets*-1   11q23–24
Wilms' tumour, aniridia deletion   11p13
IGF-II   11p15 (11p15–11p14)
Insulin   11p15
Fragile site   11q13.3
Fragile site   11q23
CD3   11q23-qter
CD5
CP03
Ti δ chain

Chromosome 12
c-*int*-1   12pter-q14
CD9   12pter-q12
c-Ki-*ras*-2   12p12.1 or 12q24.2
Fragile site   12q13.1
Diffuse mixed T lymphoma t(12;14)   12q13.1
translocation site
IGF-I   12q22-q24.1
IFN$_\gamma$ 12q24.1
CD4

Chromosome 14
IgH chains   14q32
c-*fos*   14q21-q31
Ti α chain   14pter-q21
IgH diversity region 1   14q32.3
(heavy chain genes)
Translocation sites for BL   14q32.3
t(8;14), small lymphocytic
lymphoma t(11;14), diffuse
mixed T cell lymphoma t(12;14)
follicular small cleaved cell
lymphoma t(14;18)

Chromosome 15
β$_2$ microglobulin   15q22
c-*fes/fps*   15q25-q26 (q26.1)
B$_2$ microglobulin regulator   15q13-q15
IgH diversity region 2   15q11-q12

Table 2.1. (*continued*)

Chromosome 16	
IFN production regulator	
Fragile site	16p12
Fragile site	16q22
Chromosome 17	
neu/ngl	17q21-q22
c-erb-A1	17q11-q21
growth hormone 1	17q22-q24
growth hormone 2	17q22-q24
Chromosome 18	
c-yes 1	18q21.3
IFN$_\gamma$ receptor	
bcl-2	18q21.3
Chromosome 19	
H blood group antigen	
insulin receptor	19p13.3-p13.2
TGF$_\beta$	19q13.1-q13.3
Low density lipoprotein (LDL)	
receptor	19p
Chromosome 20	
Fragile site	20p11.2
c-src-1	20q12-q13
adenosine deaminase	20q13.2-qter
Chromosome 21	
IFN$_\alpha$ receptor	21q21-qter
c-ets-2	21q22
IFN$_\beta$ receptor	
Chromosome 22	
c-sis	22q12.3–13.1 (22q13.1)
Ig λ chain	22q11
Chromosome X	
c-Ha-ras-2	Xpter-q28

Aneuploidy, departure from the normal chromosome number, is a common finding in all tumours, but the chromosomal defects showing specific cancer associations are commonly deletions and reciprocal translocations. In the specific deletions, the material lost may vary somewhat in different examples of the tumour; the loss will always include a constant band region. As more genes involved in translocations and chromosome rearrangements are recognised it is becoming increasingly likely that the chromosomal abnormalities seen in many cancers result in a gene critically important to some essential function of the cell being juxtaposed to a gene related to cell proliferation, e.g. an oncogene. The abnormal interaction of the two genes alters the expression or function of the product of one or the other and leads to malignant transformation (Rowley et al. 1986).

Trisomy is the presence of three instead of two of any given chromosome. Chromosome 8, which carries the cellular oncogenes *myc* and *mos*, is by far the commonest to be involved in trisomy. Trisomy 8 is seen in many haematopoietic disorders, ranging from relatively benign myeloproliferative disorders to acute leukaemia. Trisomy of the chromosome carrying *myc* is also found in rat tumours and mouse leukaemias induced by Rous sarcoma virus.

In the common reciprocal translocations, two chromosomes are involved in the exchange and the breakpoints are consistently at or near the same site. In a few cases the breakpoint of only one of the chromosomes appears to be disease-specific, as in chromosome 9 in CML, while either the breakage site on the second chromosome or the second chromosome itself may vary.

The first recognised specific translocation was that which resulted in the "Philadelphia" chromosome, a shortened chromosome 22. The translocation involving the q34 band of chromosome 9 and band q11 of chromosome 22 is seen in over 90% of cases of CML. Nucleotide sequencing studies have now shown that the site of breakage of 9q34 is variable. This translocation involves the proto-oncogenes c-*abl* and c-*sis*. Burkitt's lymphoma also shows translocations from chromosome 8 to chromosome 12, 14 or 2. Translocations also appear to play an important part in the oncogenic transformation of T cells.

The translocation t(8;21) (q22;q22) is associated with acute non-lymphocytic leukaemia, subgroup M2 (ANLL-M2). The breakpoint separates the oncogenes c-*mos* at band q22 and c-*ets*-2 at 21q22. The c-*mos* gene remains on the 8q-chromosome without rearrangement and the c-*ets*-2 gene is translocated to the 21q+ chromosome (Diaz et al. 1985; Rowley et al. 1986). The t(9;11)(p22;q23) common in acute monoblastic leukaemia splits the interferon genes on chromosome 9 and the *ets*-1 gene on 11q23 is translocated to 9p (Rowley 1986).

Deletions may involve sites of oncogenes. Small-cell lung cancers have a consistent deletion in the short arm of chromosome 3 (3p14–3pter). The c-*raf* oncogene is at 3p25. Deletions of portions of the short arm of chromosome 1 (1p-) are seen in about 70% of neuroblastomas. There may be a hereditary component to these tumours.

Specific genes may be amplified during adaptive responses of cells to various stresses, for example to cytotoxic drugs. Gene amplification is associated with two cytogenetic abnormalities, the double minute chromosome (dmin) and the homogeneously staining region (HSR). dmins are small spherical chromosome-like structures, usually paired, lacking centromeres. HSRs lack the bands in G- or R-banded preparations. These two abnormalities have not been found in normal cells. The disturbance caused by translocations may be associated with amplification of genes.

Susceptibility to Chromosome Damage and Cancer

Defective repair of spontaneous or mutagen-induced chromosomal damage causes chromosomal breaks, gaps and rearrangements. There is an increased susceptibility to common carcinogens in a number of rare recessively inherited syndromes, in which repair of DNA is defective. In xeroderma pigmentosum there is a deficiency of ultraviolet specific endonuclease causing inability to repair thymidine dimers induced in DNA by ultraviolet light, leading to skin cancers, including melanoma. In Fanconi's anaemia, Bloom's syndrome and ataxia telangiectasia (AT) repair enzymes are lacking. There is an increased susceptibility to common cancers, including acute myeloblastic leukaemia (AML), in Fanconi's anaemia and to ANLL in Bloom's syndrome, and a susceptibility to T cell leukaemia in AT.

In some other inherited conditions the relationship of chromosomal abnormalities to an observed predisposition to cancer is less clear. One of the number 22 chromosomes, or, less frequently, the long arm of one chromosome 22, is often absent in sporadic meningiomas. The c-sis oncogene is on the long arm of chromosome 22. Three siblings with meningioma carried a constitutional translocation, t(14;22) (14qter-cen-22qter) in peripheral blood leucocytes (Bolger et al. 1985). The surviving two siblings had a variant of the c-sis oncogene in peripheral leucocyte DNA. This variant oncogene was also present in one asymptomatic member in the third generation, whose karyotype was normal.

Constitutional Cytogenetic Abnormalities

Constitutional cytogenetic abnormalities may be associated with cancer. Such abnormalities are present from conception in every cell of the affected person These include:

1. *Klinefelter's syndrome* (XXY sex chromosomes), with increased risk of breast cancer and (possibly) some increased risk of leukaemias and lymphomas.

2. *Down's syndrome (trisomy 21)*, with a 30-fold increase in risk of leukaemia (mostly ALL).

3. *Deletion of p13 region of chromosome 11*, associated with the aniridia/Wilms' tumour syndrome. This deletion is close to the gene for the growth factor IGF-II. It results in loss of a diploid pair of regulatory genes which normally suppress the expression of a structural transforming gene named Tg.

4. *Loss of the q14.1 region of chromosome 13*, associated with retinoblastoma; a predisposition to retinoblastoma results from inheritance of a mutation known as Rb-1 at this site.

5. *Translocations involving chromosome 3*, associated with familial renal adenocarcinoma t(3;8)(p14;q24), t(3;11)(p13 or p14;p15).

Fragile Sites

A fragile site is a location where a break frequently occurs in a chromosome of cells cultured or prepared for karyotyping. Fragile sites occur in apparently normal subjects and in family members, and in some subjects with cancer. The molecular mechanism of this fragility is unknown, although fragile sites have been reported to be sensitive to the action of DNAases. Fragile sites appear either as a chromosome gap or break when cells are deprived of folic acid and thymidine during the last hours of culture. This suggests a unique DNA structure of fragile sites which renders the cell susceptible to rearrangement if the cell is deprived of DNA precursors. It has been suggested that they may be sites modified by viruses, that may be transmitted horizontally or vertically (Shabtai et al. 1984).

Most of the known fragile sites have a simple Mendelian codominant inheritance. They have a frequency of approximately 0.2% each. At least 15 heritable fragile sites have been defined (reviewed by Yunis 1984). A fragile site corresponds to the site of a specific translocation in a number of leukaemias and lymphomas. In one instance, an oncogene (c-*mos*), a fragile site and a breakpoint of a chromosome defect occur together at band 8q22. It is likely that some individuals are inherently predisposed to certain malignancies because of these inherited fragile sites.

References

Bolger GB, Stamberg J, Kirsch IR et al. (1985) Chromosome translocation t(14;22) and oncogene (c-*sis*) variant in a pedigree with familial meningioma. N Engl J Med 312: 564–567
Burnet FM (1982) Immunology, ageing and cancer. In: Isaacs B (ed) Recent advances in geriatric medicine. Churchill Livingstone, Edinburgh, pp 5–18
Cairns J (1981) The origin of human cancers. Nature 289: 353–357
Croce CM, Klein G (1985) Chromosome translocations and human cancer. Sci Am 252: 44–50
Diaz MO, LeBeau MM, Rowley JD, Drabkin HA, Patterson D (1985) The role of the c-*mos* gene in the 8;21 translocation in human acute myeloblastic leukemia. Science 229: 767–769
Harnden DG, Lindsten JE, Buckton Klinger HP (1981) (ISCN 1981) An international system for human cytogenetic nomenclature — high resolution banding. Report of the standing committee on cytogenetic nomenclature. Cytogenet Cell Genet 31: 1–32
Human Gene Mapping 8 (1985) Eighth international workshop on human gene mapping. Helsinki, Finland. 4–10 August, 1985. Cytogenet Cell Genet 40 (1–4):1–823
Mitelman F (1983) Catalogue of chromosome aberrations in cancer. Cytogenet Cell Genet 36: 1–515
Report of the 1971 Paris Conference (1972) Standardisation in human cytogenetics. Birth Defects Original Article Series VIII: 7. National Foundation, NY
Rowley JD, Le Beau CA, Westbrook CA, Diaz MO (1986) Genetic analysis of chromosomal breakpoints in human acute leukemia. XXI Congress of the International Society of Haematology, Sydney, May 1986, p 2 (abstract)
Shabtai F, Klar D, Hart J, Halbrecht I (1985) On the meaning of fragile sites in cancer risk and development. Cancer Genet Cytogenet 18: 81–85
Yunis JJ (1981) Chromosomes and cancer: new nomenclature and future directions. Hum Pathol 12: 494–503
Yunis JJ (1984) Fragile sites and predisposition to leukaemia and lymphoma. Cancer Genet Cytogenet 12: 85–88

3 Derangements of the Mechanisms Controlling Growth

Introduction

Cancer develops by the emancipation of a single cell from host control of growth. Growth has two components, proliferation and differentiation. Fetal organogenesis and wound repair are both obviously controlled according to a pattern. During embryogenesis and growth to adulthood the number of cells increases enormously. In maturity, cells are produced to replace those dying or destroyed.

To divide, a cell passes through a series of metabolic states which make up the cell cycle. Cellular proliferation is normally controlled by external factors, among which the most important are hormones, growth factors and, for many types, cell contact.

Cell Cycle

The major phases of the cell cycle are G_0, G_1, S, M and G_2 (Fig. 3.1). A resting cell is in G_0 (zero growth phase). To begin dividing, it must be induced to enter the G_1 phase. Movement to the G_1 state renders the cell competent to be driven through to the S phase by a series of specific stimuli, mostly provided by growth factors. The time from the first stimulus to onset of the S phase is at least 6 h. Stimulation by cycle-initiating factors again during the S phase results in the daughter cells being ready to respond to the factors which act during G_1. The S phase, once started, proceeds without growth factors. In some cell types, growth factors are needed again in the G_2 phase.

Each phase of the cell cycle is distinguishable by particular metabolic processes. A number of techniques yield some quantitative information about the cell cycle and its phases; these include the following:

1. Autoradiography of tritiated thymidine taken up by synthesizing cells (indicating the DNA synthesis phase, S).

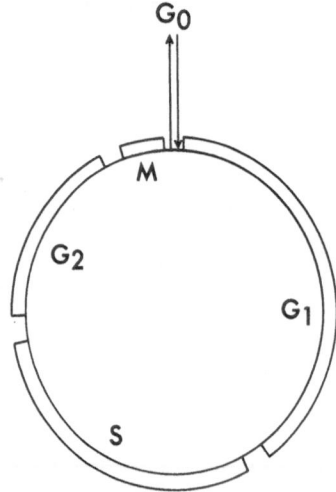

Fig. 3.1. The cell cycle. This schema depicts the sequence of events in a cell undergoing division. In the first growth phase, G_1, a pattern of gene activation leads to the synthesis of proteins essential for the process, including receptors for growth factors. In S phase, DNA is synthesised. In the second growth phase, G_2, more genes are expressed to render the daughter cells capable of mitosis, (M). A quiescent cell not undergoing division is in G_0 phase. The corresponding phases resulting from activation of a T cell and some of the specific events occurring in the phases are depicted in Figure 10–4.

2. Differential acridine orange staining of DNA and RNA (RNA increase is an early event in the transmission from G_0 to G_1 phase).
3. Incorporation of bromodeoxyuridine (BrUdR) into DNA and counting of the percentage of labelled nuclei to detect cells in S phase.

In the newly developed BrUdR technique, BrUdR incorporated into the nucleus of DNA-synthesizing cells is detected by a monoclonal antibody to BrUdR stained with an immunoperoxidase technique.

Signal Transduction

Each growth factor has a specific receptor on the surface membrane. Many of the growth factors and their receptors have been characterised and their genes have been cloned and analysed. Combination of growth factor with receptor initiates a series of events, called signal transduction, which, if effective, leads to activation of specific genes involved in growth. The term "activation", when applied to a structural gene, denotes the expression of that gene in the form of a messenger RNA (mRNA) copy. From 20 to 100 genes are induced within 20–60 min of stimulation of growth, including c-*myc*, c-*fos* and c-*myb* in lymphocytes. Yet more genes are induced within the next 12 h.

Immortalisation and Transformation

Cancer cells will multiply indefinitely in culture if the appropriate conditions are maintained. They are thus potentially immortal and the change to this state is called "immortalisation". Death is normally programmed; loss of this programme is a feature of malignancy. Cancer cells also continue to grow in culture beyond the point where they form a confluent monolayer.

"Transformation" is a term commonly applied to the assumption of malignant properties by a cell or cells in culture. It is considered to be a phenomenon distinct from immortalisation, which can occur without transformation, for example in B lymphocytes infected by Epstein–Barr virus. Criteria for transformation include the loss of anchorage dependence, the capacity to grow as spherical colonies in soft agar, disorganisation of the cytoskeleton (disorder of actin cables and microtubules) and less stringent requirements for growth factors. Loss of "contact inhibition" is a manifestation of transformation. Normal cells are inhibited by contact with each other. Transformation can be induced by viruses and oncogenes in vitro. Transformed cells may cause tumours in animal hosts, particularly if the host is immunologically incompetent. Transformation in vitro is not necessarily linked to invasiveness or metastatic potential.

Transformation appears usually to involve a loss of the ability of the transformed cells to differentiate, a phenomenon called "differentiation (or maturation) arrest". Transforming events other than those causing differentiation arrest may contribute to prolongation of life of a malignant cell. One example is the avoidance of mechanisms which remove cells from the body. This applies particularly to leukaemic cells. Memory lymphocytes possess this property of avoiding removal from the body. They recirculate by virtue of alterations of the surface membrane permitting migration from blood to lymph to blood (Reichert et al. 1983), and avoid removal from the body, presumably by not migrating to sites, which have not yet been identified, where they may be destroyed.

Despite many studies, the life span of all of the human lymphocytes is not well known. There are certainly long-lived memory cells of both T and B classes with a life of several years, but the majority of B cells, and probably of T cells, has a short life of a few days. The limit on the number of generations of non-malignant lymphocytes is probably no different from that of any other normal cell. Only immortalised lymphocytes can multiply without limit. Since 5%–10% of all B cells are newly generated each day, the same number must normally die.

Studies with malignant plasmacytomas and other lines show that malignant lymphocytes may retain susceptibility to some of the physiological influences that control their normal counterparts (see Chap. 13, p. 168).

Mechanisms Leading to Autonomous Growth

An essential requirement of malignant transformation appears to be a genetic change converting cells to a state of perpetual, if slow, uninduced replication, a state described as "constitutive for replication". For this the cell must either have growth factors, or overcome the need for them.

One likely mechanism for autonomous growth is the production of growth factors by malignant cells themselves ("autocrine" growth factor production, i.e. "constitutive" production of growth factors; Sporn and Todaro 1980). Several types of tumour do this, including neoplastic B cells of the BCL_1 line (Brooks et al.

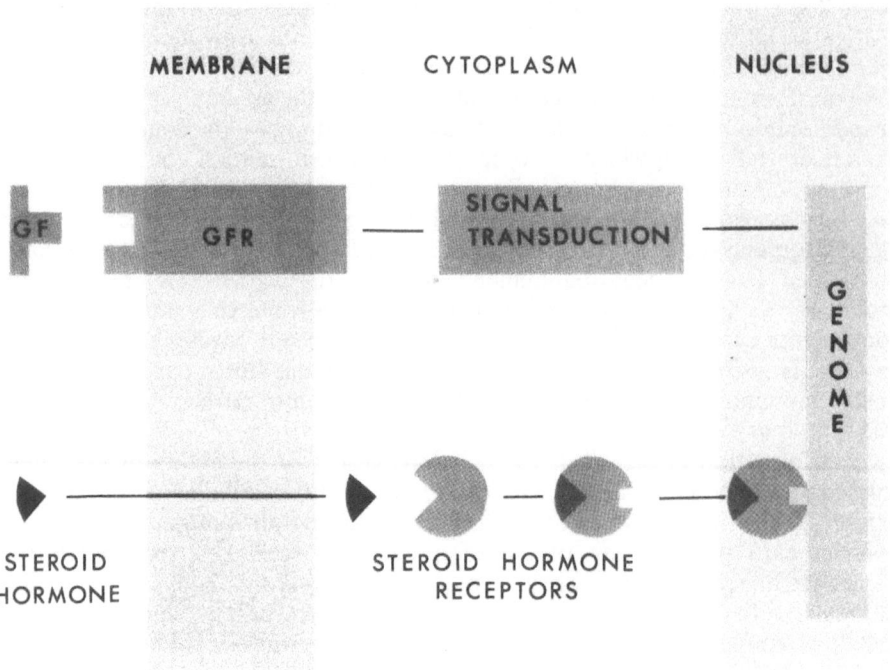

Fig. 3.2 Growth control mechanisms. Two types of growth control mechanism which may be deranged in cancer are illustrated. Binding of growth factor (GF) to its specific membrane receptor (GFR) induces a series of intracellular events, designated *signal transduction*, which lead to activation of genes involved in proliferation and differentiation. Steroid hormones diffuse across the plasma membrane, bind to and activate DNA-binding sites on specific intracellular receptors. The activated receptors bind to DNA and regulate the transcription of specific genes.

1984). Small-cell lung cancer cells produce bombesin, a growth factor for which they have receptors. Other peptide growth factors produced by cancer cells include α and β transforming growth factors (TGF_α, TGF_β) and platelet-derived growth factor (PDGF). Autocrine factors combine with specific receptors, activating a signal which leads to a growth response. Blocking, by specific antibody, of the receptors for these autologous growth factors has been shown to stop the growth of malignant cells in culture.

Another source of growth factors for malignant cells is the environment. It is conceivable that non-malignant accessory cells and T cells supply growth factors to support the growth of malignant cells in culture. Relatively mature T and B lymphocytes are under the control of specialised growth factors which are not closely related to the growth factors governing connective tissue cells. The nature of the growth factors influencing primitive lymphocytes and their precursors is unknown.

Alteration of the receptor, or modification of the signalling pathway may result in autonomous growth of tumour cells (Sporn and Roberts 1985). It has been suggested, but not proven, that unregulated expression of the receptor for interleukin 2 (IL-2) may contribute to leukaemogenesis. A cell may become independent of growth factors if it produces an abnormal receptor which initiates signal transduction spontaneously. These possibilities are discussed further in Chapter 7.

Growth of breast cells is normally stimulated by oestrogen and other hormones. This control is abnormal in cells of breast cancers. Growth of cancer cells in breast carcinoma is frequently controlled by the use of oestrogen and other hormones. Steroid hormones bind to and activate intracellular receptors. The activated receptors bind to specific sites on the genome, inducing specific genes. Two types of growth control mechanism which may be deranged in neoplasia are illustrated in Fig. 3.2.

Differentiation Arrest

Differentiation is frequently arrested in malignant cells. Normal cells of many lineages have a short life after they reach maturity. Inhibition of differentiation to full maturity is likely to prevent the corresponding malignant cells from dying early. Another suggested consequence of differentiation arrest is loss of an inhibitory control on proliferation normally exerted by mature cells.

Arrest of differentiation is possibly as important as any other characteristic for the development of a tumour. It determines many of the characteristics that distinguish different tumours arising from the same cell lineage. Chronic lymphocytic leukaemia (CLL), for example, is arrested earlier in its differentiation than multiple myeloma (see Table 11.2, p. 130).

The length of life of the malignant cells is critical to tumour formation. We can imagine that many malignancies develop which do not become evident. A clone that produces cells with a very short life, relative to the time between mitoses, will never come to notice. The fundamental requirement for the development of a tumour is that production and survival exceed the death rate.

Differentiation arrest affects malignant cells at multiple points along the differentiation pathway. What we see is the accumulation at a dominant point of maturation arrest. Differentiation arrest will have a very great impact on tumour kinetics if it operates before the tumour cells lose their capacity to multiply. If the majority of tumour cells stay immature and divide, the tumour will grow rapidly and will probably be aggressive.

The capacity to abrogate differentiation arrest could enable tumours to be controlled. We are probably controlling differentiation arrest by treating breast cancers with hormones, causing the malignant cells to mature and die.

The control of differentiation is even less well understood than control of proliferation. Differentiation is essentially an orderly, programmed, change in genome expression. It is rarely reversible and is also induced by growth factors. One oncogene product has been shown to induce differentiation under particular conditions. Rat phaeochromocytoma cells grow indefinitely in culture as round cells resembling chromaffin cells. When nerve growth factor (NGF) is added, the cells differentiate to resemble sympathetic neurons and cease growth. Microinjection of the human Ha-*ras* oncogene protein into PC12 cells results in similar differentiation (Bar-Sagi and Feramisco 1985).

Because of the availability of markers, malignant human lymphocytes are good models for the study of differentiation arrest. Mechanisms which may be involved in differentiation arrest include:

1. Lack of stimulus appropriate to the stage of differentiation arrest. Receptors are expressed at each differentiation stage for the growth factors necessary to stimulate progression to the next stage.
2. Failure to express the appropriate receptor.
3. Abnormality of the signal transduction pathway.
4. Genomic abnormality resulting in inability to switch off the expression of the programme for the current differentiation stage and switch on the programme for the next stage. Genes may be missing, abnormal or unable to be activated.
5. Abnormality of gene transcription or translation.

Terminal differentiation may be blocked by the activity of a specific oncogene, v-*erb*-A, acting on virally transformed chicken haematopoietic cells (Graf et al. 1985). When cells are transformed by the action of an oncogene such as v-*erb*-B, they still require specific growth factors, for example granulocyte-macrophage colony-stimulating factor (GM-CSF). A proportion of these cells develops into erythrocytes. The rest renew the population by division ("self-renewal"). Introduction of the v-*erb*-A oncogene completely blocks this differentiation and also abolishes the requirement for GM-CSF.

These findings show that differentiation is normally controlled, at least partly, by proto-oncogenes. Specifically, abnormalities of the *fos* and *myc* proto-oncogenes are now known to affect differentiation, as will be discussed in Chapter 6. It follows that abnormality of differentiation could result from an abnormality of these genes.

References

Bar-Sagi D, Feramisco J (1985) Microinjection of the *ras* oncogene protein into PC12 cells induces morphological differentiation. Cell 42: 841–848

Brooks KH, Kuziel WA, Tucker PW, Uhr JW, Vitetta ES (1984) Cloned neoplastic B cells release a growth factor which augments lymphokine-mediated proliferation of normal B cells. Curr Top Microbiol Immunol 113: 69–71

Graf T, Kahn P, Damm K et al. (1985) Lineage specific induction of self-renewal, differentiation arrest and growth factor independence by primary and auxiliary oncogenes in chick hematopoietic cells. Proceedings of the eleventh annual EMBO symposium on growth factors, receptors, and oncogenes, 16–19 September, 1985. European Molecular Biology Laboratory, Heidelberg, pp 23–24 (abstract)

Reichert RA, Gallatin WM, Weissman IL, Butcher EC (1983) Germinal center B cells lack homing receptors necessary for normal lymphocyte recirculation. J Exp Med 157: 813–827

Sporn MB, Roberts AB (1985) Autocrine growth factors and cancer. Nature 313: 745–747

Sporn MB, Todaro GJ (1980) Autocrine secretion and malignant transformation of cells. N Engl J Med 303: 878–880

4 Multiple Steps in the Genesis of a Cancer

Introduction

It has been suggested, on the evidence from age–incidence curves, that at least three or four successive genetic changes are necessary for emergence of leukaemias, and six to seven for carcinomas (Klein and Klein 1985). On the basis of the mouse skin model of carcinogenesis with polycyclic hydrocarbons and croton oil, three phases, initiation, promotion and progression, have been invoked to explain the phenomena of skin carcinogenesis (Fig. 4.1). These stages probably take place in the induction of cancers by most environmental agents, but they may be circumvented in viral carcinogenesis, when a virus introduces a transforming oncogene. They are presumed to occur in humans when cancer develops after a long interval in dysplastic epithelium. Carcinogenesis may occupy a major fraction of the life span of the individual, e.g. 20 years in the human (Farber 1984). The transitions between successive stages of carcinogenesis can be enhanced or inhibited in some experimental situations by different types of agent (Weinstein et al. 1984), indicating that individual phases may involve different mechanisms.

The skin model of chemical carcinogenesis (Boutwell et al. 1982) appears to be highly relevant to cancer of lymphocytes. An experimental cancer may represent in one site all the elements of a lymphoid tumour. The most basal layer contains the "immortal" malignant stem cells which divide asymmetrically to yield cells with the capacity to multiply and a limited capacity to differentiate, on the one hand, and to produce replicas of themselves, on the other. The replicas neither differentiate nor lose their capacity for unlimited proliferation. Differentiation steps have been described for keratinocytes on the basis of differential expression of keratins, just as lymphocyte differentiation can be described in terms of gene products related to each stage. For full differentiation, these cells need products from the dermis (Fusenig et al. 1985). Viral mechanisms of carcinogenesis may also be studied in epidermal cells. Immortal cell lines can be derived from human epidermis by treatment with DNA from strains of the virus SV40, and introduction of the c-Ha-*ras* oncogene by a process called "transfection" may transform them to cells capable of forming carcinomas in nude (athymic, immunologically deficient) mice.

In the classical model of tumour promotion, mouse skin is painted with a very small amount of an initiator (e.g. 3-methylcholanthrene) that causes few cancers

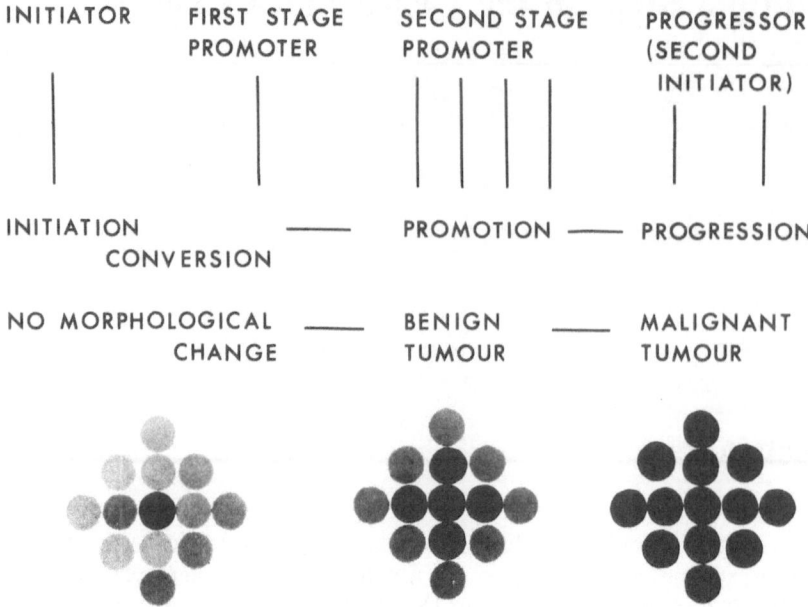

INITIATOR   FIRST STAGE   SECOND STAGE   PROGRESSOR
               PROMOTER   PROMOTER   (SECOND
                                                      INITIATOR)

INITIATION   ———   PROMOTION   ———   PROGRESSION
        CONVERSION

NO MORPHOLOGICAL   ____   BENIGN   ____   MALIGNANT
        CHANGE   TUMOUR   TUMOUR

Fig. 4.1. Stages of carcinogenesis. One exposure to an initiator induces an irreversible change in the genome of a stem cell, but no detectable change in the phenotype of the progeny. The first-stage promoter induces another essential step, also without causing detectable phenotypic change, converting a cell to a state of susceptibility to a second-stage promoter. After repeated application a benign tumour appears within the clone of cells bearing the genomic alterations induced in the first two steps. Progression of benign tumours to malignancy is enhanced by a variety of agents which damage DNA, particularly initiator-type chemicals.

itself. When the methylcholanthrene-treated mouse skin is treated repeatedly with a tumour-promoting phorbol ester, skin tumours develop rapidly. Tumour-promoting substances alone, such as phorbol esters, do not cause tumours. The delay between the application of the initiator and the promoter can be as long as a year. Some initiators, e.g. 1–2-benzanthracene have no promoting activity; a promoter must be used to induce cancers. The tumours are mostly benign papillomas, whose growth depends on further application of promoter. The longer they are treated, the more develop into carcinomas.

Initiation

At the first step, initiation, a normal cell becomes premalignant. This step is permanent and irreversible. Initiation requires only a single exposure of DNA to a carcinogen, probably causing a mutation. This exposure is frequently to a subthreshold dose of agent which is insufficient to cause a tumour by itself. Some differences between initiation and promotion are set out in Table 4.1.

Several types of chemical that initiate the cancer process yield highly reactive species or metabolites that bind covalently to cellular DNA (Miller 1978). Brief

Table 4.1. Distinctions between initiation and promotion (after Boutwell et al. 1982)

	Initiation		Promotion
1.	Single very small exposure suffices	1.	Repeated exposure essential
2.	Initiator must usually precede promoter	2.	Promoter usually has to follow
3.	Irreversible	3.	Reversible: by a prolongation of intervals or if given before initiator
4.	Additive event at subthreshold doses	4.	A theshold exists
5.	Initiators are mutagenic or metabolised to mutagen	5.	Promoters are not mutagenic
6.	Does not alter expression of genes at low, initiating doses	6.	Alters gene expression, e.g. hyperplasia, enzyme induction, induction of differentiation
7.	DNA binding and resultant repair detectable	7.	Many biochemical responses
8.	DNA amplification induced	8.	DNA amplification not induced
9.	Initiators are carcinogenic at high doses	9.	Promoters cause few, if any tumours, even after long treatment

exposure of sexually maturing female rats to nitroso-methyl-urea (NMU) induces the initiation phase of mammary cancer by bringing about a highly specific mutation affecting the *ras* proto-oncogene. The strain of animal is also a determinant in the specificity of the mutation induced by NMU.

Initiation is thought to involve gene amplification, the production of multiple copies of particular genes (Table 4.2). Agents which cause initiation also cause gene amplification in cell cultures. Since amplification of genes requires the activity of DNA polymerases, there is now much interest in studying ways in which these enzymes are activated. Oncogenes may be amplified. The amplification need not occur immediately upon exposure to the carcinogen. It may occur during cell cycles subsequent to the initiating event.

Table 4.2. Evidence for gene amplification in tumour initiation

1. Amplified sequences found near sites of translocations in several tumour cell lines
2. Amplified oncogenes are found in tumour cell lines
3. Amplification is induced by agents which damage DNA directly, or by agents which inhibit DNA replication
4. The gene for dihydrofolate reductase (DHFR) is amplified by agents that damage DNA
5. Viruses with initiator-like properties, e.g. herpes simplex virus, induce DNA amplification
6. Tumour promoters (including TPA) do not induce amplification

As mutation is a permanent event, the question arises: which cells are the targets of the initiating agents? In the skin, they must be stem cells, because they are the only permanent residents of the epidermis. Initiated cells are not different from normal cells morphologically, i.e. initiated cells are phenotypically normal.

Promotion

Tumour promoters are compounds which have virtually no carcinogenic activity themselves, but markedly enhance tumour yield when applied repeatedly following a low or suboptimal dose of a carcinogen. Promotion usually involves multiple exposures to agents that have been considered not to damage DNA directly. Promoters may induce hyperplasia of initiated cells. Pure promoters have also been considered to be non-mutagenic and non-toxic to the genome, and mitogenic for induced cells (Trosko et al. 1983). Recent studies have shown that 12-*O*-tetradecanoylphorbol-13-acetate (TPA), one of the active tumour-promoting agents in croton oil, may cause severe chromosomal aberrations, whereas the analogue 12-retinoylphorbol 13-acetate (RPA) does not (Dzarlieva-Petrusevska and Fusenig 1985). That TPA can enhance transfection with oncogenes is another hint that TPA acts in the nucleus.

Tumour promotion is a long-term process requiring at least 20 applications of promoter. All promoters of skin tumours induce epidermal hyperproliferation and inflammation in normal skin, but not all irritants which cause hyperplasia are promoters (Marks et al. 1983). TPA is no better than any other promoter at increasing the rate of conversion of papillomas to carcinomas, which is probably a manifestation of progression, not promotion. Lifelong application of TPA as the sole agent will cause some tumours to develop in particular strains. Wounding can also promote the appearance of papillomas in "initiated" mouse skin. To explain this, it has been suggested that a wound hormone may be involved. The growth factor TGF_β is suspected.

Promotion in mouse skin takes place in two phases. The first phase of promotion, also known as "conversion", renders the affected epithelium susceptible to promoters capable of inducing the second stage. The existence of two phases of promotion is known only by deduction. There are no agents that cause the first phase of promotion without causing the second. Agents with the capacity to induce the first phase of promotion are "complete" promoters, also possessing the capacity to induce the second stage if reapplied frequently. On the other hand, there are distinct agents, such as RPA, designated as "incomplete" promoters, which induce the second stage of promotion, but cannot induce the first phase. The state of conversion wears off slowly if not followed by promoting stimuli. Skin carcinogenesis has been achieved in one strain of mice by inducing conversion prior to initiation (Fürstenberger et al. 1985). Conversion requires DNA synthesis, since it is inhibited by inhibition of DNA synthesis (Kinzel et al. 1984). Stage II also requires proliferation. Although the fundamental mechanisms of promotion are unknown, evolutionary processes are probably involved. Each step probably confers a growth advantage on a modified cell, which gives rise to a new subclone capable of escaping from the control exerted on its predecessors by contact inhibition and growth factors.

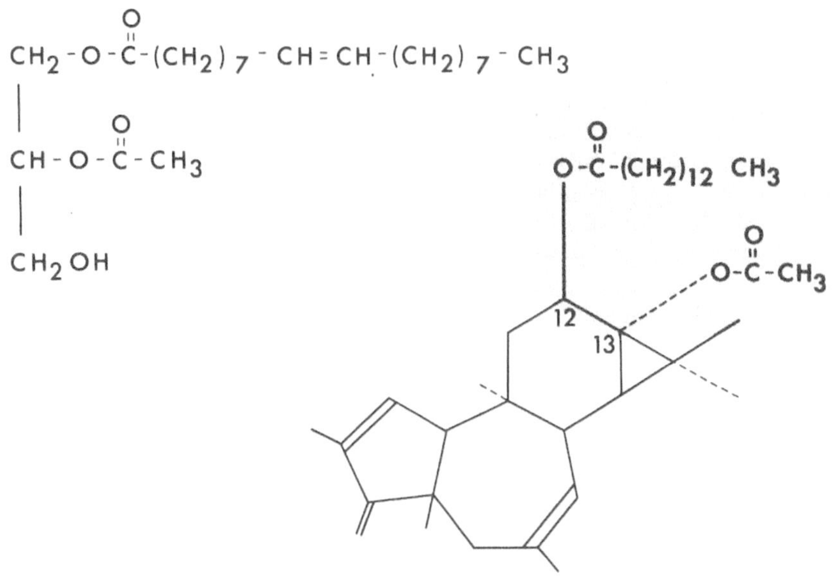

Fig. 4.2. Diacylglycerol (DAG, *left*) and 12-*O*-tetradecanoyl-phorbol-13-acetate (TPA, *right*). TPA is the most potent of the phorbol ester tumour-promoting agents. The portion of the TPA within the shaded area is the part which resembles diacylglycerol.

Tumour-promoting Phorbol Esters

The tumour-promoting phorbol esters (Fig. 4.2) have extraordinary properties and are extremely powerful. They interact widely in cellular physiological processes, and their effects on cells can be demonstrated with concentrations of TPA as low as 10^{-10} mol/litre. They mimic the action of growth factors and stimulate maturation in malignant and normal lymphocytes. Much of our knowledge of promotion comes from studies of phenomena and biochemical reactions induced by these compounds, which offer the chance of finding an essential biochemical reaction underlying the promotion of cancer. Although this goal has not been achieved, such studies have contributed greatly to our understanding of metabolic steps in cell activation and responses to hormones and growth factors.

The phorbol esters vary in their potency as tumour promoters, from the inactive phorbol to the exceedingly active TPA (also known as phorbol myristate acetate, PMA). Their relative potency as tumour promoters is generally similar to their ranking as stimuli in various cellular and biochemical systems.

Among the multiple effects of the phorbol esters are:

1. Membrane effects, such as enhancement of ion flux (Na^+, K^+), and nutrient uptake, and alteration of phospholipid metabolism.

2. Induction of specific enzymes, particularly protein kinase C.

3. Induction of changes in expression of cell surface receptors.

4. Modulation of differentiation, for example inhibition of differentiation of mouse erythroblastic cells induced by Friend virus and induction of differentiation in mouse erythroleukaemia cells induced by Rauscher virus. They cause most myeloid leukaemic cells to cease proliferation and to differentiate to mature macrophages. HL60 myeloid cells are induced to differentiate to monocyte/macrophage phenotypes by TPA, whereas dimethyl sulphoxide (DMSO) induces differentiation to granulocyte phenotypes. TPA induces terminal differentiation in epidermal keratinocytes in vitro. Transformed cells that have been changed by the initiation process respond weakly to the differentiation signal. It has been suggested that TPA stimulates the development of tumours by selecting out the keratinocytes which do not respond to differentiating signals; they have a survival advantage over those which respond, mature and die (Parkinson 1985).

5. Mimicry and enhancement of transformation. Metabolic effects of the phorbol esters are usually reversible, but enhancement by TPA of cell transformation by oncogenic viruses is irreversible.

6. Synergistic actions with growth factors and other cellular effectors.

The phorbol esters exert many of their effects by initially binding to specific receptors, inducing the phosphorylation of cellular proteins. They are thought to mimic the natural ligand, diacylglycerol (DAG, Fig. 4.2). The receptor for phorbol esters is a protein kinase C (PKC) in association with the phospholipid phosphatidylserine (PS, Fig. 4.3; Blumberg et al. 1984). Protein kinases are enzymes that phosphorylate proteins by transferring the energy-rich phosphate group of adenosine triphosphate (ATP) to them (Fig. 4.4). Binding of phorbol ester to receptor, and activation of the enzyme, occur by formation of a complex of PKC, Ca^{2+}, PS and phorbol ester. Both "complete" and "incomplete" classes of phorbol ester activate PKC. PKC phosphorylates seryl, threonyl, but not tyrosyl residues, in most tissues, including various types of human leukaemic cells. Activation dramatically increases the affinity of PKC for Ca^{2+}. Phorbol esters mimic the action of many growth factors because they induce phosphorylation of the same cellular substrates.

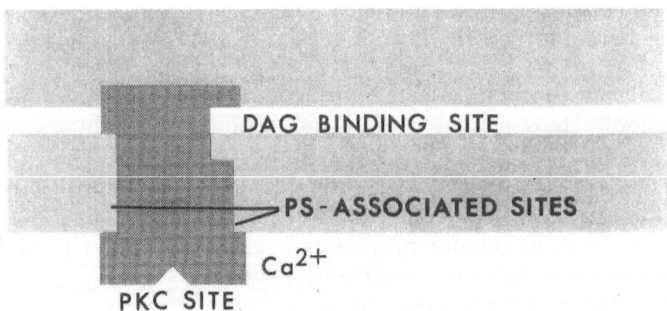

Fig. 4.3. Phorbol ester receptor. The receptor is a protein kinase C (*PKC*), in association with phosphatidylserine (PS), represented here within the lipid bilayer of the plasma membrane. Soluble PKC migrates from the cytoplasm to the membrane following an appropriate stimulus and becomes attached to the membrane. It has binding sites for Ca^{2+}, PS and diacylglycerol (*DAG*). Tumour-promoting phorbol esters bind to the same site as DAG.

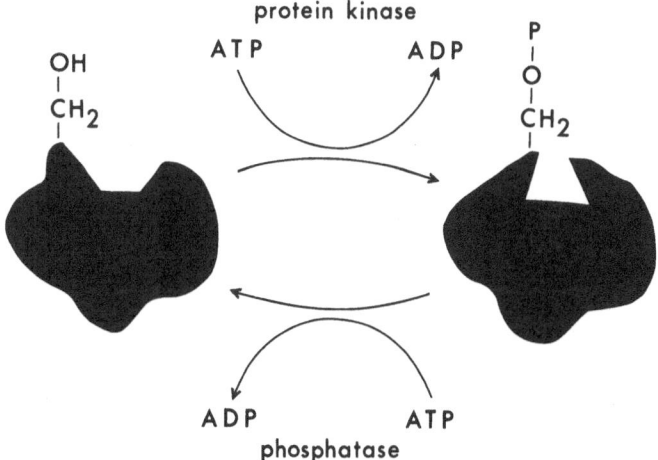

Fig. 4.4. Phosphorylation by protein kinase. The function of an enzyme, on the *left*, is regulated by protein kinase. A phosphate group from ATP is attached to a tyrosine, serine or threonine unit in the peptide chain of the enzyme. The effect is depicted here as causing a change in the shape of the catalytic site of the enzyme. This process is reversed by a protein phosphatase.

The bulk of PKC is in the cytoplasm. Here it is bound to structures which have not been identified positively; there may be more than one cytoplasmic pool. In unstimulated cells relatively little PKC is bound to the membrane. Exposure to phorbol ester causes this cytosolic protein kinase to move to the membrane (Kraft et al. 1982). The affinity with which phorbol esters bind to their specific receptors is greatly enhanced by ionophores which elevate the intracellular concentration of calcium, particularly when phorbol ester concentrations are low.

Phorbol ester receptors are present in all cells except erythrocytes, and their highest concentration is in the brain. PKC consists of a single 77 kD polypeptide chain which binds to membranes through a hydrophobic domain. The isolated 51 kD hydrophilic domain carries the catalytic site and does not bind to membranes. It is fully active without Ca^{2+}, phospholipid and diacylglycerol. It is thought that when PKC is activated, it is cleaved by an enzyme called calpain to yield this hydrophilic domain.

Phorbol esters which are active tumour promoters competitively inhibit binding of other active phorbol analogues to the specific receptor. Inactive analogues do not. In general, the more effectively a phorbol ester competes with a labelled analogue such as tritiated phorbol dibutyrate (^{3}H-PDBu) for binding to cell surface receptors, the more potently it promotes tumours on mouse skin.

There are two major classes of surface membrane receptor controlling cellular functions and proliferation, one class inducing production of cyclic adenosine monophosphate (cAMP) and the second inducing inositol phospholipid turnover, with activation of the phosphatidylinositol (PI) cycle (Fig. 4.5), elevation of the concentration of Ca^{2+} by mobilisation of cytoplasmic stores, release of arachidonic acid from the membrane and production of cyclic guanosine monophosphate (cGMP). The second class of cell surface receptors includes the receptors for a number of growth factors and hormones. These have an intramembranous segment with protein kinase activity. cGMP, often a negative messenger molecule,

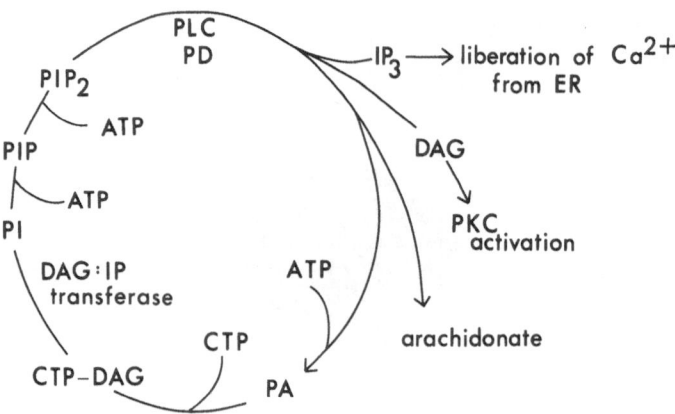

Fig. 4.5. The phosphatidylinositol (PI) cycle. Activation of membrane receptors activates phospholipase C and phosphodiesterase, leading to breakdown of PIP_2 into IP_3, which liberates calcium from the cytoplasms, and DAG, which activates PKC. PI is regenerated from DAG through PA and CTP-DAG. Hydrolysis of polyphosphoinositides also generates arachidonate, another potential messenger. *ADP*, adenosine diphosphate; *ATP*, adenosine triphosphate; *CTP*, cytidine triphosphate; *DAG*, diacylglycerol; IP_1, inositol monophosphate; IP_2, inositol diphosphate; IP_3, inositol triphosphate; *PA*, phosphatidic acid; *PD*, phosphodiesterase; *PI*, phosphatidylinositol; *PIP*, PI monophosphate; PIP_2, PI diphosphate; *PLC*, phospholipase C.

does not block the action of phorbol esters. The role of cGMP is not clearly understood. These highly complex interactions have been summarised by Nishizuka (1984). These cell surface receptors are quite distinct from a third class of receptors influencing cell growth, namely the intracellular receptors for steroid hormones (see Fig. 3.2, p. 22).

Membrane phospholipids called polyphosphoinositides help to mediate many cellular responses, including the activation of oncogenes (Marx 1985). When the PI cycle is activated, PI 4,5-biphosphate (PIP_2) is split, forming inositol 1,4,5-triphosphate (IP_3) and DAG. The enzyme phospholipase C is involved. IP_3 appears within seconds of activation of the receptor and disappears rapidly. It causes a rapid rise in intracellular calcium by releasing stored Ca^{2+} from the endoplasmic reticulum. Transient production of DAG in the membrane activates protein kinase C, greatly increasing its affinity for Ca^{2+}, without any change in Ca^{2+} levels. When DAG is added to cells in vitro it is ineffective, because it does not permeate the membrane, but its action is mimicked in vitro by addition of a soluble analogue, 1-oleoyl, 2-acetyl-glycerol, which activates protein kinase C without raising cytosol Ca^{2+} levels. There is a synergy between direct activation of PKC and the action of cell surface receptors which activate the PI cycle (Fig. 4.6). When a phorbol ester binds to PKC the enzyme becomes exquisitely sensitive to the rise in Ca^{2+}_i which follows activation of the PI cycle. The calcium ionophore A23187 can raise cytosolic Ca^{2+} concentrations, without activating PKC. A combination of individually ineffective doses of phorbol ester and A23187 acting on platelets mimics fully the rapid effects of potent platelet activators such as thrombin and platelet activating factor. Activation of the PI cycle is involved in the uncontrolled growth caused by oncogenes.

Protein kinase C is inhibited by many drugs that interact with phospholipids, including chlorpromazine, dibucaine and trifluoperazine. PKC phosphorylates a large number of proteins, including vinculin, a cytoskeletal protein linking actin microfilament bundles to the membrane. Phosphorylation of vinculin causes some of the morphological changes seen in transformation of cells by Rous sarcoma virus. The product of the Rous sarcoma virus oncogene, pp60[src], is a protein kinase which causes transformation by phosphorylating tyrosine residues on a variety of protein substrates, including vinculin, producing many of the cellular effects caused by the phorbol esters. PKC does not phosphorylate tyrosine residues itself. However, exposure of cells to TPA can enhance the phosphorylation of tyrosine residues on vinculin, by activating other protein kinases. PKC phosphorylates a site on the cytoplasmic segment of the epithelial growth factor (EGF) receptor.

It has recently been shown that PKC phosphorylates an enzyme that methylates DNA, DNA methyltransferase (De Paoli-Roach et al. 1986). This may be an important lead in understanding how abnormal activity of PKC may be involved in the neoplastic process. The activity of genes is regulated by the extent to which they are methylated, and the pattern of methylation is inherited in the progeny of

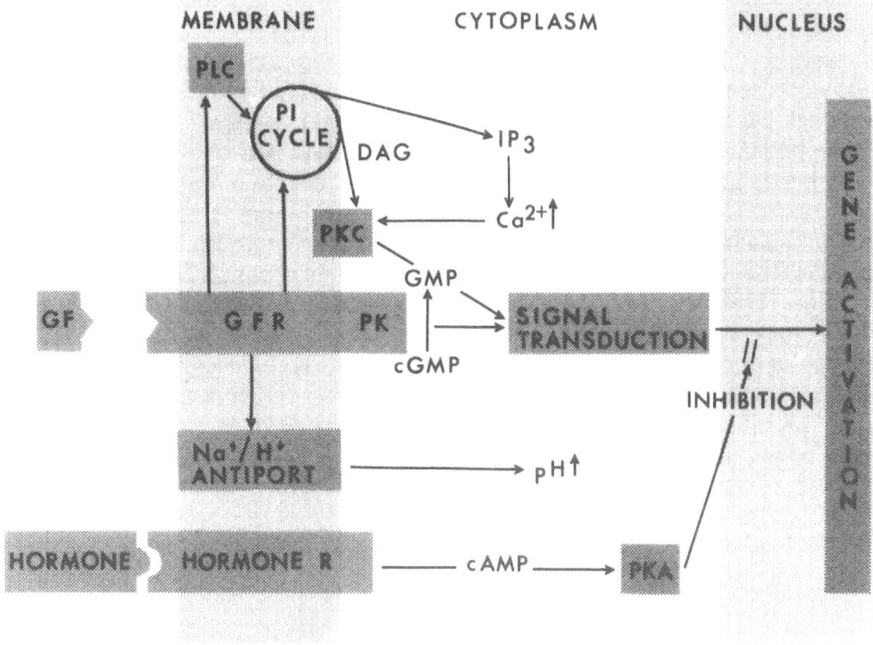

Fig. 4.6. Initiation of growth through membrane receptors. Binding of growth factor activates the phosphatidylinositol (PI) cycle (see Fig. 4.5). Inositol triphosphate (IP_3) releases Ca^{2+} from the cytoplasm. Protein kinase C (*PKC*) is activated by diacylgycerol (*DAG*), and its sensitivity to DAG is heightened by an increase in the concentration of Ca^{2+}. Phosphorylation of a number of proteins is the next step in the chain of reactions leading to activation of genes involved in cell proliferation and differentiation, including proto-oncogenes. Growth factor receptors (*GFR*) may themselves have protein kinase activity. Growth factor receptors may cause a rise in intracellular pH by influencing the $Na+/H+$ *antiport*, the membrane pump exchanging Na + for H +. Binding of hormone to receptors which cause production of *cAMP* has a negative effect on many growth factor signals. This type of receptor leads to activation of protein kinase A (*PKA*).

somatic cells. TPA can induce alterations in DNA methylation patterns, presumably by influencing the activity of DNA methyltransferase through phosphorylation of this enzyme.

As mentioned, many of the receptors for growth factors have a protein kinase segment on their intracellular portion. EGF itself causes phosphorylation of the progesterone receptor, thereby reducing its affinity for progesterone. Steroid hormone receptors may indeed be the main substrates of EGF. The progesterone receptor is also a substrate of the insulin receptor, but not of the receptor for another important growth factor, platelet-derived growth factor (PDGF).

There are analogies between the action of phorbol esters and cholera toxin. Both penetrate the plasma membrane, both cause persistent activation of a message transduction pathway common to an extensive series of hormones and cellular effectors. Cholera toxin induces the formation of cAMP, and activation of a cAMP-dependent protein kinase, whereas the phorbol esters activate protein kinase C.

Phorbol esters have become potent tools in research on normal and malignant lymphocytes, particularly since they were shown to induce activation and differentiation of lymphocytes. One important use of the phorbol esters is to reveal the sequence of expression of phenotypic markers during differentiation. Phorbol esters also have potent effects on macrophages, mainly of an inhibitory nature. TPA restores the mitogenic response to lectin of macrophage-depleted guinea pig lymph node lymphocytes, by mimicking the effect of interleukin 1 (IL-1), which is a product of macrophages. TPA replaces the macrophage requirement for induction of the T cell lymphokine interleukin 2 (IL-2; Farrar et al. 1980).

It is important to recognise that a number of effects of tumour-promoting phorbol esters cannot be ascribed to activation protein kinase C. For example, the enzyme phospholipase A_2, which splits off a fatty acid chain from phospholipids, is activated by phorbol esters by another unknown mechanism. Furthermore, the possession of phorbol receptors does not guarantee that cells will be induced to mature, at least in the case of primitive myeloid cells (Koeffler 1983). The mechanisms of other actions are not known. There is no biochemical explanation, for example, of the differences between the actions of RPA and TPA. Other tumour promoters like anthralin and benzoyl peroxide do not bind to phorbol ester receptors, indicating that they act differently. These promote skin tumours in mouse strains different from those strains in which TPA is an efficient promoter.

Progression

Progression involves the conversion of benign to malignant tumours. Each progression step may reflect the activation, mutation or loss or different genes. The process of tumour progression continues, since malignant tumours frequently continue to increase in malignancy and heterogeneity. Progressive changes in malignant tumours are due to steady emergence of new clones which have a growth and survival advantage over the others.

DNA-damaging agents are more effective than tumour promoters in enhancing the progression of papillomas to carcinomas on mouse skin (Hennings et al. 1983). This suggests that the evolution of a fully malignant tumour may involve more than one cycle of damage to DNA, not simply one hit by the initiator and subsequent non-genomic effects of the promoter. The malignant phenotype appears late in the process (Farber 1984).

Six weeks after infection with cottontail rabbit papillomavirus (CRPV) 95% of cottontail rabbits have warts. A few regress, most stay the same, but a quarter progress after a year to carcinomas which metastasise. Virus particles are no longer produced in malignant tumours. Molecular hybridisation studies show that the virus genome has undergone changes to multiple circular forms and the transcription of viral RNA is abnormal.

Little is known about the genomic abnormalities of benign tumours. c-*ras* oncogene may be abnormally activated in chemically induced benign skin papillomas in mice. DNA from these tumours can transform NIH 3T3 cells (Balmain et al. 1984; Balmain and Pragwell 1985).

It is important to consider whether the mechanisms of viral and chemical carcinogenesis are similar. At least one oncogene is capable of inducing initiation in the same way as a carcinogenic chemical. Infection of mouse skin with Harvey murine sarcoma virus (HaSV), which contains the oncogene v-Ha-*ras*, does not cause papillomas by itself, but papillomas develop if the tumour promoter TPA is then applied repetitively. The production of benign and malignant warts by the Shope virus (CRPV) in cottontail rabbits is greatly increased by the application of a number of tar products to the skin. The tar itself does not cause tumours in the doses used. It is very interesting that in this particular case the tar may be applied before the virus infection for effective tumour promotion. On the other hand, acutely oncogenic retroviruses induce cancers by introducing an oncogene, bringing about malignant transformation by a single event. Carcinogenesis by such viruses therefore appears to differ from the multistage process of chemical carcinogenesis. Acute viral carcinogenesis has been described as a "pseudo single-hit" phenomenon (Temin 1983). There may be multiple small differences between a normal cellular oncogene in situ and the homologous viral oncogene, both quantitative and qualitative, representing many steps in evolution.

Abnormal function of oncogenes may represent one mechanism of tumour progression. Other mechanisms have been suggested recently. A second group of genes, the "tumour suppressors" or "anti-oncogenes", has been proposed. There is evidence that the transforming effect of different retroviral oncogenes can be counteracted by such suppressor genes. One example is found in Wilms' tumours, involving a regulator gene acting on the gene for the growth factor IGF II. Both alleles of a gene rb-1 are lost in retinoblastoma cells (Cavanee et al. 1983). This gene may normally regulate oncogenes and may be involved in the terminal differentiation of cells.

Genes of a third group that may be involved in progression have been called modulators (Klein and Klein 1985). They affect expression of characteristics that influence tumour spread, for example the products of the major histocompatibility complex (MHC).

Progression of breast cancer results in loss of responsiveness to treatment with hormones. Many breast cancers contain subclones with and without oestrogen receptors. Although a subclone may lose these receptors, it still has the impulse to grow vigorously. It must therefore have undergone a change that causes the nucleus to be activated in the absence of the normal mechanism. Although growth control by steroid hormones clearly becomes deranged in some cancers, the derangements have not yet been related to abnormalities of oncogenes. Most normal lymphocytes have cortisol receptors. Derangements of the normal corti-costeroid hormone-receptor-DNA activation pathway have been demonstrated in mouse lymphoma cells.

Conclusions

The process of chemical carcinogenesis may be divided into the stages of induction, promotion and progression. The promotion stage has recently been dissected still further into two stages, conversion and second-stage promotion. Initiation involves a permanent, heritable change in the genome of target cells which only leads to malignancy if the initiated cells are subjected to distinct substances called tumour promoters. Further genetic damage is involved in progression.

Studies of the action of phorbol esters have helped to reveal some of the mechanisms of control of cell growth. When growth factors and hormones bind to cell surface receptors two biochemical pathways may be activated. One pathway begins with a phosphorylating enzyme, the other with activation of the PI cycle. These are interacting processes, both of which may be deranged in malignant cells.

Viral carcinogenesis may result in initiation similar to that induced by chemical carcinogens, in that promoting agents may be necessary for development of a malignant clone. Acute induction of cancer by retroviruses may circumvent the multistage process of carcinogenesis thought to occur in cancers caused by most environmental carcinogens, by introduction of an oncogene that can confer all of the genomic abnormalities necessary for the development of a fully malignant cell.

References

Balmain A, Pragnell IB (1985) Mouse skin carcinomas induced *in vivo* by chemical carcinogens have a transforming Harvey-*ras* oncogene. Nature 303: 72–74

Balmain A, Ramsden R, Bowden GT, Smith J (1984) Activation of the mouse cellular Harvey-*ras* gene in chemically induced benign skin papillomas. Nature 307: 658–660

Blumberg PM, Jaken S, Konig B et al. (1984) Mechanism of action of the phorbol ester tumor promoters: specific receptors for lipophilic ligands. Biochem Pharmacol 33: 933–940

Boutwell RK, Verma AK, Ashendel CL, Astrup E (1982) Mouse skin: a useful model for studying the mechanism of chemical carcinogenesis. In: Hecker E et al. (eds) Carcinogenesis, vol 7. Raven, New York, pp 1–12

Cavanee WK, Dryja TP, Phillips RA et al. (1983) Expression of recessive alleles by chromosomal mechanisms in retinoblastoma. Nature 305: 779–784

De Paoli-Roach A, Roach PJ, Zucker KE, Smith SS (1986) Selective phosphorylation of human DNA methyltransferase by protein kinase C. FEBS Lett 197: 149–153

Dzarlieva-Petrusevska RT, Fusenig NE (1985) Tumor promoter (TPA) enhanced chromosomal aberrations and gene amplification in mouse keratinocytes: a possible mechanism for the first stage of tumor promotion. J Cancer Res Clin Oncol A14 (abstract)

Farber E (1984) The malignant phenotype as a late expression of the carcinogenic process. J Cell Physiol [Suppl] 3: 123–125

Farrar JJ, Mizel SB, Fuller-Farrar WI, Hilfiker ML (1980) Macrophage independent activation of helper-T-cells. I. Production of interleukin 2. J Immunol 125: 793

Fürstenberger G, Kinzel V, Schwarz M, Marks F (1985) Partial inversion of the initiation-promotion sequence of multistage tumorigenesis in the skin of NMRI mice. Science 230: 76–78

Fusenig NE, Dzarlieva-Petrusevska RT, Breitkreuz D (1985) Phenotype and cytogenetic characteristics of different stages during spontaneous transformation of mouse keratinocytes *in vitro*. In: Barrett JC, Tennant RW (eds) Carcinogenesis, vol 9. Raven, New York, pp 293–326

Hennings H, Shores R, Wenk ML, Spangler EF, Tarone R, Yuspa SH (1983) Malignant conversion of mouse skin tumours is increased by tumour initiators and unaffected by tumour promoters. Nature 304: 67–69

Kinzel V, Loehrke H, Goerttler K, Fürstenberger G, Marks F (1984) Suppression of the first stage of phorbol 12-tetradecanoate 13-acetate-effected tumor promotion in mouse skin by inhibition of DNA synthesis. Proc Natl Acad Sci USA 81: 5858–5862

Klein G, Klein E (1985) Evolution of tumours and the impact of molecular oncology. Nature 315: 190–195

Koeffler HP (1983) Induction of differentiation of human acute myelogenous leukemia cells: therapeutic implications. Blood 62: 709–721

Kraft AS, Anderson WB, Cooper HL, Sando JJ (1982) Decrease in cytosolic calcium/phospholipid-dependent protein kinase activity following phorbol ester treatment of EL4 thymoma cells. J Biol Chem 257: 13193–13196

Marks F, Bertsch S, Fürstenberger G, Richter H (1983) Growth control in mouse epidermis — facts and speculation. In: Wright NA, Camplejohn RS (eds) Psoriasis: cell proliferation. Churchill Livingstone, Edinburgh, pp 173–188

Marx JL (1985) The polyphosphoinositides revisited. Science 228: 312–313

Miller EC (1978) Some current perspectives on chemical carcinogenesis in humans and experimental animals. Presidential address. Cancer Res 38: 1479–1496

Nishizuka Y (1984) The role of protein kinase C in cell surface signal transduction and tumour promotion. Nature 308: 693–698

Parkinson EK (1985) Defective responses of transformed keratinocytes to terminal differentiation stimuli. Their role in epidermal tumour promotion by phorbol esters and by deep skin wounding. Br J Cancer 52: 479–493

Temin HM (1984) Do we understand the genetic mechanisms of oncogenesis? Keynote address for Honey Harbor meeting on cellular and molecular biology of neoplasia. 2–6 October, 1983. J Cell Physiol [Suppl] 3: 1–11

Trosko JE, Jone C, Chang C-C (1983) The role of tumor promoters on phenotypic alterations affecting intracellular communication and tumorigenesis. Ann NY Acad Sci 407: 316–327

Weinstein IB, Gattoni-Celli S, Kirschmeier P et al. (1984) Multistage carcinogenesis involves multiple genes and multiple mechanisms. J Cell Physiol [Suppl] 3: 127–137

5 Multifactorial Aetiology of Cancers

Introduction

Human cancers rarely, if ever, arise through the operation of a single aetiological factor. In the controlled conditions of the laboratory many factors other than the carcinogen affect the induction of experimental cancers. 12-O-tetradecanoylphorbol-13-acetate (TPA) is an efficient promoter of skin papillomas in some strains, but not in others. Age, sex, race and nutrition all influence greatly the effect of carcinogenic agents in humans. Epidemiological studies have clarified the influence of these factors in many instances. There is constant exposure to carcinogens in the form of ionising radiation and chemicals. Viruses are undoubtedly aetiological factors in the development of cancer in animals and are now implicated in the causation of some human cancers.

As many cancers occur in later life, the relationship between ageing and the development of cancers has long stimulated speculation. There is always the possibility of error in the copying of DNA during replication of cells, but repair mechanisms appear normally to be very efficient. The accumulation of genetic errors occurring during normal division may contribute to carcinogenesis. Another suggestion is that the attachment of methyl groups to cytosine molecules in DNA is important in determining how effectively cells divide, and that it could determine the capacity for unlimited multiplication in cancer cells on the one hand, and the normal ageing process which limits the number of divisions of normal cells, on the other.

Population and Familial Factors

There are wide differences in the incidence of specific cancers, for example breast cancer, in different parts of the world. The striking variations from nation to nation in the patterns of occurrence of cancer probably reflect differences in exposure to environmental risk factors — diet and social factors. Genetic variation appears to account for only a small proportion of these differences, particularly as the incidence of many cancers in a given population has changed quite rapidly

(Muir and Parkin 1985). Women born in the USA of Japanese parents have the same high incidence of breast cancer as other women in the USA. The incidence in Japanese women in Japan is much lower. The opposite holds for stomach cancer in Japanese; the incidence is high in Japan and much lower in Japanese born in the USA. Studies of migrants show that this is a general phenomenon; descendants of people who move to another country have the pattern of cancers in their new home, within one or two generations. In 1975, stomach cancer was the most common tumour in the world, but its incidence is declining everywhere, possibly because of better methods of storing food and greater consumption of fresh vegetables, although the cause of the fall is not fully understood. A high intake of fats is suspected to be a causative factor in breast cancer. The incidence of cancer among Eskimos is low. Nasopharyngeal and bladder cancers have strong regional associations in the Far East. Oesophageal cancer occurs frequently along the shore of the Caspian Sea and in some regions of China. Food moulds and deficiency of vitamin A are suspected factors. It has been suggested that as much as 80%–90% of cancer is determined environmentally (Muir and Parkin 1985).

There are significant epidemiological differences in the incidence of lymphocytic leukaemia and of lymphoma. Regions of high incidence of Burkitt's lymphoma in Africa overlap the malaria belt, and the incidence is greatest near lakes, below an altitude of 1500 m. This has suggested a relationship to malaria. The clustering of Hodgkin's disease has been reported, and questioned. Regional differences in the incidence and sex ratio of lymphomas are reported in China. T cell lymphomas are relatively more frequent than B cell lymphomas in Japan and China. The incidence of lymphomas is strongly influenced by the human leukaemia/lymphoma virus HTLV-I in endemic areas. Epidemiological studies point to correlations between malignant lymphoma and benzene, dieldrin, phenols, phenoxyacetic acid, asbestos, immunosuppression, ionising radiation and contact with bovine lymphomas.

Diet has been implicated in the causation of carcinoma of the colon, as well as in breast cancer. Diet seems the likely explanation for the increased risk of development of breast, ovarian endometrial and prostatic cancer in migrants from low-risk countries (Berg 1976). Calorie restriction inhibits development of several types of neoplasms in mice. Underfed mice of a strain having a high incidence of leukaemia lived longer than normally fed mice and only 6.9% developed leukaemia, as compared with 55%–75% in the control group. The appearance of malignant cells in the lymph nodes of underfed mice was delayed until 14–16 months of age, as compared with 5–8 months in control mice (Saxton et al. 1944).

Genetic bases for different incidences of most cancers among different populations are yet to be discovered. No striking associations have emerged between cancer susceptibility and expression of genes of the major histocompatibility complex (MHC). A weak, but statistically significant association between HLA-Cw5 and myeloma has been reported in American blacks (Leech et al. 1983). The G3m(g5) immunoglobulin allotype is also significantly associated with multiple myeloma (Leech et al. 1985).

Familial cancers are relatively rare. Some are associated with constitutional chromosomal abnormalities (see Chap. 2, p. 17). Numerous inherited syndromes confer an increased susceptibility to the development of cancer, for example tuberous sclerosis, familial intestinal polyposis and neurofibromatosis. If these subjects have chromosomal lesions, they are well below the limits of sensitivity of the most refined method of cytogenetic study. With von Recklinghausen neurofibromatosis, brain tumours, including meningiomas, may occur in several members of the family.

A clear-cut pattern of dominant inheritance exists for a number of cancer syndromes: childhood retinoblastoma, basal cell naevus syndrome, neurofibromatosis, multiple endocrine neoplasia syndromes, dysplastic naevus syndrome and intestinal polyposis. The dominant genes involved do not affect multiple systems, and the lesions associated with cancer are focal in the affected organs (Harnden et al. 1984). It is presumed that the primary effect on the gene does not cause malignant transformation; a subsequent event or events are required. Alternatively, the inherited abnormality could, as in cancers associated with defective DNA repair, predispose to malignancy, but the tissue specificity is hard to explain.

Other inherited or congenital conditions predisposing to leukaemia are Down's syndrome, Klinefelter's syndrome and ataxia telangiectasia. The Wiskott–Aldrich syndrome and X-linked immunodeficiency syndrome are two others. The Cancer Family Syndrome of Lynch is characterised by the frequent occurrence of different types of cancers, often adenocarcinomas of the colon, endometrium, and breast, at early ages. In one family, rare cancers, six primary cancers and a case of B cell leukaemia associated with Burkitt's lymphoma were recorded (Love 1985).

Very little is known about inherited susceptibility to common cancers. High concordance of childhood leukaemia has been reported in identical twins (McMahon and Levy 1964).

Carcinogens

The term "carcinogen" is commonly used to describe an agent that leads to an increased incidence of cancers in exposed subjects. This usage allows for the fact that unexposed populations may spontaneously develop certain cancers. We refer to "causation" of cancer in this sense: induction of an increased incidence.

Many experts consider that chemical carcinogens in the environment, in the diet, or in the form of drugs are the major causes of cancer. Epidemiological evidence certainly supports this contention. The formulae of some carcinogenic chemicals are shown in Fig. 5.1. Tobacco smoke is the major causative factor in carcinoma of the bronchus, and tobacco is probably the most important carcinogen, globally speaking (Muir and Parkin 1985). World annual production of tobacco exceeds 5 million tonnes. The risk of cancers of larynx, oesophagus, bladder and pancreas is also increased by cigarette smoking. Many carcinogens are associated with occupation (Table 5.1). Vast quantities of polycyclic hydrocarbons are released into the atmosphere by the burning of fossil fuels. Metals carcinogenic in humans are arsenic, nickel and chromium.

Other carcinogens are found in food. Peanut meal contaminated with the fungus *Aspergillus flavus*, when introduced into the UK in 1960, killed more than 100 000 turkeys. This led to the identification of aflatoxin, which causes liver tumours in experimental animals and is suspected of causing liver cancer in southern Africa. Compounds carcinogenic for experimental animals can be extracted from bracken, cycad nuts, sassafras root and golden ragwort. Nitrosamines are highly carcinogenic in animals and readily formed in the body from nitrates (Fig. 5.1).

There is a strong relationship between analgesic abuse and transitional cell carcinoma of the renal pelvis and bladder. Compound analgesics containing

Table 5.1. Some occupational carcinogens

Substance	Site	Industry
Mineral oil	Skin, scrotum, lung	Machine tool
Aniline	Bladder	Dye
β-naphthylamine	Bladder	Rubber
Asbestos	Bronchus, serosa	Brakes, insulation
Vinyl chloride monomer	Liver: angiosarcoma	Plastics
Polycyclic aromatic hydrocarbons	Lung, kidney	Coke, gas, steel
Benzene	Bone marrow: myeloid leukaemia	Petrochemical
Chromates	Lung	Plating
Cadmium	Prostate	
Nickel	Lung, paranasal sinuses, larynx	
Arsenic	Lung, skin	

aspirin, caffeine and phenacetin are implicated (Mahoney et al. 1977). Myeloge-nous leukaemia may be induced in experimental animals by a number of chemical compounds, but benzene is the only substance implicated in the induction of acute and chronic myelogenous leukaemia in man.

Is there a common thread to the causation of cancer by diverse insults to DNA? Some rules relating to the chemical interaction of substances with DNA and carcinogenesis have been formulated (Hathaway and Kolar 1980). There appears to be a reasonable correlation between the distortion to the double helix, caused by the chemical reaction, and carcinogenic potency. Many chemical carcinogens

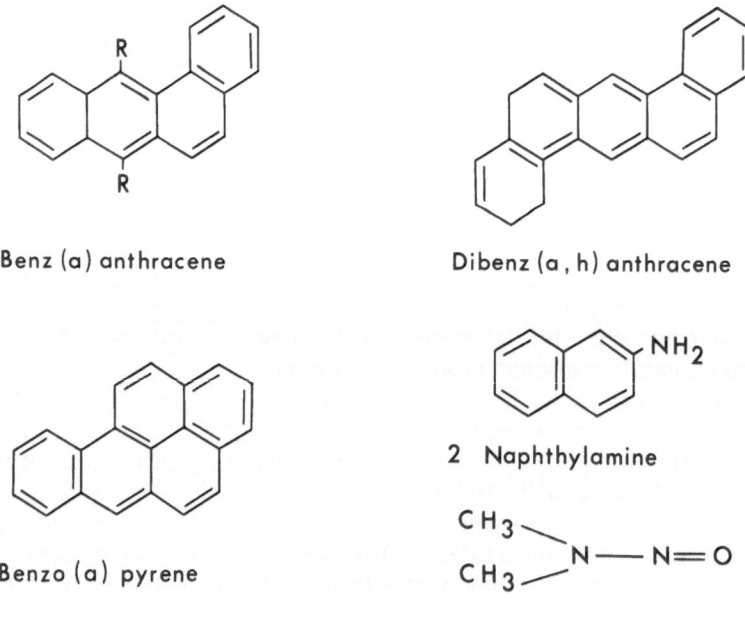

Benz (a) anthracene

Dibenz (a, h) anthracene

Benzo (a) pyrene

2 Naphthylamine

Dimethylnitrosamine

Fig. 5.1. Formulae of some carcinogenic chemicals.

bind covalently to DNA. Many require to be activated in the body. Damage to DNA, whether caused by irradiation or chemical carcinogens, is normally repaired rapidly. Impairment of repair mechanisms is implicated in the susceptibility to cancer in Fanconi's anaemia and Bloom's syndrome.

Oncogenic viruses may introduce new genes into cells, but chemical carcinogens cannot. However, genes, including oncogenes may be rearranged and amplified in chemically induced tumours. Induction of leukaemias and lymphomas in mice and rats, whether by chemical agents or ionising radiation, is due to activation of dormant leukaemogenic viruses of the murine leukaemia virus (MuLV) class.

Carcinogenesis by nitroso-methyl-urea (NMU) during sexual development in female rats (Barbacid 1985) illustrates some very important principles in chemical carcinogenesis.

1. Since NMU is very unstable under physiological conditions, its mutagenic activity is confined to the first few hours after it has been administered. Therefore, initiation occurs within a very short time of administration of the drug.

2. The mutation affects an oncogene. A single dose of NMU activated the *ras* locus in 61 out of 72 tumours. Furthermore, this mutation was in the same part of the c-*ras* proto-oncogene in all 61 (the second nucleotide of the twelfth codon of the Ha-*ras*-1 locus).

3. The mutation is highly specific. NMU changes the nucleic acid base guanine to adenosine. Dimethylbenzanthracene (DMBA) induces a different mutation. Mammary cancers that arise from treatment with DMBA do not have mutations of the Ha-*ras* gene. Ethylnitrosourea induces rat neuro/glioblastomas, in which the *neu* oncogene is activated.

4. The change associated with initiation persists, and promotion does not have to follow until later.

5. The experiment shows that a specific hormonal status is required for promotion of the tumour. When pregnant rats were treated with NMU on day 17 of gestation, all mothers developed benign breast tumours (fibroadenomas), none of which contained activated Ha-*ras*-1 oncogenes. Cancers develop in mammary cells bearing the specific mutation induced by NMU, but only during the time when the breast is developing. Two female offspring of NMU-treated mothers developed mammary cancer 10–12 weeks after reaching sexual development. One of them contained an activated Ha-*ras*-1 oncogene with the guanine to adenine mutation. Other offspring had neural tumours, and several contained transforming oncogenes with sequence homology to the *erb*-B oncogene.

Radiation

Ionising radiation knocks electrons out of atoms of the DNA itself. The interaction of radiation with water generates highly reactive chemical species — free radicals and active oxygen species. These have a lifetime measured in picoseconds. They damage DNA and are the main agents of the carcinogenic action of radiation. High energy ionising radiation is the most hazardous, but non-ionising radiation, such as ultraviolet light, can cause skin cancers.

Electromagnetic and particulate irradiation are used in medicine. Both can damage DNA by creating reactive ions. The higher the ionisation per unit distance the greater the damage to DNA, resulting most frequently in breaks to one or both strands of the helix. These breaks are mostly repaired without permanent damage.

Ionising radiation can be delivered in the form of radioactive substances, as exemplified by the painters of luminous watch dials in New Jersey during the 1920s, who absorbed traces of luminous paint. Of 800 women using paint containing radium and mesothorium, 9 died from osteogenic sarcoma. Other notorious evidences of the carcinogenic potential of ionising radiation are the high incidence of skin cancers among the early radiologists and the after-effects of the atomic bombs. The risk of developing leukaemia is increased nearly ten times as a result of irradiation for the treatment of ankylosing spondylitis (Hirohata 1976).

Ionising radiation apparently plays no part in the causation of chronic lymphocytic leukaemia (CLL). CLL did not occur in the Hiroshima population, but this disease is relatively rare in Japan. Chronic myelogenous leukaemia (CML) was the predominant leukaemia, developing after a latent period of 5 years, in heavily irradiated middle-aged survivors of the Hiroshima atomic bomb. Acute leukaemia developed in those irradiated in their first year of life or after age 60. CML may occur after therapeutic irradiation. An increased incidence of melanoma appeared 20 years after the Hiroshima bombing. Many reports suggest that ionising radiation may induce multiple myeloma (Cuzick 1981).

In mice, ionising radiation produces thymic lymphomas, which sometimes develop into generalised lymphomas and leukaemias. Irradiation of both the thymus and bone marrow is essential, and the tumours do not arise from a mutation, but by facilitation of carcinogenesis by viruses of the MuLV type already present in the cells.

Most carcinogenic ultraviolet radiation comes from the sun. Although most of the short-wavelength ultraviolet radiation is filtered out by the atmosphere, there is sufficient to cause skin cancer in susceptible persons who have significant exposure, particularly those with fair skin. Ultraviolet radiation causes dimerisation of thymidine, which is particularly carcinogenic in patients with xeroderma pigmentosum, because their cells lack the enzyme necessary to excise such dimers.

Viruses

Viruses cause cancer in animals under natural and experimental conditions. The oncogenic viruses in animals are of the following types:

1. DNA viruses:
   papovaviruses
   adenoviruses
   herpesviruses
   hepatitis B virus
2. RNA viruses: oncornaviruses (retroviruses)
   a) "acutely transforming", containing an oncogene
   b) "chronically transforming", not containing an oncogene
   c) HTLV-type retroviruses

Oncogenic adenoviruses adsorb to virus receptors on the cytoplasmic membrane, enter the cell, replicate their DNA in the nucleus and transcribe virus messenger RNA for cytoplasmic biosynthesis of virus proteins. New virus particles assemble in the nucleus and are released following cell lysis. As a general rule, transformation is accompanied by repression of late steps in virus replication, with no release of infectious virus. Herpesviruses adsorb to cell-specific receptors and the virus envelope and cell membrane fuse. The synthesis of host DNA is shut down and replication of the viral DNA begins. Virus bodies, nucleocapsids, are assembled in the nucleus and, after acquisition of a lipid envelope from the nuclear membrane, the virus particles exit through the endoplasmic reticulum.

Papovaviruses include simian vacuolating virus 40 (SV40), polyomavirus and papillomaviruses. They contain circular DNA. SV40, first found in monkey kidney tissue cultures, does not cause tumours in monkeys or man (it was present in early poliomyelitis vaccines), but readily induces tumours in hamsters. SV40 encodes three extensively studied oncogenes, the T oncogenes, which transform cells in tissue culture.

Papilloma viruses include Shope cottontail rabbit papillomavirus (CRPV), which is transmitted to rabbits by mosquitoes and induces benign fibrous papillomas. When injected into domestic rabbits, the virus induces tumours that progress to carcinomas and the virus is no longer found, whereas it is recoverable from tumours of wild-type cottontail rabbits. Warts of squamous epithelium are induced by specific types of human papillomavirus (HPV).

Many *adenoviruses* are pathogenic in man, but none is known to cause human cancer. Some, for example human adenovirus type 12, are oncogenic in experimental animals, readily inducing cancers in neonatal hamsters. Adenoviruses can transform cells in vitro. Transforming adenoviruses contain the A oncogenes.

Herpesviruses are large viruses containing linear, double-stranded DNA surrounded by a lipid and glycoprotein coat, generally giving rise to life-long infections. Productive herpesvirus infection is accompanied by cell death. Cells that have undergone malignant transformation are infected with virus, but the infection does not result in production of virus and the cells are able to grow and divide. It is interesting that peripheral blood leucocytes are a preferred site for some herpesviruses and some lymphomas are associated with herpesviruses. Herpesviruses cause Lucké's renal adenocarcinoma in frogs, Marek's disease in chickens and cancers in rabbits, monkeys and guinea pigs. A non-pathogenic herpesvirus of turkeys (HVT) immunises chicks against Marek's disease. Epstein–Barr virus (EBV) is a herpesvirus.

Retroviruses (Fig. 5.2) are 100–115 nm spherical particles with a central dimeric RNA nucleoid and an outer envelope of two or three shells. They are natural pathogens in all classes of vertebrates, including man. The retrovirus life cycle is illustrated in Fig. 5.3.

A number of avian sarcoma retroviruses stem from Rous sarcoma virus (RSV). The development of tumours depends on the age of the animal at infection. Sarcomas develop in immature birds with great rapidity (within 48–72 h) at the site of application, whereas mature birds make an immune response which protects them.

The mouse leukaemia viruses are related to the leukosis viruses of the fowl and to RSV. They belong to the MuLV family of closely related RNA viruses, of which the Gross/AKR and the RadLV viruses exist in virtually all strains of mice (and probably other species) and are propagated vertically from one generation to the

phospholipid bilayer

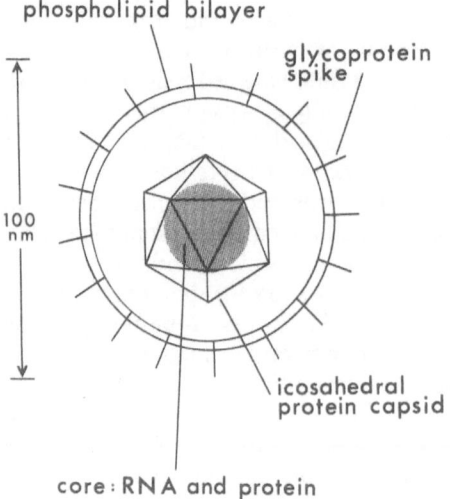

glycoprotein
spike

100
nm

icosahedral
protein capsid

core: RNA and protein

Fig. 5.2. Structure of a retrovirus. The ripe retrovirus (a type C particle), possesses an electron-dense central nucleoid surrounded by membranes. The core contains two copies of single-stranded RNA complexed with two virus-specific basal proteins, group-specific antigens and DNA-dependent RNA polymerase (reverse transcriptase). The envelope is a phospholipid bilayer, derived from the host, containing protein derived from the virus.

next. Mouse sarcoma viruses come from experimental tumours that were produced by passage of the mouse leukaemia viruses. They are similar in structure and mode of replication to the leukaemia viruses (Fig. 5.3).

Four types of retrovirus particles can be distinguished on electron microscopy. Type A particles are ring forms with membrane and nucleoid. Type B are intermediate forms with an eccentric nucleoid and spikes on the outer membrane. Type C are the mature budding viruses, having dense central nucleoids and spikes or knobs on the outer membrane (the lipid of which is derived from the host). Type D particles are rod forms of primate retroviruses.

Leukaemia and sarcoma retroviruses have the following genes (Fig. 5.4):

1. *gag* (group-specific antigen), for the 30 000 dalton viral core protein, which is the group-specific antigen.

2. *pol*, for reverse transcriptase (RNA-dependent DNA polymerase), by which they copy their genetic information into the double-stranded DNA of the host. A complementary strand is first made on the viral RNA template, then the RNA is degraded. A second (positively complementary) strand of DNA is then synthesised on the template of the first DNA strand (see Fig. 5.3).

3. *env*, for the 70 kD envelope glycoprotein.

4. Long terminal repeat (LTR) region, on both ends of the integrated provirus.

5. Retroviruses may have acquired oncogenes from their hosts during their evolution.

The LTR region controls transcription of viral and possibly of cellular genes. The LTR genes are unusually long in HTLV. The genes are arranged from the 5′ to the 3′ end in the order *gag*, *pol*, *env*, and separated by non-coding sequences.

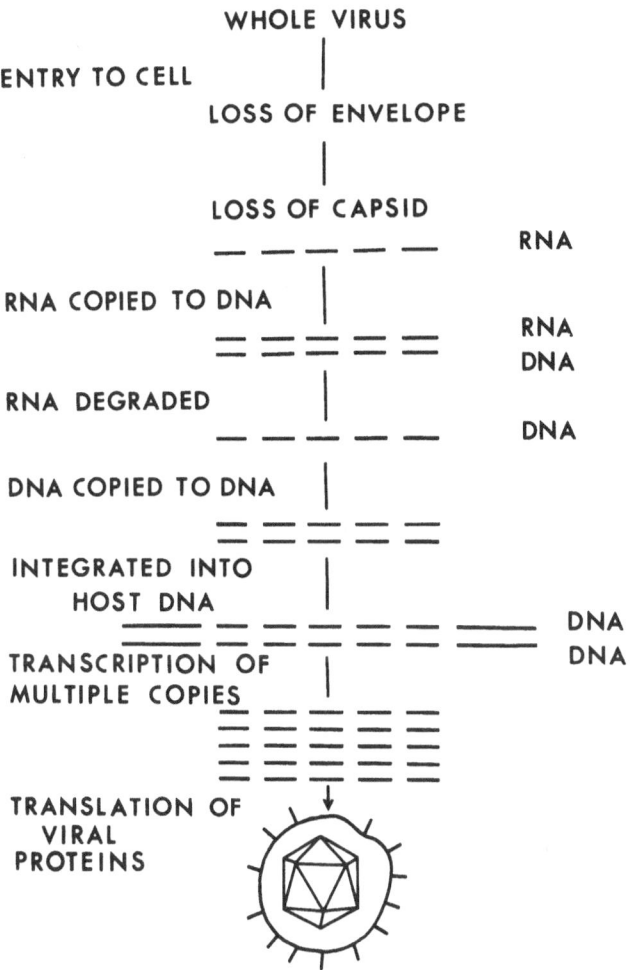

WHOLE VIRUS

ENTRY TO CELL

LOSS OF ENVELOPE

LOSS OF CAPSID

RNA COPIED TO DNA

RNA DEGRADED

DNA COPIED TO DNA

INTEGRATED INTO
HOST DNA

TRANSCRIPTION OF
MULTIPLE COPIES

TRANSLATION OF
VIRAL
PROTEINS

RNA

RNA
DNA

DNA

DNA
DNA

Fig. 5.3. Life cycle of a retrovirus. The virus enters a cell, loses its envelope and capsid coat. The enzyme reverse transcriptase first makes a DNA copy of the viral RNA. The viral RNA is then degraded. A second DNA copy is made of the first DNA strand. The incorporation of the double-stranded DNA copy of the RNA genome is catalysed by host enzymes. New viral RNA molecules are transcribed from the proviral DNA.

Amongst the retroviruses, only HTLV have introns. Introns are loops of DNA not encoding protein. Exons are the intervening segments. They join up to form the template for the mRNA copy.

Acute leukaemia viruses are usually incapable of replication, because they have lost essential genes. For replication and the development of malignancy they generally require coinfection with a non-defective helper virus. They arose by recombination between a helper virus and host genes that function in cell proliferation and differentiation, now known as proto-oncogenes. These viruses transform cells in vitro. The defective retroviruses have part of the *gag* gene, part of the *env* gene, the LTR region and an oncogene sequence. RSV, which is not replication defective, has the gene arrangement 5'-*gag-pol-env-src*-3'. The latent

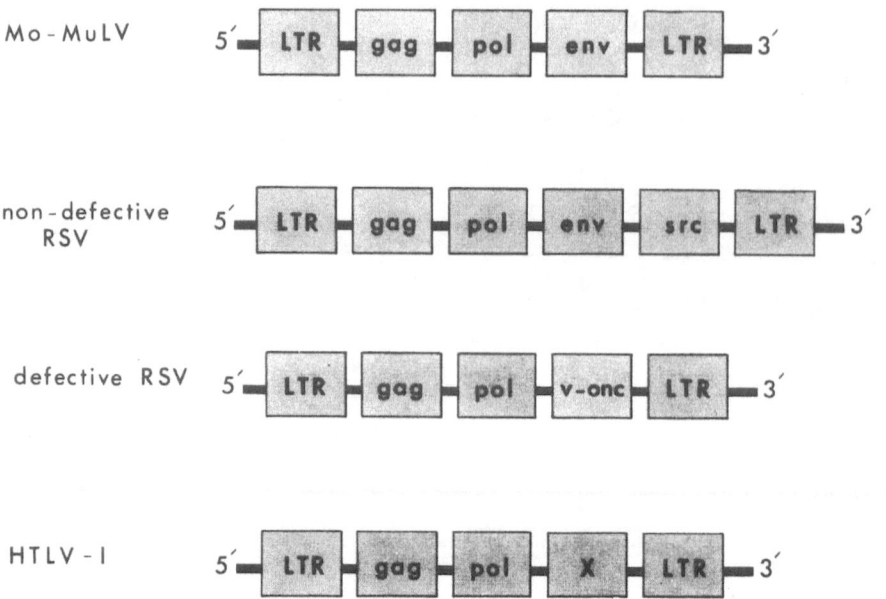

Fig. 5.4. RNA genomes of some of the retroviruses. Non-defective retroviruses, e.g. Moloney murine lymphoma virus (Mo-MuLV) and Rous sarcoma virus (RSV) have the three essential genes *gag*, *pol* and *env*, with long terminal repeats (*LTR*) at each end. Most acute transforming viruses are defective, being dependent on helper viruses for replication. Transforming viruses may have an oncogene, e.g. *src*, *abl*, *mos*, *fos*, *fms*, or a mutant gene, in the place of *env*.

period of induction of leukaemia by acutely transforming retroviruses is usually short, and the neoplasia is polyclonal.

Chronic leukaemia viruses are exogenous retroviruses which do not carry an *onc* gene. The chronic leukaemia viruses associated with naturally occurring lymphomas and leukaemias are replication competent and require a long incubation period to induce malignancy. They cause erythroid and myeloid leukaemias as well as lymphoid neoplasms, but infection does not always result in development of disease, as in adult cats infected with feline leukaemia virus.

Transmission of retroviruses may be either (1) endogenous (vertical) or (2) exogenous (horizontal). Probably every type of retrovirus can be transmitted vertically through the germline, and vertically transmitted retroviruses may induce tumours. Most retroviral tumours in outbred animals are caused by horizontal, exogenous infections. Transmission in this case is called epigenetic, i.e. by transmission of virus particles not incorporated into a cellular genome. Some retrovirus-induced tumours are overtly contagious under natural conditions, for example avian and bovine leukosis and feline leukaemia.

Direct effects of the viruses on the cells can be classified (Fig. 5.5) as:

1. Insertion of a viral oncogene by an acute leukaemia virus. This may code for proteins which induce transformation, act as receptors for growth factors or disturb the transmission of signals from growth factors. These viral proteins are *trans*acting (i.e. by diffusing to a distant site) and the virus does not need to be integrated in any particular site in the genome.

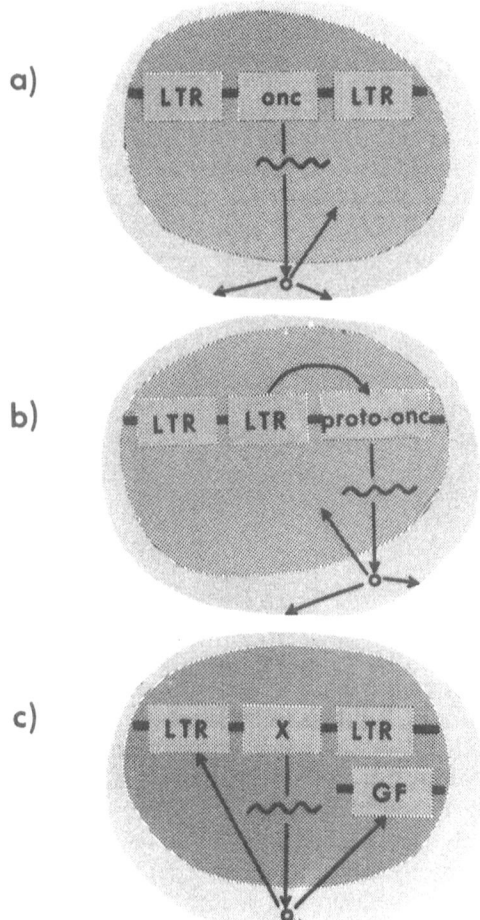

Fig. 5.5. Mechanisms of carcinogenesis by viruses. **a** Acute leukaemia viruses have captured oncogenes which encode proteins capable of inducing transformation. No constant ("conserved") site of insertion is necessary. **b** Chronic leukaemia viruses integrated at a particular site activate cellular oncogenes abnormally. This mechanism is called *cis*-activation, i.e. acting on the same DNA strand, in close proximity. **c** HTLVs make a nuclear protein TAT, encoded by the gene *X* (also known as *tat* and *lor*). TAT *trans*activates, inducing expression of distant genes promoting growth (depicted here as growth factor *GF*), either through its own products, or through action on the *LTR*. The *wavy line* represents mRNA, which is translated into protein. The gene products are shown as *circles*, and the *arrows* indicate the direction of action of products. (Adapted from Wong-Staal and Gallo 1985).

2. Activation of a cellular oncogene by insertion of a viral genome proximally, resulting in disordered regulation of the oncogene. Chronic leukaemia viruses act this way.

3. HTLV and related monkey and bovine leukaemia/lymphoma viruses (STLV and BLV) make a nuclear protein (TAT) which *trans*activates transcription, possibly of lymphocyte growth-promoting genes (Fig. 5.5). A specific site of integration is not necessary.

Viruses in the Causation of Animal Cancers

Viruses causing murine lymphoid neoplasms include the Moloney leukaemogenic virus (Mo-MuLV), murine sarcoma virus (MSV), polyomavirus and adeno-12 viruses. Oncogenic viruses in mice usually remain latent and innocuous throughout the entire life span of the host unless the host–virus relationship is disturbed. The disturbance precipitating the emergence of leukaemia or lymphoma may be injury to the thymus, bone marrow, or impairment of immune competence. Tumours arise spontaneously in some strains having a high incidence of leukaemia, notably AKR and C58. AKR mice usually die of spontaneously occurring T cell leukaemia.

In most strains the malignancy usually arises in the thymus and spreads to other lymphoid tissues, bone marrow and viscera. Frank lymphocytic leukaemia develops preterminally in those animals which survive long enough. Development of this disease is related to the presence of endogenous Gross C-type virus. Intrathymic injection of Abelson virus (AMuLV) into nude mice induces thymomas. Tumour cell lines derived by transformation in vitro of bone marrow or spleen cells by this agent are predominantly pre-B or B cells. These transformed lines may become independent of growth factors and may grow as tumours in animals (Cook et al. 1984).

Leukaemia/lymphoma viruses also occur naturally in chickens (avian leukosis virus, ALV) and cats (feline leukaemia virus, FeLV, and the closely related feline sarcoma virus, FeSV). A high incidence of cat lymphomas occurs when FeLV is introduced into households with large numbers of cats. Kittens do not produce antibodies, but develop a viraemia and a high incidence of leukaemias and lymphomas. Infected older cats develop protective antibodies against the virus. A syndrome resembling acquired immunodeficiency syndrome (AIDS) has also been described in association with FeLV infection. Malignant lymphoma of cattle (enzootic bovine leukosis) is caused by an RNA virus (bovine leukaemia virus, BLV) and can be transmitted experimentally to sheep and goats.

In chickens susceptible to ALV, lymphomas develop primarily in the bursa of Fabricius, 8–12 weeks after virus infection and eventually metastasise to spleen, liver and kidneys, resulting in death of the animal.

Retroviruses are also involved in the causation of neoplasms in gibbons. Malignant lymphoma epidemics, associated with retroviruses and herpes type viruses, occur in New World and Old World monkeys.

Some viruses are oncogenic in species other than those in which they occur naturally. Herpesvirus ateles and Herpesvirus saimiri induce lymphomas in marmosets. Experimental induction usually requires immunosuppression, or the use of tumour promoters, e.g. TPA. EBV, a human virus, also produces malignant lymphomas when injected into marmosets.

Viruses in the Causation of Human Cancers

Until recently the evidence for a viral aetiology of human neoplasms has been lacking. Now there is increasing evidence that viruses are involved in the pathogenesis of human cancers, and some are believed actually to cause them. Adult T cell leukaemia/lymphoma (ATL) is the first human cancer which can, with confidence, be attributed to the effects of an infectious virus, HTLV-I. HTLVs are a family of related T lymphotropic retroviruses.

HTLVs share some structural features with the other retroviruses and manifest important differences (see Fig. 5.4). Although the HTLVs all lack cell-derived oncogenes, they have the usual viral replicative genes *gag*, *pol* and *env* present in the mammalian type C viruses. They have a region at the 3′ end (*X* in HTLV-I, tat in HIV[1]) encoding proteins that increase the efficiency of expression of genes at distant sites on the genome either by direct action on those genes, or by activating the LTR sequences flanking the virus genome which cause increased expression of distant genes (Rosen et al. 1986). This activation of genes at a distance is called "transactivation" (see Fig. 5.5). The genes affected may encode lymphocyte growth factors or viruses. Induction of increased expression of these genes by the integrated virus could lead to immortalisation and subsequently to malignant transformation (Wong-Staal and Gallo 1985). It has been suggested that HIV acts like a tumour promoter, inducing cancer in association with other occasionally oncogenic viruses.

ATL was first reported as a new disease in Japan, where it is the predominant lymphoid neoplasm, with a marked clustering of the disease in the southwest of the country. The disease is also endemic in the Caribbean islands, and occurs in many parts of Africa. The HTLV-I virus itself has a unique geographical distribution. It is widespread in Africa and may have originated there (Vogt 1985). Simian T leukaemia/lymphoma virus-I (STLV-I), a virus very similar to HTLV-I, is associated with lymphomas in some Old World monkeys, particularly African green monkeys. HTLV-I occurs in the Caribbean, in areas of Central and South America, Southwestern Japan, Africa, the Middle East, the Indian subcontinent and areas of the Far East other than Japan. It is not indigenous to Europe or North America, although HTLV-I antibodies and integrated virus sequences were recently found in a few cases of T cell leukaemia in Italy (Pandolfi et al. 1985a, b)

The transmission of the virus and the induction of T cell malignancy are partly understood from epidemiological studies and molecular biological investigations. Antibodies to p19 and p24 proteins of HTLV-I are found in patients and in their healthy relatives (Hinuma et al. 1981). In endemic areas of Japan and the Caribbean basin, up to 15% of normal blood donors have antibodies to these core proteins, contrasting with less than 1% of normal donors from non-endemic areas of the world. In Japan, anti-HTLV-I is more common in adults than in children. Transmission of HTLV-I is common among family members, apparently because infection requires prolonged close contact. It occurs from mother to offspring and between couples, more frequently from male to female than in the other direction. The mode of transmission is still unknown, although transplacental transmission has been demonstrated. Children who have received a positive blood transfusion become seropositive after 50 days but apparently do not develop ATL, and virus is not found in the genomes of circulating lymphocytes in these patients. Children

[1]It has recently been decided to rename HTLV-III. This virus is now known as the human immunodeficiency virus (HIV).

who have apparently acquired the disease from their parents in early life may not become seropositive until the late teens. The development of a malignant clone of lymphocytes evidently takes many years after infection. ATL has been observed to develop in previously healthy HTLV-I carriers who had had serum antibodies against HTLV-I for at least 10 years before the onset of ATL.

HTLV-I proviral DNA (i.e. viral DNA integrated into the host genome) is present in peripheral blood cells of all patients with overt ATL, including those with a smouldering type of disease. HTLV-I-carrying clones can also be obtained from cultures of peripheral blood leucocytes of HTLV healthy carriers (Sugamura and Hinuma 1985). The virus has also been found in patients with malignant lymphoma, who are seropositive but do not show clinical features characteristic of ATL. The HTLV-I provirus can integrate into many chromosomal loci in the DNA of the host cell. In any one tumour the viral sequence is integrated in the same place in every cell, indicating the origin of each neoplasm from a single cell. Even different chromosomes are involved in different patients. Since only one clone is found in patients with ATL, the emergence of fully malignant cells must be very infrequent.

HTLV-I can be grown in helper T cells of the CD4+ phenotype in the presence of the lymphocyte growth factor IL-2, and the virus can be transmitted from cell to cell, most likely using the CD4 cell surface molecule as receptor. HTLV-I "immortalises" these T cells. Human T cell cultures immortalised by HTLV-I in vitro also develop into clonal lines as shown by the unique integration site of the provirus in each line. These cell lines grow autonomously, without IL-2, although they have IL-2 receptors and their growth is inhibited by IL-2 (Sugamura et al. 1985). The leukaemic cells freshly obtained from patients with ATL do not immediately express viral RNA or proteins, but subsequently produce viral particles in culture and release type C particles in culture.

The possibility has been raised that HTLV-I may be indirectly involved in other types of lymphoid neoplasm. In a survey of lymphoid malignancies in Jamaica, antibodies to HTLV-I were found in 6 of 17 patients with CLL of the B cell variety (Clark et al. 1985). Analysis of the malignant B cells of one patient with an HTLV-I genomic probe showed no integrated virus, but HTLV-I was integrated into the genome of a T cell line cultured from the patient. The authors suggested that B lymphoid malignancy may occur by an indirect mechanism, for example as a result of a primary T cell abnormality. In support of this idea, abnormality of B cell function, with the production of monoclonal immunoglobulin, has been found in much higher frequency in patients with ATL than in control groups (Matsuzaki et al. 1985).

HTLV-I, like HIV, may involve the nervous system. Antibodies to HTLV-I have recently been found in patients in Martinique suffering from tropical spastic paraparesis, a slowly progressive degeneration of white matter (Gessain et al. 1985).

HIV, a lymphotropic retrovirus related to HTLV-I and causing the acquired immunodeficiency syndrome (AIDS), is associated with a wide range of malignancies, particularly Kaposi's sarcoma, non-Hodgkin's lymphoma, and carcinoma of tongue and rectum. Non-Hodgkin's lymphoma has been reported in 90 homosexual men, presumably carriers of the virus (Ziegler et al. 1984). Hodgkin's disease is also associated with AIDS-related generalised lymphadenopathy in homosexual men (Schoeppel et al. 1985).

There are viruses similar to HIV in *Macaca* species, African green monkeys and baboons. The prevailing impression is that the AIDS epidemic originated in Africa, either through mutation of a pre-existing HIV virus, or through escape from an acclimatised population.

HIV is not directly involved in AIDS-related neoplasms, as viral genetic material is found only in a small fraction of cells in Kaposi's sarcoma or B cell lymphomas. It may be concluded that HIV is also only indirectly involved in the pathogenesis of HIV-related lymphadenopathy syndrome for the same reason, namely, that virus is found in the genome of only a small fraction of the cells of lymph nodes of these patients. In the AIDS patients with Kaposi's sarcoma, the virus is found in blood, bone marrow, lymph nodes, spleen, semen and saliva. Kaposi's sarcoma appears to be associated with HIV infection almost exclusively in homosexual males. Kaposi's sarcoma is uncommon in those who acquire infection with HIV via blood transfusions or drug addiction. Cytomegalovirus (CMV) and use of amyl nitrite may be co-factors. Profound immunodeficiency is thought to be a significant factor in the pathogenesis of cancers in AIDS patients. It is not, however, an essential factor in the development of lymphoma. EBV infection, on the other hand, is possibly a co-factor in the genesis of malignant lymphomas in AIDS patients. Similarly, papillomavirus infection may cooperate in the induction of anal carcinoma in homosexual males.

Antibodies to other potentially oncogenic viruses, including CMV, hepatitis B virus (HBV) and EBV have also been detected in patients with AIDS (Sarin and Gallo 1984) and there is some evidence of CMV gene sequences in DNA from Kaposi's sarcoma tumour cells (Boldogh et al. 1980). It is interesting that B cell lines from these patients secrete large amounts of γ interferon (IFN$_\gamma$). Macrophages can also be infected by the virus, and HIV has been cultured in high frequency from brain tissue of those infected.

HIV enters CD4+ helper T cells via the CD4 antigen, which acts as receptor and is then modulated. Infected CD4+ cells grow for only 2–3 weeks and then perish when the virus is expressed. There is a profound decrease in the ratio of CD4+ to CD8+ cells in the blood of persons affected by AIDS. Reported abnormalities of lymphocytes in these patients include decreased blast formation to mitogens and antigens, IL-2 production, B lymphocyte helper capacity and expression of receptors for IL-2. However, when individual subsets of lymphocytes were examined, blast transformation and lymphokine production appeared to be normal, but there was a severe defect in the capacity to recognise and respond to soluble antigen (Lane et al. 1985).

EBV has been implicated in the development of Burkitt's lymphoma (BL) and nasopharyngeal carcinoma. It is the causative agent of infectious mononucleosis, which represents the reaction to primary EBV infection during adolescence. In the countries where BL and nasopharyngeal carcinoma are endemic, primary infection occurs during the first year of life, and perinatal infection may be related to the development of BL (de Thé 1977). EBV eventually infects virtually all people in technologically advanced as well as in non-advanced countries. EBV antibody titres are high in patients with BL, and the EBV genome has been demonstrated within the genome of the cancer cells.

Antibodies are formed to three EBV antigen systems: (1) early antigens, mainly viral enzymes; (2) viral capsid antigen; and (3) nuclear antigens (EBNA), synthesised during the quiescent or latent phase. Two of the nuclear antigens have been designated M and K. Of Chinese and North African patients with nasopharyngeal carcinoma, 90% have antibody to M. Patients with the X-linked immunodeficiency syndrome, who have diffuse lymphoproliferative syndromes caused by EBV, have impaired antibody responses, particularly to EBNA.

In African children, EBV DNA and EBNA are found in tumour cells; 97% of African BL patients carry multiple copies of the EBV genome in their cells; high-titre antibodies to viral capsid antigen, EBNA and other antigens appear in the sera of BL patients. EBV from BL and infectious mononucleosis patients seem to be of the same strain (Purtilo 1980). The exact significance of this association in the pathogenesis of cancer is not clear. Non-African BL cases are often not associated with EBV (Lenoir et al. 1984).

EBV causes a polyclonal B cell proliferation in infectious mononucleosis, which is controlled by T and natural killer (NK) cells and by antibodies to EBV-specific antigens (Tosato and Blaese 1985). EBV is a B cell mitogen and is mitogenic for CLL B cells (Gahrton et al. 1979). It "immortalises" cultured lymphoblasts. It activates production of B cell growth factor (BCGF), creating an autocrine mechanism, i.e. the cell itself produces a growth factor essential for its own growth. Cell lines obtained by transformation of normal B cells are dependent on BCGF, but BL cells are not.

Immunosuppressive therapy reactivates latent EBV. The simultaneous occurrence of fatal infectious mononucleosis and immunoblastic sarcoma in a renal transplant recipient suggested that EBV may have initiated the lymphoma (Briggs et al. 1978), although the patient also had infection with herpes simplex virus. Patients with X-linked immunodeficiency syndrome are particularly susceptible to infection with EBV. Males with this syndrome may develop immunoblastic sarcoma following EBV infection. EBV has also been associated with a lymphoma developing in a patient with ataxia telangiectasia (Saemundsen et al. 1981). Patients with AIDS may develop BL and the tumours carry EBV and may have chromosomal translocations characteristic of BL (Klein and Klein 1985).

There is a clear association between primary hepatocellular carcinoma and chronic infection with HBV. The excess risk, at least in Taiwan, among carriers of HBV is at least 100-fold. This relationship is probably causal. If HBV does indeed cause hepatocellular carcinoma, more than 80% of all primary liver tumours — one of the commonest forms of human cancer — can be attributed to it.

In a prospective study of 22 707 male government employees in Taiwan with a follow up of 75 000 man-years, 3454 (15.2%) had the surface antigen of hepatitis B (HBsAg) in the blood, of whom 40 subsequently died of hepatocellular carcinoma (Beasley et al. 1981). Of 19 253 negative controls only 1 has died of liver cancer. This gives a relative risk of 223 for the development of hepatocellular carcinoma in HBsAg carriers. The follow-up of this study has now been extended to 97 000 man-years (Beasley 1982). No further cases of hepatocellular carcinoma have occurred in the control group, but there have been 70 cases in the group with circulating HBsAg — a relative risk of 390.

In contrast to the Taiwan experience, a study of Greenland Eskimos, a population with a high prevalence of hepatitis carriers, revealed no excess of mortality from hepatocellular carcinoma (Skinhoj et al. 1978), in keeping with the low incidence of other cancers in this race. A British survey also found evidence against a relationship to HBsAg. In a prospective study of 613 patients with cirrhosis of different aetiological types, seropositivity for HBsAg was not related statistically to the development of liver cancer (Zaman et al. 1985). Such contradictory evidence in different races strongly suggests that other factors than HBV are very important in the aetiology of hepatocellular carcinoma. There is indeed evidence of other factors. Males have a higher incidence of hepatocellular carcinoma than females, all over the world. The contributions of alcohol, α_1-antitrypsin deficiency and aflatoxin to causation of hepatocellular carcinoma are not clear.

The DNA of HBV is integrated into the genome of tumour cells. HBV-DNA has also been demonstrated in chronic hepatitis antigen carriers with and without liver disease in the absence of hepatocellular carcinoma. In carriers of less than 2 years' duration, only "free", i.e. non-integrated HBV-DNA, is found in liver cells.

Woodchuck hepatitis virus, ground squirrel hepatitis virus, and the Chinese domestic duck hepatitis B virus all closely resemble the human virus in morphology and molecular biological characteristics. Woodchuck hepatitis virus is associated with chronic active hepatitis and hepatocellular carcinoma, particularly in captive animals with persistent woodchuck virus infection, and the DNA of the virus is integrated into the genome of the cancer cells in the same way as the human hepatitis virus is integrated into the genome of the human liver cancer cells.

Specific strains of human papillomavirus (HPV) — types 16 and 18 — are associated with carcinoma of the vulva, cervix and penis. Carcinoma in situ developed in 30 out of 846 women within 6 years of finding cytological evidence of HPV infection in smears of cervical epithelium, compared with an expected number of 1.9, representing a overall relative risk of 15.6, and a 38.7-fold risk in women younger than 25 years (Mitchell et al. 1986). DNA from different types of papillomaviruses is found in some cervical cancer biopsy specimens and in premalignant lesions, but types 16 and 18 are found almost exclusively in severe dysplasia, carcinoma in situ and invasive carcinoma (Gissmann 1984). In cervical warts and dysplasia, papillomavirus is present in an episomal ring form, whereas in the cancers and in cell lines derived from them it is integrated into the host cell genome. DNA sequences homologous with HPV types 16 and 18 are present in over 80% of invasive squamous cancers of cervix, vulva and penis and in the higher grades of intraepithelial neoplasms of the cervix and vulva. In contrast, HPV types 6 and 11 are often associated with benign genital warts or mild dysplasia. Papillomavirus is not associated with endometrial carcinoma. The period of latency to the time of malignant transformation could be as long as 30 years.

The mechanism of causation of cancer by the papillomaviruses is unknown. These viruses can transform cells in culture, but no oncogenes have been identified in them.

In conclusion, in ATL and carcinoma of the cervix the neoplasms are, in the majority of cases, related to infection with the specific virus. The relationship of HBV to hepatocellular carcinoma is similar to the relationship of BL to EBV, where all the cases in the endemic areas have the virus, but the sporadic cases in non-endemic areas do not. What takes the place of the virus in non-endemic areas? We await further evidence from studies of the integration of the viral genome into normal and cancer tissues. EBV, CMV, herpes simplex virus and others all seem to be passengers in various cancers.

Immunodepression and Immunosuppression

The popularity of theories linking immunodeficiency to cancer has waned considerably in the past decade, but the effect of immunodeficiency or the competence of immunological mechanisms in immune surveillance (Kirchner 1984) cannot be dismissed from considerations of the aetiology of cancer. The high incidence of cancers in AIDS sufferers has again focused on the relationship of immunodeficiency to neoplasia. It is argued that failure of immune recognition and rejection of antigenically distinct tumour cells may be restricted mainly to virally induced tumours, particularly those caused by DNA viruses. Most of the spontaneous tumours, if they arise by non-viral mechanisms, may not provide an immunological target for immunological rejection processes. If, for example, they arise by activation of oncogenes as a result of a chromosomal translocation, they may not bear tumour-specific antigens.

The activity of NK cells may be at least as important as rejection by specifically sensitised T cells. Their action is not restricted to virally or chemically induced tumours. Diminished expression of MHC class I antigens, caused, for example, by the activity of adenovirus oncogenes, may enable cells to avoid rejection by specifically sensitised MHC-restricted cytotoxic T cells, but this increases the probability of their elimination by NK cells.

The increased incidence of malignant disease in congenitally immunodeficient or immunosuppressed patients is limited to a small and unusual group of tumours, which includes lymphomas, other lymphoproliferative diseases, Kaposi's sarcoma, skin papilloma and carcinoma. B cell lymphomas which develop after transplantation are mostly extranodal. About 13% of recipients of cardiac transplants who have received cyclosporin develop a B cell lymphoma, diffuse large cell immunoblastic type. These tumours may be polyclonal, since they express both light chain classes and various heavy chain classes. Different clonal immunoglobulin arrangements have been shown within single tumours, suggesting that the tumours must at least be oligoclonal, not monoclonal. These lesions almost always contain EBV (Hanto et al. 1983), which is incorporated into the tumour cell DNA. They may regress when immunosuppressive therapy is reduced. Chemotherapy and irradiation are not helpful in controlling these lymphomas (Starzl et al. 1984).

Polymorphic B cell lymphomas occur in patients receiving renal transplants (Frizzera et al. 1981). Within a year of renal transplantation the risk of lymphoma is increased 35 times and continues for at least 5 years. Soft tissue and hepatobiliary malignancy is 2.5 times more common, in men. Other cancers include carcinomas of cervix uteri, skin and of the lip (Sheil et al. 1981). This greater risk of other cancers appears later than that for the lymphomas and becomes more pronounced as the interval after transplantation increases (Hoover and Fraumeni 1973).

Skin malignancies are a frequent problem in Australian patients with long-standing renal allografts receiving azathioprine and prednisolone (Hardie et al. 1980), apparently because of the high exposure to ultraviolet light. Cyclosporin may also increase this risk (Thompson et al. 1985), whereas this drug has not been shown to be associated with serious risk of true monoclonal lymphomas and other cancers.

Patients surviving Hodgkin's disease (HD) are at high risk of developing second tumours, most commonly acute non-lymphocytic leukaemia. This is usually attributed to combination chemotherapy or combined modality treatment (Coltman and Dixon 1982). HD itself is associated with cellular and humoral immunodeficiencies (Twomey and Rice 1980). Of 1405 patients with HD, 6 developed malignant melanoma (Tucker et al. 1985).

Viral warts are common in recipients of renal transplants, both children and adults. In epidermodysplasia verruciformis, a rare disease in which numerous flat warts occur, several types of HPV may be found, but only types 6 and 18 are found in warts transforming to squamous cell carcinoma. Malignant tumours are found only in areas of the skin exposed to sunlight. Immunosuppression has been documented in this condition (Dymock et al. 1977). Multiple viral warts have also been reported in a patient with immunological deficiencies resembling those found in the Wiskott–Aldrich syndrome (Ormerod et al. 1983), an X-linked recessive disorder associated with an abnormality in platelet and lymphocyte plasma membranes. This disorder has similarities to the X-linked immunodeficiency *xid* of the CBA/N strain of mice, which lack B cells bearing the Lyb5 differentiation antigen and cannot make antibodies to polysaccharide antigens. The patients with Wiskott–Aldrich syndrome also have a specific inability to respond to polysaccharide antigens and have a T cell defect associated with the progressive depletion of T cell zones in the paracortex of lymph nodes. Preliminary reports suggest that the T cells may lack receptors for IL-1 and IL-2.

X-linked immunodeficiency syndrome is a rare sex-linked disorder with unrestrained proliferation of lymphocytes, resembling infectious mononucleosis, resulting from EBV infection. The victims die in the acute phase of the disease with heavy infiltrates of B lymphoid cells in many internal organs. There is a subtle combined T and B cell immunodeficiency in this syndrome (Purtilo et al. 1978). The males cannot mount effective EBV-specific immune responses, so that polyclonal B cell proliferation persists. Death occurs in 1–4 weeks. Males with marginal immune competence show persistent B cell proliferation. Immunoblastic sarcoma, a polyclonal B cell malignancy, or histiocytic lymphoma, may develop. Prospective studies of patients with common variable immunodeficiency (CVID) surviving the first 2 years after diagnosis, showed a 5-fold increase of cancer caused mainly by large excesses of stomach cancer (47-fold) and lymphomas (30-fold) (Kinlen et al. 1985).

Prolonged Antigenic Stimulation

An oncogenic effect of prolonged antigenic stimulation has been demonstrated in mice (Metcalf 1961). Stimulation by an unrelated antigen actually inhibited the viral induction of tumours (Siegel et al. 1967). Chronic graft versus host reactions (GVHR) induce pleomorphic histiocytic lymphomas and lymphocytic lymphomas in mice. GVHR, like ionising radiation and chemical leukemogens activate replication of MuLV dormant in most mice. MuLVs are also activated by mixed lymphocyte reactions (MLRs) in vitro. There is anecdotal evidence that chronic antigenic stimulation may induce multiple myeloma in man, as it does in mice.

In summary, the HIV-induced acquired immunodeficiency syndrome (AIDS) has shown that failure of helper T cells allows viral and perhaps other factors to increase very substantially the risk of cancers. It is not possible to dismiss the theory of immune surveillance of cancer, but it is still impossible to prove or disprove it. The fact that cancers arise despite putative immune surveillance speaks against it. If the immune system can not deal with a tumour when it is small, how can it deal with it when it has become relatively massive? Although it has been considered unlikely, there is increasingly convincing evidence that immune mechanisms can be utilised to treat established cancers (see Chap. 20, p. 348).

References

Barbacid R (1985) Oncogenes and chemical carcinogenesis In: Proceedings of the eleventh annual EMBO symposium on growth factors, receptors and oncogenes, 16–19 September, 1985. Heidelberg, p 1 (abstract)

Beasley RP (1982) Hepatitis B virus as the aetiologic agent in hepatocellular carcinoma — epidemiologic considerations. Hepatology 2: 21S-26S

Beasley RP, Hwang LY, Lin CC, Chien CS (1981) Hepatocellular carcinoma and hepatitis B virus. A prospective study of 22,707 men in Taiwan. Lancet II: 1129–1133

Berg JW (1976) Nutrition and cancer. Semin Oncol 3: 17–23

Boldogh I, Beth E, Huang ES, Kyalwazi SK, Giraldo G (1980) Kaposi's sarcoma IV. Detection of CMV DNA, CMV RNA and cDNA in tumour biopsies. Int J Cancer 28: 469–474

Briggs JD, Hamilton DNH, MacSween RNM, Pennington TH (1978) Infectious mononucleosis, herpes simplex infection and diffuse lymphoma in a renal transplant recipient. Transplantation 25: 227–228

Clark JW, Hahn BH, Mann DL et al. (1985) Molecular and immunologic analysis of a chronic lymphocytic leukemia case with antibodies against human T-cell leukemia virus. Cancer 56: 495–499

Coltman CA Jr, Dixon DO (1982) Second malignancies complicating Hodgkin's disease: a Southwest Oncology Group 10-year follow up. Cancer Treat Rep 66: 1023–1033 (abstract)

Cook WD, Fazekas de St Groth S, Miller JFAP (1984) In vitro transformation of a peripheral T cell line by Abelson murine leukaemia virus. Australian Society for Immunology fourteenth annual meeting, Perth, 5–7 December, 1984 (abstract)

Cuzick J (1981) Radiation-induced myelomatosis. N Engl J Med 304: 204–210

de Thé G (1977) Is Burkitt's lymphoma related to perinatal infection by Epstein-Barr virus? Lancet I: 335–338

Dymock RB, Forbes IJ, Simmons I, Weldon M (1977) Epidermolysis verruciformis — investigation of immune function in two cases. Aust J Dermatol 18: 4–9

Frizzera G, Hanto DW, Gajl-Peczalska KJ et al (1981) Polymorphic diffuse B-cell hyperplasias and lymphomas in renal transplant recipients. Cancer Res 41: 4262–4279

Gessain A, Barin F, Vernant JC (1985) Antibodies to human T-lymphotropic virus in patients with tropical spastic paralysis. Lancet II: 407–410

Gissmann L (1984) Papillomaviruses and their association with cancer in animals and in man. Cancer Surveys 3: 161–181

Gahrton G, Zech L, Robèrt K-H, Bird AG (1979) Mitogenic stimulation of leukemia cells by Epstein-Barr virus. N Engl J Med 301: 438–439

Hanto DW, Gaijl Peczalska KJ, Frizzera KJ et al (1983) Epstein-Barr virus induced polyclonal and monoclonal B-cell lymphoproliferative diseases occurring after renal transplantation: clinical pathologic and virologic findings and implications for therapy. Ann Surg 198: 356–369

Hardie IR, Strong RW, Hartley LCJ, Woodruff PWH, Clunie GJA (1980) Skin cancer in Caucasian renal allograft recipients living in a sub-tropical climate. Surgery 87: 177–183

Harnden D, Morsten J, Featherstone T (1984) Dominant susceptibility to cancer in man. Adv Cancer Res 41: 185-255

Hathaway DE, Kolar GF (1980) Mechanisms of reaction between ultimate chemical carcinogens and nucleic acid. Chem Soc Rev 9: 241–264

Hinuma Y, Nagata K, Hanaoka M et al. (1981) Adult T cell leukaemia: antigen in an ATL cell line and detection of antibodies to the antigen in human sera. Proc Natl Acad Sci USA 78: 6476–6480

Hirohata T (1976) Radiation carcinogenesis. Semin Oncol 3: 25–34

Hoover R, Fraumeni JF (1973) Risk of cancer in renal-transplant recipients. Lancet II: 55–57

Kinlen LJ, Webster ADB, Bird AG et al. (1985) Prospective study of cancer in patients with hypogammaglobulinaemia. Lancet I: 263–266

Kirchner H (1984) Immunologic surveillance and human papillomaviruses. Immunol Today 5: 272–276

Klein G, Klein E (1985) Evolution of tumours and the impact of molecular oncology. Nature 315: 190–195

Lane HC, Depper JM, Greene WC, Whalen G, Waldmann TA, Fauci AS (1985) Qualitative analysis of immune function in patients with the acquired immunodeficiency syndrome. N Engl J Med 313: 79–84

Leech SH, Bryan CF, Elston RC et al. (1983) Genetic studies in multiple myeloma: I Association with HLA-Cw5. Cancer 51: 1408–1411

Leech SH, Brown R, Schanfield MS (1985) Genetic studies in multiple myeloma. II. Immunoglobulin allotype associations. Cancer 55: 1473–1476

Lenoir GM, Philip T, Sohier R (1984) Burkitt-type lymphoma: EBV association and cytogenetic markers in cases from various geographic locations. In: Magrath IT, O'Conor GT, Ramot B (eds) Pathogenesis of leukaemias and lymphomas: environmental influences. Raven, New York, pp 283–295

Love RR (1985) Small bowel cancers, B-cell lymphatic leukemia and six primary cancers with metastases and prolonged survival in the Cancer Family Syndrome of Lynch. Cancer 55: 499–502

Mahoney JF, Storey BG, Ibañez R, Stewart JH (1977) Analgesic abuse, renal parenchymal disease and carcinoma of the kidney or ureter. Aust NZ J Med 7: 463–469

Matsuzaki H, Yamaguchi K, Kagimoto T, Nakai R, Takatsuki K, Oyama W (1985) Monoclonal gammopathies in adult T-cell leukemia. Cancer 56: 1380–1383

McMahon B, Levy M (1964) Prenatal origin of childhood leukemia: evidence from twins. N Engl J Med 270: 1082

Metcalf D (1961) Reticular tumors in mice subjected to prolonged antigenic stimulation. Br J Cancer 15: 769–779

Mitchell H, Drake M, Medley G (1986) Prospective evaluation of risk of cervical cancer after cytological evidence of human papillomavirus infection. Lancet I: 573–575

Muir CS, Parkin DM (1985) The world cancer burden: prevent or perish. Br Med J 290: 5–6

Ormerod AD, Finlay AY, Knight AG, Mathews N, Stark JM, Gough J (1983) Immune deficiency and multiple viral warts: a possible variant of the Wiskott-Aldrich syndrome. Br J Dermatol 108: 211–215

Pandolfi F, Manzari V, De Rossi G et al. (1985a) T-helper phenotype, chronic lymphocytic leukaemia and "adult T-cell leukaemia" in Italy. Endemic HTLV-I-related T-cell leukaemias in southern Europe. Lancet II: 633–636

Pandolfi F, de Rossi G, Semenszato G (1985b) T-helper phenotype leukaemias: role of HTLV-I. Lancet II: 1367–1368

Purtilo DT (1980) Epstein-Barr-virus-induced oncogenesis in immune-deficient individuals. Lancet I: 300–303

Purtilo DT, Szymanski I, Bhawan JM et al. (1978) Epstein-Barr virus infections in the X-linked recessive lymphoproliferative syndrome. Lancet I: 798–801

Rosen CA, Sodroski JG, Goh W-C, Dayton AI, Lippke J, Haseltine WA (1986) Post-transcriptional regulation accounts for the *trans*-activation of the human T-lymphotropic virus type III. Nature 319: 555–559

Saemundsen AK, Purtilo DT, Sakamoto K et al. (1981) Documentation of Epstein-Barr virus infection in immunodeficient patients with life-threatening lymphoproliferative diseases by Epstein-Barr virus complementary RNA/DNA hybridisation. Cancer Res 41: 4237–4242

Sarin PS, Gallo RC (1984) Human T-lymphotropic retroviruses in adult T-cell leukemia-lymphoma and the acquired immune deficiency syndrome. J Clin Immunol 4: 415–423

Saxton JA, Boon MC, Furth J (1944) Observations on the inhibition of development of spontaneous leukemia by underfeeding. Cancer Res 4: 401

Schoeppel SJ, Hoppe RT, Dorfman RF (1985) Hodgkin's disease in homosexual men with generalised lymphadenopathy. Ann Intern Med 102: 68–70

Sheil AG, Mahoney JF, Horvath JS et al (1981) Cancer following successful cadaveric renal transplantation. Transplant Proc 13: 733–735

Siegel BV, Mahoney JF, Horvath JS et al. (1967) Influence of immunologic hyperstimulation in murine viral leukemogenesis. Blood 29: 585–593

Skinhoj P, Hart V, Hansen JPH, Nielson NH, Mikkelson F (1978) Occurrence of cirrhosis and primary liver cancer in an Eskimo population hyperendemically infected with hepatitis B virus. Am J Epidemiol 108: 121–125

Starzl TE, Nalensik MA, Porter KA et al. (1984) Reversibility of lymphoma and lymphoproliferative lesions developing under cyclosporin-steroid therapy. Lancet I: 583–587

Sugamura K, Hinuma Y (1985) Human retrovirus in adult T-cell leukemia/lymphoma. Immunol Today 6: 83–88

Sugamura K, Nakai S-I, Fujii M, Hinuma Y (1985) Interleukin 2 inhibits in vitro growth of human T cell lines carrying retrovirus. J Exp Med 161: 1243–1248

Thompson JF, Allen R, Morris PJ, Wood R (1985) Skin cancer in renal transplant patients treated with cyclosporin. Lancet I: 158–159 (letter)

Tosato G, Blaese RM (1985) Epstein-Barr virus infection and immunoregulation in man. Adv Immunol 37: 99–147

Tucker MA, Misfeldt D, Coleman CN, Clark WH, Rosenberg SA (1985) Cutaneous malignant melanoma after Hodgkin's disease. Ann Intern Med 102: 37–41

Twomey JJ, Rice L (1980) Impact of Hodgkin's disease upon the immune system. Semin Oncol 7: 114–125

Vogt PK (1985) Human T-cell leukemia lymphoma viruses — an introduction. Curr Top Microbiol Immunol 115: 1–5

Wong-Staal F, Gallo RC (1985) Human T-lymphotropic retroviruses. Nature 317: 395–403

Zaman SN, Melia WM, Johnson RD et al. (1985) Risk factors in development of hepatocellular carcinoma in cirrhosis: prospective study of 613 patients. Lancet I: 1357–1360

Ziegler JL, Beckstead JA, Volberding PA et al. (1984) Non-Hodgkin's lymphoma in 90 homosexual men. Relation to generalized lympadenopathy and the acquired immunodeficiency syndrome. N Engl J Med 311: 565–570

6 Oncogenes

Introduction

Oncogenes are essential genes encoding proteins involved in cell replication and differentiation. The cellular oncogenes, also known as proto-oncogenes, comprise a set of distinct genes which are normal components of the cell. They behave as classic Mendelian loci, occupying constant positions within the genomes of each species. These genes are often actively transcribed ("expressed") at particular times during the cell cycle, or during particular phases of ontogeny and otherwise may be expressed at very low levels. The known chromosomal locations of human cellular oncogenes are set out in Table 6.1 and Table 2.1 (see p. 13). The evolutionary conservation of oncogenes attests to their fundamental importance to cells. The oncogenes have been found in organisms from yeasts to man, representing a presence over a billion years of evolution.

When oncogenes were first recognised in retroviruses and in malignant cells they were not thought of as normal cellular components. The original concept that they were transferred to cells by retroviruses had to be revised when representatives of the different classes of viral oncogenes were found in normal cells. It is now believed that retroviruses have picked up these cellular genes from cells they have infected and have introduced molecular changes in them. Cellular oncogenes are denoted by the prefix "c-" and viral counterparts of oncogenes are designated by "v-".

The term "oncogene" is justified by the capacity of viral oncogenes and altered cellular oncogenes to transform susceptible cells to malignancy. They may do this by deregulating or dysregulating the control of growth normally exerted by growth factors. Such oncogene-bearing retroviruses may transmit a viral oncogene back to a mammalian cell. When the retrovirus infects host cells, it uses its reverse-transcriptase enzyme to transcribe viral RNA genome into viral DNA that becomes integrated into the genome of the host. Acquisition by a cell of an oncogene that has undergone multiple evolutionary changes may confer, in a single event, the equivalent of many of the multiple steps generally regarded as necessary for the development of malignancy. Point mutations may also occur in cellular oncogenes, disturbing the cell sufficiently to lead to the development of cancer, even though the expression of the oncogene has not apparently been disturbed or its position changed.

Normal cellular oncogenes would be more appropriately named "mitogenes" (Gordon 1985), as their protein products are normally involved in control of cell proliferation and differentiation, in the form of growth factors, receptors for growth factors on the plasma membrane and proteins involved in transmitting signals to the nucleus and activating specific genes (Fig. 6.1).

Cellular oncogenes contain introns from a few to thousands of base pairs, but their viral counterparts do not, and viral oncogenes may differ considerably from

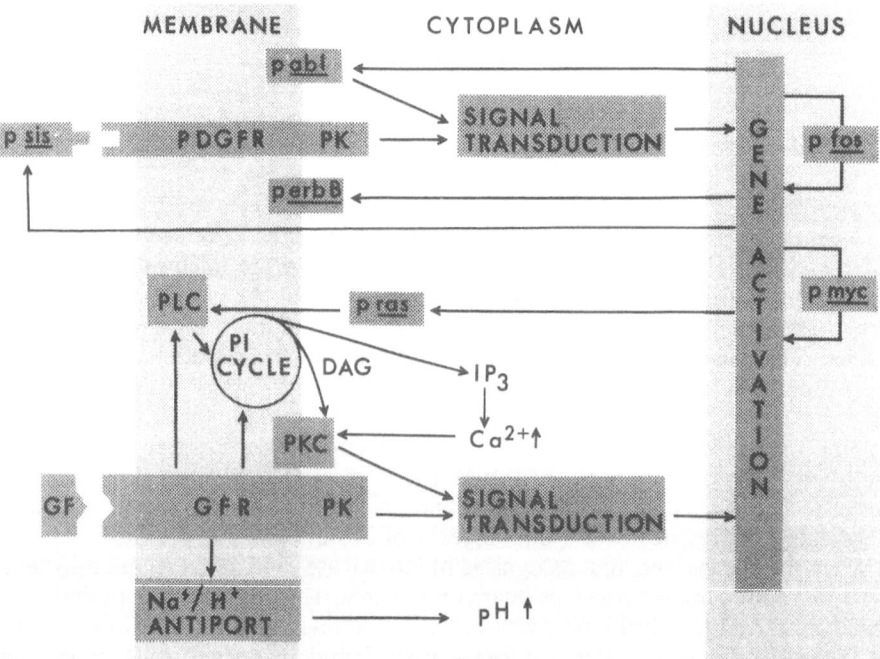

Fig. 6.1. Effects of oncogene products on cell growth. The product of *sis* is PDGF. The product of *erb-B* is substantially the same as the protein kinase segment of the EGF receptor. The *ras* family of proteins appear to be involved in activation of phospholipase C, releasing DAG and IP$_3$. At least six oncogenes are protein kinases whose activity affects the function of numerous enzymes. Others, e.g. *myc* and *fos* make products that affect gene expression, i.e. the transcription of RNA or subsequent steps. *DAG*, diacylglycerol; *GF*, growth factor; *GFR*, growth factor receptor; *PK*, protein kinase; *PKC*, protein kinase C; *PLC*, phospholipase C; *IP$_3$*, inositol triphosphate; p^{sis}, p^{ras} etc., products of the respective oncogenes.

their cellular homologues. When viral oncogenes are integrated into host DNA they are usually flanked by segments of DNA called long terminal repeats (LTRs), in contrast to the proto-oncogenes. LTRs contain promoters, sequences of DNA that initiate transcription. Many of the viruses oncogenic for experimental animals cannot replicate; a non-defective helper virus is often needed for replication. An exception is Rous sarcoma virus (RSV).

The acutely transforming retroviruses can rapidly induce a broad spectrum of tumours in animals, with a latent period of 2–3 weeks, and can transform cells in culture. Most of these viruses carry transformation-specific oncogenes; the slow-transforming avian leukosis and murine leukaemia viruses, with a latent period of 4–12 months, do not contain an oncogene and do not induce transformation in tissue culture cells.

The proof of the oncogenic nature of these genes was obtained by showing that malignant transformation of a cell could be induced by the introduction of a single gene. Virus strains were discovered which transform cells only after incubation at specific temperatures — temperature-sensitive mutants. Strains were developed in which the capacity to induce malignant transformation of cells was shown to reside in one gene (Kawai and Hanafusa 1978). Transformation by the temperature-sensitive oncogene can be induced by incubating the cells at the appropriate temperature. Later, some oncogenes of tumour cells were identified by their capacity to induce transformation to malignant phenotype of tissue culture cells by "transfection". Transfection is the introduction of exogenous DNA, usually in multiple copies, into new locations in the genome of the recipient cells, by infecting the cells with bacteriophages or plasmids into which the exogenous DNA has been incorporated. Normal cellular DNA introduced in this way cannot transform cells. The commonest cell used as target in transfection experiments is the NIH 3T3 line, which is probably not representative of normal cells, because it has already undergone one or more steps towards malignancy.

Translation Products of Oncogenes

More than 30 oncogenes have been isolated and almost all of them have been mapped to the human genome (Table 6.1; see also Table 2.1, p. 13). The list continues to lengthen. In every case in which the function of an oncogene product has been established, it is related in some way to proliferation and progression through the cell cycle. The oncogenes may be classified on the basis of the biochemical activity of their products (Table 6.1):

Class 1.   Protein kinases: *src*, *abl*, *fes/fps*, *yes* and *ros*

Class 2.   Guanosine triphosphate-binding proteins (G proteins): oncogenes of the *ras* class; Ha-*ras*-1, Ha-*ras*-2, Ki-*ras*-1, Ki-*ras*-2 and N-*ras*

Class 3.   DNA-binding proteins: *ets*, *fos*, *myc*, N-*myc*, *myb* and *ski*

Class 4.   Growth factor: *sis*

Class 5.   Growth factor receptors: *erb*-B, *fms*, *mos*, *neu*

Class 6.   Products whose nature and function are uncertain: *erb*-A, B-*lym*, *met*, *raf*-1, *raf*-2

Table 6.1. Properties of some of the oncogenes

Name	Chromosome (human)	Product mol. wt. (kD)	Site	Class
abl	9q34.1	120	Membrane	1
erb-A	17q11-q21	75	Cytoplasm	6
erb-B	7p14-p122	65	Membrane	5
ets-1	11q23-q24		Nucleus	3
ets-2	21q22		Nucleus	3
fes/fps	15q25-q26	98/92	Cytoplasm	1
fms	5q34	170	Membrane	5
fos	14q21-q31	55	Nucleus	3
int-1	12q14-pter			
B-*lym*-1	1p32	8–10	Nucleus	6
mil/raf-1	3p25-p24		Cytoplasm	6
raf-2	4			
met	7p11.4–7qter			6
mos	8q11-q22	37	Cytoplasm	5
myb	6q15-q24	48k	Nucleus	3
myc	8q24	58	Nucleus	3
N-*myc*	2p24–23		Nucleus	3
myc-L	1p32		Nucleus	3
neu (*ngl*)	17q21-q22	185	Membrane	5
Ha-*ras*-1	11pter-p15.6	21	Membrane	2
Ha-*ras*-2	Xpter-q28	21	Membrane	2
Ki-*ras*-1p	6p23-q12	21	Membrane	2
Ki-*ras*-2	12p12.1 or 12q24.2	21	Membrane	2
N-*ras*	1p22 and/or 1p12-p11	21	Membrane	2
rel	2p11-q14		Cytoplasm	6
ros			Membrane	1
sis	22q12.3-q13.1	p28	Secreted	4
ski	1q22-qter		Cytoplasm	3
c-*src*-1	20q12-q13	60	Membrane	1
c-*src*-2	1p36–34	60	Membrane	1
yes-1	18q21.3	90	Membrane	1
yes-2	6			

Class 1: encoding tyrosine protein kinases.
Class 2: encoding proteins binding guanosine triphosphate.
Class 3: encoding DNA-binding proteins.
Class 4: encoding growth factor.
Class 5: encoding growth factor receptors.
Class 6: encoding products of unknown function.
Note: *fps* and *fes* are homologous genes from chicken and rat, respectively.
Data from Gordon (1985) and Human Gene Mapping 8 (1985).

Oncogene Products with Protein Kinase Activity

The phosphorylating oncogenes cause deregulation of many cellular functions, particularly those involved in biochemical pathways which transmit signals, from activated membrane receptors to the nucleus, which activate specific genes. The products of class 1, excluding *abl*, form a complex with a 90 kD protein called a "heat shock protein", one of a number whose synthesis is stimulated by heat shock and metabolic stresses. Receptors of four steroid hormones (progesterone, oestrogen, androgen and glucocorticosteroid) also form complexes with this 90 kD protein.

src is the first oncogene for which a function was identified. Its viral counterpart, v-*src*, is the transforming oncogene in RSV. Expression of c-*src* is increased during organogenesis, and decreases thereafter. It is expressed at relatively high levels in brain tissue. It is expressed during metamorphosis in frogs and during TPA-induced differentiation of HL60 cells to macrophages. It is concluded that its expression is related more to differentiation than to proliferation.

pp 60^{src}, the product of *src*, is localised in adhesion plaques on the surface of a variety of cells. pp 60^{src} phosphorylates tyrosine residues in a number of proteins. Malignant transformation by *src* is thought to be caused by excessive or abnormal phosphorylation of proteins involved in regulation of cell proliferation. In cells that have been transformed by the action of *src*, phosphorylation of tyrosine residues is considerably increased. Vinculin is a protein in adhesion plates at the termination of actin filaments, just inside the plasma membrane. Vinculin is phosphorylated 20 times more in transformed than normal cells through the action of pp 60^{src}. Disruption by phosphorylation of the linkage of vinculin with actin would explain the disorganisation of actin bundles characteristic of transformed cells. Other proteins which are phosphorylated abnormally in RSV-transformed cells are a 36 kD protein on the inner face of the plasma membrane of many cells, whose function is unknown, as well as three important glycolytic enzymes — enolase, phosphoglycerate mutase and lactate dehydrogenase. The abnormal function of v-*src* is due to an abnormality of the amino acid sequence at the carboxyl end of its protein product.

v-*abl* is the oncogene of the Abelson murine leukaemia virus (A-MuLV), which was originally derived from the Moloney virus (Mo-MuLV). A-MuLV was isolated from a corticosteroid-treated BALB/C mouse that had been inoculated with Mo-MuLV, a virus that is capable of replicating. A-MuLV cannot replicate, because its genome, which is made up of part of the Mo-MuLV and the oncogenic *abl* sequence, is defective. Abelson virus induces lymphomas of pre-B cell origin and T cell lymphomas in mice and transforms fibroblasts, lymphocytes and myeloid cells in vitro. Unrestrained growth may result from the transformed myeloid cells producing the growth factor GM-CSF, permitting them to become independent of exogenous growth factor.

The v-*abl* tyrosine kinase (p120^{abl}) is located on the cytoplasmic side of the plasma membrane. The c-*abl* gene is on human chromosome 9 and is translocated from chromosome 9 to 22 in the formation of the Philadelphia chromosome. The transformation fuses c-*abl* to another gene in such a way that a novel hybrid polypeptide can be made (Adams 1985). c-*abl* is expressed during embryogenesis.

fes is associated with the cat viruses — feline sarcoma virus (FeSV) and feline leukaemia virus (FeLV). FeSV causes fibrosarcomas in cats. FeLV are transmitted horizontally between domestic cats and are associated with a wide range of neoplastic and non-neoplastic diseases. FeLV and FeSV cause T cell lymphosarcomas after short latent periods when inoculated into newborn cats. *fps* is the avian counterpart of *fes*. The *fes* protein kinase differs from that of *src* by using ATP instead of GTP as phosphate donor. *fgr* is the oncogene of the feline sarcoma retrovirus GR-FeSV. Its product is a protein kinase in the cytoplasm and inner membrane containing sequences homologous to actin.

GTP-binding Oncogene Products

Several viruses contain oncogenes of the *ras* family, including Harvey murine sarcoma virus (HaSV), Kirsten murine sarcoma virus (KiSV), Rasheed (rat) sarcoma virus (RaSV) and BALB mouse sarcoma virus (BALB-MSV). These viruses induce sarcomas, extrathymic lymphomas and erythroblastosis in mice after a short latent period, usually 2–3 weeks. The human genome contains two genes homologous to v-Ha-*ras* (c-Ha-*ras*-1 and c-Ha-*ras*-2, the latter lacking introns), two homologous to c-Ki-*ras* and another homologue named N-*ras*.

ras proto-oncogenes are expressed throughout the mitotic cycle. Both c-Ha-*ras* and c-Ki-*ras* are expressed during embryogenesis. The normal cellular counterparts of the viral *ras* family encode the 21 kD α subunit of a protein on the inner face of the plasma membrane which binds guanosine diphosphate (GDP) and guanosine triphosphate (GTP). These so-called G proteins, consisting of α, β and γ subunits, hydrolyse GTP and phosphorylate a threonine residue of their own protein with GTP as phosphate donor. The G proteins participate in the transduction of signals from membrane receptors through the cytoplasm to the nucleus. The oncogenic capacity of viral *ras* products is related to their poorer function as GTPases. Their transforming capacity is proportional to the loss of GTPase activity. The cellular content of the *ras* product is enhanced by insulin and epithelial growth factor (EGF). In yeast, p21^{ras} is thought to activate adenylate cyclase, but there is no evidence for this function in mammalian cells. It has recently been reported that antibodies against p21^{ras} inhibit cells from entering S phase.

In addition to their capacity to cause sarcomas, *ras*-containing retroviruses induce proliferation of chicken erythroid cells both in vivo and in tissue culture. DNA from benign papillomas and from transplantable mouse skin carcinomas induced by chemical carcinogens has the capacity to transform cells in tissue culture. The gene responsible for the transformation is an activated form of c-Ha-*ras* (Balmain et al. 1984).

Oncogenes Whose Products Bind to DNA

v-*fos* is a gene of the FBJ osteosarcoma virus (FBJ-MSV), isolated from a spontaneous murine osteosarcoma. This virus produces cancers of bones and cartilage in newborn mice, and transforms fibroblasts in vitro. The 55 kD product of the human c-*fos* gene can be demonstrated in the nucleus after a stimulus which activates a cell to enter into cycle, by the use of fluorescent monoclonal antibodies to *fos* protein. The v-*fos* product is defective, lacking a segment in the carboxy terminus.

c-*fos* appears to be a key proto-oncogene in normal cellular growth and differentiation. It is activated soon after a resting cell receives an appropriate stimulus to enter G1. Exposure of mouse fibroblasts to platelet-derived growth factor (PDGF) induces mRNA from the c-*fos* proto-oncogene within 10 min, followed by synthesis of nuclear c-*fos* protein. Activation of c-*myc* is a later event (Müller and Verma 1984). c-*fos* is differentially expressed in placenta and the fetus during fetal development, suggesting a role in differentiation. High levels are also found in differentiated macrophages. The c-*fos* gene can be turned into a transforming gene by manipulating it, for example by adding transcriptional enhancer elements or by putting viral sequences at its 3' end.

ets is the cellular equivalent of v-*ets*, the transforming oncogene of avian reticuloendotheliosis virus. Besides the recognised site on chromosome 11 (Table 6.1), another locus has been detected on chromosome 21q22 (Jacobson et al. 1986). The oncogene has been shown to be involved in a translocation t(2;11)(p13;q23) in leukaemic cells of a case of immunoblastic lymphadenopathy.

myb (also known as *amv*) is a viral oncogene in avian myeloblastosis virus (AMV). AMV causes acute myeloblastic leukaemia in chickens and transforms specific haematopoietic cells in vitro. DNA rearrangements and altered expression of *myb* have been reported in mouse lymphoid tumours, human acute myeloblastic leukaemia (AML), chronic myelogenous leukaemia (CML), colon, breast and lung tumours. *myb* proteins act in the nucleus, but their action is little understood. The viral oncogene has lost substantial portions of both ends of the cellular oncogene, resulting in the generation of a truncated gene product that is responsible for the transforming capacity of the virus (Rosson and Reddy 1986).

The *myc* (myelocytomatosis) oncogene is perhaps the most studied, and certainly one of the most interesting in the search for the disturbance of function of oncogenes basic to cancer. The cellular *myc* proto-oncogene is homologous to the transforming gene of the acute avian myelocytomatosis retrovirus MC29 and several other strains (Table 6.2). c-*myc* is transcribed at a very high rate and the cellular level of *myc* RNA is regulated to a considerable extent by consumption and breakdown (Blanchard et al. 1985). Rises are probably largely due to reduction in turnover, since inhibitors of protein synthesis cause a rise in c-*myc* mRNA levels, presumably by affecting the level of an enzyme which breaks it down. In general, c-*myc* mRNA levels are low in resting cells and rise in response to growth factors, for example PDGF, and a variety of other stimuli, including TPA and avian, murine and feline leukaemia viruses not containing the *myc* oncogene. Cytoplasmic c-*myc* RNA levels increase enormously (e.g. 20–40 fold) in lymphocytes within 2–4 h of activation by virtually any effective stimulus. The increase in c-*myc* expression which follows activation precedes by 6 h the overall increases in RNA synthesis associated with cell enlargement and precedes by 13 h the onset of DNA synthesis. *myc* RNA levels peak between 2 and 9 h after stimulation of murine spleen cells by bacterial lipopolysaccharide (LPS) and concanavalin A, remain elevated for approximately 48 h and subsequently drop to near background levels. The protein product of *myc* binds to DNA or to DNA-associated nuclear proteins, regulating the transcription of particular genes

Table 6.2. Oncogenes associated with tumours

Oncogene	Retrovirus		Species	Tumours
abl	A-MuLV	Abelson murine leukaemia virus	Mouse, cat	T and B leukaemia
B-lym			Man, chicken	lymphomas including Burkitt's
erb-A	AEV-ES4	Avian erythroblastosis virus	Chicken	Leukaemia
erb-B	AEV-ES4 AEV-H	Avian erythroblastosis virus	Chicken	Erythroblastosis, sarcoma
ets	REV	Avian reticuloendotheliosis virus	Chicken	
fgr	GR-FeSV	Feline sarcoma virus	Cat	Sarcoma
fms	SM-FeSV	Feline sarcoma virus	Cat	Sarcoma
fos	FBJ-MSV	FBJ osteosarcoma virus	Mouse	Colon, ovarian, breast carcinoma
fes/	FuSV	Fujinami sarcoma virus	Chicken	Sarcoma
fps	ST-FeSV GA-FeSV	Feline sarcoma virus	Cat	Leukaemia, lymphoma
int-1	MMTV	Mouse mammary tumour virus	Cat	Mammary tumours
met			Man	Osteosarcoma
mos	Mo-MSV	Moloney mouse sarcoma	Mouse	Rhabdomyosarcoma
myc	MC29,OK10, CMII, MH2 FeLV	Avian myelocytomatosis virus	Chicken	Carcinoma, lymphoma
myb	AMV	Avian myeloblastosis virus	Chicken	Myeloblastosis, erythroblastosis
myc-L			Man	Small cell lung carcinoma
N-myc			Man	Neuroblastoma
neu (ngl)			Rat	Neuroblastoma
mil/ raf	MH2V, 3911-MSV	Murine sarcoma virus	Mouse	Fibrosarcoma
Ha-ras/ bas (has)	Ha-MSV	Harvey sarcoma virus	Rat, mouse	Erythroleukaemia, sarcoma
Ki-ras (kis)	Ki-MSV	Kirsten sarcoma virus	Rat	Erythroleukaemia
N-ras			Man	Neuroblastoma
ros	UR-2V		Chicken	Sarcoma
sis	SSV	Simian sarcoma virus	Monkey	Sarcoma
ski[a]	SKV 770		Cat	
src	RSV	Rous sarcoma virus	Chicken	Sarcoma
rel	ARV	Avian reticuloendotheliosis virus		
yes	Y-73	Yamaguchi sarcoma virus	Chicken	Sarcoma
yes1		Yamaguchi sarcoma virus homologue 1		
yes2		Yamaguchi sarcoma virus homologue 2		

[a] Oncogene of defective virus generated in vitro.

(Moelling et al. 1984). The regions of the genome to which the *myc* protein binds are presumed to be regulators of the activity of genes. *myc* protein is thought to inhibit the action of these regulatory structures. The regulation and activation of *myc* are reviewed by Cole (1985).

c-*myc* mRNA seems to drop to very low levels when a cell has made a step in differentiation. The lymphocyte line WEHI 231 is a model; when these cells are exposed to anti-Ig they divide once, then stop. A rapid increase of c-*myc* mRNA occurs 2 h after stimulation, then falls. Further stimulation with anti-Ig induces neither activation nor elevation of c-*myc* mRNA.

The locus on chromosome 8 containing the *myc* oncogene is the site of an extraordinary number of rearrangements, amplifications and retroviral insertions, of which perhaps the most notable are the translocations associated with Burkitt's lymphoma (BL).

Oncogene Product with Growth Factor Activity

Only one oncogene, *sis*, has been identified as encoding a growth factor. *sis* is the proto-oncogene encoding the growth factor PDGF and its viral oncogene counterpart, v-*sis*, is the transforming oncogene of simian sarcoma virus (SSV). Infection of cells by SSV leads to secretion of a growth factor resembling PDGF which results in unregulated autostimulation. Antibodies to PDGF inhibit the induction of proliferation and transformation by SSV (Johnsson et al. 1985) and partially inhibit growth of some SSV-transformed lines. c-*sis* is on human chromosome 22, and is translocated to chromosome 9 in the reciprocal translocation producing the Philadelphia chromosome.

Oncogenes Encoding Receptors for Growth Factors

v-*erb*-B is the transforming oncogene of the avian erythroblastosis virus (AEV), specifically subtypes AEV-ES4 and AEV-H. These viruses transform chicken marrow erythroblasts. The product of v-*erb*-B resembles a truncated epidermal growth factor (EGF) receptor, lacking the EGF-binding region, retaining the transmembrane segment and the intracellular catalytic domain of the protein kinase of the EGF receptor. There are two genes related to the viral *erb*-B gene in the human genome. c-*erb*-B1 is the same as the gene for the EGF receptor and c-*erb*-B2 encodes a receptor-like protein very similar to, but distinct from, the EGF receptor. The c-*erb*-B2 gene was found to be amplified in 5 of 63 adenocarcinomas and none of 38 other types of tumour, whereas the c-*erb*-B1/EGF receptor gene was amplified in only 1 of 8 squamous cell carcinomas (Yokota et al. 1986). c-*erb*-B has also been reported to be highly expressed in glioblastomas. The c-*erb*-B2 gene was amplified in a metastasis from breast carcinoma, but not in the primary tumour, suggesting that the amplification of this gene is involved in the progression of the tumour (Yokota et al. 1986). The *erb*-B product is presumed to act by uncoordinated, ill-timed or abnormal phosphorylation of substrates of the EGF receptor, resulting in irregular transduction of a signal resembling the EGF signal to the nucleus. One result of this signal is activation of c-*myc*. Another result is independence from GM-CSF, a growth factor which has its own receptor, distinct from the EGF receptor. It is now suspected that *ras* products are also involved in transduction of signals from the EGF receptor.

The product of the *fms* oncogene of the McDonough strain of FeSV is closely related to the receptor for the monocyte growth factor M-CSF (CSF-1) (Sherr et al 1985), which has tyrosine kinase activity. *fms* is expressed in utero and has tyrosine kinase activity.

neu (also known as *ngl*) is an oncogene found in rat neuroblastomas. It has similarities to *erb*-B, and its 185 kD growth factor-like product is antigenically related to the c-*erb*-B gene product. It has protein kinase activity. Growth of transformed cells under the influence of *neu* can be controlled by an antibody to its p185 product (Drebin et al. 1985). A proto-oncogene similar to *neu* has been found in the human genome.

v-*mos* is the viral oncogene of the Moloney murine sarcoma virus (Mo-MSV). The protein products of *mos* (Moloney sarcoma) and *raf* (murine sarcoma) oncogenes also have structural resemblances to the *erb*-B product. The 37 kD protein product of *mos* (p37^{mos}) controls, in an unknown way, the synthesis of the growth factor TGF$_\alpha$.

Oncogenes Whose Products have Undefined Function

v-*erb*-A is found as a second oncogene in avian erythroblastosis virus AEV-ES4, the acute leukaemia type retrovirus causing erythroblastosis in chickens. It is an important oncogene because it gives clues to the understanding of differentiation arrest. It blocks terminal differentiation in the leukaemic cells of affected chickens. *erb*-A by itself is not able to trigger transformation. This oncogene can modulate the activity of c-*src*. The recent finding of extensive homology between the product of v-*erb*-A and the human oestrogen receptor (Green et al. 1986) gives impetus to research on the abnormal expression of c-*erb*-A on chromosome 17 in breast cancer. The v-*erb*-A protein is approximately the same size as the oestrogen receptor and binds oestrogen.

B-*lym*, first identified in a human B cell lymphoma is also the transforming gene of chicken B cell lymphoma. The product of B-*lym* may be homologous to some extent with proteins of the transferrin family (Lane et al. 1984). B-*lym* has been isolated from many kinds of B lymphocyte neoplasms in animals. It is activated in BL, as well as *myc*. *int*-1 is the gene activated in many mouse mammary tumours when the mouse mammary tumour virus becomes inserted into the genome. The oncogene encodes a 370 amino acid protein. The c-*int*-1 human proto-oncogene is closely homologous. *int*-1 transforms rat embryo fibroblasts in vitro, if complemented by a *ras* gene, to cells tumorigenic in nude mice.

Some Important Non-human Oncogenes

It is necessary to mention the adenovirus oncogenes *E1A* and *E1B*, although their action is complex and poorly understood, because some adenoviruses can cause transformation. No cellular counterparts of the adenovirus oncogenes have been found. Transformation requires the combined action of two domains, known as *E1A* and *E1B*. One very interesting feature of *E1A* is that its products may inhibit expression of major histocompatibility complex (MHC) class I genes. Tumours not expressing MHC class I product could escape recognition by T cells.

The *T* oncogenes of the papovaviruses are also most complex. The transforming region of polyomavirus SV40 encodes three proteins, large T (100 kD), middle T (55 kD) and small T (22 kD) antigens. Large T induces indefinite growth in cells (immortality) and middle T induces, or at least contributes to the induction of, transformation. The action of small T has yet to be clarified. Large T antigens act in the nucleus of the infected cell, binding to a specific 36 base pair sequence. Middle T antigen exists in combination with the protein kinase pp $60^{c\text{-}src}$, the product of the *src* oncogene, and its action is to prevent phosphorylation of a regulatory site on pp $60^{c\text{-}src}$. This has the effect of enhancing the activity of pp 60^{src} (Courtneidge, 1985). This is an example of synergy between two oncogenes. Middle T may also phosphorylate phosphatidylinositol.

Aberrations of Oncogenes in Cancer

Oncogenes may be faulty and make a defective product or make it at the incorrect time or in the incorrect amount. To understand how their expression may be faulty, knowledge of the normal mechanisms controlling their expression is needed. Some of the DNA sequences (enhancers and promoters) involved in control of gene expression are known, but knowledge of the ways in which these controls may become deranged so as to cause malignant transformation is still rather rudimentary.

Several mechanisms may cause increased activity, or abnormally timed activation:

1. Overexpression of an oncogene product, through interference with normal control of expression, e.g. when the normal controlling genes are lost through translocation. The *myc* gene may lose its own regulatory sequences and acquire normally unlinked sequences involved in immunoglobulin production in the translocations found in BL, but this is not commonly the case. *abl* may be deregulated in the Philadelphia chromosome of CML.

2. Gene amplification may cause overexpression. Amplification is an increase in the number of copies of a particular gene within the genome. Amplification of a number of oncogenes has been found in human cancers: Ki-*ras*, *myc* (in a colon carcinoma), N-*myc* (in human neuroblastomas) and c-*abl*. Some squamous cell carcinomas express high levels of EGF receptor, probably as a result of amplification of the *erb*-B gene. The mechanism of oncogene amplification is not well understood. Interruption of DNA synthesis apparently leads to repetitive copying

of a gene near the point of interruption, possibly by a disturbance of the function of DNA polymerase. Gene amplification is induced in vitro by chemical and physical agents, particularly hypoxia, and is enhanced, but not caused by, TPA. Double minute chromosomes and homogeneously staining regions of chromosomes are cytological manifestations of gene amplification, which can be seen in tumours.

3. LTR sequences of retroviruses may play a part in carcinogenesis by enhancing transcription of neighbouring genes. Normal murine cells contain a large number of copies of DNA sequences homologous to the LTR sequence of murine retrovirus proviral DNA. Damage to cellular DNA causing rearrangement or activation of these endogenous LTR sequences could lead to the constitutive expression of host genes whose products may contribute to malignant cell transformation. Insertion of LTR sequences near oncogenes may also cause amplification of oncogenes.

4. One interesting possibility is the abnormal expression or loss of expression of MHC products preventing immunological recognition of tumour cells. This may be caused by the product of the adenovirus oncogenes E1A.

5. Genes which normally control the activity of oncogenes ("anti-oncogenes") may be defective. Loss of a controlling segment on chromosome q13 is thought to underlie the hereditary form of retinoblastoma (Green and Wyke 1985). The existence of anti-oncogenes is supported by cell-fusion experiments. Fusion of transformed or tumorigenic cells with normal cells often results in hybrids with a normal phenotype. Multiple copies of an oncogene may swamp normal regulation by anti-oncogenes.

6. Alteration in the structure of the oncogene protein may have innumerable effects, unrelated to abnormalities of the level or timing of expression. The simple point mutation in *ras* is a good example. It is quite remarkable that in cases in which the sequence of the abnormal *ras* oncogene has been analysed, it differs from its normal allelic counterpart by a single critical nucleotide. One mutation alters p21 by converting the 12th amino acid (glycine) to valine. The amino acid position 59 is occupied by alanine in products of all cellular *ras* genes, but by threonine in both Harvey and Kirsten viral p21^{ras}. Change of adenine to thymine also results in the substitution of leucine for glutamine at amino acid 61. The carcinogen nitroso-methyl-urea (NMU) induces a specific point mutation of the *ras* gene in rat mammary tissue. A much grosser abnormality has arisen in v-*erb*-B, resulting in a truncated version of the EGF receptor, whose function is evidently so abnormal as to cause malignant transformation. An oncogene may be fused to another gene so that a novel peptide is made. This occurs with the formation of the Philadelphia chromosome, when c-*abl* fuses to another gene to encode a large protein with tyrosine kinase activity (Adams 1985).

Proteins Homologous to Oncogene Products

A clue to the action of a gene may be obtained by comparing the amino acid sequence of its product with other known sequences. Thus we know of homologies between products of *sis* and PDGF, *erb*-B and EGF receptor, *erb*-A and oestrogen receptors, *fms* and M-CSF and *ras* and the α subunit of GTP-binding proteins. Other suggested homologies are *mos* product with EGF precursor, *src* with insulin receptor and with catalytic chain of cAMP-dependent protein kinase, *fes/fgr* with actin, and one of the *lym* family with an MHC subunit.

Transgenic Mice

An oncogene or hybrids of an oncogene with a controlling or promoter gene can be inserted into the germline genome. Lines of mice carrying such inserts ("transgenic mice") have been established. For example, the oncogene large T of SV40 can be placed under the control of DNA from the rat insulin gene. The mice develop normally but die at 9–12 weeks. The large T antigen is expressed in β cells of the pancreas. The pancreatic islets become hyperplastic and some develop β-cell tumours. Insertion of a hybrid of c-*myc* and the LTR of hormone-dependent mouse mammary tumour virus leads to mammary cancer in multiparous mice in their first or second pregnancies.

The most interesting example of oncogenesis in transgenic mice, from the point of view of lymphoid tumours, is the production of B cell tumours in mice by c-*myc* coupled to DNA segments which enhance the transcription of immunoglobulin μ or κ genes (Adams et al. 1985). More than 85% of mice carrying these additional genes develop B cell lymphomas, of either early or relatively mature phenotype, mostly with aggressive leukaemia. The tumours are mostly monoclonal. The enhancer-*myc* gene is taken up by all cells, but it only leads to tumours of B lymphocytes. More importantly, only one malignant lymphoid clone emerges in most animals, although it is likely that more premalignant clones exist. This model offers new ways to study the premalignant state.

Oncogenes in Human Tumours

Some human and animal tumours associated with the activity of oncogenes, many from viruses, are listed in Table 6.2. Activated transforming genes have been detected in many human tumours, particularly lymphoid tumours and cell lines derived from them. The oncogenes most frequently isolated by transfection of human tumours are homologues of the retroviral oncogene Ha-*ras*. Tumorigenic Ha-*ras* and Ki-*ras* genes have been detected in many human tumours, particularly of lung and colon, by transferring genes from DNA of tumours into cells in tissue culture. Using morphological transformation of NIH-3T3 cells as an assay, it has been estimated that 10%–30% of human tumours have an activated *ras* gene. The cellular gene N-*ras*, which has no close viral counterpart, has been found in active form in the DNA of a variety of haematopoietic tumours, including promyelocytic and acute lymphocytic leukaemia and CML.

A number of other oncogenes, including c-*erb*-B, c-*myc* and c-*fos*, are commonly expressed in human tumours, probably as a result of abnormal activation. Some, c-*abl*, c-*fms* and c-*myb*, are expressed infrequently. c-*fes* is actively expressed in some leukaemias and CML. c-Ha-*ras* is expressed in acute and chronic leukaemias, whereas *src* and *erb* are not. The significance of expression of an oncogene in tumour cells is not always clear, because the pattern of oncogene expression in the corresponding normal cells may not have been established.

fos is actively expressed in a range of human tumours (of kidney, ovary, lung and breast; Slamon et al. 1984). Abnormalities of the c-*myc* gene or its distant relatives N-*myc* and L-*myc* are found in virtually all lymphoid tumours, as well as a variety of other cancers, including neuroblastomas, retinoblastomas and terato-carcinomas (N-*myc*), and small cell carcinomas of lung (L-*myc*). L-*myc* is always expressed in the acute leukaemias, but the gene is not necessarily translocated or rearranged. *myc*, on chromosome 8, is translocated to one of the chromosomes bearing immunoglobulin genes (14, 2 or 22) in BL, but it is not necessarily very close to an immunoglobulin gene.

Multiple Oncogene Expression

Multiple oncogene expression appears to be important in malignancy. Multiple genes are activated in a wide variety of cancers, lymphomas and leukaemias. This concept is hard to evaluate because expression of proto-oncogenes in normal tissue is also complex, making proper comparisons difficult. Two or more oncogenes (e.g. *myc* and *ras*) may have to cooperate to transform cells. Neither *ras* nor *myc* can cause transformation by transfection singly into rat embryo fibroblasts, but they do so if transfected together. Many other synergisms are now known, suggesting that activation of specific oncogenes, probably in specific sequence, is essential for carcinogenesis. The *myc* oncogene may immortalise a cell, and the *ras* may act to complete the malignant transformation. Sequential activation of multiple transforming genes could correspond to the multiple steps in the evolution of a cancer.

When oncogenes are synergistic, they may be classified as primary and secondary. The primary oncogene may induce transformation of target cells in vitro, and the secondary oncogene may induce further changes, principally the inhibition of differentiation of the cell (Graf et al. 1985). In the case of avian erythroid cells, *erb*-A can be the secondary oncogene to *erb*-B. *erb*-A can also be secondary to *src*, *fps* and *ras*. In avian myeloid cells, *myc* may be the primary oncogene and *erb*-B, *fps*, *yes* and *ras* may be secondary.

Conclusions

Oncogenes were discovered in retroviruses that cause cancer in animals. It is now known that every eukaryotic cell has many genes, closely related to the cancer-causing genes, as essential elements of the genome related to control of prolifer-ation and differentiation. The action of these genes is to provide the cell with the proteins necessary to undergo the cellular changes involved in growth and differentiation.

Each event in the preparation of a cell for division must be controlled and coordinated. A resting cell is induced to enter the cell cycle by a primary stimulus, then synthesises in correct order the proteins necessary to proceed through the cycle and to divide. The cell expresses receptors for growth factors sequentially and transmits signals from these receptors, when they are occupied, to the genome. The whole process depends on orderly activation of a set of genes, to which the oncogenes belong.

Oncogenesis results from derangements of this complex mechanism. At last, with the growing knowledge of these genes, the growth factors, their receptors and the metabolic pathways connecting them, it is becoming possible to construct coherent schemes of the abnormalities fundamental to the neoplastic process. Good reviews of oncogenes are to be found in the following articles: Bishop (1983, 1985), Blick et al. (1984), Champlin (1986), Cory (1983), Gordon (1985), Hunter (1984), Land et al. (1983), Ratner et al. (1985), Weinberg (1984) and Weiss 1984). The history of the oncogene concept is reviewed by Lacey (1986).

References

Adams JM (1985) Oncogene activation by fusion of chromosomes in leukaemia. Nature 315: 542–543

Adams JM, Harris AW, Pinkert CA et al. (1985) The c-*myc* oncogene driven by immunoglobulin enhancers induces lymphoid malignancy in transgenic mice. Nature 318: 533–538

Balmain A, Ramsden M, Bowden GT, Smith J (1984) Activation of the mouse cellular Harvey-*ras* gene in chemically induced benign skin papillomas. Nature 307: 658–660

Bishop JM (1983) Cellular oncogenes and retroviruses. Annu Rev Biochem 52: 301–354

Bishop JM (1985) Viral oncogenes. Cell 42: 23–38

Blanchard J-M, Piechaczyk M, Dani C et al. (1985) c-*myc* gene is transcribed at high rate in Go-arrested fibroblasts and is post-transcriptionally regulated in response to growth factors. Nature 317: 443–445

Blick M, Westin E, Gutterman et al. (1984) Oncogene expression in human leukemia. Blood 64: 1234–1239

Champlin R (1986) Chronic leukemias: oncogenes, chromosomes, and advances in therapy. Ann Intern Med 104: 671–688

Cole MD (1985) Regulation and activation of c-*myc*. Nature 318: 510–511

Cory S (1983) Oncogenes and B cell neoplasia. Immunol Today 4: 205–207

Courtneidge SA (1985) Activation of pp 60[c-src] kinase activity by middle-T antigen binding or by dephosphorylation. Eleventh EMBO annual symposium on growth factors, receptors and onco-genes, 16–19 September, 1985. European Molecular Biology Laboratory, Heidelberg, pp 10–11 (abstract)

Drebin JA, Link VC, Stern DF, Weinberg RA, Greene MI (1985) Down modulation of an oncogene protein product and reversion of the transformed phenotype by monoclonal antibodies. Cell 41: 695–706

Gordon H (1985) Oncogenes. Mayo Clin Proc 60: 697–713

Graf T, Kahn P, Beug H (1985) Lineage specific induction of self-renewal differentiation arrest and growth factor independence by primary and auxiliary oncogenes in chick haematopoietic cells. Proceedings of the eleventh annual EMBO symposium on growth factors, receptors and oncogenes, 16–19 September, 1985. European Molecular Biology Laboratory, Heidelberg, p 23 (abstract)

Green AR, Wyke JA (1985) Anti-oncogenes A subset of regulatory genes involved in carcinogenesis? Lancet II: 475–477

Green S, Walter P, Kumar V et al. (1986) Human oestrogen receptor cDNA: sequence, expression and homology to v-*erb*-A. Nature 320: 134–139

Human Gene Mapping 8 (1985) Eighth international workshop on human gene mapping, Helsinki, Finland, 4–10 August, 1985. Cytogenet Cell Genet 40 (1–4): 1–823

Hunter T (1984) The proteins of oncogenes. Sci Am 251: 60–69

Jacobson RJ, Sacher RA, Rovigatti U (1986) Human *ets* oncogene amplification and rearrangement in clonal hematologic malignancy. XXI Congress of the International Society of Haematology, Sydney, May 1986, p 629 (abstract)

Johnsson A, Betsholtz C, Heldin C-H, Westermark B (1985) Antibodies against platelet-derived growth factor inhibit acute transformation by simian sarcoma virus. Nature 317: 438–440

Kawai S, Hanafusa H (1978) The effects of reciprocal changes in temperature on the transformed state of cells infected with a Rous sarcoma virus gene product. Proc Natl Acad Sci USA 75: 2021–2024

Lacey SW (1986) Review: oncogenes in retroviruses, malignancy, and normal tissues. Am J Med Sci 291: 39–46

Land H, Parada LF, Weinberg RA (1983) Cellular oncogenes and multistep carcinogenesis. Science 222: 771–778

Lane M-A, Stephens HAF, Doherty KM, Tobin MB (1984) *Tlym-1*, a stage specific transforming gene shares homology with MHC I regions genes. Curr Top Microbiol Immunol 113: 31–33

Moelling K, Benter T, Bunte T et al. (1984) Properties of the *myc*-gene product: nuclear association inhibition of transcription and activation in stimulated lymphocytes. Curr Top Microbiol Immunol 113: 198–207

Müller R, Verma IM (1984) Expression of cellular oncogenes. Curr Top Microbiol Immunol 112: 73–115

Ratner L, Josephs SF, Wong-Staal F (1985) Oncogenes: their role in neoplastic transformation. Ann Rev Microbiol 39: 419–449

Rosson D, Reddy EP (1986) Nucleotide sequence of chicken c-*myb* complementary DNA and implications for *myb* oncogene activation. Nature 319: 604–606

Sherr CJ, Rettenmier CW, Sacca R, Roussel MF, Look AT, Stanley ER (1985) The c-*fms* proto-oncogene product is related to the receptor for the mononuclear phagocyte growth factor CSF-1. Cell 41: 665–676

Slamon DL, de Kernion JB, Verma IM, Cline MJ (1984) Expression of cellular oncogenes in human malignancies Science. 224: 256–262

Weinberg RA (1984) *ras* oncogenes and the molecular mechanisms of carcinogenesis. Blood 64: 1143–1145

Weiss RA, Marshall CJ (1984) DNA in medicine: oncogenes. Lancet II: 1138–1142

Yokota J, Yamamoto T, Toyoshima K et al. (1986) Amplification of c-*erb*-B2 oncogene in human adenocarcinomas in vivo. Lancet I: 765–766

7 Growth Factors

Introduction

Growth factors are proteins which are essential for the growth of normal cells. They act at extraordinarily low concentrations, inducing cells to proceed from the resting phase, G_0, through the cell cycle, by binding to specific high-affinity receptors. They induce a series of metabolic events which lead to expression of specific genes whose products are necessary for each stage of the growth cycle. The group of genes which are involved in growth include the known oncogenes. At least one growth factor, platelet-derived growth factor (PDGF), and several receptors for growth factors are the products of proto-oncogenes. Known chromosomal locations of some of the genes for growth factors are set out in Table 2.1 (see p. 13). Growth factors are also involved in differentiation, although less is known about this aspect of their action. Activation of some oncogenes, for example c-*fos*, leads to proliferation in some cells and to differentiation in others.

The autonomy of malignant cells is largely based on independence from exogenous growth factors. Where the growth requirements of tumour cells have been elucidated, they have usually been simpler than the requirements of normal cells for growth in vitro. However, many human tumours cannot be cultured, because the growth factors they require are not known. It is now well established that endogenous production of growth factor can induce malignant transformation. Some viruses, e.g. human T cell leukaemia/lymphoma virus I (HTLV-I) are thought to transform cells by this means.

The best understood growth factors act on mesenchymal and haematopoietic cells. Whereas much is known of the factors controlling the growth and differentiation of immunologically competent lymphocytes, an understanding of the factors controlling the early phases of lymphocyte growth and differentiation is rudimentary. Nevertheless, it would be surprising if such factors do not exist. The factors that are described in this chapter may well be models of the factors yet to be discovered for the lymphoid system.

Mechanisms of Action of Growth Factors

Growth factors induce transition from G_0 to G_1, by combining with specific receptors, activating a series of biochemical reactions constituting a "signal transduction pathway", leading to expression of "competence" genes, including cellular oncogenes. Among the gene products resulting from this activity are specific receptors for growth factors subsequently required for cells to proceed to DNA synthesis, i.e. S phase. Self-renewing stem cells of haematopoietic and epithelial tissues do not appear to be influenced by any of the growth factors which have been purified to date (Burgess 1985a). PDGF induces competence in fibroblasts to go through cell cycle. Epidermal growth factor (EGF) and insulin-like growth factors (IGFs) are required for progression of cells through a later stage of G_1. Growth factors do not always induce mitosis; some B cell growth factors induce resting B cells to differentiate without proliferation.

The number of signal transduction pathways appears to be limited. The initiation or propagation of a signal may be affected at numerous points, for example by inhibition of enzymes, or by deficiency or excess of substrates. The absolute dependence of some cell lines on growth factors can be overcome by infection with a transforming retrovirus if a product of the oncogenic virus enters into the signal pathway of the growth factor.

When membrane-associated receptors are activated by combining with growth factors specific for them, intracellular proteins are phosphorylated. In many cases one of the targets is the intracellular domain of the receptor-kinase itself. Phosphorylation of the internal domain of a receptor modulates its capacity to bind its specific ligand. The activity of many enzymes is regulated by phosphorylation and they may be dysregulated by abnormal phosphorylation, e.g. on serine instead of on tyrosine. Regulatory phosphorylation is reversed by the action of phosphatases. Binding of growth factor to receptor causes "down regulation" of the receptor, which means that it is then less able to transmit signals by subsequent stimuli. Down regulation results from reduction in the numbers of available receptors or loss of binding power ("affinity"). It generally results from clustering and internalisation of the receptors into vesicles, where they may be either destroyed by association with lysosomes or recycled into the plasma membrane.

Some of the insights into the action of the growth factors have come from analysis of the action of the tumour-promoting phorbol esters, because these agents mimic many effects of growth factors. They possess insulin-like activity (stimulation of glucose transport and oxidation) in a number of cell types and they facilitate the growth-promoting action of insulin on 3T3 fibroblastic cells. Phorbol esters mimic EGF and insulin by phosphorylating the same substrates as do the receptors for these growth factors. Phorbols inhibit further action of growth factors by phosphorylating their receptors.

The known biochemical pathways of signal transduction activated by growth factors include:

1. Activation of protein kinases, the enzymes which phosphorylate proteins.

2. Activation of the phosphatidylinositol (PI) cycle, as with PDGF. Active products of this cycle are diacylglycerol (DAG), inositol triphosphate (IP_3) and

metabolites of arachidonic acid. These may themselves lead to activation of protein kinases.

3. Mobilisation of calcium from endoplasmic reticulum, as with PDGF.

4. Increased influx of Ca^{2+}, as with EGF.

5. Activation of the Na^+/H^+ exchange pump, called the Na^+/H^+ antiport, resulting in a sustained rise in intracellular pH from $\sim$ 7.0 to 7.2–7.3 within 10 min (Moolenaar et al. 1985), by exchange of external $Na+$ for internal $H+$. This pump is activated by the action of protein kinase C and blocked by amiloride. Intracellular Na^+ is also under the influence of the Na^+,K^+ dependent ATPase. Elevation of intracellular pH by exposure of cells to an alkaline environment stimulates an increase in protein synthesis but not DNA synthesis. The action of growth factors is inhibited by an intracellular pH below 7.0.

6. Release of secondary chemical messengers, such as cyclic AMP (cAMP) and prostaglandins. Type E prostaglandin synthesis may be induced, e.g. by the growth factor bombesin, leading to an accumulation of the secondary messenger cAMP.

Successful stimulation and signal transduction result in activation of one or more genes, with an increase in specific mRNA by 20-fold or more. mRNAs for c-fos and c-myc rise rapidly in many cell types. This rise has been considered to indicate activation of the gene, i.e. enhanced mRNA transcription, but it is now known that in the case of c-myc it results mainly from reduced turnover. c-fos is usually activated first, and often transiently. The maintenance of the ability to respond to growth factors acting later in the cell cycle does not require a sustained activation of these oncogenes. Both of these oncogenes can be restimulated in S phase, but not during M, to reinduce competence in the daughter cells to respond in the next cycle.

Some growth factors stimulate DNA synthesis in suitable target cells only in synergistic combinations (Rozengurt et al. 1985). Others, like PDGF and bombesin do not require assistance from other factors. This suggests that there are multiple signals, and DNA synthesis will only proceed when all of the necessary signals have been transduced.

Growth Factors in Malignant Transformation

A number of growth factors (EGF, transforming growth factors and PDGF) induce changes associated with transformation — loss of anchorage dependence, growth in soft agar in the presence of serum, and, in some cases, morphological changes associated with malignant cells in monolayer culture. These morphological effects are reversible upon removal of the factor from the medium. Insulin, the insulin-like growth factors (IGF-I, IGF-II) and nerve growth factor stimulate confluent quiescent cells in monolayer culture to synthesise DNA in the presence of serum or plasma proteins. Some of the growth factors are clearly involved in the manifestations of non-lymphomatous human cancers. For example, receptors for EGF are present in high density in anaplastic breast carcinomas. The best known growth factors, for example PDGF and EGF, are not known to be involved in lymphoid cell growth and differentiation.

Growth Factors for Haematopoietic Cells

Growth factors for granulocytes and macrophages were originally called colony-stimulating factors (CSFs) and many other names (Table 7.1). Four different murine factors have been characterised: Multi-CSF, granulocyte-macrophage CSF (GM-CSF), macrophage CSF (M-CSF) and granulocyte CSF (G-CSF), which are produced by a variety of mesodermal cells, including monocytes (Burgess 1985a, b). Receptors have also been identified for each. Genes of the human equivalents are being identified and cloned.

Table 7.1. Nomenclature of haematopoietic growth factors

Currently accepted name	Other names
Multi-CSF	CSF, IL-3, HCCF, Hp2
GM-CSF	Granulocyte-macrophage CSF, CMGF, CSF-2, hCSFα
M-CSF	Macrophage CSF, CSF-1
G-CSF	Granulocyte CSF hCSFβ

These factors induce proliferation of immature macrophages and haematopoietic cells. When stem cells differentiate they produce committed progenitor cells which are restricted in their development to only one or two lineages. These committed cells can still proliferate, but they normally differentiate to non-dividing end cells. In the absence of growth factors haematopoietic cells die rapidly in vitro, unless they are co-cultivated with stromal cells (Metcalf 1985). The myelomonocytic leukaemia cell line WEHI-3B has overcome the reliance of corresponding normal cells on external growth factor by producing its own multi-CSF. This constitutive production, i.e. production in the absence of external stimuli, is caused by the insertion of a retroviral genome near the gene for multi-CSF, and malignant growth of these leukaemic cells is due to an autocrine mechanism (Ymer et al. 1985).

Multi-CSF is produced by T lymphocytes and T lymphoma cells after stimulation by antigen, mitogens and phorbol esters. Multi CSF acts on early progenitor cells, as well as more mature progeny (Fig. 7.1). GM-CSF acts upon a slightly more mature colony-forming cell capable of differentiation into an end cell of different haematopoietic classes. The actions of G-CSF and M-CSF are more restricted (Stanley et al. 1985).

GM-CSF appears to act by stimulation of glucose uptake and anaerobic glycolysis. Phosphorylation is also induced, probably of the glucose transport protein. GM-CSF induces the differentiation of pluripotent stem cells into progenitor cells committed to the granulocyte-monocyte lineage that are then dependent on additional growth factors for further division. TPA can mimic the early events in differentiation of cells induced by GM-CSF.

M-CSF (CSF-1) is particularly interesting because it is the product of a gene which is closely related to the oncogene c-*fms*. It is a 45–80 kD glycosylated protein, consisting of a pair of polypeptide chains, which regulates the survival,

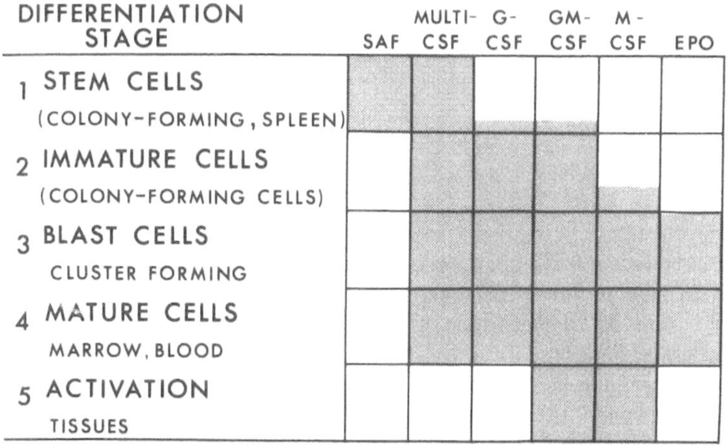

DIFFERENTIATION STAGE	SAF	MULTI-CSF	G-CSF	GM-CSF	M-CSF	EPO
1 STEM CELLS (COLONY-FORMING, SPLEEN)						
2 IMMATURE CELLS (COLONY-FORMING CELLS)						
3 BLAST CELLS CLUSTER FORMING						
4 MATURE CELLS MARROW, BLOOD						
5 ACTIVATION TISSUES						

Fig. 7.1. Haematopoietic growth factors. The growth factors function in stages of haematopoiesis. *Multi-CSF* stimulates different lineages. Stem cell activating factor(s) (*SAF*) influence early erythroid cell generation. The others are more specific for particular types. *G-CSF* and *GM-CSF* both stimulate some cells during differentiation, but multi-CSF or the lineage-specific growth factors, e.g. erythropoietin (*EPO*), are required for the final stages of proliferation and differentiation. (After Burgess 1985b).

proliferation and differentiation of mononuclear phagocytes. The variation in its molecular weight is due to variation in the degree of glycosylation, i.e. the number of sugar molecules attached to the protein chains. It binds to specific receptors of a single class of molecular weight 160 kD.

Day-to-day production of erythrocytes is sustained by progenitor cells recognised in vitro as colony-forming cells (CFU-E), which are dependent on circulating erythropoietin (Goldwasser et al. 1985). More primitive erythroid stem cells, burst-forming cells (BFU-E), are under the influence of stem cell activating factor(s) (SAF). The most primitive erythroid progenitors are under the influence of unidentified cells in the marrow, which probably produce a number of growth factors.

Transforming Growth Factor α

The transforming growth factors (TGFs) are low molecular weight, acid-stable polypeptides, present in the culture medium of chemically and virally transformed cells, human tumour cell lines, embryonic mice and rats, fetal calf serum, the urine of normal pregnant or tumour-bearing humans, and platelets. They are structurally related to (but distinct from) EGF.

TGF_α (also known as TGF 1) induces the formation of small colonies of normal rat kidney cells in soft agar. It binds to the receptor for EGF as well as to its own receptor. Many human cancer cells produce and release TGF_α and have functional receptors for it. Although it is produced by virally transformed cells, TGF_α is not encoded by the virus. Viral transformation activates the TGF_α gene. It can be shown, using temperature-sensitive rodent sarcoma viruses, that TGF_α is only released by cells grown at a temperature permitting transformation. Products of the oncogene v-*mos* (p37^{mos}) or Ki-*ras* (p21^{ras}) of the temperature-sensitive mutants control synthesis of TGF$_α$, by influencing either transcription of TGF$_α$-specific mRNA or translation of it into protein.

Transforming Growth Factor β

TGF$_β$ is quite different from TGF$_α$ in structure and function. It is a 50 kD dimer. TGF$_β$ induces precocious eyelid opening in newborn mice and induces tissue culture cells to form large colonies in agar, whether or not EGF is present. The richest source is the granules of platelets, which also contain PDGF. It is found in many tissues, normal and neoplastic, and is produced in vitro by many transformed and untransformed cells. Specific cell membrane receptors for TGF$_β$ are widely distributed. In serum, TGF$_β$ is bound to an undefined carrier, from which it is released by treatment with acid. TGF$_β$ shares many properties with EGF, but one property which distinguishes it is a greater activity than EGF in inducing growth of new blood vessels.

TGF$_β$ is made by mammary, squamous and adrenal carcinomas and by cells transformed by Moloney, Harvey and Kirsten murine sarcoma viruses. The proto-oncogene *myc* controls the responsiveness to TGF$_β$ and cells transfected with c-*myc* are rendered very sensitive to its action (Moses and Loef 1985). There is a suspicion that *ras* is involved in the transduction of the TGF$_β$ signal. TGF$_β$ activates c-*sis*, c-*fos* and the actin gene. It may produce some of its effects by inducing c-*sis* to synthesise PDGF.

TGF$_β$ does not stimulate any epithelial cells and is a potent inhibitor of the growth of many cells. It may even be an autocrine growth inhibitor, i.e. an inhibitor of the growth of the cells which produce it. It inhibits the growth of several human carcinoma lines growing in soft agar and inhibits proliferation of T and B lymphocytes. Under some circumstances it inhibits the effect of the mitogenic growth factors PDGF and EGF. It causes normal, but not transformed, bronchial epithelium to differentiate in vitro. TGF$_β$ is released in deep wounds, and is possibly a wound hormone. It has been suggested that TGF$_β$ may mediate the tumour-promoting effect of wounding in skin which has been treated with a carcinogen capable of tumour initiation (Parkinson 1985).

Epidermal Growth Factor

EGF is a single chain polypeptide of molecular weight 6045 daltons found in milk, cerebrospinal and pancreatic secretions and urine (the 53 amino acid sequence of EGF is almost identical to the 52 amino acid sequence of urogastrone). The main source is the submaxillary gland of the adult mouse. EGF derives from a 130 kD precursor which may give rise to seven EGF-like peptides. Its gene is on chromosome 4.

The exact physiological functions of EGF are unknown. It accelerates fetal and post-partum growth and maturation, promoting, for example, the growth of hair and teeth in immature mice. When added to a culture of non-dividing cells, the cells are stimulated to divide a single time. The effect of EGF on DNA synthesis is highly synergistic with insulin.

EGF binds to a 170 Kd specific plasma membrane receptor with an extracellular domain (621 amino acids) that binds EGF, a segment of 23 amino acids spanning the membrane, and a tyrosine-specific protein kinase domain (542 amino acids) inside the cell (Fig. 7.2). This type of structure is commonly seen in growth factor receptors. The EGF receptor phosphorylates itself on specific tyrosine residues. Serine and threonine residues of the EGF receptor are also phosphorylated in vivo, as a result of activation of other protein kinases, such as pp 60^{src}. The gene for the EGF receptor is on chromosome 7.

The EGF receptor phosphorylates the intracellular receptor for progesterone. Other steroid hormone receptors may also be targets (Fox et al. 1985). Many other proteins are phosphorylated by the EGF receptor, including vinculin, as well as an unidentified 34 Kd protein, and possibly also gastrin and growth hormone.

The EGF receptor is down regulated from a high- to a low-affinity state by a number of agents, such as PDGF, bombesin, vasopressin, TPA and soluble analogues of diacylglycerol. The change in affinity is due to phosphorylation of the receptor.

The erb-B oncogene product mimics the tyrosine kinase domain of the EGF receptor. It lacks the EGF-binding domain, but retains most of the cytoplasmic region with intrinsic tyrosine kinase activity. It phosphorylates EGF receptors. This may amount to an autocrine mechanism, activation of the receptor being independent of the normal interaction of growth factor with receptor.

EGF receptors have been demonstrated on human breast cancers, squamous cell carcinomas, non-neuronal (glial) brain tumours and cultured breast and bladder carcinoma cell lines. A higher than normal density of EGF receptors has been found on poorly differentiated and invasive bladder tumours (Neal et al. 1985), and an increase in receptors seems to correlate with resistance to drugs. In breast cancers there is an inverse ratio between receptors for EGF and oestrogen, and EGF receptors are found more frequently on metastases than on the primary tumour (Sainsbury et al. 1985a, b). A molecule closely related to the EGF receptor is encoded in the neu oncogene found in gliomas induced in rats by ethylnitrosourea. One of the five domains of the receptor for human low-density lipoprotein is also homologous with the EGF receptor.

Platelet-derived Growth Factor

PDGF is one of a family of growth factors. One of the most potent mitogens known, it is the major mitogen in serum for cells derived from connective tissue. PDGF is a 31 kD protein composed of two polypeptide chains, α and β. The amino acid sequence of the β chain is almost the same as the sequence of p28^{sis}, the transformation-inducing product of the oncogene v-sis of simian sarcoma virus (SSV), which also resembles PDGF in function.

PDGF is probably synthesised as a much larger precursor protein, in which form it may be stored. It is released into the serum from the α granules of platelets when blood clots. Connective tissue cells are among the normal targets, and their growth is stimulated by PDGF. PDGF is thought to be involved in the normal growth of muscle cells in the aorta.

PDGF binds to a 185 kD high-affinity cell surface receptor protein with tyrosine kinase activity. Formation of a PDGF-receptor complex activates the kinase, leading to autophosphorylation of its internal domain. Binding of PDGF to its receptor leads to activation of about 30 cell cycle genes (the "competence" gene family), in fibroblasts and other cells, amongst which *fos* is one of the earliest to be activated. The range of genes activated varies considerably with the cell type. In 3T3 cells the IFN_β gene is activated, rather later in the course of events. Interferon may exert a negative effect on activation of genes by PDGF, representing a kind of feed-back control mechanism.

PDGF and similar proteins are strongly implicated in various models of neoplastic transformation. Tumour cells lines from some human osteosarcomas, gliomas and rhabdomyosarcomas, as well as various cell lines transformed by SSV, Mo-MSV, Ki-MSV and *ras* produce PDGF-like molecules. All of these cells probably have receptors for PDGF. There is good evidence of autocrine receptor activation in some of these cell lines. Antibodies to PDGF inhibit both proliferation and transformation of human fibroblasts by SSV.

PDGF may be involved in the pathogenesis of atherosclerosis. Factors very like PDGF, made by endothelial cells, smooth muscle cells and macrophages, are found in atherosclerotic lesions. Macrophages themselves respond to exogenous PDGF by chemotaxis and activation. Endothelial cells and smooth muscle respond to PDGF by release of prostaglandin, a potent inhibitor of platelet aggregation.

Bombesin

Bombesin is a tetradecapeptide made in large amounts by most lung carcinomas of the anaplastic small cell type. It is a member of a family of related peptides which includes gastrin-releasing peptide. The cells which produce bombesin also have receptors for this product. Bombesin permits the growth of small cell carcinoma cells in vitro in plasma-free media, and specific antibody to bombesin blocks bombesin-dependent growth, by blocking bombesin from binding to its receptor.

Binding of bombesin to its receptor causes changes similar to those caused by PDGF. Protein kinase C activity causes phosphorylation of an 80 Kd protein (Rozengurt et al. 1985). Intracellular calcium is mobilised, the Na^+/H^+ exchange mechanism is affected, the Na^+/K^+ pump is activated and intracellular pH is raised. EGF receptors are transmodulated. Bombesin stimulates the synthesis of E-type prostaglandins, which, in turn, bind to their own receptors and induce cAMP accumulation. Thus, bombesin activates a number of different signal transduction pathways.

Insulin

Insulin binds to an integral membrane glycoprotein receptor composed of two α subunits and two β subunits, with ATP-binding sites and tyrosine kinase activity, very similar to the IGF-I receptor and to the single chain EGF receptor (Fig. 7.2; Ullrich et al. 1985). T and B lymphoblasts possess insulin receptors (Lee et al. 1986). The α and β subunits of the insulin receptor derive from a single glycosylated polypeptide precursor. Tyrosine residues of the β subunit are autophosphorylated after exposure to insulin or anti-insulin receptor antibodies.

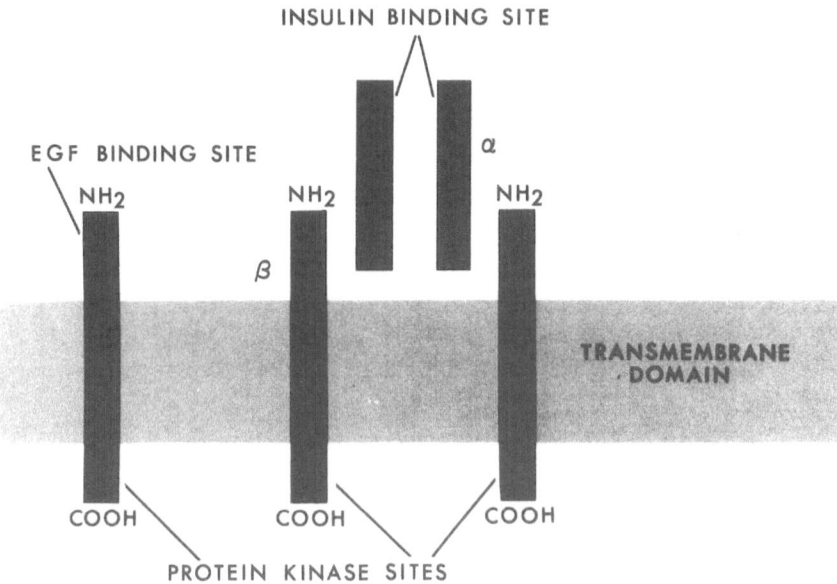

Fig. 7.2. Receptors for EGF (*left*) and insulin (*right*). The EGF receptor has the simplest structure to meet the requirements, with an extracellular domain containing the growth factor binding site, a hydrophobic transmembrane segment and an intracellular segment with tyrosine kinase activity. The receptor for insulin has two α and two β subunits. The receptor is on the extracellular α subunits and protein kinase activity is on the intracellular domain of the β subunits. The receptor for IGF-I is similar to the insulin receptor. (After Ullrich et al. 1985).

The insulin-dependent protein kinase of the receptor has a specificity similar to that of the EGF receptor kinase and tyrosine-specific protein kinases of a number of oncogenes, e.g. *src*. The progesterone receptor is one of its targets. The insulin receptor gene may logically be considered to be a cellular proto-oncogene, because of its protein kinase function, but no corresponding viral oncogene or abnormal cellular gene has yet been identified in malignant or transformed cells.

Insulin-like Growth Factor I

Growth hormone (somatotropin) induces the liver to secrete a number of protein hormones, including those formerly known as somatomedins, which stimulate the growth of muscle and cartilage cells. Infants with deficient somatotropin become dwarfs; those who produce too much become giants. IGF-I (formerly somatomedin-C) is synthesised in response to somatotropin in the form of a precursor protein. It occurs in the blood as a 70-amino-acid peptide which mediates actions of growth hormone. It has some insulin-like activity on adipocytes and muscle cells and stimulates fibroblasts and chondrocytes to divide. IGF-I is needed by target cells for the last 6 h in G_1. As receptors for IGF-I are present on T and B lymphoblasts, it has been suggested that IGF-I may play a part in lymphocyte differentiation and metabolism (Lee et al. 1986), but this has not yet been demonstrated.

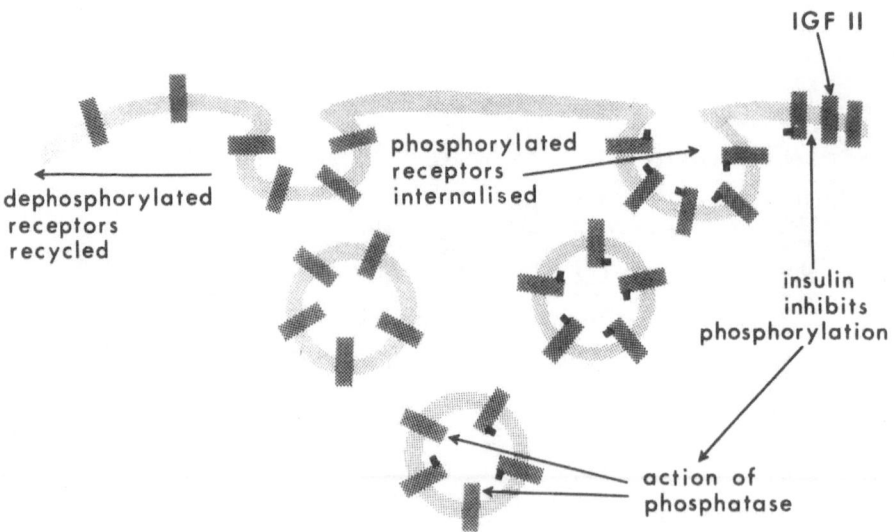

Fig. 7.3. Recycling of IGF-II receptors. Receptors are internalised when they are phosphorylated, as a result, for example, of their specific growth factor binding to them. Insulin inhibits this process, either by inhibiting phosphorylation or by increasing phosphatase activity. Dephosphorylation occurs in the internalised vesicles, and the dephosphorylated receptors are returned to the surface.

Insulin-like Growth Factor II

IGF-II is a growth factor widely produced during fetal development. The gene for IGF-II is on chromosome 11, band p14–15. A deletion of band p13 of chromosome 11, found in all cells of subjects with the aniridia/Wilms' tumour syndrome, removes a regulator gene. In the sporadic form of Wilms' tumour a similar deletion is found in the tumour cells. These deletions may lead to overexpression of IGF-II. The IGF-II gene is also overexpressed in rhabdomyosarcomas.

The IGF-II receptor is a 250 kD glycoprotein having high affinity for IGF-II, lower affinity for IGF-I and none for insulin. Receptors cycle from cell surface into cytoplasm and back. Phosphorylated receptors are internalised. Insulin, by binding to its own receptor, causes a rapid decrease in phosphorylation of membrane IGF-II receptor, inhibiting the movement of IGF-II receptors into the cytoplasm (Fig. 7.3). It does this either by inhibiting a protein kinase or by activating a phosphatase (Czech et al. 1985).

Nerve Growth Factor

Nerve growth factor (NGF) is most abundant in the male salivary gland, and its production in this gland is stimulated by testosterone and thyroxine. It is necessary for the survival of neural cells in vitro. It is taken up by developing nerves and produces hypertrophy of neurons. It is produced by Schwann cells, and there are receptors for it on axons. In motor neuron disease there is an antibody to NGF in the blood. NGF acts by allowing Na^+, K^+ -dependent ATPase to function. It is not a mitogen.

A clue to the action of NGF (and incidentally to the product of the *ras* oncogene) comes from injection of minute quantities of this growth factor into individual cells of a phaeochromocytoma line in culture (Feramisco and Bar-Sagi 1985). Microinjection of NGF into PC12 phaeochromocytoma cells causes them to differentiate into cells with characteristics of neurons. In the absence of NGF, microinjection of human *ras* protein into PC12 cells results in similar differentiation.

Chalones and Other Antiproliferative Factors

Stimulatory growth factors certainly do not constitute the whole mechanism of growth control. A strong inhibitory control is exerted by contact with neighbouring cells (contact inhibition). Soluble factors called chalones inhibit proliferating cells. They are still not fully characterised. In the skin, the G_1 chalone inhibits transition from G_1 to G_2. The G_2 chalone interacts with cells at the G_2-M transition (Marks et al. 1985). They are highly specific for cell type but are not species specific.

Conclusions

The grand pattern of control of growth and differentiation of animal cells is gradually becoming clearer. Growth depends on the orderly expression of genes specifically involved in mitosis and expression of characteristics appropriate to the mature specialised cell. Growth from the fertilised ovum to maturity may be thought of as resulting from the operation of sets of programs, analogous to, but more complicated than, computer programs, directing the activity of the gene repertoire. The genome is programmed to integrate incoming signals and select the appropriate, specific response to each set of information from the environment of the cell.

From this analogy it may be predicted that malignant behaviour can develop if the program is scrambled, or if the incoming line of communication or outgoing line of execution are falsified. Some biological equivalents in this analogy are now known. Growth factors are environmental information, which can be dispensed with if the cell synthesises its own growth factors. The line into the program is represented by the biochemical pathway which transduces the signal arising from the interaction of the growth factor and its receptor. The program itself is written in units (genes, including oncogenes) that are concerned either with integration of the program or with production of the effector (protein) product. The program can be dislocated or falsified by the insertion of false units in the form of viral oncogenes, by rearranging the order of the program (by chromosomal translation), or by changing the letters in the program (by chemical mutagenesis). Any alteration in the sequence of execution of the program may have dire results for the harmonious coordination of growth and for the production of cellular products. Certain patterns of disruption constitute neoplasia.

Reviews of growth factors not already cited are to be found in Heldin and Westermark (1984), Kelly (1985), Newmark (1985), Sporn and Roberts (1985), Strosberg (1985) and Evan (1986).

References

Burgess AW (1985a) Growth factors and oncogenes. Immunol Today 6: 107–112

Burgess AW (1985b) Hematopoietic growth factors In: Ford RJ, Maizel AL (eds) Mediators in cell growth and differentiation. Raven, New York, pp 159–168

Czech MP, Davis RJ, MacDonald RG, Corvera S (1985) The role of phosphorylation in regulating the recycling of receptors for insulin-like growth factor. Proceedings of the eleventh annual EMBO symposium on growth factors, receptors and oncogenes, 16–19 September, 1985. European Molecular Biology Laboratory, Heidelberg, p 14 (abstract)

Evan G (1986) Growth factors, receptors and oncogenes. Trends Genet 2: 2–3

Feramisco JR, Bar-Sagi D (1985) Microinjection of the ras oncogene into PC12 cells induces neuronal differentiation. Proceedings of the eleventh annual EMBO symposium on growth factors, receptors, and oncogenes, 16–19 September, 1985. European Molecular Biology Laboratory, Heidelberg, p 9 (abstract)

Fox CF, Sarup J, Woo D et al. (1985) Actions of tyrosine kinases on steroid hormone receptors and steroid hormone receptor properties. Proceedings of the eleventh annual EMBO symposium on growth factors, receptors and oncogenes, 16–19 September, 1985. European Molecular Biology Laboratory, Heidelberg, p 21 (abstract)

Goldwasser E, Krantz SB, Wang FW (1985) Erythropoietin and erythroid differentiation In: Ford RJ, Maizel AL (eds) Mediators in cell growth and differentiation. Raven, New York, pp 103–107

Heldin C-H, Westermark B (1984) Growth factors: mechanisms of action and relation to oncogenes. Cell 37: 9–20

Kelly K (1985) Growth factors short-circuited. Nature 317: 390

Lee PD, Rosenfeld RG, Hintz RL, Smith SD (1986) Characterisation of insulin, insulin-like growth factors I and II, and growth hormone receptors on human leukemic lymphoblasts. J Clin Endocrinol Metab 62: 28–35

Marks F, Bertsch S, Fürstenberger G, Richter H (1985) Growth control in mouse epidermis — facts and speculations. In: Wright NA, Camplejohn RS (eds) Psoriasis: cell proliferation. Churchill Livingstone, Edinburgh, pp 173–188

Metcalf D (1985) The granulocytic-macrophage colony stimulating factors. Minireview. Cell 43: 5–6

Moolenaar WH, Defize LHK, van der Saag PT, de Laat SW (1985) Ionic signal transduction by growth factors. Proceedings of the eleventh annual EMBO symposium on growth factors, receptors and oncogenes, 16–19 September, 1985. European Molecular Biology Laboratory, Heidelberg, p 33 (abstract)

Moses HL, Loef EB (1985) Transforming growth factor β. Proceedings of the eleventh annual EMBO symposium on growth factors, receptors and oncogenes, 16–19 September, 1985. European Molecular Biology Laboratory, Heidelberg, p 34 (abstract)

Neal DE, Marsh C, Bennett MK et al. (1985) Epidermal-growth-factor receptors in human bladder cancer: comparison of invasive and superficial tumours. Lancet I: 366–368

Newmark P (1985) Events at the surface of the cell. Nature 317: 380

Parkinson EK (1985) Defective responses of transformed keratinocytes to terminal differentiation stimuli. Their role in epidermal tumour promotion by phorbol esters and by deep skin wounding. Br J Cancer 52: 479–493

Rozengurt E, Zachary I, Mendoza SA, Sinnett-Smith JW (1985) Early signals and synergistic effects in mitogenesis: effects of bombesin and structurally related peptides. Proceedings of the eleventh annual EMBO symposium on growth factors, receptors and oncogenes, 16–19 September, 1985. European Molecular Biology Laboratory, Heidelberg, p 49 (abstract)

Sainsbury JRC, Farndon JR, Sherbet GV, Harris AL (1985a) Epidermal-growth-factor receptors and oestrogen receptors in human breast cancer. Lancet I: 364–366

Sainsbury JR, Malcolm AJ, Appleton DR, Farndon JR, Harris AL (1985b) Presence of epidermal growth factor receptor as an indicator of poor prognosis in patients with breast cancer. J Clin Pathol 38: 1225–1228

Sporn MB, Roberts AB (1985) Autocrine growth factors and cancer. Nature 313: 745–747

Stanley ER, Kawasaki ES, Ladner MB et al. (1985) The colony stimulating factor, CSF-1 and its receptor. Proceedings of the eleventh annual EMBO symposium on growth factors, receptors and oncogenes, 16–19 September, 1985. European Molecular Biology Laboratory, Heidelberg, p 56 (abstract)

Strosberg AD (1985) Receptors and recognition: from ligand binding to gene structure. Trends Biochem Sci 9: 166–169

Ullrich A, Bell JR, Chen EY et al. (1985) Human insulin receptor and its relationship to the tyrosine kinase family of oncogenes. Nature 313: 756–761

Ymer S, Tucker WQJ, Sanderson CJ, Hapel AJ, Campbell HD, Young IG (1985) Constitutive synthesis of interleukin-3 by leukaemia cell line WEHI-3B is due to retroviral insertion near the gene. Nature 317: 255–258

8 The Lymphoid Tissues

Introduction

The cells of the lymphoid tissues primarily involved in the generation of specific immune responses are the lymphocytes. As well as the lymphocytes, cells of the monocyte-macrophage series, which are collectively called accessory cells (ACs) are essential for generation of both cellular and humoral (antibody) responses. They play a large part in regulating immune responses, by presenting antigen to T and B cells, by degrading antigen and by release of mediators.

The lymphocytes are classified into three types:

1. T (thymus-derived) lymphocytes concerned both with the regulation of T and B cell responses and with the execution of cellular immune responses.

2. B (bursal in birds, bone marrow in mammals) lymphocytes, involved in the synthesis of antibody.

Resting lymphocytes of T and B classes are small cells, 6–10 μ diameter in smears, with a high ratio of nucleus to cytoplasm. Small T and B lymphocytes are morphologically indistinguishable. They have few organelles in the cytoplasm and the nucleus is dense.

3. Null, non-T non-B, or "third population" lymphocytes. Lymphocytes with antibody-dependent cytotoxic capacity (ADCC) and natural killer (NK) activity are the major cell types in this category. They are somewhat larger than resting T and B lymphocytes and usually contain granules.

Monocytes, circulating cells of the macrophage-accessory cell family, are somewhat larger than lymphocytes in smears of peripheral blood, frequently having an indented "horseshoe-shaped" nucleus and abundant cytoplasm containing lysosomal acid hydrolases and peroxidase. Macrophages are phagocytic cells in tissues. Their enzyme-rich cytoplasm may be extended widely in numerous processes. The mononuclear phagocytes have many subclasses, including Kupffer cells in the liver, histiocytes in connective tissues, Langerhans cells in skin, microglial cells in nervous tissue, osteoclasts in bone and macrophages in pulmonary alveoli, peritoneal and pleural spaces.

Origin of Lymphocytes

T and B cells develop from precursors that have differentiated from pluripotential haematopoietic cells in the yolk sac. They are first present between the 21st and 28th days of gestation. From this point onwards, the developmental pathways of B and T cells are quite distinct.

In postnatal life myeloid cells are derived from a stem cell that is more primitive than stem cells which give rise to lymphocytes. Chronic myelogenous leukaemia (CML) probably involves a pluripotential stem cell common to the lymphocyte and the myelocyte. In some patients with CML, blastic transformation involves cells with morphological, antigenic and enzymatic characteristics of lymphocytes.

T Lymphocytes

T lymphocytes were originally distinguished by their capacity to form rosettes with sheep erythrocytes (E). Several non-lymphoid human cell types, such as fibroblasts and parenchymal cells of the liver, lung and parathyroid have also been shown to form E rosettes (Woda et al. 1977). T cells may express receptors for the Fc part of IgM or IgG (Grossi et al. 1978) and a number of enzymes which can be used as markers (Table 8.1).

Cells of the immune system are now classified by the use of a bewildering array of monoclonal antibodies. Fortunately, two international workshops have made progress in systematic classification of these. The CD (clusters of differentiation) system developed at these workshops will be used whenever possible, in keeping with usage in the recent literature, to overcome an otherwise insuperable confusion. The important T cell monoclonal antibodies are listed in Tables 8.2 and

Table 8.1. T lymphocyte markers

T receptor gene rearrangement	
Surface membrane antigens	CD1, CD2 (ER), CD3, CD5, CD6, CD7
	CD4 ($T_{helper/inducer}$),
	CD8 ($T_{suppressor/cytotoxic}$)
Receptors	IL-2 receptor (activated T)
	Transferrin receptor (activated T)
	$Fc_\gamma R$ T cell subset
	$Fc_\mu R$ T cell subset
	$Fc_\alpha R$ T cell subset
MHC product	Class I
	Class II, on some, particularly activated T cells
Enzymes	α-naphthyl acid esterase (ANAE),
	acid hydrolase (AH),
	acid phosphatase (AP),
	β-glucuronidase (BG),
	terminal deoxynucleotidyl transferase (TdT)

Table 8.2. Commonly used anti-T cell monoclonal antibodies

Cluster	MW	OK antibody	LEU antibody	Specificity
CD1	p21/48	T6	Leu-6	Cortical thymocytes, Langerhans cells
CD2	p50	T11	Leu-5b	E receptor
CD3	p20/20/15	T3	Leu-4	Mature T cells
CD4	p55	T4	Leu-3a	T helper/inducer
CD5	p76	T1	Leu-1	Pan T, B CLL, WDLL B cell subpopulation
CD6	p120	T12		Mature T cells
CD7	p41		Leu-9	Pan T
CD8	p30/45	T8	Leu-2a	T suppressor/cytotoxic
CD25	p50–55			Activated T and B cells. Receptor for IL-2 recognised by anti-Tac
CD45	p220/205 p190/180			Leucocyte common antigen (T and B)
T10[a]	p12/46	T10		Early thymocytes and activated lymphocytes
T17[a]				Thymocytes, circulating lymphocytes

[a] Not assigned by the international workshop.

8.3 and some of the B cell monoclonal antibodies are listed in Table 8.5. The most commonly used T cell antibodies belong to the commercially available OKT and Leu series (Table 8.2).

Several monoclonal antibodies are available which detect the so-called leucocyte common antigen (LCA). This antigen is expressed on all normal lymphoreticular cells, as well as cells of bone marrow origin. Although these antibodies are not useful in the subclassification of the lymphoid malignancies, they are useful markers to differentiate malignant lymphomas from other non-lymphoid neoplasms such as carcinomas and sarcomas. (Table 8.3).

Eight antibody clusters are specific or selective for cells of the T cell lineage. T cells express either CD4 or CD8 and a small percentage expresses both. The E (sheep erythrocyte) receptor is detected by CD2 antibodies. Of the anti-T monoclonal antibodies, those of specificity CD2, CD3 and CD5 react with nearly all normal peripheral blood T lymphocytes (reviewed by Janossy and Prentice 1982). CD5 antibodies label a minority population of normal B cells and also label neoplastic lymphocytes of chronic lymphocytic leukaemia (CLL) and related low-grade lymphomas (Schroff et al. 1982; Burns et al. 1983). CD4 antibodies, usually assumed to indicate helper/inducer activity, label 55%–65% of circulating T lymphocytes. T17 is a pan-T cell marker which is apparently distinct from other recognised T cell markers. As it recognises an antigen found on T-acute lymphoblastic leukaemia (ALL) cells and most T cell malignancies it is thought to be expressed on T cells from the earliest thymic stage onwards (Matutes et al. 1985). T17 has not yet been assigned a CD designation. None of these monoclonal antibodies are markers of distinct T cell clones. CD4 is detected on 45%–60% of normal circulating lymphocytes and a wide variety of monocytes, macrophages

Table 8.3. Catalogue of monoclonal antibodies reacting with T cells, granulocytes and monocytes[a]

A. Monoclonal antibodies reacting with T cells

CD 1   C-47, T411E1, M-241, NA1/34, SK9/Leu-6, 4A76, 10D12.2, NU-T2, I-19

CD 2   9–1, MT 1110, S2/Leu-5b, MT910, 9.6, MT26, T11/7T4–7E10, T411B5, T11/3Pt2H9,
        T11/3T4–8B5, 35.1, T57, 9–2, 8961, 39C1.5, T11/7T4–7A9, 6F10.3, NU-T1,
        T11/ROLD2–1H8

CD 3   SK7/Leu-4, T3/2Ad2A2, BW242/55, 39H7.3, 41F2.1, T3/RW2–4B6, T3/RW2–8C8, X35–3,
        G19–4.1, BW264/56, KOLT-2, T10B9, CRIS-7, BW239/347, T10C5, T3/2Y8–2F4

CD 4   G19–2, 91D6, 94b1, 13B8.2, T4/12T4DU, T4/18T3A9, MT310, MT151, T4/19THY5D7,
        EDU-2, 66.1, BW264/123, MT321, T4/2T8–2F4, 9.3

CD 5   H65, G19–3.1, 6–2, L17F12/Leu-1, MT61

CD 6   T12/3Pt12B8, 12.1.5, SJ10–2H10, MT421, G3–5, T12A10, MT211

CD 7   3A1A, 3A1B-4G6, MT215, G3–7, 4H9/Leu-9, 8H8.1, I21, 4A, 1–3, T55, 5A12, WT-1

CD 8   M236, T8/21thy2D3, G10–1.1, C12/D3, MT415, 4D12.1, 8E-1.7, T8/7PE3F9, T8–2T8–1C1,
        T41D8, 66.2, MT122, BW135/80, T8/2T8–2A1, T8/25T8-H7, 14, MT1014, BW264/162,
        10B4.6

B. Monclonal antibodies reacting with monocytes and granulocytes

CD11   M01, B2.12, M522,   (reacting with monocytes, granulocytes and other cells)

CDw12   20.2, M67   (as above)

CDw13   MY7, DU-HL60–4, MCS.2   (as above)

CDw14   20.3, 5F1, MOP15, M02,   (typically reacts with monocytes)
        MOS1, MY4, MOS39, FMC17
        TM18, MOP9,

CDw15   80H3, B13.9, MCS.1, FMC12,
        FMC13, WM37, DU-HL60–1, FMC10,
        W27, WM30, G1120, TG8, WM38,
        TG1, DU-HL60–3, G2, B4.3, VIMD5, WM41, 1G10, Leu-M1

[a] Data from sundry sources, including Reinherz et al. (1986)

and dendritic cells (Wood et al. 1983). CD8 is present on 25%–30% of normal circulating lymphocytes.

Terminal deoxynucleotidyl transferase (TdT) is expressed during T cell differentiation (see Table 10.3, p. 118). Activated T cells express high- and low-affinity receptors for interleukin 2 (IL-2) detected by monoclonal antibodies of the CD25 cluster. Although some fetal thymocytes possess receptors for complement, most mature T lymphocytes do not. Activated T cells may express major histocompatibility complex (MHC) class II antigens. T cells can be classified into subsets by functional tests and surface markers. The definitive marker of T cells is rearrangement of the genes encoding the T cell receptor. The technology to determine rearrangement of these genes in cells of tissue samples is now becoming available for application to diagnosis and classification of lymphoid neoplasms.

B Lymphocytes

The standard marker of B cells is immunoglobulin (Table 8.4). The definitive marker is rearrangement of immunoglobulin genes, by gene hybridisation tech-

Table 8.4 B lymphocyte markers

Immunoglobulin chain rearrangement
Cytoplasmic immunoglobulin
Surface immunoglobulin
MHC class II product
Surface membrane antigens: CD5, CD19, CD20, CD21, CD22, CD23, CD24
Fc receptors: Fc_μ, Fc_γ, Fc_α, Fc_ϵ
MER (mouse erythrocyte receptor)
Complement receptors: CR1 (C3b), CR2 (C3d, recognised by CD21), CR3 (inactivated C3b)
Epstein–Barr virus receptor
Enzymes: acid hydrolases (AH), peroxidase (POX), non-specific esterase (NSE), alkaline phosphatase (AP)
Others: receptors for interferon (IFN), macrophage activating factors (MAFs), migration inhibition factor (MIF)

niques. Antibodies can be used to detect common epitopes on immunoglobulin, or to detect idiotypes, the specific epitopes on the antibody synthesised by a particular clone of B lymphocytes. IgM is the most common heavy chain on circulating B lymphocytes, and the ratio of cells expressing κ light chains to those expressing λ is about 2: 1 (Black et al. 1980). Following antigenic stimulation, B cells may switch from synthesis of IgM heavy chain to that of IgG or IgA. The mouse erythrocyte receptor, another B cell-specific marker, is discussed on p. 97.

Table 8.5 lists anti-B cell monoclonal antibodies in common use. The monoclonal antibodies having broadest reactivity, which could be termed pan-B cell antibodies, belong to the cluster CD20, perhaps the best known being B1 (Stashenko et al. 1980). These antibodies bind to nearly all B lymphocytes from blood and lymphoid organs but binding is lost at the plasma cell stage (see Fig. 11.1, p. 131; Table 11.2, p. 130). Monocytes, resting and activated T cells, null cells and tumours of T cell and myeloid origin are CD20-negative (Stashenko et al. 1980).

Antibodies of the cluster CD24 (perhaps best represented by BA1) are also useful for identification of cells of human B cell lineage. The determinant detected by these antibodies is found primarily in peripheral blood lymphocytes and is lost when these cells undergo terminal differentiation (Abramson et al. 1981). CD24 antibodies react with sIg +ve CLL, pre-B ALL, most non-Hodgkin's lymphomas and most non-T non-B ALL. BA1 also reacts weakly with peripheral blood granulocytes and B lymphoblastoid cell lines.

CD21 (e.g. B2) antibodies are also relatively B cell specific. However, less than 100% of normal B lymphocytes in peripheral blood and lymphoid tissue react with CD21, and the determinant is absent at very early stages of B cell differentiation and is lost before CD20 during plasma cell differentiation (Nadler et al. 1981). CD21 detects the receptor for the C3d component of complement (CR2).

Other markers commonly found on B lymphocytes include MHC class II antigens and receptors for complement and for the Fc segment of Ig heavy chains (FcR). Complement receptors (CRs) may play a part in regulating the activation of B cells. B lymphocytes may bind antigen-antibody complexes through the FcR.

J chain, a polypeptide around which IgA and IgM molecules polymerise, is produced by B cells synthesising these immunoglobulin classes. Staining for this polypeptide is a useful marker of normal B cells and of B cell lymphomas (Isaacson 1979).

Table 8.5 Anti- B cell monoclonal antibodies

Cluster	Mol. wt. (kD)	Antibodies	Specificity
A. CD classification of monoclonal antibodies reacting with B cells			
CD19	p95	B4, HD37, 4G7, SJ 25-C1	Pan B
CD20	p35	B1, 2H7, 1F5	Pan B
CD21	p140	B2, HB5, BL13 (RFB-1[a])	Resting B (C3d = CR2, EBV receptor)
CD22	p135	HD6, HD39, 29–110, SJ10–1H11, SHCL-1 (RFB4, To15[a])	Resting B (cell surface), pan B (cytoplasm)
CD23	p45	B-LAST-2, NMN6, PL-13	Activated B, DRC
CD24	p45,55,65	BA1, HB8, HB9	Pan B/ myeloid cells
CD9	p24	BA2, DU-ALL-1, J2 CLB-thromb	B-CLL, Non B/T ALL monocytes, platelets, B cells
CD10	p100	J5, BA3, NL-1, 24.1, VIL-A1, CLB-CALLA	CALLA cALL, pre-B cells, polymorphs, follicular centre cells, activated B
B. Other antibodies reacting with B cells			
μ chain antibody			B cell
Transferrin receptor Ab (e.g. OKT9, 5E9)			Binds to activated T and B
CD45			Binds "Leucocyte common" antigen on T and B lymphocytes
9.4, AB-1			Activated B. Putative antigen is BCGF receptor
4F2, B-LAST-1, B5, BB-1			React with activated B
Tü1			Same distribution as CD23
FMC 1, Y29/55			Generally follow sIg. Expression does not correlate with formation of rosettes with mouse erythrocytes
PC-1, PCA-1			Expressed at the plasma cell stage of B cell differentiation
FMC 3			Reacts with some B cells, only some B CLL, most T cells and monocytes
FMC7			Distinguishes HCL and PLL from CLL. Delineates a subpopulation of B lymphocytes in normal blood. Expression of the FMC7 antigen appears to be maturation-linked
PI 153/3			Reacts with neuroblastoma, B cells, non-T non-B ALL
BB 5, EC3			β_2-microglobulin.
CD25, Tac			IL-2 receptor, present on activated B (and T) cells
Anti-MHC class II gp 29, 43 complex			Most monoclonal antibodies to Ia-like antigens react with HLA/DR associated non-polymorphic antigens. Some react with polymorphic determinants, for example FMC 2 (reacting with some HLA/DRw4). Genox .353 reacts with HLA-DRw1, 2 and 6

[a] Not assigned by international workshop.

B cells can be classified into subsets on the basis of differentiation stage, by tests of function or by surface marker phenotype. Markers on B cells may be classified into five groups:

1. Pan B cell antigens (MHC class II, CD 19 and CD20 molecules) appear in B cell development before cytoplasmic μ chains and persist until terminal differentiation.

2. CD22 appears in the cytoplasm at the pre-B cell stage, then on the cell surface of resting B cells, and disappears with activation; sIgD and CD21 are present on resting B lymphocytes and are lost with activation.

3. BB1, B5, IL-2 receptors, B-LAST-1 and CD23 appear following activation.

4. T10, PCA-1 and PC-1 appear late in B cell differentiation.

5. CD10 (CALLA) appears early in B cell ontogeny and on a subpopulation of activated B cells.

Until the advent of monoclonal antibodies to B cell surface molecules, formation of rosettes with mouse erythrocytes was one of the few specific markers of human B lymphocytes, apart from surface immunoglobulin. This marker is, in addition, a marker of B cells in common B CLL (Stathopoulos and Elliott 1974). The subpopulation expressing the mouse erythrocyte receptor (MER) is also increased in rheumatoid arthritis. The cause of this is unknown.

From 1%–12% of peripheral blood lymphocytes are MER+ in normal subjects. MER is distinct from other markers such as MHC class II (Ia), receptors for Fc and complement, and sIg. Most MER+ cells have sIg and CR (Forbes and Zalewski 1976), but only a proportion of sIg+ cells form mouse erythrocyte rosettes. Anti-Ig and C3b inhibit rosetting. This may result from steric hindrance, since rosetting with mouse erythrocytes is not inhibited when MER+, sIg- B cells are treated with anti-Ig. Alternatively, anti-Ig and C3b may act as triggers to modulation of expression of MER.

MER is a lipid-protein complex, deriving its specificity from the membrane lipid phosphatidylethanolamine, which in the micellar state selectively agglutinates mouse erythrocytes. The proteins in the complex include albumin and other unidentified proteins, one of which is a glycoprotein. Albumin is also a hidden component of mouse (Sidman 1981) and guinea pig (Owen et al. 1978) B and T lymphocyte plasma membranes. MER can be removed from B cells by gentle trypsinisation, and the receptor-rich preparation obtained in this way will confer the capacity to form mouse erythrocyte rosettes on B cells that cannot form MER. The presumed ligand of MER is albumin, since pure undenatured serum albumin prepared under non-damaging conditions inhibits the agglutination of mouse erythrocytes by soluble preparations of the receptor or by phosphatidylethanolamine itself.

MER has to be distinguished from a second receptor, R2, which mediates rosetting with pronase-treated mouse erythrocytes (Forbes et al. 1982). Treatment of mouse erythrocytes with proteolytic enzymes (trypsin, papain or pronase) or with the enzyme neuraminidase, which splits off the carbohydrate sialic acid, raises the percentage of rosette-forming lymphocytes to 15%–20%. The receptor mediating this type of rosettes is distinct from MER and also from MHC class II antigens, Fc_γ, Fc_μ and CR (Forbes et al. 1982). As R2 is lost later in the differentiation pathway of B cells, most of the circulating B cells expressing this receptor belong to a MER-, R2+ population. It must be stressed that the use of protease-treated lymphocytes to obtain a higher yield of cells rosetting with mouse erythrocytes results in the measurement of a different population of B lymphocytes.

NK, ADCC and Lymphokine-activated Killer Cells

A population of lymphocytes, also referred to as "null" or "third population" cells, was distinguished originally by lack of markers of either T or B cells. The majority of such cells are recognisable as "large granular lymphocytes" (LGLs, Table 8.6) because of their intracytoplasmic azurophilic granules. Some null cells lacking Fc receptors are erythroid and myeloid precursors (Ferrarini and Grossi 1984).

Table 8.6. Markers of large granular lymphocytes (LGLs)

Surface antigens	CP03, M1, CD3±, CD4±, CD8±
Function	Tests for ADCC and NK activity
Receptor	$Fc_\gamma R$ (Fc receptor for IgG)
MHC product	Class II

Note: It is not known whether the NK receptor is the CP03 antigen and whether the ADCC receptor is $Fc_\gamma R$.

LGLs are mainly NK or ADCC, distinguished by the capacity to kill target cells in vitro. NK cells kill a range of tumour cells. The recognition mechanism is unknown. They have also been thought to be involved in the normal regulation of immune responses. LGLs may release lymphocyte growth factors (reviewed by Pistoia et al. 1985). ADCC attach via the Fc segment of the antibody (which consists of the second and third heavy chain constant domains; see Fig. 11.2, p. 136) which has bound specifically to the target cell. The azurophilic granules, well developed in human NK cells, but difficult to demonstrate in mouse NK cells, are electron dense and peroxidase negative. They are found close to the Golgi apparatus and also scattered in the cytoplasm.

Blood LGLs express a myeloid antigen CD11, and some subpopulations express T cell antigens (CD2, CD3, CD4, CD5 and CD8). They also express T10, which is an antigen of unknown function on thymocytes and plasma cells. NK cells in splenic red pulp express CD11, but those in tonsils, lymph nodes and the white pulp of the spleen do not. One-quarter of blood LGLs express MHC class II products. LGLs are also recognised by monoclonal antibodies of the CP03 cluster, including HNK-1 and Leu-7. Unfortunately, characterisation of NK cells by CP03 antibodies is not very satisfactory, because antibodies having the specificity of this cluster recognise non-killer cells within the LGL population, and also a glycoprotein in myelin (reviewed by Burns et al. 1985). The highest NK activity is associated with the CP03+, CD3−, CD11+ fraction of LGLs (Abo et al. 1982). The maturation sequence CP03+, CD3+, CD11− (the phenotype in bone marrow) to CP03+, CD3−, CD11+ (in blood) has been proposed (Abo et al. 1983).

The origin of NK cells is still not certain (Robertson 1985): they may represent a distinct lineage, or may derive from either myeloid or lymphoid stem cells. They are not found in thoracic duct lymph. One strong piece of evidence that NK cells belong to the T cell lineage is the demonstration of rearranged genes for the β chain of T cell receptors in some, although the rearrangement is incomplete, and genes for the α chain have not been rearranged.

The association of NK-like (CP03+) cells with tumours is beginning to be explored, on the supposition that these cells form part of the natural defence against malignancy. A greater infiltration of NK cells has been reported in non-Hodgkin's lymphomas of low and intermediate grade of malignancy than in those of high grade (Greil et al. 1986).

NK cells require activation to exert their cytotoxic effect in vitro and in vivo. Upon activation they lose their granules. Interferons (IFNs) of all types, at very low concentration, activate NK cells. Indomethacin potentiates this effect. IFNs also recruit pre-NK cells in vivo. Whether they can be activated directly by viruses is not yet settled. NK cells are also activated by IL-2 and by antibodies against CD2. They possess the receptor for IL-2 and they proliferate in response to this factor without the requirement for another stimulus such as a lectin.

A number of types of lymphoid cells lyse tumour cells in vitro, including cytotoxic T lymphocytes (CTLs), cells named "anomalous killer cells" and lymphokine-activated killer (LAK) cells. There is still some uncertainty as to the definition of these categories. The name "lymphokine-activated killer" has recently been given to a type of cell recognised through studies on the growth of autologous lymphocytes having anti-tumour activity obtained from patients with cancer (reviewed by Rosenberg 1985). The aim of such studies is to grow large numbers of cells with anti-tumour activity which can then be reinjected. LAK cells grow in vitro when peripheral blood lymphocytes are cultured in the presence of IL-2. They can lyse fresh tumour cells that are resistant to NK cells; they do not lyse normal cells. LAK precursors are also found in lymph nodes, bone marrow and thoracic duct lymph. LAK cells lack antigens recognised by CP03 and CD11 monoclonal antibodies.

Accessory Cells

The term "accessory cell" (AC) has been used to designate a group of cells which control the amount of antigen to which lymphocytes are exposed and carry out certain effector functions of the immune system, such as destruction of pathogens after phagocytosis. These cells are essential in cellular interactions involved in the induction of immune responses. Such cells are referred to in the literature as "adherent cells", "antigen-presenting cells", "macrophages" and " monocytes". Dendritic monocytes, Langerhans cells and histiocytes in tissues are included in this category. These cells present large numbers of receptors for the Fc segment of IgG and have complement receptors primarily for C3b and C4b. Activated monocytes also appear to bear receptors for C3b.

There are two types of AC, the macrophages which destroy antigen, and the antigen presenting cells (APCs). A number of cell types may function as APCs.

APCs take up, process and present antigen to immunologically competent T and B lymphocytes. They stem principally from the monocyte-macrophage series.

Follicular dendritic reticulum cells (DRCs) are non-phagocytic APCs of the B lymphocyte system in the lymphoid follicles. Their counterparts in the T lymphocyte system (also non-phagocytic) are the interdigitating dendritic reticulum cells (IDRCs) of the paracortex of lymph nodes and other T-zones and the Langerhans cells of the epidermis. IDRCs are found in the corticomedullary junction and the area adjacent to lymphatic sinusoids, sites in lymph nodes which have substantial numbers of B cells (MacLennan and Gray 1986). IDRCs are involved in T-dependent B cell activation. DRCs and IDRCs express MHC class II antigens and Fc receptors (Table 8.7).

Table 8.7. Macrophage markers

Complement receptors	CR1 (C3b), CR3 (inactivated C3b)
Fc receptors	$Fc_\gamma R$, $Fc_\epsilon R$, $Fc_\mu R$
MHC products	Class I, Class II (variable, must be present for antigen presentation)
Surface antigens	Monoclonal antibodies reacting with monocytes and granulocytes: CD11, CDw12–15
Enzymes	Acid hydrolases (AH), peroxidase (POX), lysozyme, α-1-antitrypsin, α-1-anti-chymotrypsin, esterases
Others	Receptors for interferon (IFN), macrophage activating factors (MAFs), migration inhibition factor (MIF)

Most monoclonal antibodies which react with monocytes and macrophages also react with cells of the granulocyte series. Included in this category are the monoclonal antibodies M01 and Leu-M1. Leu-M1 stains histiocytes, monocytes, granulocytes and IDRCs (Hsu et al. 1985). This antibody is particularly interesting because it stains Reed–Sternberg cells and their mononuclear variants in paraffin sections (Hsu et al. 1985; Pinkus et al. 1985). CD4 antibody, which reacts with helper T cells, has recently been shown to react with a wide variety of monocytes, macrophages and dendritic cells (Wood et al. 1983).

Monocytes and macrophages have been identified by the histochemical demonstration of intracellular lysozyme (Mason and Taylor 1975) and the enzymes α-1-antitrypsin (Isaacson et al. 1981) and α-1-anti-chymotrypsin (Papadimitriou et al. 1978). Specific antibodies can stain these enzymes in routinely processed paraffin-embedded tissue using any of the immunocytochemical techniques.

Few specific reagents are available to distinguish APCs from phagocytic cells. The monoclonal antibody KiM1 recognises monocyte-macrophages, cells of the phagocytic system and IDRCs. It does not react with other human tissues or other haematopoietic cells, including granulocytes (Radzun et al. 1984). The antibody R4/23 stains DRCs (Naiem et al. 1983). Staining for S100 protein is seen in both DRCs (Cocchia et al. 1983) as well as in IDRCs (Takahashi et al. 1981; Wood et al. 1985).

APCs must express compatible MHC products (usually class II) for effective presentation of antigen. They are found principally in lymphoid tissues and skin. Vascular endothelial cells may also act as APCs. Many kinds of epithelial cells, including thyroid cells, may express class II MHC products when activated to enter the mitotic cycle. This may lead to presentation of autoantigen, inducing an autoimmune response. Langerhans cells of the skin contain characteristic racquet-shaped Birbeck granules which appear after antigenic stimulation. Langerhans cells migrate through afferent lymphatics to the paracortical area of the regional lymph nodes, where they become IDRCs which make intimate contact with surrounding T cells. Their function is to activate T cells which have specific receptors for the antigen which they present. IDRCs in the thymus probably express self antigens, thereby causing self-reactive T cells to be aborted or to become anergic.

Cells of the macrophage system are derived from progenitors in the bone marrow. Their generation and differentiation are controlled by the growth factors multi-CSF and GM-CSF. They circulate as monocytes and migrate into various tissues to become macrophages. Tissue macrophages constitute the reticuloendothelial system (RES).

Activation of Macrophages

Macrophages must themselves be activated to function efficiently. Activation enhances their metabolism and their capacity to destroy ingested cells and micro-organisms. They enlarge, become more motile and increase their content of cytoplasmic organelles.

Macrophages are activated by various products of activated T lymphocytes, including IFN_γ and other macrophage activating factors (MAFs) (Krammer et al. 1985), and by endotoxin. The agent often referred to as MAF may turn out to be IFN_γ.

Activated macrophages have been shown to kill tumour cells. IFN_γ alone does not activate macrophages sufficiently to kill tumour cells; a second signal is necessary. Killing of tumour cells may be dependent on specific antibody, or independent of antibody.

Macrophages are activated during immunisation, particularly by organisms, such as *Listeria monocytogenes* and mycobacteria, which can survive within the macrophages. Peritoneal monocytes from mice immunised with soluble antigen proliferate in response to the same antigen, but may not be activated as a result (Forbes 1963).

Macrophages interact with T cells through special surface molecules, lymphocyte-function-associated-1 (LFA-1) and macrophage-1 (Mac-1). These molecules are also involved in spreading, phagocytosis of particles and killing of target cells. They share common segments with the C3b receptor.

Lymphoid Organs and Immunological Function

Primary lymphoid organs generate "virgin" cells with specific immunological potential. Secondary lymphoid organs are sites of generation of immune responses, i.e. activation, proliferation and differentiation of clones of lymphocytes with individual specificities.

Primary lymphoid organs are the yolk sac, the liver, the thymus and the bone marrow. All lymphoid cells originate in the yolk sac. The first recognisable T lymphocytes are found in the thymus. The first recognisable B cells are found in the fetal liver.

The lymphocytes generated in the primary lymphoid organs emerge in a virgin or resting state. The term "resting" is also applied to quiescent memory cells. Rearrangement of T cell receptor genes to encode a T cell receptor of unique specificity takes place in primitive T lymphocytes in the thymus, and the immunoglobulin genes of primitive B lymphocytes are rearranged in the liver of the early fetus and later in the bone marrow. The primary lymphoid organs are thus the site of the generation of immunological diversity.

Secondary lymphoid organs are the encapsulated organs (the lymph nodes and spleen) and unencapsulated lymphoid tissues associated with mucosae (pharynx, gut and respiratory tract, gut- or mucosa-associated lymphoid tissues). Secondary lymphoid tissue can be formed in granulomas and sites of chronic inflammation.

Vast numbers of lymphocytes, estimated to be of the order of 10^9 in humans, are produced daily. The majority of these are short lived. The half-life of most B cells is 24 h or less. Long-lived T and B cells live for a year or more (Ottesen 1954; Buckton et al. 1967). They are evidently the "memory" cells, ready to respond to activation by a stimulus corresponding to their immunological specificity.

Lymphocyte Circulation

Lymphocytes circulate from blood to lymph to blood (Gowans and Knight 1964; Perry et al. 1967). The majority of recirculating lymphocytes are long-lived T small lymphocytes. They pass from the blood through the white pulp of the spleen and back into the blood, and from the blood to the lymph node cortex via specialised post-capillary high-endothelial venules (Jalkanen and Butcher 1985) and thence through the efferent lymphatics to the blood. They can also go from the blood directly into the tissues, returning via the afferent lymphatics and thence through the efferent lymphatics to the blood. B lymphocytes recirculate to a far lesser extent than T lymphocytes and are shorter lived.

Studies of radiolabelled lymphocytes have demonstrated long- and short-lived recirculating pools. Intravascular and readily accessible extravascular pools are also described. The kinetics of B cell production in the marrow are also discussed in Chapter 11 (see p. 128).

Organisation of Immunological Function

The architecture of the lymphoid tissues allows the selection of lymphocytes with immunological specificity appropriate to the antigenic challenge and the proliferation of these cells to form clones. The formation of such clones is controlled with beautiful precision in health. The body must also be able to suppress an immunological response when it has answered the challenge, or if the response is inappropriate, for example when it would lead to autoimmunity.

Lymph nodes may be divided into different anatomical compartments (Fossum and Ford 1985), and the cells within these compartments may be classified according to functional and morphological criteria and current concepts of their ontogeny. Lymph nodes are composed of the cortex, which is a B cell area, the paracortex, containing T cells and a medulla. Most of the lymphocytes are in the cortex and paracortex. The superficial cortex contains follicle centre cells within primary and secondary follicles and perifollicular mantle zones rich in B lymphocytes with surface immunoglobulin of the IgD class. Primary follicles contain collections of lymphocytes which appear to be unstimulated. The majority of follicle centre cells in primary follicles are recirculating B cells (centrocytes) with cleaved or irregular, indented nuclei, varying in size up to twice that of a normal lymphocyte. They have surface immunoglobulin of both IgM and IgD classes, but the cytoplasm does not contain stainable immunoglobulin. Follicles are surrounded by a mantle of small lymphocytes which is broadest over the pole of the follicle centre closest to the lymph node capsule. Secondary follicles differ from primary follicles by possessing germinal centres containing activated and mitotic lymphocytes (centroblasts). They also contain DRCs, macrophages, a few T cells and NK cells. Germinal centres arise within lymphoid follicles a few days after immunisation, with the appearance of a focus of centroblasts shortly after antibody production commences, although their formation is dependent upon antigen. Centroblasts have non-cleaved nuclei with one to three nucleoli. They arise in large numbers from activated centrocytes after antigenic stimulation and soon enter mitosis, accumulating in the dark basal layer of the follicle. They have the morphology of activated B lymphocytes but have no surface membrane immunoglobulin, although one-third of them have cytoplasmic immunoglobulin. These events are followed by the appearance of cleaved cells which mostly accumulate beneath the mantle zone, producing a light upper zone in the follicle centre. Centroblasts are presumed to leave the germinal centres as large lymphoblasts (immunoblasts). The morphology of lymphoid follicles is discussed in greater detail in Chapter 17 (see p. 244).

The deep cortex contains recirculating small lymphocytes and immunoblasts within cortical sinuses. Many of the T cells of the paracortex are found in close apposition to the IDRCs which present antigen to them. Cords of lymphoid tissue, containing both T and B cells, extend into the medulla along strands of connective tissue. The medullary cords are separated from one another by large lymphatic sinuses. Most of the plasma cells in the node are in the medullary sinuses, as are most of the phagocytic cells.

There are two main types of tissue in the spleen, red and white pulp. The main function of the red pulp is to destroy effete erythrocytes. The white pulp contains the lymphoid tissue, which is mainly located in the periarteriolar sheath surrounding the central arteriole. T cells are found around the central arteriole, B cells are more peripheral and may be in primary or secondary follicles. The lymphoid tissue is surrounded by a mantle zone of recirculating B cells, APCs and macrophages.

It will become apparent that the control of immune responses is exceedingly complex. Much of the control results from interactions between T cells, B cells and ACs. These cellular interactions are guided, to a large extent, by molecules of the MHC. Antibody exerts an inhibitory feedback control, and complement molecules can either inhibit or facilitate an antibody response.

An understanding of these regulatory mechanisms is a prerequisite to finding ways to control the autonomous growth of malignant lymphocytes. While relatively little is known about the growth factors influencing proliferation and differentiation of the earliest cells in the lymphoid series, which proceeds in the absence of antigenic stimulation, a great deal has been learnt in recent years of the control of growth and differentiation of immunologically competent lymphocytes in immune responses. These mechanisms are the subject of subsequent chapters. Antigen-dependent B cell differentiation occurs in secondary lymphoid tissue, particularly in the lymph nodes. Lymphocytes enter nodes from the blood through high endothelial venules and migrate through the cortex. If a virgin or memory B cell of appropriate specificity meets antigen in the cortex, in association with an IDRC and a helper T cell, it may be activated to a short-lived plasma cell, which migrates to the medulla. On the basis of experiments in rats, MacLennan and Gray (1986) propose that memory B cells may be activated in the mantle zone of lymphoid follicles, with three possible outcomes: they may become centroblasts, long-lived plasma cells or memory cells. These cellular reactions are dealt with in greater detail in Chapter 11 (see p. 244).

References

Abo T, Cooper MD, Balch CM (1982) Characterization of HNK-1 + (Leu 7) human lymphocytes. I Two distinct phenotypes of human NK cells with different cytotoxic capacity. J Immunol 129: 1752–1757

Abo T, Miller CA, Gartland L, Balch CM (1983) Differentiation stages of human natural killer cells in lymphoid tissues from fetal to adult life. J Exp Med 157: 273–284

Abramson CS, Kersey JH, LeBien TW (1981) A monoclonal antibody (BA-1) reactive with cells of human B lymphocyte lineage. J Immunol 126: 83–88

Black RB, Leong AS-Y, Cowled PA, Forbes IJ (1980) Lymphocyte subpopulations in human lymph nodes. The normal range. Lymphology 13: 86–90

Buckton KE, Court Brown WM, Smith PG (1967) Lymphocyte survival in men treated with X-rays for ankylosing spondylitis. Nature 214: 470

Burns BF, Warnke RA, Doggett RS, Rouse RV (1983) Expression of a T-cell antigen (Leu-1) by B-cell lymphomas. Am J Pathol 113: 165–171

Burns GF, Begley GG, Mackay IR, Triglia T, Werkmeister JA (1985) 'Supernatural' killer cells. Immunol Today 6: 370–373

Cocchia D, Tiberio G, Santarelli R, Michetti F (1983) S100 protein in "follicular dendritic": cells of rat lymphoid organs. An immunochemical and immunocytochemical study. Cell Tissue Res 230: 95–103

Ferrarini M, Grossi CE (1984) Definition of the cell types within the "null lymphocyte" population of human peripheral blood: an analysis of phenotypes and functions. Semin Hematol 21: 270–286

Forbes IJ (1963) Mitosis in macrophages. Lancet II: 1203–1204

Forbes IJ, Zalewski PD (1976) A subpopulation of human B lymphocytes that rosette with mouse erythrocytes. Clin Exp Immunol 26: 99–107

Forbes IJ, Zalewski PD, Valente L, Gee D (1982) Two maturation-associated mouse erythrocyte receptors of human B cells. I. Identification of four human B cell subsets. Clin Exp Immunol 47: 396–404

Fossum S, Ford WL (1985) The organization of cell populations within lymph nodes: their origin, life history and functional relationships. Histopathology 9: 469–499

Gowans JL, Knight EJ (1964) The route of recirculation of lymphocytes in the rat. Proc R Soc Lond [Biol] 159: 257–282

Greil R, Gattringer C, Knapp W, Huber H (1986) Growth fraction of tumour cells and infiltration density with natural killer-like (HNK$^+$) cells in non-Hodgkin lymphomas. Br J Haematol 62: 293–300

Grossi CE, Webb SR, Zicca et al. (1978) Morphological and histochemical analyses of two human T-cell subpopulations bearing receptors for IgM or IgG. J Exp Med 147: 1405–1417

Hsu S-M, Yang K, Jaffe ES (1985) Phenotypic expression of Hodgkin's and Reed-Sternberg cells in Hodgkin's disease. Am J Pathol 118: 209–217

Isaacson P (1979) Immunochemical demonstration of J chain: a marker of B-cell malignancy. J Clin Pathol 32: 802–807

Isaacson P, Jones DB, Millward-Sadler GH, Judd MA, Payne S (1981) Alpha-1-antitrypsin in human macrophages. J Clin Pathol 34: 982–990

Jalkanen SP, Butcher EC (1985) In vitro analysis of the homing properties of human lymphocytes: developmental regulation of functional receptors for high endothelial venules. Blood 66: 577–582

Janossy G, Prentice HG (1982) T cell subpopulations, monoclonal antibodies and their therapeutic applications. Clin Haematol 11: 631–660

Krammer PH, Gemsa D, Hamann U, Kaltmann B, Kubelka C, Müller W (1985) Heterogeneity of macrophage-activating factors (MAFs) and their effects in vivo. In: Ford RJ, Maizel AL (eds) mediators in cell growth and differentiation. Raven, New York, pp 193–197

MacLennan ICM, Gray D (1986) Antigen-driven selection of virgin and memory B cells. Immunol Rev 91: 61–85

Mason DY, Taylor CR (1975) The distribution of muramidase (lysozyme) in human tissues. J Clin Pathol 28: 124–132

Matutes E, Parreira A, Foa R, Catovsky D (1985) Monoclonal antibody OKT17 recognises most cases of T-cell malignancy. Br J Haematol 61: 649–656

Nadler LM, Stashenko P, Hardy R et al. (1981) Characterisation of a human B-cell specific antigen (B2) distinct from B1. J Immunol 126: 1941–1947

Naiem M, Gerdes J, Abdulaziz Z, Stein H, Mason DY (1983) Production of a monoclonal antibody reactive with human dendritic reticulum cells and its use in the immunohistological analysis of lymphoid tissue. J Clin Pathol 36: 167–175

Ottesen J (1954) On the age of human white cells in peripheral blood Acta Physiol Scand 32: 75–93

Owen MJ, Barber BH, Faulkes RA, Crumpton MJ (1978) Albumin is associated with the inner surface of the lymphocyte plasma membrane. Biochem Soc Trans 6: 920–922

Papadimitriou CS, Stein H, Lennert K (1978) The complexity of immunohistochemical staining pattern of Hodgkin and Sternberg-Reed cells — demonstration of immunoglobulin albumin α-1 antichymotrypsin and lysozyme. Int J Cancer 21: 531–541

Perry S, Irvin GL III, Whang J (1967) Studies of lymphocyte kinetics in man. Blood 29: 22–28

Pinkus GS, Thomas P, Said JW (1985) Leu-M1 — a marker for Reed-Sternberg cells in Hodgkin's disease. An immunoperoxidase study of paraffin-embedded tissues. Am J Pathol 119: 244–252

Pistoia V, Cozzolino F, Ferrarini M (1985) More about NK cells and regulation of B cell activity. Immunol Today 6: 287

Radzun HJ, Parwaresch MR, Feller AC, Hansmann M-L (1984) Monocyte/macrophage-specific monoclonal antibody Ki-M1 recognizes interdigitating reticulum cells. Am J Pathol 117: 441–450

Reinherz EL, Haynes BF, Nadler LM, Bernstein ID (eds) (1986) Leucocyte typing II, vols 1, 2 and 3. Proceedings of the second international workshop and conference on human lymphocyte differentiation antigens. Springer, Berlin Heidelberg New York

Robertson M (1985) T cell receptor. The present state of recognition. Nature 317: 768–771

Rosenberg S (1985) Lymphokine-activated killer cells: a new approach to immunotherapy of cancer. J Natl Cancer Inst 75: 595–603

Schroff RW, Foon KA, Billing RJ, Fahey JL (1982) Immunologic classification of lymphocytic leukemias based on monoclonal antibody-defined cell surface antigens. Blood 59: 207–215

Sidman CL (1981) Lymphocyte surface receptors and albumin. J Immunol 127: 1454–1458

Stashenko P, Nadler LM, Hardy R, Schlossman SF (1980) Characterisation of a human B lymphocyte-specific antigen. J Immunol 125: 1678–1685

Stathopoulos G, Elliott EV (1974) Formation of mouse or sheep red blood cell rosettes by lymphocytes from normal and leukaemic individuals. Lancet I: 600–601

Takahashi K, Yamaguchi H, Ishizeki J, Nakajima T, Nakazato Y (1981) Immunohistochemical and immunoelectron microscopic localisation of S-100 protein in the interdigitating reticulum cells of the human lymph node. Virchows Arch (Cell Pathol) 37: 125–135

Woda BA, Fenaglio CM, Nette EG, King DW (1977) The lack of specificity of the sheep erythrocyte-T lymphocyte rosetting phenomenon. Am J Pathol 88: 69–80

Wood GS, Warner NL, Warnke RA (1983) Anti-Leu-3/T4 antibodies react with cells of monocyte/macrophage and Langerhans lineage. J Immunol 131: 212–216

Wood GS, Turner RR, Shiurba RA et al. (1985) Human dendritic cells and macrophages. In situ immunophenotype definition of subsets that exhibit specific morphologic and micro-environmental characteristics. Am J Pathol 119: 73–82

9 The Major Histocompatibility Complex

Introduction

The basis of all immunological activity is interaction between members of different populations which constitute the lymphoid system. When one cell touches another, it responds according to its own state and its interpretation of the identity and state of the other. The existence of the major histocompatibility complex (MHC) was revealed when the difficulty of transplanting tissues between genetically different individuals was explored. It was natural to conclude that the primary function of the system was to enable the body to recognise foreign cells and to keep them out. Thoughts then turned towards the recognition of different cells arising within the body. There are two needs: to preserve normal cells, and to destroy aberrant, potentially dangerous cells. When cells are infected by a virus they can be destroyed, together with the virus, by cytotoxic T cells only if the T cells and the target cells express the same MHC class I product on their surface membranes. Whether immunological surveillance is effective against potentially malignant mutants is still not clear. The MHC is essential for recognition of one cell of the immune system by another, for recognition of genetically foreign cells and for regulation of immunological activity.

All vertebrates possess one MHC, containing three major classes of histocompatibility genes. In addition, there are many minor histocompatibility systems. The MHC in man was originally called the human leucocyte A (HLA) system. The genes of the MHC system are clustered together in a very small segment of the short arm of the sixth human chromosome (Fig. 9.1).

The genes and their protein products are as follows:

Class I: A, B and C loci, coding for A, B and C class I MHC proteins,

Class II: D region genes comprising DP (formerly SB), DQ (formerly DC and MB) and DR loci, encoding DP, DQ and DR proteins, respectively. Products of these genes are often referred to in the literature as Ia, HLA-D or HLA-DR antigens.

Class III: Genes coding for the complement system proteins C2, Factor B (Bf), C4a and C4b.

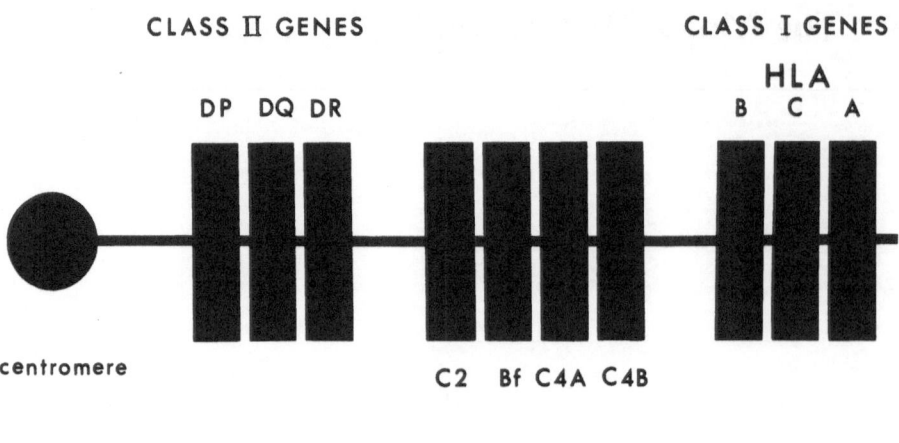

Fig. 9.1. Arrangement of MHC genes on chromosome 6.

The genes for the complement system seem to be placed among the MHC by chance. They are not on the same chromosome as the MHC in some species and apparently have no functional connection or structural relationship. However, components of the complement system not known to be coded on chromosome 6 do influence B cell activation.

An individual distinguishes his own tissues from tissues of another individual ("foreign or non-self" tissues) through immunological processes, which depend on the recognition of differences between the MHC on his own and foreign cells. As well as its role in distinguishing self from non-self, the MHC has a major influence on immunological responsiveness to antigens through the requirement for MHC matching in cell–cell interactions. In one form of congenital severe combined immunodeficiency (SCID) in man, which is generally lethal, MHC class II antigens are not expressed on peripheral blood lymphocytes, so that they cannot collaborate with T cells or antigen-presenting cells (APCs) to generate immune responses (de Préval et al. 1985).

The basis for the individuality of the tissues of members of mammalian species is the mode of inheritance of MHC genes and the variability (polymorphism) of the individual genes of the MHC complex. An outbred population has many alternative genes (alleles) at each locus of the MHC. The result of this is that the products of each MHC gene locus may differ greatly from individual to individual. MHC genes inherited from one parent constitute an MHC haplotype (from Greek *haplous*, single + *typos*, impression, model). Each individual inherits a haplotype from each parent. Each haplotype carries one gene for each MHC locus. The MHC genes are inherited as codominants, so that an individual will express a pair of allelic variants for each locus, one transmitted from the mother and one from the father. These factors ensure that histocompatibility is only complete between identical twins.

Tissue Distribution of MHC Products

Although all nucleated cells have been thought to express class I antigens, studies with monoclonal antibodies show little or no class I antigens on a number of tissues, including myocardial and skeletal muscle. However, it seems that class I antigens can be expressed on dystrophic skeletal muscle and on the transplanted heart. A transplanted tissue cannot be rejected if it does not express MHC antigens. One solution to homograft rejection would be to stop the grafted organ from expressing its MHC genes. Similarly, autoimmune activity can only occur against cells which express MHC antigens.

MHC class II antigens are on the surface of B lymphocytes, on activated T lymphocytes and on antigen-presenting macrophages of all kinds, some vascular epithelia and sperm, to name the most important. The paucity of class II-bearing cells within the central nervous system may be an important factor in its freedom from immunological activity. Different genes of the MHC class II complex are expressed at different stages of development. Class II MHC products are found on progenitor cells of the erythroid and granulocyte series, but not on their stem cells, and are lost before the cells reach functional maturity. They may also be expressed at particular stages of the cell cycle and may be induced in a number of tissues in which they are not expressed on resting cells. Comparison of the expression of class II MHC antigens in acute lymphoblastic leukaemia (ALL) and chronic lymphocytic leukaemia (CLL), peripheral B cells and TPA-treated CLL, suggests a distinct sequence of expression of the MHC genes encoding class II products, namely, DP (SB) followed by DR and DC (DQ). This postulated sequence follows the order of the genes on chromosome 6. The most undifferentiated type of ALL invariably lacks sIg, but expresses MHC class II. This places these cells very early in the differentiation sequence, MHC class II being expressed before sIg.

MHC Gene Products and Their Specificities

Class I MHC glycoproteins can make up as much as 1% of the plasma membrane protein (about 5×10^5 molecules/cell). Their structure is illustrated in Fig. 9.2. β_2-microglobulin does not form part of the antigenic site of class I molecules, but is somehow necessary for these molecules to be expressed. In congenital absence of β_2-microglobulin, the class I antigenic determinants are not expressed.

The genes that code for these glycoproteins are the most polymporphic known. There may be more than 50 alleles at the same locus, and there may be a 25% difference in the amino acid composition of the products. Polymorphism is largely due to variability in certain sites in the first two domains. The mechanism of generation of polymorphism is unknown. One possibility is a process called gene conversion, which is exchange of nucleotides from one gene to another. Another possible process is point mutation.

The class II (HLA-D) region encodes two gene products: glycopeptides of 33 kD (α) and 28 kD (β), which combine to form a two-chain molecule. The α

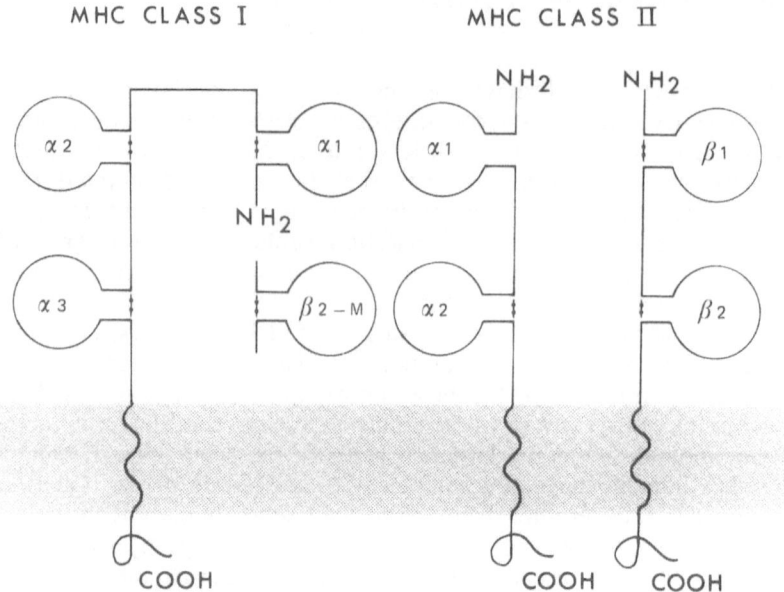

Fig. 9.2. Structures of the MHC gene products. Class I glycoproteins (45 kD) have a short internal segment, a hydrophobic transmembrane segment and three extracellular domains (α_1, α_2 and α_3). Each polypeptide contains two intra-chain disulphide loops (only one is illustrated) similar to the disulphide loops in each domain of Ig chains. Non-covalently associated β_2-microglobulin (β_2-M) constitutes the fourth domain. Class II glycoproteins consist of two chains, α (33 kD) and β (28 kD), with intracellular, transmembrane and extracellular segments. The extracellular segments are folded into two domains (α_1, α_2; β_1, β_2). The α_1 domain lacks stabilising disulphide bridges.

chain of HLA-DR is invariable and the β chain is polymorphic, whereas in DQ both the α and β chains are known to be variable.

A number of surface molecules show a clear relationship to immunoglobulin. They all seem to have a function related to recognition of cell surfaces. Members of this immunoglobulin superfamily include MHC class I and II products, the T cell receptor and CD4 and CD8 molecules (Williams 1985). Certain domains of these molecules are very similar in structure to the constant domains of Ig.

The HLA-A, -B, and -C gene products (often referred to as "antigen") can be recognised by serological techniques. The HLA-D antigens were first recognised in the mixed lymphocyte reaction (MLR) and the specificities so recognised are designated Dw. Many MHC class II products can now be recognised serologically, in which case they are called HLA-DR (as a group), or HLA-DP, -DQ and -DR, although the serological definition of DP antigens is difficult. The relationship between HLA-D recognised by cellular techniques and DR and DQ recognised serologically is complex. It is likely that the MLR results from recognition of a combination of DR, DQ and perhaps DP molecules.

Since class I and class II molecules carry several variable parts, many different antigenic determinants may be expressed on each MHC molecule, some being recognised by B cells, others mainly by T cells. Antisera recognise "private" and "public" specificities. A public specificity is shared by a number of distinct MHC products. A private specificity belongs to only one particular MHC antigen.

Immunoregulatory Function of the MHC

MHC products serve as recognition signals between cells of the immune system, facilitating interactions between cells collaborating in immune responses. To a large extent, cells of the immune system only "see", or interact with, antigen when it is intimately associated with molecules of the MHC. Only accessory cells (ACs) expressing the same class II MHC product as the T cells can present antigen to T cells. Class II molecules apparently guide the appropriate sub-population of T cells to the antigens held on the surface of ACs or B cells. Each class of MHC molecules associates with specific classes of antigen; e.g. viral antigens associate only with class I MHC glycoproteins. Also, some classes of lymphocyte interact with class I-associated antigens, others with class II-associated molecules.

Helper T cells (CD4+) are stimulated by antigen-presenting cells (APCs) that bear antigen in association with class II MHC product. A stable trimolecular complex of antigen, MHC product and T cell receptor must be formed for effective T cell triggering. Similarly, helper T cells activate B cells through an antigen-MHC class II bridge. In the activation of macrophages, T cells triggered by APCs through an antigen-MHC class II bridge release macrophage activating factor (MAF) and other lymphokines which bind to receptors on the macrophages.

Cytotoxic T cells (CD8+) interact with cell-associated viral antigens if the T cell and the target cell share class I MHC antigens. Killing of a target cell by a cytotoxic T lymphocyte will be blocked by antibody to the specific class I MHC molecules on the target cells. Killing will also be blocked by antibodies to the CD3 or CD8 antigens on the cytotoxic T cell, because these are associated with the T cell receptor. Interaction of suppressor T cells with other immune cells is largely restricted to cells which bear class I MHC product.

MHC matching between helper T cell and B cell is required for the first step in activation of the B cell, but after the B cell has begun the activation process, T cells expressing non-matching MHC molecules can support progression to later stages of activation by delivering appropriate lymphokines.

Whether interactions involving T cells result in an immunogenic or tolerogenic outcome depends on the circumstances of this T-B-antigen-MHC interaction. There has been intense debate about the nature of the interaction of class II MHC product and antigen. Among the outcomes which can be envisaged are:

1. Helper T cells recognise an association of class II MHC product with antigen, possibly a complex of the two. This interaction sets in train a sequence of events leading to an immune response.

2. Cytotoxic T cells may recognise a specific antigen in association with class II MHC product on the lymphocyte surface. This leads to deletion of the clone of lymphocytes (clonal deletion), a mechanism for inducing tolerance.

3. Cells from persons who do not respond to a particular antigen, i.e. are tolerant of the antigen, may be unable to form an immunogenic complex of MHC product and antigen.

4. A complex may be formed, but is not recognised by helper T cells, because they have matured in an environment causing them to be tolerant to such complexes.

5. Helper T cells capable of recognising the complex of MHC product and antigen may be lacking from the T cell repertoire.

Expression of class I and class II MHC products by T cells is determined by the thymus in which they mature. If murine T cells of one genotype are allowed to mature in a thymus of another genotype, they express only MHC products of the host genotype. Such T cells then recognise only these MHC antigens as self. The mechanism of this process is unknown.

Mixed Lymphocyte Reaction

Lymphocytes from subjects identical at the MHC class I locus but differing at the class II locus stimulate each other to divide. In this reaction the class II MHC product on B cells and macrophages stimulates genetically different T cells which lack a class II antigen expressed by the stimulator cells. If the responder cells also differ at the class I locus, cytotoxic responder T cells will be induced in this reaction, which, in turn, react against the stimulator cells through the class I MHC product (Fig. 9.3). The killing of target cells by these cytotoxic cells is called cell-mediated lympholysis (CML). Two potent humoral mediators, the lymphokines

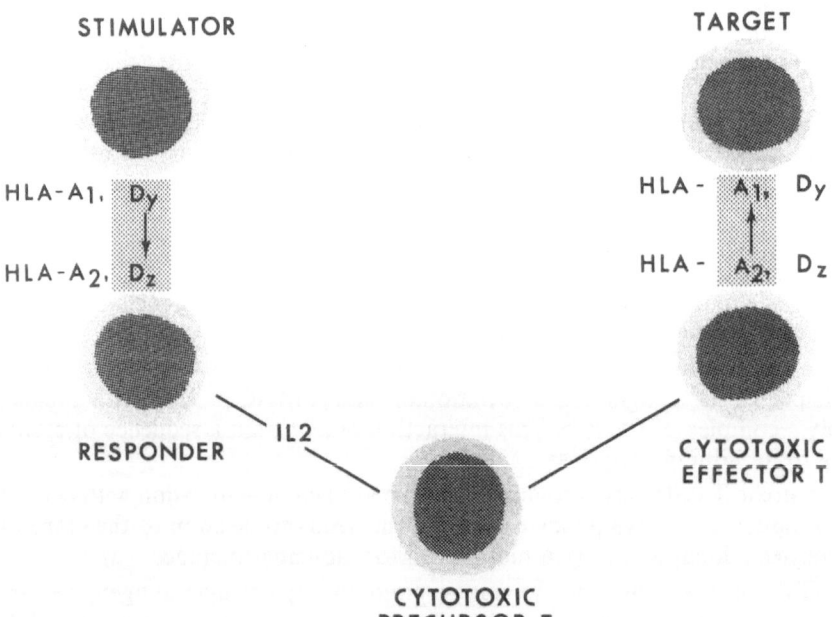

Fig. 9.3. Cell responses in the one-way MLR. The stimulator cells of HLA phenotype A_1, D_y are treated to prevent them responding. T helper cells of the responder population of phenotype A_2, D_z, stimulated by the difference at the D locus, multiply and release lymphokines. Cytolytic cells are activated and react against the MHC class I product ($HLA\text{-}A_1$) of the stimulator cells.

IFN$_\gamma$ and interleukin 2 (IL-2), are produced by activated T cells in this reaction. These two lymphokines have potent effects on the function of lymphocytes.

A one-way MLR is carried out by preventing the lymphocytes from one subject (the stimulator cells) from dividing (by treatment with an antimitotic drug or X-rays), allowing only the lymphocytes from the second subject to respond. The lymphocytes respond if they lack a class II MHC product expressed by the stimulator lymphocytes. The mechanism whereby an MHC class II product on a cell stimulates a T cell of a different MHC class II constitution to react against the MHC class I product of the stimulator cell is not clear. The receptor on the responding T cell may be the T cell receptor for antigen in association with its own MHC class I or II complex. It may recognise the class I product on the stimulating cell in association with a foreign class II molecule.

Graft Versus Host Reaction

If a graft of immunologically competent foreign lymphoid cells is not rejected by the host, either because the host is immunologically incompetent, or because the engrafted lymphoid cells are not recognised as foreign, the graft will mount an immune response against the host. If the graft has all the MHC antigens expressed by the cells of the host, it will not be recognised as foreign. If the host expresses additional class II specificities, the graft will see these as foreign, and will be induced to proliferate and to mount a cytotoxic reaction. The graft versus host reaction (GVHR) is frequently seen after transplantation of bone marrow when the tissue matching is not perfect — the situation in virtually all cases except when marrow is exchanged between identical twins. The response causes symptoms and signs according to the target: anaemia (erythrocytes or marrow stem cells), rash (epidermis), and diarrhoea (gut). There are also manifestations with complex pathogenesis, such as fever, wasting and splenomegaly. Graft versus host reactions in young experimental animals cause runting.

Association of Diseases with MHC Phenotype

There is a remarkable association of MHC specificities with susceptibility or resistance to a variety of diseases. As to the mechanism underlying this association, not much is known. It may be related to the mechanism which controls HLA expression: poor expression of MHC products could lead to poor collaboration in immune responses.

HLA-DR2 is associated with low IFN$_\alpha$ and IFN$_\beta$ responses (Abb et al. 1983). Interferon is involved in the control of expression of both classes of genes. IFN$_\gamma$ increases the expression of class II MHC product on monocytes and macrophages, B lymphocytes and myeloid cell lines. Anomalous expression of MHC products may also result from the action of adenovirus oncogenes. Anomalous expression of MHC antigens has been proposed as a mechanism leading to autoimmunity. The thyroid cells in glands affected by Hashimoto's disease express class II antigens, whereas normal thyroid epithelium does not (Hanafusa et al. 1983). Immunodeficiency associated with absence or incomplete expression of class I or II products on B cells, monocytes and other APCs has been described. It is interesting that few cancers have an association with the MHC phenotype. A relationship of HLA cw5 to multiple myeloma has been proposed.

Conclusions

The MHC genes on chromosome 6 encode two families of proteins which are essential for cellular interactions in the lymphoid system. All immune responses require complex interactions of lymphocytes and APCs. The basis of these interactions is contact through these MHC molecules. Most antigens will only activate immunologically competent cells if combined in an unknown way with the appropriate MHC product on the surface of a lymphocyte or APC. In addition to this requirement, the cell receiving the stimulus must express matching MHC molecules.

This intricate system is fundamental to the control of immune responses. It is the basis for lack of immunological reactivity against the non-immunological tissues of the host, and also the basis for recognition of foreign or non-self molecules, of an inanimate, microbial or homograft nature. Any theory of immunological surveillance of mutant and neoplastic cells must take the MHC into account. As monoclonal antibodies become available, a knowledge of the distribution of MHC products among different lymphoid cells and their expression during ontogeny is finding increasing practical application in determining the phenotypes of lymphoid neoplasms.

For reviews of the MHC see Accolla et al. (1984), Bach (1985), Bodmer (1984), Giles and Capra (1985) and Rose (1985).

References

Abb J, Zander H, Abb H, Albert E, Deinhardt F (1983) Association of human leucocyte low responsiveness to inducers of interferon α with HLA-DR 2. Immunology 49: 239–244

Accolla RS, Moretta A, Carrel S (1984) The human Ia system: an overview. Semin Hematol 21: 287–295

Bach FH (1985) The HLA class II genes and products: the HLA-D region. Immunol Today 6: 88–94

Bodmer J, Bodmer W (1984) Histocompatibility 1984. Immunol Today 5: 252–254

de Préval C, Liskowska-Grospierre B, Loche M, Griscelli C, Mach B (1985) A trans-acting class II regulatory gene unlinked to the MHC controls expression of HLA class II genes. Nature 318: 291–293

Giles RC, Capra JD (1985) Structure, function and genetics of human class II molecules. Adv Immunol 37: 1–71

Hanafusa T, Pujol-Borrell R, Chiovato L, Russell RCG, Doniach D, Botazzo GF (1983) Aberrant expression of HLA-DR antigen on thyrocytes in Graves' disease: relevance for autoimmunity. Lancet II: 1111–1115

Rose ML (1985) Immunoregulation of MHC antigen expression. Immunol Today 6: 297–298

Williams AF (1985) Immunoglobulin-related domains for cell surface recognition. Nature 314: 579–580

10 T Cell Differentiation

Introduction

All lymphocytes are derived from an unidentified multipotent precursor (Fig. 10.1). T cell precursors migrate from the liver and bone marrow in fetal life and from the bone marrow in adult life, to the thymus. It is unknown whether the stem cells become committed to T cell differentiation before or after they have entered the thymus.

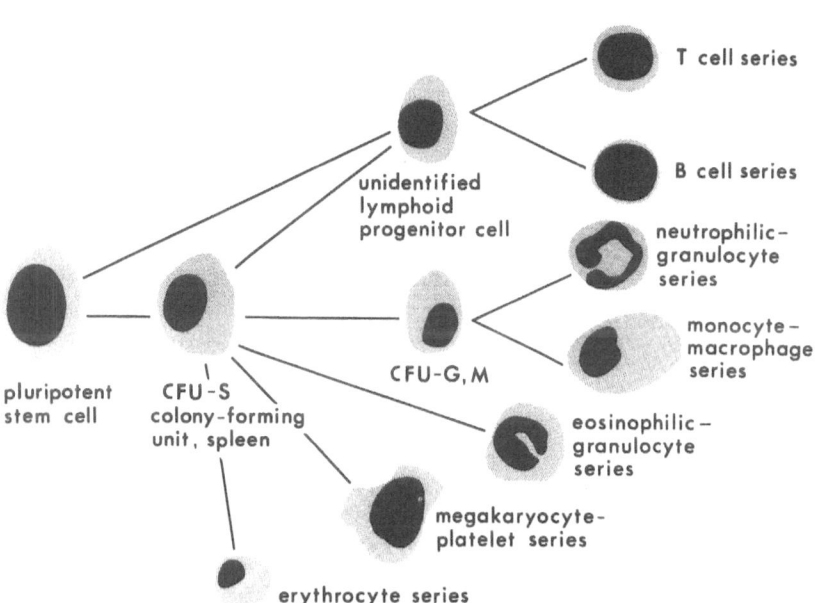

Fig. 10.1. Origin and differentiation of haematopoietic cells. Lymphocytes are derived originally from an unidentified precursor that has the potential to differentiate into haematopoietic cells of the erythrocyte, polymporphonuclear leucocyte, megakaryocyte or monocyte series. After birth the stem cells for T and B lymphocytes are restricted to lymphoid differentiation.

The Thymus

The thymus develops by fusion of elements from the third pharyngeal pouch (ectoderm) and cleft (endoderm). The epithelial anlage of the thymus appears on day 40 of fetal life and lymphocytes appear in perithymic mesenchyme at 50 days (Lobach et al. 1985). Haematopoiesis begins in the liver at about day 45 and lymphocytes appear in the thymus at day 70 (Table 10.1). The thymus has three anatomical and functional regions, the peripheral subcapsular region, the cortex and the medulla. Ectodermal epithelial cells are found mainly in the cortex, and endodermally derived cells in the medulla. Both express MHC class I and II antigens, the medullary epithelial cells strongly expressing class II antigens. Connective tissue is derived from the mesoderm.

Table 10.1. Timetable of T and B cell development in utero (Stutman and Calkins 1977)

Site	Time (days)
Yolk sac haematopoiesis	21–28
Epithelial thymus anlage	40
Liver haematopoiesis	42
Lymphocytes in the thymus	70
B lymphocytes in liver	65–68
Lymphocytes in lymph nodes	70–130
Spleen haematopoiesis	90–100
B lymphocytes in bone marrow	105
Thymus medulla distinct from cortex	105–110
Hassal's corpuscles in thymus	105–110
Lymphocytes in Peyer's patches	120 (?)
Lymphocytes in blood	120–130
B lymphocytes in spleen	140
Marrow haematopoiesis	140

The peripheral subcapsular region of the thymus contains large blast cells which derive from the bone marrow. Gangliosides in the subcapsular epithelial cells (probably antigen-binding cells) bind tetanus toxin and are recognised by a monoclonal antibody designated A2B5. These cells also contain thymosins and thymopoietin (Table 10.2).

The cortex contains the non-dividing small cortical thymocytes, which are probably generated from cells in the subcapsular region and mostly die within the cortex. It also contains MHC class II-expressing thymic "nurse" cells, which seem to have a role in the differentiation of thymocytes. These nurse cells contain large numbers of lymphocytes. Whether the lymphocytes are actually within the cytoplasm, or have invaginated the surface membrane of the nurse cells is not clear. The T lymphocytes within the nurse cells may represent a distinct population, being unresponsive to activation stimuli by the plant mitogen concanavalin A (con A). One speculation is that the lymphocyte population within the nurse cells may be spared destruction within the thymus and be allowed to pass on to the medulla.

Table 10.2. Some well-defined thymus factors

Factor	Size (kD)	Amino acid sequence	Function
Thymosin$_{\alpha 1}$	3.1	Known	Modulates TdT, increases MIF production, influences corticosteroid levels by a CNS action
Thymosin$_{\alpha 7}$	2.5	Unknown	Increases suppressor T cell count
Thymosin$_{\beta 4}$	4.9	Known	Induces TdT in mouse marrow cells
Thymosin fraction 5	10–15	Unknown	Induces T cell differentiation and immunocompetence in man
Thymic humoral factor (THF)	3.2	Known	Increases splenic lymphocyte responses to con A and PHA
Thymopoietin	5.6	Known	Induces myasthenia, induces T cells to mature in the thymus
Facteur Thymique Sérique (thymulin)	0.8	Known	Increases count of cytotoxic T cells in vitro and in vivo

The medulla contains T cells, marrow-derived dendritic cells and macrophages, both expressing MHC class II antigens, and Hassal's corpuscles, whose origin and function are unknown. The latter contain keratin and thymosin$_{\alpha 7}$ (Tridente 1985), and are probably involved in the pathogenesis of myasthenia gravis, as they bind α-bungarotoxin and express acetylcholine receptors. Neuroendocrine cells with properties of amine precursor uptake and decarboxylation (APUD) also occur predominantly in the medulla. Their function is unknown. Thymocytes leave the thymus from the medulla. The development of the thymus and the ontogeny of thymocytes are well discussed by Ceredig et al. (1984) and Haynes (1984).

A number of hormone-like substances have been purified from the thymus (Table 10.2), e.g. thymopoietin and Facteur Thymique Sérique (now known as thymulin); others like ubiquitin (ubiquitous immunopoietic polypeptide) are less well characterised. They can all induce maturational changes in thymocytes. Thymosin fraction 5, so named because there are five purification steps, contains more than a dozen active peptides. Thymosin$_{\alpha 1}$ is reported to increase the frequency of cells capable of producing interleukin 2 (IL-2; predominantly CD4 + helper T cells). Thymopoietin increases T cell proliferative responses in vitro at optimal concentrations and suppresses at suboptimal concentrations. The precise actions of these hormones within the thymus are not known. Many of the thymic polypeptides are found in the brain, where they are thought to be biologically active.

Cells are thought to enter the subcapsular area of the thymus, where they proliferate and differentiate. Subcortical early blast cells, termed prothymocytes (Stage I, Table 10.3), comprising less than 5% of thymocytes, are the precursors of both cortical and medullary thymocytes. The CD2 antigen, on the same molecule as the sheep erythrocyte (E) receptor, is the earliest recognised marker of thymocyte ontogeny. However, early fetal thymocytes do not form E rosettes, probably because the molecule is not complete at this stage. Terminal deoxynucleotidyl transferase (TdT), a DNA polymerase present in some precursors of B and T cells, is present in subcapsular and cortical thymocytes. Prothymocytes also express CD7 and T10 (a marker of activated and/or immature lymphocytes).

Table 10.3. T cell differentiation

Stage		Site	Phenotype
I	(Early, prothymocyte)	Subcapsular	CD2+, transferrin receptor+, T10+, (CD5+), CD7+, TdT+
II	(Common)	Cortex	CD1+, CD2+, CD4+, CD5+, CD7+, CD8+, transferrin receptor+, T10+, TdT+, PNA+
III	(Mature)	Medulla	CD2+, CD3+, CD4+, CD5+, CD8+, T10
IV	(Peripheral) (Helper)	Blood	CD2+, CD3+, CD4+, CD5+, MHC class I+
IV	(Peripheral) (Suppressor)	Blood	CD2+, CD3+, CD5+, CD8+, MHC class I+

Prothymocytes migrate to the cortex, where CD1 is expressed on 80% of thymocytes but is absent from circulating T cells. The pathway from cortex to medulla is not known. The genes of β and α chains of the T cell receptor are rearranged at this stage. Peanut agglutinin (PNA) binds to a 110 Kd glycoprotein on cortical thymocytes, but not medullary thymocytes or blood T cells.

Cortical thymocytes are not functional and most of them probably die, although necrotic cells are not seen. The death and disappearance of thymic cells could be due to the process of apoptosis characterised by condensation and fragmentation of nuclei, caused by endonucleases, and phagocytosis (Duvall and Wyllie 1986). Apoptotic bodies are commonly observed in involuting thymuses in young infants and neonates subject to various stresses, and can be induced experimentally by adrenocorticotrophic hormone (ACTH) and other steroids (Wyllie et al. 1984).

Final maturation takes place in the medulla, where the lineages divide into helper/inducer and suppressor/cytotoxic. CD3 is expressed in the medulla and is present on 90% of circulating T cells. The 37 kD T10 antigen and the transferrin receptor are also expressed on a proportion of thymocytes. Cells recently migrated from the thymus resemble medullary thymocytes in phenotype and function.

Unidentified cells in the thymus are responsible in some way for determining the MHC-restricted recognition repertoire of T cells. The cells which determine MHC restriction are known to come from the bone marrow. They are sensitive to ionising radiation.

All thymocytes (except possibly the prothymocytes) express CD5, although in different amounts. CD4 and CD8 antigens are expressed on more than 85% of thymocytes. Ninety-five per cent of thymocytes are CD2+, medullary cells staining only weakly and subcapsular cells staining strongly. All thymocytes express MHC class I products, the medullary thymocytes most strongly. Thymocytes do not express class II antigens. Only stage III thymocytes (see Table 10.3) are responsive to antigen, since the genes of the T cell receptor are rearranged in stage II, and the rearranged gene is expressed as the receptor at stage III.

Lobach et al. (1985) studied the appearance of antigens on thymic cells from 50 days of gestation to birth. The CD7 antigen was already present on lymphocytes in perithymic mesenchyme at 50 days, before lymphocytes were found in the thymus. T cell antigens are acquired sequentially, CD4, CD5 and CD8 being found in thymic tissue by 70 days and CD1, CD2 and CD3 by 100 days of gestation.

T Lymphocytes in Bone Marrow

T lymphocyte populations in bone marrow appear to consist of two groups; (1) the T lymphocyte precursors, and (2) those having the phenotype of peripheral T cells. The putative precursor T cells react with T10 monoclonal antibody, which also reacts with early haematopoietic stem cells and cells derived from them. No transitional forms are detectable. The situation is, however, not quite clear; after bone marrow transplantation, T cells appear to be reconstituted from cells having a mature phenotype.

T Cells in Lymph Nodes

T cells are located in the paracortical or interfollicular regions of lymph nodes and in the lymphoid tissues of the intestine and tonsil, in a ratio of CD4+ (helper) to CD8+ (suppressor) of approximately 2:1, similar to that in blood. B cells are found mainly in follicular areas and medullary cords. T cells occur primarily in the periarteriolar region of the Malpighian corpuscles of the spleen.

T cells make up 5%–15% of the lymphocyte population of germinal centres. Some CD4+ helper/inducer T cells are found amongst the sIgM+ B cells in primary follicles and immediately beneath the mantle zone in germinal centres. Helper T cells are involved in the generation of secondary follicles. Their presence in germinal centres may indicate a role in B cell proliferation. The topographical arrangements within tonsils are similar, with paracortical T helper/inducer cell areas and well-defined germinal centres containing B cells.

Interdigitating reticular cells (IDRCs) are MHC class II positive CD1+ cells found in the paracortex surrounded by a corona of CD4+ helper T lymphocytes. Their origin is unclear. Their function is believed to be the presentation of antigen. A CD8+ T cell population surrounds these aggregates of IDRCs and CD4+ helper T cells.

T Cell Subsets

T cell subsets may be defined by functional capacities or by phenotype. The functions of T cells subsets include:

1. Helper activity, inducing B cell proliferation, differentiation and synthesis of antibodies to thymus-dependent antigens.

2. Helper/inducer activity affecting other T cells via the release of IL-2 through direct contact or through soluble factors that function polyclonally, inducing T or B cell proliferation and/or differentiation. The main producers of IL-2 are CD4+ cells. T cells, including CD8+ suppressor cells, must have IL-2 to proliferate; if they cannot make it for themselves, they must be provided with it. CD4+ helper T

cells expressing MHC class II product are needed for the induction of CD8 + cells capable of suppressing synthesis of antibody in vitro.

3. Activation of macrophages by release of lymphokines. This is an essential component of delayed type hypersensitivity (DTH) reactions, which are involved in immune responses to many infections and in homograft and autoimmune reactions. In DTH reactions, antigen must be presented by macrophages to T cells in association with MHC class II product. The T cells so activated release lymphokines which induce inflammatory reactions and attract and activate macrophages.

4. Regulation of the growth of haematopoietic cells by production of the granulocyte and macrophage colony-stimulating factor multi-CSF.

5. Lysis of foreign or "non-self" (allogeneic) cells or modified "self" cells. Cytotoxic T cells (T_c) may destroy grafted allogeneic cells, tumour cells and cells infected by viruses, thereby terminating viral infections.

6. Suppressor activity inhibiting the induction (activation) of both T and B lymphocytes. Two functionally distinct T cell subsets (T_μ and T_γ), defined by the possession of receptors either for the Fc portion of IgM or of IgG respectively, are of historical interest. The T_μ subset was found to promote polyclonal B cell activation and IgG synthesis in response to pokeweed mitogen (PWM) in vitro, whereas T_γ cells suppressed in this system. However, the correlation between Fc receptor expression and function is not rigorous, and these markers are now superseded by antigens recognised by monoclonal antibodies. T cells express Fc receptors when they are activated. The T_γ subset includes most of the NK cells.

T Cell Subsets Defined by Monoclonal Antibodies

Virtually all T cells express the CD3 surface molecule. Mature T cells express either CD4 or CD8, occasionally both (Blue et al. 1985). In general, CD4 + cells have helper/inducer capacity, whereas CD8 + T cells manifest cytotoxic or suppressor activity.

The CD4 + subset comprises 60% of peripheral T cells. When they are cloned, 70%–80% of CD4 + cells give rise to progeny producing IL-2, indicating a potential to exert helper activity. By contrast, 15%–20% of CD8 + cells give rise to clones producing IL-2. Occasional CD4 + cells give rise to cytotoxic T cells (T_c) capable of both lysing specific target cells and producing IL-2. The CD4 + subset does not correspond closely to the T_μ subset. A relatively small proportion of T_μ cells are CD4 +.

The CD8 + subset amounts to 30% of normal peripheral blood T cells. A proportion of them has cytotoxic activity which can be inhibited by antibody to CD8. It is not yet clear whether suppressor and cytolytic T cells belong to a separate lineage, or conversely, whether T cells may express either or both activities, depending on environmental conditions.

Three types of T_c are produced in the mixed lymphocyte reaction (MLR):

1. Cytotoxic T lymphocytes with specificity for MHC class I allotypes. These cells can lyse target cells expressing antigens for which the cytotoxic cells have a specific receptor.

2. Natural killer (NK) cells.

3. ADCC cells.

T cell clones produced in the MLR may have the following phenotypes: CD8 + / CD4-, CD8-/CD4+ and CD8-/CD4-. When circulating CD8+ cells are cloned, virtually all of them give rise to cytotoxic T cells. Other studies have shown that individual T cell clones may or may not produce IL-2, B cell growth factors (BCGFs) and B cell differentiation factors (BCDFs).

These studies show that the T cell subsets are not yet fully clarified. Surface marker studies of circulating T cells are beset with two difficulties (1) because they may not reflect the functional activity of the lymphoid tissues and (2) because the surface markers do not necessarily reflect the functional state of the T cells in vivo. A review of these problems may be found in Moretta et al. (1984). T cell differentiation antigens are discussed by Emmrich and Meuer (1985).

The T Cell Receptor

The elucidation of the structure of the T cell receptor, which has been a puzzle for many years, is a very considerable achievement (Acuto and Reinherz 1985; Robertson 1985). It was long known that T cells had antigen-specific receptors, because they bind radiolabelled antigen and are activated specifically by antigen.

The human T cell receptor is a surface complex of the Ti receptor, the three polypeptides, γ (20 kD), δ (20 kD) and ε (25 kD), of the CD3 (T3) protein and either a CD4 (T4) or a CD8 (T8) molecule (Fig. 10.2). The specific part of the

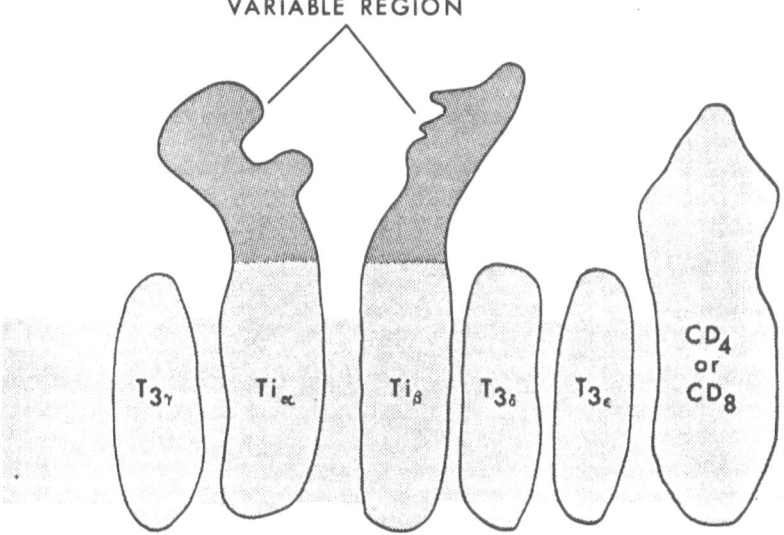

Fig. 10.2. The T cell receptor complex. Two chains of the clonogenic receptor (Ti) are illustrated and the three parts of the CD3 (T3) molecule with which Ti is associated. The Ti_γ chain is also expressed on some T cells. The Ti molecules are also associated with either a CD4 (T4) or a CD8 (T8) molecule.

receptor is the Ti molecule, called a clonogenic molecule because it is individual to each specific clone of T cells. It has two glycoprotein chains, α (43 kD) and β (51 kD). Each chain has extracellular, transmembrane and intracellular portions. The external (N-terminal) part has a distal variable (V) region and a proximal constant (C) region. Monoclonal antibodies against CD3 co-precipitate Ti, but monoclonal antibodies against the specific Ti do not co-precipitate the CD3 molecules. CD4 antigen combines with the constant portions of MHC class II molecules and CD8 antigen with the constant part of MHC class I molecules, apparently facilitating cell contact for triggering B cells and for lysing target cells. CD4 and CD8 are not essential for T cell activation.

Genetic Mechanisms in T Cell Differentiation

Elucidation of the genetic mechanisms for generation of the diversity of immunological specificity is one of the triumphs of modern biology. The diversity of the T cell receptor and of antibody must be generated by somatic mutation in precursor cells, i.e. by a random mechanism which changes the somatic genes, since there is no way by which antigen could alter the genes to make them encode molecules complementary to antigen. The rules which govern translation and transcription of all other proteins apply to the synthesis of antibody. The immune response is necessarily based on a selective mechanism, i.e. a mechanism that generates a clone from a cell with the correct specificity. These ideas, so hard to accept at first, have now been confirmed by unravelling the molecular mechanisms.

Genes for T receptors and antibody are created by similar processes. In the germline form, i.e. in the form in which they are inherited, numerous discrete segments of T and B receptor genes are distributed quite widely. Genes encoding the different chains which comprise the complete molecule may even be on different chromosomes. The functional gene arises by a process of selection and rearrangement. In each cell units are selected for each component of the functional gene, brought together and joined. Unwanted intervening segments are excised.

Three gene families, α, β and γ, encode subunits of the antigen-specific T cell receptor (Fig. 10.3). The formation of the T receptor gene is best understood in the case of the β chain. The β chain genes on chromosome 7 consist of V, D, J and C segments, similar to the genes encoding immunoglobulin heavy chains. These are rearranged in stage II thymocyte differentiation within the chromosomes of individual T cells to form a fully mature gene. T cells also have a complete set of germline immunoglobulin genes which are not normally rearranged. Rearrangement of T receptor β chain genes has been demonstrated in a number of T cell malignancies and T cell lines.

The α chain genes on chromosome 14 have been partially analysed. V, J and C genes exist. The number of J α genes appears to be very much greater than the number of J segments of the immunoglobulin or T receptor β chain gene families. Ti_γ genes are also assembled from V, J and C genes resembling the corresponding Ig genes. They are expressed early in T cell development, followed by expression of the Ti_β chain genes and lastly by expression of the Ti_α genes. Helper and cytotoxic cells use the same pool of V gene segments in their rearranged and expressed α and β genes. The γ gene family is rearranged in cytolytic T cells, but not in most helper T cells.

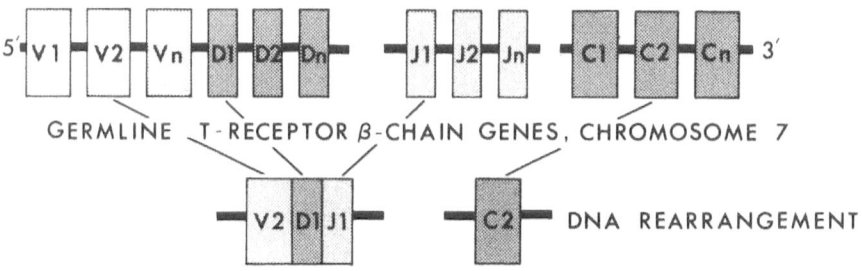

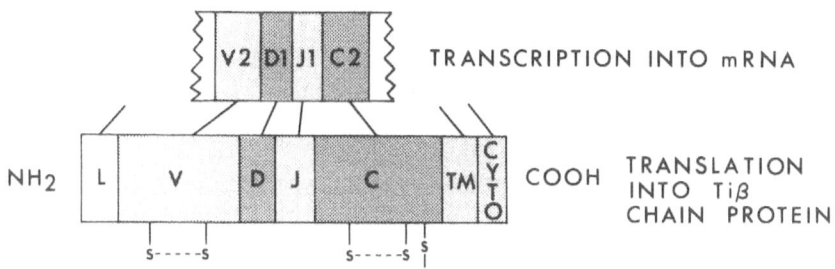

Fig. 10.3a,b. Generation of the clonogenic T cell receptor. **a** The germline β chain genes are in distinct V, D, J and C pools. The β chain gene of a newly emerging T cell is formed by a rearrangement resulting in the joining of one segment from each of these pools. **b** The gene product, the T cell receptor itself, has a short leader segment (*L*), *V*, *D*, *J* and *C* segments, transmembrane (*TM*) and cytoplasmic segments (*CYTO*). Disulphide bridges give the V and C segments a looped structure similar to that seen in immunoglobulin and members of the immunoglobulin superfamily.

T Cell Activation

Activation of T cells is the process leading to proliferation, differentiation to specialised function and generation of memory cells. The corresponding process in B cells leads to the generation of clones of antibody-secreting cells or memory cells.

In general, T cells need two signals for activation: antigen (correctly presented) together with IL-1 and IL-2 (Fig. 10.4). Under some circumstances, which are not well understood, T cells may proliferate and release B cell growth factors in response to the presence of IL-2. However, IL-2 cannot induce some effects, such as activation of B cells, unless the T cells themselves have received an inducing stimulus.

The T cell activation steps are:

1. Binding of antigen, usually in association with a matching MHC molecule, on an accessory cell (AC). A trimolecular complex of MHC product, T cell receptor and antigen must be formed. IL-1, secreted by macrophages, is generally needed for triggering of T cells when antigen is presented by ACs. B lymphocytes, like

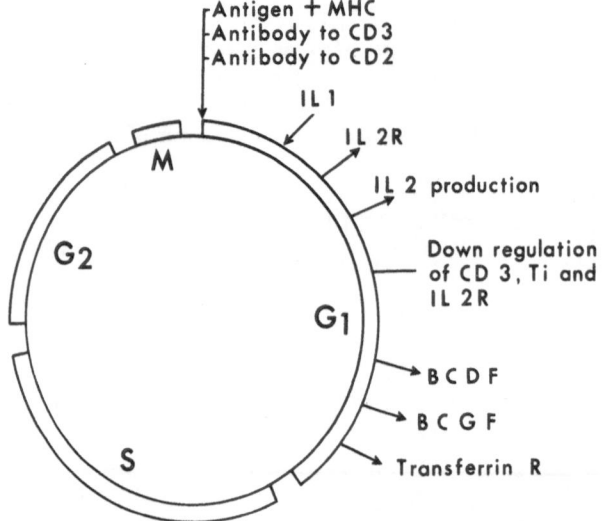

Fig. 10.4. T cell activation. Antigen, correctly presented with MHC product, induces the cell to enter the mitotic cycle. Other stimuli may by-pass this requirement, e.g. antibody to membrane molecules CD2 or CD3. The antigen receptor is down regulated, IL-2 receptors (*IL-2R*) and then IL-2 are synthesised. The cells synthesising IL-2 may respond to their own lymphokine, or to lymphokine produced by other helper T cells. IL-2 receptors are, in turn, down regulated. The T cell expresses receptors for transferrin and must have adequate concentrations of transferrin in its environment, for binding to the receptor (*R*), to proceed to S phase.

macrophages, may take up, process and present antigen to T cells. This combination leads to entry into the G_1 phase of the cell cycle.

2. Rapid reduction of expression (modulation) of the T cell receptor-CD3 complex.

3. Rapid increase in expression of IL-2 receptors and CD4 or CD8 molecules. There are high- and low-affinity IL-2 receptors. The function of the low-affinity receptors is not clear. Only the high-affinity receptors are internalised when they combine with IL-2. Anti-CD25 binds to both. Anti-Tac antibody (of the CD25 cluster) and IL-2 bind to separate sites on the IL-2 receptor.

4. Production and secretion of IL-2

5. Binding of IL-2 to receptors

6. DNA synthesis and mitosis.

In the absence of continued antigenic stimulation, the antigen receptor-CD3 complex is re-expressed and the number of IL 2 receptors is reduced.

Resting T cells can be activated by antibody either to the CD3 complex or the Ti molecules. Activation of T cells can also be initiated by T cell mitogens and metallic ions (mercury, nickel and zinc). Phytohaemagglutinin (PHA) binds to the T cell receptor and to CD2. Concanavalin A and lentil lectin bind to both the T cell receptor and CD3.

It is of interest that IL-2 receptors are also induced by HTLV-I virus. Adult T cell leukaemia/lymphoma (ATL) cell lines which are infected with HTLV-I all express large numbers (300–500 000/cell) of IL-2 receptors. They constitutively make large amounts of IL-2 mRNA but do not synthesise much IL-2.

Pretreatment of T cells with antibodies to CD3 blocks the induction phase in mixed lymphocyte culture, blocks the effector phase of cell-mediated lympholysis and inhibits T lymphocyte proliferative responses to soluble antigen.

T and NK cells can also be activated through CD2 (Siciliano et al. 1985). CD2 has three epitopes (antigen-binding sites). Antibodies must bind to more than one epitope to be mitogenic. Epitope 1 contains the sheep erythrocyte-binding site. Since sheep erythrocytes bind only through this one epitope they do not induce mitosis.

Signal Transduction in T Cell Activation

The initial events in T cell activation involve essentially the same processes of signal transduction as those induced by many hormones and growth factors, which are described in greater detail in Chapters 7 and 12 (see pp. 78, 154). The first step in T cell activation is associated with a rapid rise of intracellular Ca^{2+}. One of the CD3 molecules may actually form the calcium channel of the T cell receptor. Activation will not proceed following this event alone; accessory cells or IL-1 must also be present.

IL-2 synthesis stops during during S phase. The daughter cells require another activation stimulus, via the antigen receptor, for IL-2 production during the next cell cycle. IL-2 can also be stimulated by molecules which activate the common signal receptor transduction pathways, such as diacylglycerol (DAG), phospholipase C, PHA and 12-O-tetradecanoylphorbol-13-acetate (TPA). IFN_γ is produced under virtually all conditions known to cause activation of T cells. Proliferation is not necessary for IFN_γ production.

Expression of the transferrin receptor and binding of transferrin is also necessary for T cells to proceed to S phase. The final stage, T cell replication, can be induced only by IL-2 interacting with its receptor.

Since the description of cytokines in the activation of T and B cells, the search has begun for conditions associated with failure of expression of the cytokines or their receptors. Absence of receptors for IL-1 and reduced expression of CD25 with poor T cell function have been described in ataxia telangiectasia and the Wiskott–Aldrich syndrome.

References

Acuto O, Reinherz EL (1985) The human T-cell receptor. Structure and function. N Engl J Med 312: 1100–1111

Blue M-I, Daley JF, Levine H, Schlossman SF (1985) Coexpression of T_4 and T_8 on peripheral blood T cells demonstrated by two-color fluorescence flow cytometry. J Immunol 134: 2281–2286

Ceredig R, Lopez-Botet M, Moretta L (1984) Phenotype and functional properties of mouse and human thymocytes. Semin Hematol 21: 244–256

Duvall E, Wyllie AH (1986) Death and the cell. Immunol Today 7: 115–119

Emmrich F, Meuer S (1985) Human T-cell clones find ever wider application. Immunol Today 6:
    197–228
Haynes BF (1984) The human thymic microenvironment. Adv Immunol 36: 87–142
Lobach DF, Hensley LL, Ho W, Haynes BF (1985) Human T cell antigen expression during the early
    stages of fetal thymic maturation. J Immunol 135: 1752–1759
Moretta A, Pantaleo G, Maggi E, Mingari C (1984) Recent advances in the phenotypic and functional
    analysis of human T lymphocytes. Semin Hematol 21: 257–269
Robertson M (1985) T-cell receptor. The present state of recognition. Nature 317: 768–771
Siciliano RF, Pratt JC, Schmidt RE, Ritz J, Reinherz EL (1985) Activation of cytolytic T lymphocyte
    and natural killer function through the T_{11} sheep erythrocyte binding protein. Nature 317: 428–430
Stutman O, Calkins CE (1977) Ontogenic aspects In: Altmann HW, Büchner F, Cottier H et al. (eds)
    Transplantation. Springer, Berlin Heidelberg New York, pp 169–193 (Handbuch der allgemeinen
    Pathologie, volume 6, part 8)
Tridente G (1985) Immunopathology of the human thymus. Semin Hematol 22: 56–67
Wyllie AH, Morris RG, Smith AL, Dunlop D (1984) Chromatin cleavage in apoptosis: associated with
    condensed chromatin morphology and dependence on macromolecular synthesis. J Pathol 142:
    67–77

11   B Cell Differentiation

Introduction

The B cell differentiation pathway extends from the most primitive stage represented by the earliest recognisable B cells to the most differentiated plasma cell stage. B cell differentiation may be divided into two phases: antigen-independent and antigen-dependent differentiation. The first detectable step in B cell differentiation is rearrangement of the heavy chain immunoglobulin genes. Rearrangement of immunoglobulin genes is the physical basis of the generation of antibody diversity, incorporating the somatic mutation predicted by Burnet (1959).

A distinct organ, the bursa of Fabricius, is the site of development of B cells in birds. In mammals, B cells are produced in a series of haematopoietic organs in fetal life. In humans, after birth, they are produced exclusively in the bone

Table 11.1. Timetable of B cell ontogeny

Weeks	Phenotypes	Site
7–9	cIg_μ, MER	Liver
11	sIg_μ, sIg_δ, $Fc_\gamma R$	
12	TdT, CD10 (cALLA), MHC class II, CD24, RFB1	
15–16	Population 1: TdT+, sIg_μ+ Population 2: TdT–, sIg_μ+, sIg_δ–CD20–, CD24–	Bone marrow
16–21	sIg_μ++, sIg_δ++, CD5–, CD21+, CD22+	Spleen
16–17	sIg_μ++, sIg_δ++, CD5–, CD21+, CD22+	Lymph nodes
18–20	sIg_μ+, sIg_δ+, CD5+, CD20+, CD21+, CD22+, CD24+, RFA-1+	Lymph nodes, primary nodules
22	sIg_μ+, sIg_δ+, CD5+, CD20+, CD21+ CD22+, CD24+, RFA-1+	Spleen, primary nodules
22+	sIg_μ++, sIg_δ++, CD5–	Lymph node, paracortex
22	sIg_μ++, sIg_δ++, CD5–	Spleen, marginal zone
40	sIg_μ+, sIg_δ+, CD5–, CD20+, CD21+, CD22+, CD24+, Y29/55+, RFA+	Peripheral blood

marrow, which they leave when they are immunologically competent. After activation by antigen, under appropriate conditions, they may differentiate to plasma cells. A timetable of B cell ontogeny is presented in Table 11.1.

Antigen-independent B Cell Differentiation

In the mouse embryo the placenta is the first site of B cell development, which peaks at day 12, when blood islands develop in the yolk sac (Melchers 1977). This is followed by waves of B cell development in the fetal liver, then spleen and bone marrow. Explants of liver and spleen from 12- to 14-day mouse embryos give rise to Ig+ B cells. The early events are unknown; the pluripotential stem cell is thought to give rise to a lymphoid progenitor, the common ancestor of T and B lymphocytes.

Large pre-B cells with convoluted nuclear margins have been detected in the human fetal liver at 80 days or earlier. They are identified by having immunoglobulin μ chains, but not light chains, in the cytoplasm (Gupta et al. 1976). They also express the mouse erythrocyte receptor (MER), terminal deoxynucleotidyl transferase (TdT), and antigens CD9, CD10, major histocompatibility class II (MHC II), CD20 and CD24 (Bofill et al. 1985). Some bind peanut agglutinin (PNA) and express receptors for the complement component C3d (CD21) and receptors for the Fc part of the IgM molecule. PNA also binds to germinal centres in lymph nodes in later life. Pre-B cells in fetal liver and bone marrow, and in adult bone marrow are large and small. Only small pre-B cells are found in fetal spleen, blood and lymph nodes.

B cells in the liver express sIgD at about 80 days of gestation. Small populations of cells expressing either sIgG or sIgA appear within the next 10–20 days. By 90 days the number of B cells exceeds the number of pre-B cells.

The development and kinetics of B cells are better known in mice than in humans. About 5×10^7 B cells are produced daily in the bone marrow of the adult mouse (Opstelten and Osmond 1983). The number of B cells produced each day is equal to about 20% of the number of B cells in the peripheral lymphoid tissues (Opstelten and Osmond 1985). Large dividing parent cells, with rearranged heavy chain genes, which do not produce either heavy or light chains of immunoglobulin, give rise to large daughter cells which can be identified positively as pre-B cells by having μ chains in their cytoplasm ($c_\mu+$ cells). A proportion of these transforms directly to small non-dividing $c_\mu+$ cells (non-cycling pre-B cells). The rest (cycling pre-B cells) divide only once. Thus normal marrow pre-B cells probably do not renew themselves.

Maturation in the marrow from large pre-B cells to small sIg+ cIg– cells takes from 12 h to 3 days (Landreth et al. 1984). Maturation from sIg– small lymphocytes to functional B cells can also occur in vitro (Stocker 1977), provided appropriate humoral factors and/or adherent regulatory cells are present (Kincade et al. 1984). There is some evidence that antigen-independent maturation of pre-B cells is controlled by T cells.

The pool of B cell precursors is thought to be very large, constituting 25% or more of normal adult bone marrow (Coffman and Weissman 1981). Pre-B cells comprise approximately 5% of nucleated cells in adult bone marrow. Progeny of these B cell precursors are seeded to peripheral lymphoid tissues at rates sufficient to replace 5%–10% of all mature B cells each day (Osmond and Nossal 1974). In the human infant bone marrow, TdT +, CD10 + and MHC class II + cells appear to be precursors of the first recognisable pre-B cells. Some TdT +, c_μ + cells are present, probably intermediates on the way to becoming TdT–, c_μ +, then sIg_μ +, sIg_δ-cells. TdT + pre-B cells, and sIg_μ +, sIg_δ– B cells express CD22 in the cytoplasm. They also express an antigen AL-1, not present on peripheral B cells (Campana et al. 1985).

Little is known about the control of B cell production in the marrow. There is presumably a mechanism to regulate the entry of stem cell progeny into the B cell lineage.

Bone marrow B cells migrate from bone marrow primarily to the spleen and, to a lesser extent, to the lymph nodes. The spleen is thought to be a major site of antigen-independent differentiation of B cells. The sIg is less dense on B cells in the spleen than in the lymph nodes, in keeping with the finding that B cells acquire sIgD before activation, which takes place principally in the lymph nodes. After leaving the marrow, the majority of B cells die within a half-time of 24 h (Freitas and Coutinho 1981; Freitas et al. 1982). The life span of such cells, if stimulated, apparently cannot exceed the time required for an additional 30–50 replications, unless they are converted to memory B cells by a process which is not understood.

The first B cells in lymph nodes, at 110–120 days of gestation express sIg_μ and sIg_δ strongly, CD21 and CD22, but lack the T cell-associated marker CD5 (Table 11.2). The same cells are seen in the spleen from 110 to 150 days and they persist in the paracortical region of the lymph nodes in succeeding weeks. The second population to reach the lymph nodes expresses MER, weak sIg_μ and sIg_δ, and CD5. At this time the lymph nodes lack germinal centres, and a mantle zone of lymphocytes, but follicular dendritic reticular cells (DRCs) are seen. Primary nodules develop around the DRCs after 150 days. These contain a pure population of B cells with the following markers: CD20, CD21, CD22, CD24, RFA-1 (Bofill et al. 1985). The MER +, CD5 +, sIg_μ +, sIg_δ + cells are a minor population in the paracortical region of adult lymph nodes, which may represent the normal equivalents of malignant lymphocytes in B CLL and centrocytic lymphoma, and a prominent subpopulation in rheumatoid arthritis.

In the spleen, B cells of the sIg_μ +, sIg_δ +, CD5 + type appear at about 155 days in smaller numbers. Cells of the splenic marginal zone are sIg_μ +, sIg_δ–, and express CD21 and CD22 (Campana et al. 1985).

After birth, the proportion of immature cells in the marrow decreases, and the proportion expressing sIgM, sIgD, CD21, and Y29/55 increases, partly reflecting the accumulation of memory B cells (Benner et al. 1981). Y29/55 is a unique B cell antibody reacting with a 70 kD protein antigen that appears during the sIg_μ +, sIg_δ– stage (Campana et al. 1985).

B Lymphocyte Differentiation in Postnatal Life

MHC class II antigens, MER, CD10 and TdT are present from the pre-B stage. Surface CD19 and CD20 and cytoplasmic CD22 molecules appear before cytoplasmic μ chains and persist until terminal differentiation. CD21 appears later

Table 11.2. Phenotypes of B cell subsets during differentiation

Normal B cell phenotype	Corresponding malignant subtype	Marker
Pre-pre-B	Acute lymphoblastic leukaemia (ALL)	MHC class II+ CD19+ CD20± CD22+ (cytoplasm) CD24± TdT+ CD10±
Pre-B	Pre-B-ALL	c_μ+ MHC class II+ CD10+ CD19± CD20+ CD22+ (cytoplasm) CD24+ (MER+)
Early B	B-ALL	sIgM MHC classII+ CD10± CD19+ CD20+ CD21+ CD22+ (cytoplasm) CD23+ CD24+ MER+
Intermediate B	Chronic lymphocytic leukaemia (CLL) Diffuse well-differentiated lymphocytic lymphoma	sIgM+, D± MHC class II+ CD10± CD19+ CD20+ CD21+ CD22+ (cytoplasm and surface) CD23+ CD24+ MER+ Y29/55+
Mature B	Hairy cell leukaemia Diffuse poorly differentiated lymphoma Nodular lymphoma	sIg++ MHC class II+ CD19+ CD20+ CD21+ CD22+ (cytoplasm and surface) CD23+ CD24+ MER± Y29/55+
Activated B cell	Hairy cell leukaemia B lymphomas	T10+ MER− CD23+ sIg+/++ MHC class II+ CD19+ CD20+ CD24+

Table 11.2. (*continued*)

Early plasma cell	Waldenstrom's macroglobulinaemia	sIg + MHC class II + CD19 ± CD20 + CD24 + T10 + PCA-1 + PC-1 + cIg +
Terminally differentiated	Multiple myeloma	cIg + PCA-1 + PC-1 + MHC class II ± CD10 ±

(Fig. 11.1). The order of expression of markers is: intracellular μ chains, MER and TdT, receptors for the Fc moiety of Ig, and then receptors for C3b and C4. Free light chain synthesis occurs at this stage (Hannam-Harris and Smith 1981). Synthesis of membrane heavy chains follows. The IgM, as the first class of Ig to be expressed on the B cell surface, is the 8S ($\mu_2 L_2$) molecule.

Antigen-independent B lymphocyte differentiation has been considered to stop with the formation of cells expressing sIgM and sIgD. This is not necessarily so, since studies on mice kept under germ-free conditions suggest some progression to

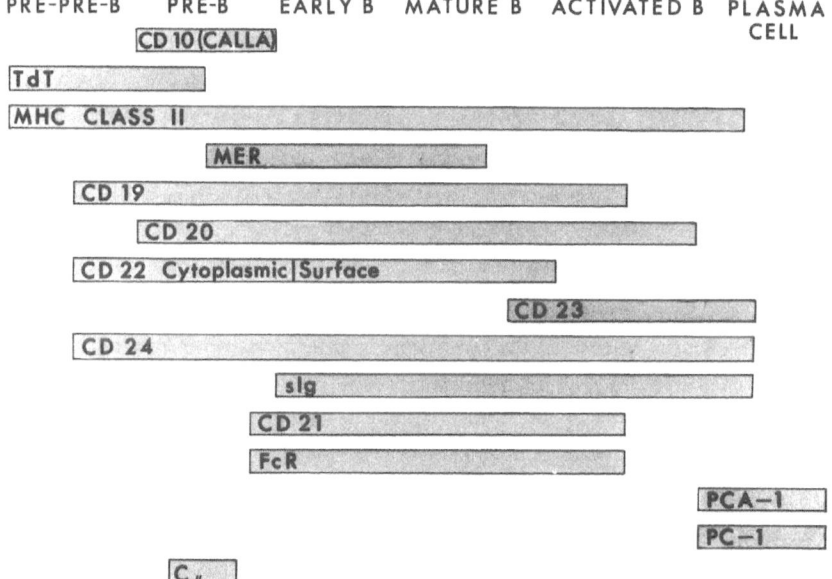

Fig. 11.1. Human B lymphocyte differentiation. This schema shows markers which may be used to identify the stages. The CD monoclonal antibody markers are defined in Table 8.5. *TdT*, terminal deoxynucleotidyl transferase; *MHC*, major histocompatibility complex; *MER*, mouse erythrocyte receptor; *FcR*, receptor for the Fc moiety of Ig; *PCA-1* and *PC-1* monoclonal antibodies; C_μ, cytoplasmic μ chains.

a stage of antibody secretion occurring independently of antigenic stimulation. Of course, these antibody-producing cells may have an anti-self antigen specificity. The same question arises in explaining the differentiation of malignant lymphocytes.

Antigen-dependent B Cell Differentiation

Antigen-dependent B cell differentiation begins with activation by antigen. Phenotypic changes on activation involve shifts in surface Ig phenotype, from IgM+ to IgM+, IgD+, then to IgM+, IgD–, and loss of MER and CD22, while BB1, B5, IL-2 receptors, B-LAST-1, and CD23 appear with activation. These antigen-dependent processes are regulated by T cells and occur predominantly within germinal centres in the lymph nodes and Peyer's patches.

Synthesis of mRNA for secretory μ chain begins shortly after activation, preceding proliferation. Expression of J chain RNA and amplification of J chain and secretory μ chain mRNA coincide with a phase of rapid proliferation and with the secretion of pentamer IgM antibody, although pre-B cells, which do not secrete Ig, contain J chain (see Fig. 11.2).

The mature B cell may retain sIgM or sIgD, or acquire sIgG, sIgA, or sIgE as it becomes a recirculating memory B cell or an antibody-producing cell. Change to expression of these additional isotypes is called the "isotype switch". The additional isotypes have the same heavy chain variable region, the same light chain, and hence the same antigen specificity as the IgM on a particular B cell. Genetic rearrangements leading to heavy chain class switch occur in the germinal centres of lymph nodes.

B lymphocytes from neonatal humans may bear three or more sIg isotypes simultaneously, whereas sIgG+ and sIgA+ B lymphocytes in adult blood usually express only the single isotype. It is rare to find more than one of the IgG subclasses expressed at the same time, and cells expressing IgG rarely express IgA. Only one IgA subclass is expressed at a time. sIgM+, sIgD+ cells appear to be the major precursors of the primary antibody response to thymus-dependent antigens, whereas sIgM+, sIgD– cells may be precursors for the primary IgM response to thymus-independent antigens.

As the B cell passes through its terminal differentiation steps to become a plasma cell it loses most of the surface markers, including sIgD, sIgM and class II MHC, and gains the surface antigens T10, PCA-1 and PC-1, while continuing to express cytoplasmic immunoglobulin.

B Cell Subsets

B cells are subdivided into subsets on the basis of their maturation stage, not on lineage, because it is not known if there are distinct lineages of B cells in man.

The following are designated subsets:

1. *Unidentifiable precursors*. These are B stem cells with the property of self renewal. The designation "pro-B cell" has been used. The immunoglobulin genes

of these cells have not been rearranged from the germline state, and they therefore also lack immunoglobulin markers.

2. *Ig-negative pre-B cells* or "pre-pre-B cells". These are cells with rearranged heavy chain genes, which are not yet expressing cIg. It is believed, but not yet proven, that they express TdT.

3. *Pre-B cells.* These cells have cIg but no sIg and are unable to respond to antigen. Pre-B cells are demonstrable by possession of rearranged heavy, but not light, chain genes. Two subgroups have been described within this category: (a) cycling pre-B cells in fetal liver, and a proportion of B cells in adult bone marrow that may undergo one division; and (b) non-cycling pre-B cells. Pre-B cells express CD10, MER, TdT, CD19, CD24 and MHC class II, but lack FcR.

4. *Early B cells.* These cells have acquired sIg_μ, but not sIg_δ. They do not express CD10. Cells of acute lymphoblastic leukaemia (ALL) and Burkitt's lymphoma (BL) may have this phenotype.

A B cell is designated as immature by its reaction to antigen. Immature B cells are exquisitely sensitive to antigen, being made tolerant by very low concentrations of antigen. Mature B cells are activated by anti-Ig reagents, whereas newly formed B cells are inactivated by cross-linking of their sIg (Raff et al. 1975). This may be related to the development of tolerance.

5. *Virgin, primary or mature B cells.* These are functional B cells which have not interacted with antigen, have sIgM and usually sIgD, but no cIg. Virgin lymphocytes responding to thymus-dependent antigens have the phenotype sIgM+, sIgD+, whereas those responding to thymus-independent antigens bear sIgM, but frequently lack sIgD. Under physiological conditions, most B cells recently formed in the bone marrow have a short life span. Newly formed B cells can be activated by antigen in secondary lymphoid organs and in some cases give rise to long-lived clones (MacLennan and Gray 1986). Virgin B cells are recruited only in the first few days after antigenic challenge. After this the response is sustained by long-lived memory B cell clones. Primary B cells enter secondary lymphoid organs through high endothelial venules. Virgin lymphocytes having the appropriate rearrangement of immunoglobulin chains, encoding antibody of the correct specificity, are activated by the corresponding antigen presented on interdigitating reticular cells (IDRCs) in extrafollicular areas, in association with T cells in the case of T-dependent antigens. The activated cells may become either short-lived antibody-producing plasma cells or memory B cells. The majority of peripheral blood lymphocytes are probably recirculating mature cells, both virgin and memory. Most of them express CD21.

The term "resting B cell" is used to designate a B cell which is not secreting Ig, in the G_0 phase of the cell cycle. Resting lymphocytes do not express the receptors for growth factors which act in the G_1 phase.

6. *Activated B cells.* The majority of B cells in primary lymphoid follicles express class II MHC products. When activated, they undergo cell division, lose sIgD, but retain sIgM. This alteration in isotype expression may be necessary for entry into the germinal centre. Activation induces loss of MER and CD22, while BB1, B5, IL-2 receptors, B-LAST-1 and CD23 appear. After further divisions they secrete IgM and IgG. *Centroblasts* are activated B cells in germinal centres of lymph nodes; they have non-cleaved nuclei and are derived from follicular centrocytes. (Centrocytes are distinguished by having cleaved nuclei).

7. *Memory B cell (secondary B cell).* Memory B cells are typical small to

medium-sized lymphocytes that cannot be distinguished from other B cells on morphological grounds. Memory B cells are heterogeneous with regard to Ig isotype expression. A proportion bears sIgM after primary immunisation, and switches the isotype after secondary immunisation. Many bear sIgG of the subclass to which they are committed and may also express sIgM and sIgD. Mature memory B cells found some time after an immune response do not usually express sIgM or sIgD.

Memory B cells are produced in lymphoid tissues, as a result of stimulation by antigen, in association with T cells and accessory cells. Memory B cells enter secondary lymphoid organs from the blood through high endothelial venules. They may be activated to become centroblasts on contact with DRCs presenting the antigen corresponding to the specificity of their sIg. Memory B lymphocytes activated by DRCs may give rise to plasma cells which migrate to other lymphoid tissue, or to recirculating memory cells. Germinal centre cells have a high density of surface molecules recognised by PNA (Kraal et al. 1982), which contrasts with the low density of PNA-binding glycoprotein on plasma cells. They also express CD10. Germinal centre cells lack sIgD. The possible differentiation sequences in germinal centres are discussed in greater detail in Chapter 17 (see p. 244)

The phenotype of mantle B cells is MHC class II +, CD21 +, CD20 +, CD24 +, sIgM +, sIgD +. sIg_μ + cells in the interfollicular area may be in transit from the subcapsular region to the medullary cords, where IgM-secreting plasma cells are found. Some sIg_μ + B cells found outside the lymphoid follicles are activated by T-independent antigens. These do not switch isotypes.

Memory B cells recirculate, by virtue of an undefined alteration of surface membranes that allows the migration from blood to lymph to blood (Reichert et al. 1983). They may also seed back to the bone marrow. It has recently been suggested that memory cells may be identifiable by the phenotype CD20–, CD24 + (Patrick et al. 1984).

8. *Immunoblasts*. The term "immunoblast" is used as a general designation for activated B or T lymphocytes in a proliferating and differentiating phase. In histopathology immunoblasts are considered to be at a later stage than centroblasts of lymphoid follicles. *Plasmablasts* are proliferating and differentiating activated Ig-secreting B cells, having both sIg and cIg. They share some phenotypic markers with mature B cells (MHC class II, CD20, CD24) and plasma cells (PCA-1, PC1), and a marker of activated B cells (T10).

9. *Plasma cells*. These cells, which secrete Ig and have cIg but no sIg, are the end cells of an immune response. Mouse plasma cells generated early in immune responses have an average life span of less than 3 days. Plasma cells generated in established responses appear to have an average life span in excess of 20 days (MacLennan and Gray 1986). Plasma cells have lost most surface markers of B cells, including sIg, receptors for B cell growth and differentiation factors and transferrin and they express the surface markers PCA-1, PC-1 and T10.

Immunoglobulin

Immunoglobulin molecules are composed of two identical light (L) chains and two identical heavy (H) chains consisting of the amino-terminal variable (V) region (V_L

or V_H) and the carboxy-terminal constant (C) region (C_L or C_H) (Fig. 11.2). V and C regions are encoded by separate genes in germline cells which are rearranged and joined during lymphocyte development. The highly variable V regions contain the antigen-binding sites. They make up about half of a light chain and about one-quarter of a heavy chain.

There are two types of light chain, κ and λ. Each light chain type, and subtypes (e.g. $λ_1$ and $λ_2$) are defined by unique C_L region sequences. The C_H region is composed of three or four similar domains, C_{H1}, C_{H2}, etc. A cysteine-rich hinge region separates C_{H1} and C_{H2} of γ chains. The C regions define the types or classes. They are responsible for a variety of effector functions, such as complement fixation, binding to Fc receptors and passage through the placenta. Allotypic variations are found here.

The IgG class is subdivided into four subclasses (Table 11.3). IgM usually exists as a pentamer in the free state (Fig. 11.2b). IgA is secreted by plasma cells as a dimer, trimer or pentamer, its Ig chains bound to a J chain (Fig. 11.2c). IgA passes from the inner side of an epithelial cell through the cytoplasm, where it acquires a "secretory piece", and is secreted on the epithelial surface.

Genetic Mechanisms in B Cell Differentiation

The genetic mechanisms which result in the generation of each unique antibody-producing cell, are similar to the more recently discovered gene rearrangements which result in the formation of the T cell receptor for antigen.

Organisation of Immunoglobulin Genes

Immunoglobulin heavy chain genes are on chromosome 14; κ light chains are encoded on chromosome 2 and λ light chains on chromosome 22. In their embryonic or germline form they are organised as separate DNA segments scattered along their respective chromosomes. Mature B cells produce an immunoglobulin from only the maternal or paternal allele, containing only κ or λ light chains.

To code for Ig molecules there are separate variable (V), joining (J), diversity (D) constant (C), and signal or leader (L) peptide gene subsegments (Fig. 11.3). The leader gene codes for a short hydrophilic amino acid sequence involved in transporting the antibody molecule through the endoplasmic reticulum during translation. The peptide chain is then cleaved off. In addition, there are indepen-

Table 11.3. The subclasses of IgG

	IgG$_1$	IgG$_2$	IgG$_3$	IgG$_4$
Proportion	0.67	0.24	0.06	0.03
Half-life (days)	23	23	8	23
Complement binding	+ +	+	+ + +	–
Binding to macrophages	+	–	+	–
Passing placenta	+	+	+	+

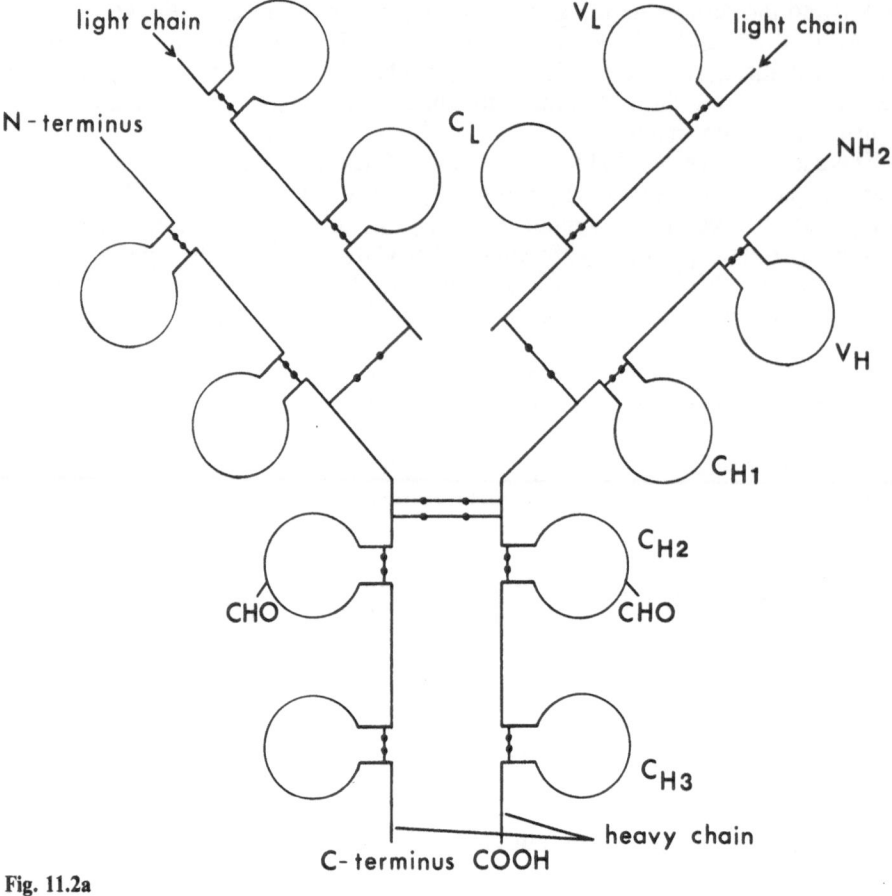

Fig. 11.2a

dent exons for the hinge regions of the γ chains, for each of the C_H segments, and the hydrophilic segments particular to surface immunoglobulins which lie within the surface membrane.

Rearrangement of B Cell Genes During Ontogeny

During the development of B cells the gene segments are recombined into a complete gene. The chromosome is actually broken, the DNA rearranged and the chromosome rejoined. This process is one of the mechanisms for the generation of antibody diversity (combinatorial diversity). Others are the occurrence of single point mutations at a high rate in the amino-terminal region (somatic mutational diversity), and junctional insertion diversity, occurring only in the V_H-D and D-J_H junctions, where one to several extra nucleotides may be inserted. Junctional site diversity occurs because, after chromosomal rearrangement, the points at which rejoining occurs are not precise. It is estimated that these mechanisms could generate 2×10^{10} different antibody molecules from a few hundred different genetic elements in the embryonic DNA.

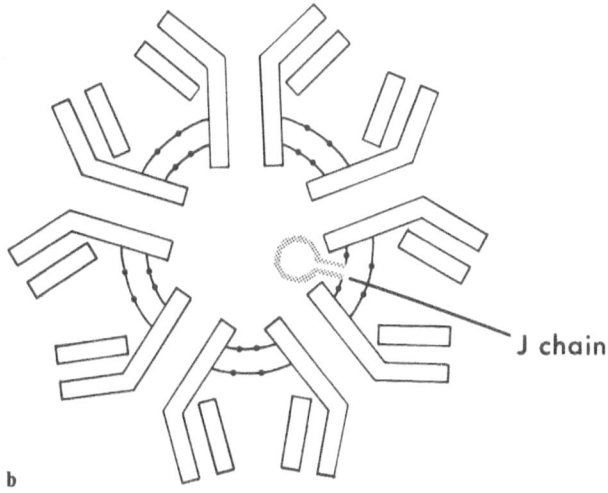

J chain

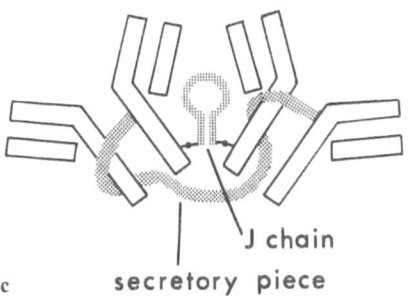

J chain

secretory piece

c

Fig. 11.2a–c. Structure of immunoglobulin molecules. a shows a heavy chain with three constant domains, C_{H1}, C_{H2} and C_{H3}, and one variable domain, V_H, and a light chain with one constant C_L and one variable domain V_L. The C_{H2} and C_{H3} domains form the Fc segment. b shows the usual pentameric form of IgM and c illustrates an IgA molecule. Disulphide bridges are illustrated by —●—●—.

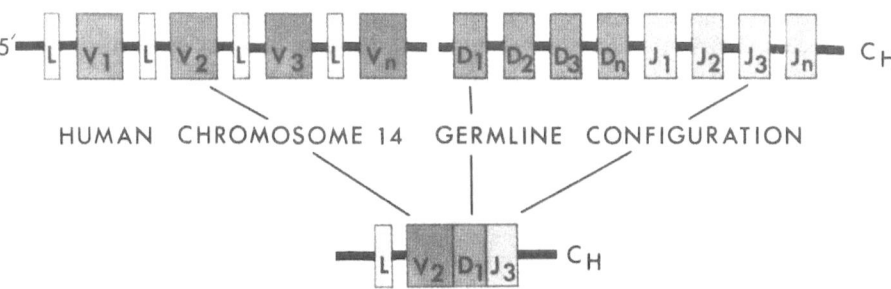

HUMAN CHROMOSOME 14 GERMLINE CONFIGURATION

REARRANGED HEAVY CHAIN CONFIGURATION

Fig. 11.3. Heavy chain gene rearrangement. In the germline genes of the lymphopoietic stem cells there are multiple V_H genes, each preceded by a leader (L) sequence, and multiple D_H and J_H segment genes. The rearrangement consists of a recombination of one of the V_H genes with one of the D_H genes and one of the J_H genes to encode the variable segment of the heavy chain. This rearranged gene is joined to the genes for the constant regions (C_H).

Immunoglobulin expression reflects the rearrangements occurring first for the μ gene, and subsequently for κ and λ genes of the light chains. If rearrangement of κ genes is effective, the cell may mature into a sIg$_μ$, $_κ$-bearing B cell. If the κ gene recombinations are aberrant or lead to deletion, λ gene rearrangement follows.

Human Heavy Chain Gene Organisation

The heavy chain V region is formed by selection of one of several hundred V segments to join one of several dozen D segments, and then to one of five or six J segments. Recombination must occur between a V_H and a D_H segment and between that D_H and a J_H subsegment.

Because the V_H region is encoded in three gene segments (V, D and J) which join in various combinations, whereas the V_L region has only V and J genes, the diversity is potentially much greater for heavy chains than for light chains. Enhancer sequences are present between the J and the switch regions in the heavy chain gene, and between the J and constant regions in the κ chain gene. Enhancer sequences are necessary for activation of the V region-associated promoters in B cells. They markedly increase the transcription of genes into mRNA. Unlike the promoters, they can act at a distance from the beginning of the gene.

Co-expression of membrane-bound and secretory heavy chains arises by differential splicing of RNA. In plasma cells, at the terminal stage of B cell differentiation, the V-D-J complex is translated to lie adjacent to a particular C_H gene, through one of the switch sites located on the 5′ side of each of the C_H genes, and the intervening sequence is deleted.

Light Chain Organisation

The light chain genes are arranged discontinuously in multiple germline variable regions (V_L), with alternative joining (J_L) segments and single or multiple constant (C_L) regions. They lack a D segment. The genome is rearranged to form the $V_L J_L$ sequences encoding the light chain variable regions after the heavy chain gene rearrangements have taken place. Light chain synthesis occurs soon after the onset of light chain rearrangement, and surface expression of complete immunoglobulin molecules occurs very soon after the onset of light chain synthesis.

Kappa light chains are used in approximately 60% of Ig molecules. From 50 to 200 different $V_κ$ segments encode the first 95 amino acids of the variable portion. The remaining 13 amino acids are encoded by one of 5 alternative $J_κ$ segments. A long intervening sequence (IVS) separates the variable portion from the $C_κ$ region. Gene rearrangements during differentiation result in one of the $V_κ$ regions coming together with one $J_κ$ segment of the germline DNA. This rearranged allele is then transcribed into RNA and the remaining IVS is removed by RNA splicing, before the mature mRNA is translated into a complete κ chain (Fig. 11.4).

Kappa-producing B cells have no remaining germline κ genes, but retain their λ genes in the germline configuration. By contrast, λ-producing B cells have either deleted or rearranged their κ germline genes so that they are ineffective. These processes occur in both normal and malignant B cells.

The λ gene locus varies more in size than the κ locus, because of the variable number of the $C_λ$ genes. It is comprised of six distinct $C_λ$ regions, each associated

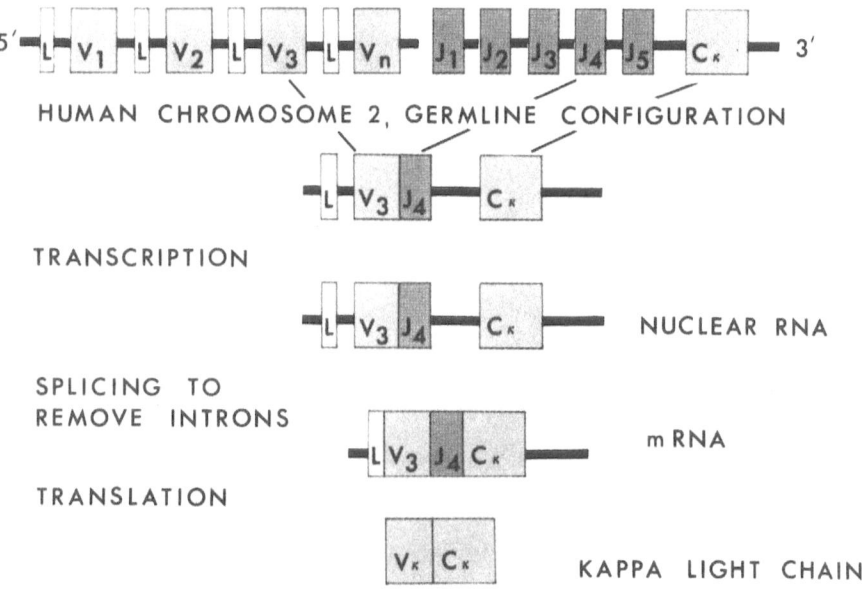

Fig. 11.4. Kappa chain production. One of the V_κ genes recombines with a J_κ segment. The primary RNA transcript is a copy of the rearranged gene, including the long intervening sequence (IVS) between the J_κ and C_κ segments. The primary transcript is converted to mRNA by splicing the exons together.

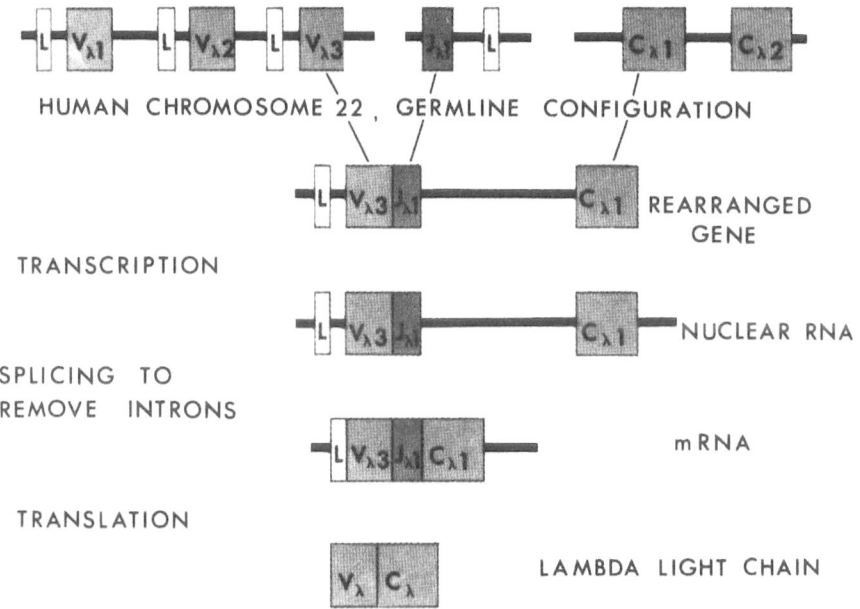

Fig. 11.5. Lambda chain production. If κ chain rearrangement is unsuccessful, λ chain rearrangement proceeds. There is a small number of V_λ genes, each preceded by its L segment. Similarly, there are a few C segments, each having a corresponding J segment. These differ from the J chains of heavy and κ genes, but the basic pattern of the rearrangement is the same as for heavy and κ chains.

with a particular J_λ segment. λ genes undergo a rearrangement that joins a V_λ and a J_λ segment. The rearranged VJ sequence is not joined with the C gene at the level of DNA, but at the RNA stage by splicing out intervening RNA, including unused J genes (Fig. 11.5).

Isotype Switch

As an antibody response proceeds, differentiation occurs through switching of the class of immunoglobulin produced. Primary immune responses generate clones of IgM-producing B cells. The $C\mu$ and C_δ genes are co-expressed during a segment of B cell differentiation. Initially a complete section of DNA is transcribed, including the recombined V_H region through the μ and δ C regions. Then, by differential splicing two messenger RNA molecules are produced, each with the same V_H, but having either μ or δ C regions.

In the secondary immune response, following a strong primary response or resulting from a further dose of antigen, selected clones switch from IgM to IgA, or possibly to IgE production. This occurs through a distinct type of rearrangement. The heavy chain switch involves joining of the completed V genes to another of the the heavy chain genes. Distally located C regions may be moved closer to a previously assembled V_H-D_H-J_H complex by deletion of intervening segments, by the activity of a switch site at the 5' side of each of the C region genes, except the δ gene. The rearranged V gene is still a significant distance from the C gene region. The isotype switch is induced by signals from isotype-specific T cells or T cell factors.

Pre-B cells can be detected by the immunoglobulin gene rearrangements that they have undergone. There is rearrangement of μ chain genes, and they have almost totally lost their germline J_H fragment because of very early rearrangement at the J_H locus. Rearrangement at the J_κ locus occurs later. Significant rearrangement is seen in small, more mature pre-B cells, but κ rearrangement is not complete in B cells expressing κ. Most retain one germline κ gene. Tumours induced in mice by Abelson virus usually consist of large pre-B cells with heavy chain rearrangements on both chromosomes. A few have light chain rearrangements.

Soon after rearrangement of the genes, both large and small pre-B cells synthesise significant amounts of μ heavy chain but little if any light chain. Secretory heavy chain production begins during early B cell differentiation, but the product is degraded intracellularly in the absence of a secretory apparatus.

Membrane or surface Ig (sIg) has a different tail (C-terminal segment) from secreted Ig. The terminal segment of sIg contains a hydrophilic, lipophilic segment that anchors it in the membrane. There are a further three hydrophilic amino acids beyond the membrane segment protruding into the cytoplasm.

The astonishing progress in demonstrating immunoglobulin gene rearrangement during B cell differentiation has rapidly found clinical application. Detection of a unique rearrangement in a B cell population is very strong evidence of B cell malignancy. The stage of differentiation of early malignant B cell populations can be determined by the extent of rearrangement of the immunoglobulin genes.

B cell differentiation is well reviewed by Calvert et al. (1984) and Zola (1985). Reviews of immunoglobulin gene rearrangement may be found in Morrison (1984), Rabbits (1984) and Waldmann (1985).

References

Benner R, Hijmans W, Haajiman JJ (1981) The bone marrow: the major source of serum immunoglobulins but still a neglected site of antibody formation. Clin Exp Immunol 46: 1–8

Burnet FM (1959) The clonal selection theory of immunity. Vanderbilt University Press, Nashville, Tennessee

Bofill M, Janossy G, Janossa M et al. (1985) Human B cell development. II. Subpopulations in the human fetus. J Immunol 134: 1531–1538

Calvert JE, Maruyama S, Tedder TF, Webb CF, Cooper MD (1984) Cellular events in the differentiation of antibody-secreting cells. Semin Hematol 21: 226–243

Campana D, Janossy G, Bofill M et al. (1985) Human B cell development. I. Phenotypic differences of B lymphocytes in the bone marrow and peripheral lymphoid tissue. J Immunol 134: 1524–1530

Coffman RL, Weissman IL (1981) A monoclonal antibody that recognises B cells and B cell precursors in mice. J Exp Med 153: 269–279

Freitas AA, Coutinho A (1981) Very rapid decay of mature lymphocytes in the periphery. J Exp Med 154: 994–999

Freitas AA, Rocha B, Forni L, Coutinho A (1982) Population dynamics of B lymphocytes and their precursors: demonstration of high turnover rates in the central and peripheral lymphoid organs. J Immunol 128: 54–60

Gupta S, Pahwa R, O'Reilly R, Good RA, Siegal FP (1976) Ontogeny of lymphocyte subpopulations in human foetal liver. Proc Natl Acad Sci USA 73: 919–922

Hannam-Harris AC, Smith JL (1981) Free light chain synthesis by human fetal liver and cord blood lymphocytes. Immunology 43: 417–423

Kraal G, Weissman IL, Butcher EC (1982) Germinal centre B cells: antigen specificity and changes in heavy chain class expression. Nature 298: 377–379

Kincade PW, Jyonouchi H, Landreth KS et al. (1984) Factors affecting normal and malignant B lymphocyte precursors. Curr Top Microbiol Immunol 113: 104–108

Landreth KS, Kincade PW, Lee G, Harrison DE (1984) B lymphocyte precursors in embryonic and adult W anemic mice. J Immunol 132: 2724–2729

MacLennan ICM, Gray D (1986) Antigen-driven selection of virgin and memory B cells. Immunol Rev 91: 61–85

Melchers F (1977) Murine embryonic B lymphocyte development in the placenta. Nature 277: 219–221

Morrison C (1984) Rearranging pre-B cell genes. Immunol Today 5: 37–38

Opstelten D, Osmond DG (1983) Pre-B cells in mouse bone marrow: immunofluorescence stathmokinetic studies of cytoplasmic mu chain-bearing cells in normal mice. J Immunol 131: 2635–2640

Opstelten D, Osmond DG (1985) Regulation of pre-B cell proliferation in bone marrow: immunofluorescence stathmokinetic studies of cytoplasmic mu chain-bearing cells in anti-IgM-treated mice, hematologically deficient mice and mice given sheep red blood cells. Eur J Immunol 15: 599–605

Osmond DG, Nossal GJV (1974) Differentiation of lymphocytes in mouse bone marrow. II Kinetics of maturation and renewal of antiglobulin-binding cells studied by double labelling. Cell Immunol 13: 132–141

Patrick CW, Harrison KA, Libnoch JA et al. (1984) Monoclonal antibody studies in human B cell lymphoproliferative disorders suggest B1 negative B4 positive lymphocytes may identify B memory cells. Proceedings of the second international conference on malignant lymphoma, Lugano, Switzerland, 1984, p 110 (abstract)

Rabbitts TH (1984) DNA in medicine. DNA juggling in the immune system. Lancet II: 1086–1088

Raff MC, Owen JJT, Cooper MD, Lawton AR, Megson M, Gathings WE (1975) Differences in susceptibility of mature and immature mouse B lymphocytes to anti-immunoglobulin-induced immunoglobulin suppression in vitro. Possible implications for B cell tolerance to self. J Exp Med 142: 1052–1064

Reichert RA, Gallatin WM, Weissman IL, Butcher EC (1983) Germinal center B cells lack homing receptors necessary for normal lymphocyte recirculation. J Exp Med 157: 813–827

Stocker JW (1977) Functional maturation of B cells in vitro. Immunology 32: 275–281

Waldmann TA (1985) Immunoglobulin gene rearrangements and antibody diversity. In: Waldmann TA (moderator) Molecular genetic analysis of human lymphoid neoplasms. Immunoglobulin genes and the c-myc oncogene. Ann Intern Med 102: 497–510

Zola H (1985) Differentiation and maturation of human B lymphocytes: a review. Pathology 17: 365–381

12 B Cell Activation

Introduction

The term "B cell activation" describes processes by which small resting B cells, in G_0 phase, are stimulated to divide and produce large amounts of secretory Ig molecules. If they are not activated, virgin B cells have a short life and memory B cells remain dormant.

Resting B cells may be activated by T-dependent antigens, T-independent antigens and polyclonal B cell activators (PBAs). A number of steps are recognised. The first, ("induction", "triggering" or "excitation"), resulting from the first effective "signal" received by the B cell, involves transition from the G_0 to the G_1 phase of the cell cycle. Requirements for induction differ according to whether the antigen is protein or polysaccharide, or contains lipid, and whether it is large or small. Antigen in an aggregated state more readily induces an immune response, whereas soluble antigen may exert a negative, tolerogenic effect. It is usually necessary for antigen to be taken up by accessory cells (ACs). ACs process antigen by limited proteolysis to smaller peptides which are returned to the cell surface for "presentation" in association with major histocompatibility complex (MHC) class II gene products. Activation of helper T cells may be necessary before the B cell is activated by T-dependent antigens.

After induction, B cells express receptors for growth and differentiation factors sequentially. Increased expression of class II MHC antigens and insulin receptors (Helderman and Strom 1978), and loss of sIgD are early consequences of B cell activation. Later, receptors for transferrin are expressed. The cycle is arrested if transferrin is lacking and iron deficiency inhibits both proliferation and antibody synthesis, although T cell function is affected more than other arms of the immune response (Brock and de Sousa 1986).

G_1 to S transition is induced by signals which are distinct from those required for excitation (G_0 to G_1 transition). Clonal expansion is mediated by soluble growth factors produced by monocytes and T lymphocytes. Soluble factors may not be essential in some responses, at least in vitro, for example those produced by powerful signals from anti-Ig. B cells cease to divide after 10–15 divisions, even if adequately supplemented with all of the factors and transferrin.

The final step, differentiation to the plasma cell or memory B cell stage is induced by B cell differentiation factors (BCDFs). These act polyclonally, through specific receptors, directing the switch from IgM to another immunoglobulin isotype.

Activated human B lymphocytes appearing in the blood after antigenic stimulation are large cells, refractory to further activation by antigen or anti-Ig, but responsive to B cell growth factors (BCGFs). They express sIgG or sIgM and surface markers (CD23, BB1, 4F2) of activated cells (Kehrl and Fauci 1983). Activated and resting populations can also be distinguished in tonsil B cells.

T Cells in B Cell Activation

Activation of resting B cells usually requires interactions with T helper cells (Coutinho et al. 1984). Depending on the conditions and the characteristics of the antigen, antigen can both stimulate and tolerise specific lymphocytes. More than one antigenic determinant appears to be necessary on immunogenic molecules. A hapten is a small molecule which can combine with specific antibody but cannot induce an immune response unless it is combined with a larger carrier molecule, which is usually a protein. To induce a secondary response to a hapten, the hapten must be on the same carrier in the second immunisation as was used in the primary immunisation, unless the subject has also been immunised separately to the second carrier.

This requirement for the antigen to be on the same carrier in a secondary immune response is explained by the phenomenon of linked recognition, the joining of a helper T cell with the responding B cell by an antigen bridge (Fig. 12.1a). Linked recognition involves recognition of antigenic determinants on the carrier by the T cell, and B cell recognition of haptenic determinants. It has recently been shown that a B cell can capture antigen through its 10^5 Ig receptors, digest and present it in the form of peptide fragments to MHC-restricted helper T cells (Lanzavecchia 1985). B cells can accumulate and present immunologically significant antigen when the external concentration of antigen is in the range of 10^{-12} mol/litre. A B cell which has taken up about 10 molecules can activate a T cell (Fig. 12.1b). Recycling of antigen receptors from cytoplasm back to surface membrane could act as an antigen pump, greatly increasing the efficiency of the process. Activated B cells present antigen to T cells more efficiently than resting B cells.

Requirements for activation of virgin and memory cells may differ. In experimental situations, immature B cells encountering antigen for the first time have a much lower activation threshold, and are suppressed by relatively low concentrations of antigen.

The isotype switch, i.e. from synthesis of IgM class antibody to antibody having another class of heavy chain, occurring during maturation of an antibody response, is regulated by T cells. These T cells act regardless of the antibody specificity of the B cell clones (i.e. they are not clonally restricted), by elaboration of BCDFs (Bergstedt-Lindqvist et al. 1984), or possibly by direct contact with the B cells.

Although activation by antigen may occur without the need for T cell help in the case of T cell independent antigens (TI antigens), both T cell-dependent (TD) and

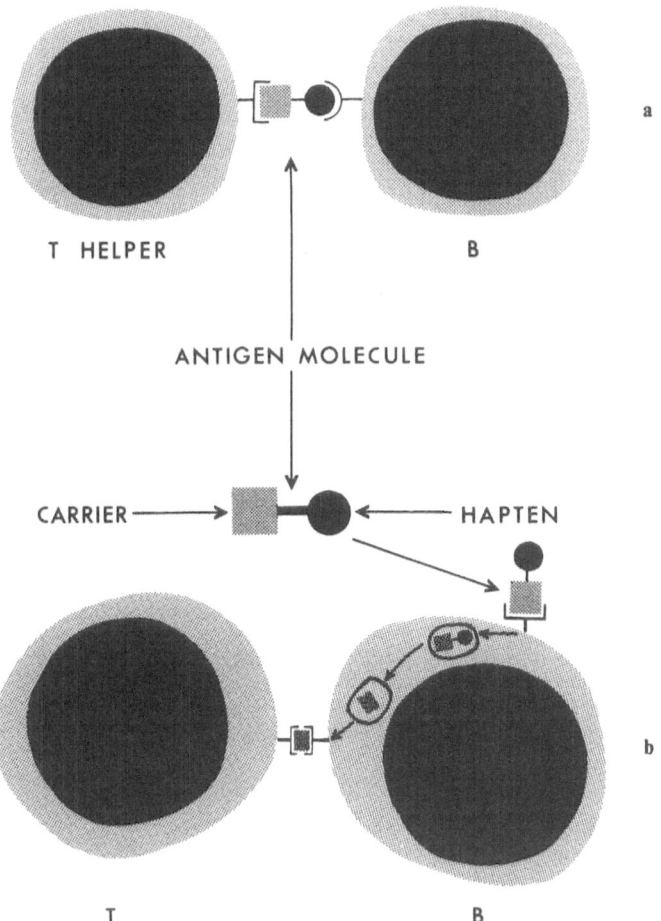

Fig. 12.1a,b. Two types of T–B interaction through antigen. **a** Linked recognition. For activation of B cells by a strongly antigenic epitope on a large protein, corresponding to a hapten on a carrier molecule, the B cell may bind the hapten through its sIg receptor and the T cell receptor binds specifically to an epitope on the carrier, forming an antigen bridge. The T cell may need to be activated first by an AC presenting the carrier antigen to it in association with a MHC class II product. **b** B cells can take up antigen specifically, i.e. through sIg receptors, and degrade it enzymatically. Fragments of antigen (bearing either the hapten or the carrier epitopes) can then be presented to T cells in association with a MHC class II product.

TI B cell responses require ACs. Some cellular interactions in B cell activation are illustrated in Fig. 12.2. Studies of single hapten-specific B cells (Nossal and Pike 1984) have shown that antigens can be classified into at least four categories:

1. Antigens that cannot trigger the B cell without T cell help, even when B cell growth factors are present

2. Antigens that can only stimulate B cells when BCGFs are present

3. Antigens partially dependent on exogenous BCGFs

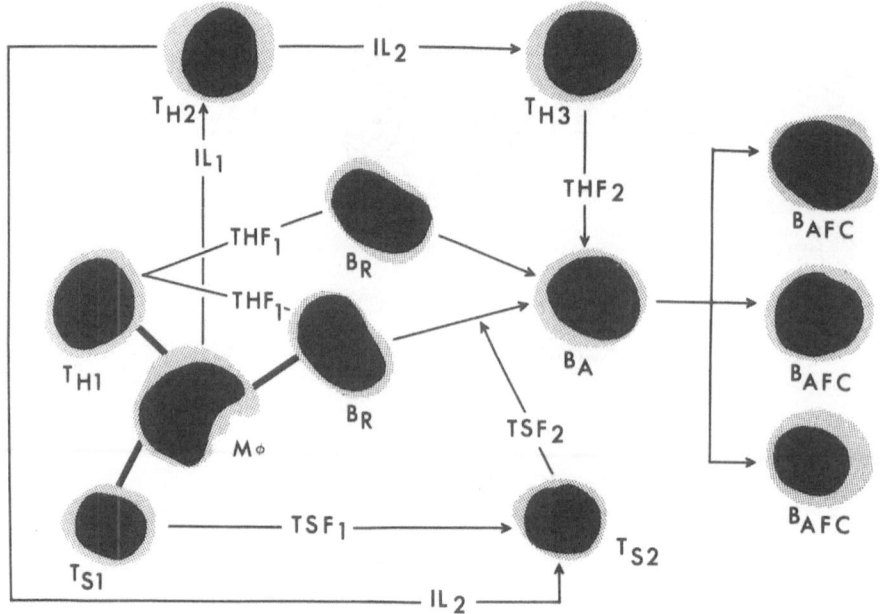

Fig. 12.2. Activation of B cells. A helper T cell (T_{H1}) is activated by an antigen-presenting macrophage (M_ϕ). A resting B cell (B_R) contacts this activated T cell through an antigen-MHC class II product bridge, receiving a chemical signal (THF_1), becoming an activated B cell (B_A). Two other sorts of helper T cell are depicted. T_{H2} is activated by IL-1 from the activated antigen-presenting macrophage to produce IL-2, which is necessary for the proliferation of both helper and suppressor T cells. T_{H3} produces a second lymphokine (THF_2). The reaction is influenced by two sets of suppressor T cells (T_{S1} and T_{S2}), producing T suppressor factors TSF_1, TSF_2. The response of the B cell may be modified by interaction with the antigen-presenting macrophage through an antigen-MHC class II product bridge. The end result of activation is differentiation of B cells to antibody forming cells (B_{AFC}).

4. Antigens that stimulate highly efficient B cell responses without the presence either of specific helper T cells or T-cell derived, antigen-non-specific factors. TI antigens are also PBAs, i.e. they activate B cells other than those with specific receptor for the antigenic epitope in the PBA. TI antigens are usually polymeric and are resistant to enzymatic degradation. The response is relatively weak and does not switch to IgG production.

Mitogens activate B cells polyclonally by binding to key molecules on the B cell surface. Some mitogens have to interact with ACs and/or T cells to induce B cell activation (Bruszewski et al. 1984). *Nocardia* water-soluble mitogen (Brochier et al. 1976), formaldehyde-killed *Salmonella paratyphi B* (Chen et al. 1981), antibody to β_2-microglobulin and *Staphylococcus aureus* Cowan strain (SAC) are TI B cell mitogens acting directly on human B lymphocytes. B cell mitogenesis by phyto-haemagglutinin (PHA) and pokeweed mitogen (PWM) requires T cells. Epstein–Barr virus (EBV) is another polyclonal B cell activator (Rosen et al. 1977), which can also "immortalise" B cells in vitro, i.e. they can go on replicating indefinitely. EBV enters B cells via the CR2 (C3b) receptor, recognised by CD21 antibodies.

B cells may also be activated by CD20 antibodies (Clark et al. 1985) without the need for T cells, but the activation is augmented by T cell factors. CD20 may be a key molecule in triggering of B cell activation. Conversely, antibodies to class II products inhibit the proliferation of small, resting B cells in response to any stimulus, but activated B cells are not affected (Clement and Tedder 1985).

Accessory Cells in B Cell Activation

Debate continues as to whether ACs are always necessary for B cell growth and maturation (Persson et al. 1977, 1978; Rosenberg and Lipsky 1981, 1982; Biozzi et al. 1984; Corbel and Melchers 1984). Responses in vitro which have been shown to require ACs are set out in Table 12.1. ACs promote the numbers and effector functions of helper T cells by secreting growth and maturation factors. Significant B cell responses are detected upon interaction with primed helper T cells under conditions of extreme macrophage depletion. However, the problem is that it is almost impossible to remove macrophages from most preparations of lymphoid cells.

ACs control the amount of antigen and process it. They activate T cells, which then activate B cells, or they may secrete inhibitory molecules, including prostaglandins E_1 and E_2, which suppress the production of interleukin 2 (IL-2), as well as cytokines affecting cells of other lineages (Fig. 12.3). Monocytes can suppress B cell responses in vitro if present in excess. Class II MHC molecules are usually necessary on macrophages for activation of B cells. However, macrophages in the marginal zone of lymphoid follicles apparently activate B cells despite the fact that they lack class II MHC products, by forming a bond to B cells through antigen-antibody-complement complexes via Fc or C3 receptors.

ACs are necessary for the activation of B cells by TI antigens, by soluble antigen and by plant lectins. Interleukin 1 (IL-1) is an essential factor in this process for most lectins, but not for activation by PWM. Macrophages bind and present mitogens to T cells and are effective even when they differ from the T cells in their class II MHC expression, i.e. they are not MHC-restricted in this activity. The stimulatory function of antigen-presenting cells (APCs) is radioresistant. Histocompatible ACs have been found necessary for B cell activation by antigen-specific helper factors.

The T cell signal generated in the presence of IL-1 is relatively weak, and can be enhanced by a third component, a thiol-reducing agent such as 2-mercaptoethanol

Table 12.1. Responses in vitro requiring ACs

Response	Requirement	Reference
PWM-induced lymphocyte proliferation.	Intact ACs, syngeneic or allogeneic	Rosenberg and Lipsky (1981)
PWM-induced B lymphocyte differentiation to Ig-secreting cells	Intact ACs, + IL-1	Rosenberg and Lipsky (1982)
TD proliferative responses to soluble antigens	Intact ACs?	Alpert et al. (1981) Bruszewski et al (1984)
B responses to dextran sulphate	Intact ACs or 2 ME	Persson et al. (1977, 1978)

2 ME, 2 mercaptoethanol.

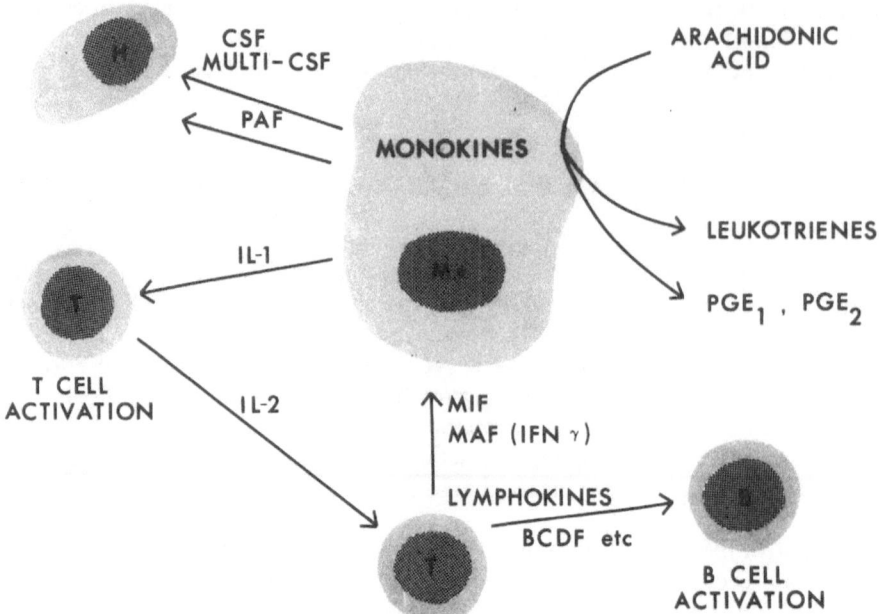

Fig. 12.3. Regulation of cellular activity by macrophages. Macrophages (M_ϕ) produce a wide range of short-range factors (monokines) affecting the activity of lymphoid (T and B) and blood cells (H). Amongst these are leukotrienes and prostaglandins (PGE_1, PGE_2), the latter inhibiting B cell activation. *PAF*, platelet activating factor; *CSF*, colony-stimulating factor. CSF and *multi-CSF* are growth factors for macrophages and granulocytes. Interleukin 1 (*IL-1*) and antigen (not shown) initiate activation of T cells, resulting in production of interleukin 2 (*IL-2*), inducing further steps in T cell activation and necessary for production of lymphokines. *MIF*, migration inhibitory factor; *MAF*, macrophage activating factor = *IFN$_\gamma$*, acting back on macrophages; *BCDF*, B cell differentiation factor. Macrophages are necessary for activation of B cells by T-dependent antigens and facilitate B cell activation by all classes of antigen.

(2 ME). Thiols are adjuvants in many immune responses in vitro, such as activation of B cells by agents which cross-link sIg. Their action is poorly understood. Macrophages secrete thiols, such as cysteine, which evidently play a part in their function. For example, they enhance the activation of lymphocytes when the proportion of macrophages is severely reduced, but not when they are absent. 2 ME will not replace macrophages essential for PHA-induced activation of T cells, but acts synergistically with IL-1. 2 ME-treated fetal calf serum has properties similar to 2 ME itself (Opitz et al. 1977). Many B cell tumour lines will not grow without 2 ME; conversely, a requirement for 2 ME is a strong indication of the lymphoid origin of a cell line.

B Cell Activation by Cross-linking Immunoglobulin

Because of the relative rarity of B cells specific for any particular antigen in most lymphoid populations, much of the understanding of B cell activation has come through the use of PBA. The signal induced by cross-linking of sIg by anti-immunoglobulin antibody or by SAC is presumed to reproduce the signal engendered by antigen. Anti-Ig stimulates rabbit B cells to proliferate; 2 ME must also be present for anti-Ig antibodies to induce proliferation of human B cells (Sieckmann et al. 1978; Sidman and Unanue 1978). A pulse of anti-Ig induces, in general, one round of proliferation. Anti-Ig is needed directly after mitosis for daughter cells to be excited. Excitation leads to the appearance of receptors for BCGFs and for transferrin.

Results with anti-Ig in human systems have been variable and controversial, probably because of the various types of anti-Ig antibodies used and the differing cellular requirements for activation. Low concentrations of anti-μ antibody (10 μg/ml) result in little or no proliferation, but activate B cells to a state of responsiveness in the G_1 phase to cytokines produced by T cells and macrophages. Anti-μ must be present in culture for a prolonged period for progression to the S phase, and removal terminates the activation process.

Besides the activating effects, both anti-μ and anti-δ can have suppressive effects on B lymphocytes in vitro. Anti-μ and anti-isotype antibodies may have a profound inhibitory effect on mitogen-induced maturation and proliferation of B cells induced by bacterial lipopolysaccharide, whereas anti-δ antibodies can enhance such responses.

Fetal and newborn B lymphocytes are very sensitive to the inhibitory effect of anti-Ig. Tolerance follows treatment of newborn mice with antigen and anti-μ antibodies, because of the destruction of specific clones ("clonal abortion"). Anti-μ antibodies do not influence the generation of pre-B cells. Anti-idiotype antibodies induce B lymphocytes to secrete specific antibody in the absence of antigen and T lymphocytes, if the B lymphocytes are obtained from mice previously primed in vivo with the antigen.

Staph. aureus Cowan strain 1 binds to the Fc as well as the Fab portion of sIg, inducing B cell proliferation and high numbers of immunoglobulin-secreting cells. Under some conditions SAC induces Ig secretion without the help of T cells or ACs. SAC-stimulated B cells do not require BCDFs for maximal generation of immunoglobulin-secreting cells until 48 or 72 h after stimulation, whereas cells activated by PWM need BCDFs from the beginning. Conflicting reports concerning the requirement for T cell factors to induce Ig secretion after SAC, as with anti-Ig stimulation, are probably explained by the variation in strength of the original stimulus through the Ig receptor.

Staphylococcal protein A (SPA), itself a B cell mitogen and polyclonal B cell activator of antibody synthesis for human lymphocytes (Scouros et al. 1983), requires T cell help. Although it binds to the Fc segment on Ig molecules, it acts through a separate site on the membrane as a polyclonal B cell activator. Reviews of B cell activation by agents cross-linking sIg are found in Cooper et al. (1980), DeFranco et al. (1982), Fauci and Ballieux (1982) and Fauci (1983).

Soluble Factors in B Cell Activation

Cytokines, soluble cell products influencing cells of the immune system, offer new therapeutic possibilities. Many are well characterised only in murine systems. A

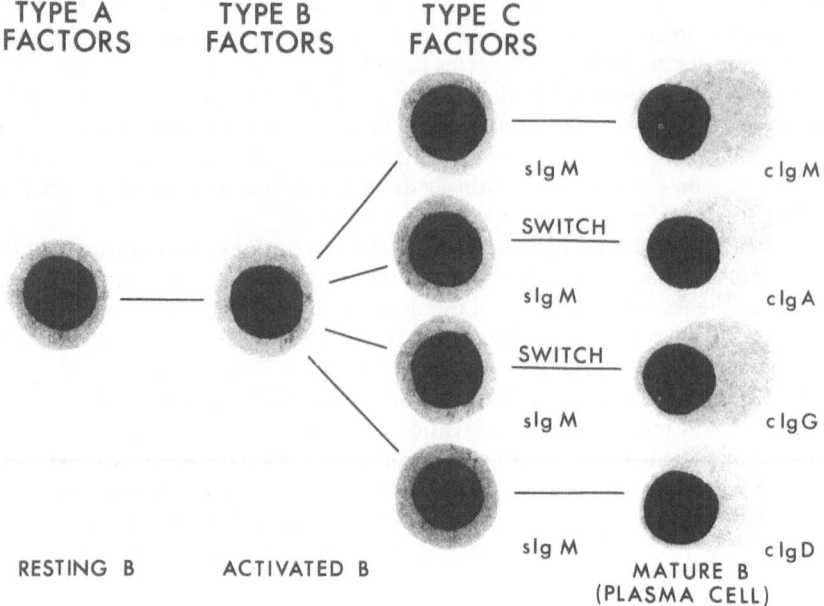

TYPE A
FACTORS

TYPE B
FACTORS

TYPE C
FACTORS

s Ig M

c Ig M

SWITCH

s Ig M

c Ig A

SWITCH

s Ig M

c Ig G

s Ig M

c Ig D

RESTING B   ACTIVATED B   MATURE B
(PLASMA CELL)

Fig. 12.4. Soluble factors in B cell activation. Type A factors act on virgin or resting B cells. Type B factors, acting on B cell blasts are necessary for proliferation. Type C factors induce secretion of immunoglobulin by cells already in cycle. They may be isotype-non-specific, or they may induce a switch to production of a particular immunoglobulin isotype.

number of these powerful, short-range-acting substances have been purified and some are being synthesised. Clinical trials are in progress with some (e.g. thymic cytokines and IL-2) for manipulation of immunological responsiveness. Many will be produced by recombinant gene technology in the near future and will become available for clinical use. At this stage there is a lack of conformity in the description of the factors involved in B cell maturation and differentiation because of the use of different assay systems.

Growth- and maturation-inducing factors acting on B lymphocytes may be classified into types A, B and C (Fig. 12.4):

Type A factors act on resting or virgin B cells.

Type B factors (BCGFs) stimulate proliferation of B cell blasts, after they have been induced into cycle.

Type C factors (BCDFs) induce the secretion of immunoglobulin by cells already in cycle. Factors involved in the activation of B cells have been reviewed by Howard and Paul (1983), Howard et al. (1984), Muraguchi et al. (1984) and Mayer et al. (1984).

Type A Factors

Type A factors (BMF, $BCDF_\mu$, BCPF, BCSF) have been described as acting on virgin or resting B cells to drive them through to the antibody-forming stage, without the addition of antigen, mitogen, anti-Ig or other non-specific B cell triggering agent. Resting B cells are thought to respond to factors of this type by differentiating without replication, whereas cells which are already excited are stimulated both to proliferate and differentiate. There is some doubt that truly quiescent cells can respond to such factors without first receiving a signal from helper T cells.

Antigen-specific soluble helper factors reported to induce the proliferation and differentiation of clones to produce a specific antibody (Webb 1983) have been produced by murine spleen cells primed in vitro, cloned murine helper T cells and T cell hybridomas. They may react with antisera specific for V_H-framework determinants. Many also react with anti-idiotype-specific antisera.

Antigen specific T cell suppressor factors have also been reported. It has been suggested that virtually every type of immune response results in the generation of suppressor T cells that may release antigen-specific T suppressor factors. T suppressor factors may also be idiotype specific. Some also react with antisera to MHC class II products. While such factors would undoubtedly be important in the control of immune responses, it is too early to be sure if they exist, or to present a clear account of them.

Type B Factors (BCGFs)

IL-1 is the only well-characterised α (macrophage-derived) factor acting on B lymphocytes. Originally known as lymphocyte activating factor (LAF) and as endogenous pyrogen, IL-1 is a strongly hydrophobic 15–20 kD protein. Two human genes encoding IL-1, α and β, have been cloned (review by Oppenheim et al. 1986). Either IL-1 or similar monokines stimulate the release of acute phase reactants (C-reactive protein, α-1-antitrypsin, serum amyloid A protein) from the liver, and prostaglandins from synovial cells and fibroblasts. These compounds induce fever, perhaps through prostaglandins acting on the hypothalamus, and stimulate the production of plasminogen activator. IL-1 also stimulates the growth of fibroblasts and the breakdown of muscle. IL-1 is thought to induce polyclonal B cell proliferation, by acting in the late G_1 phase. It does not induce Ig synthesis. It has a less potent effect on human than on murine B cells.

Molecules of the IL-1 family are also produced by the monocyte line P388D$_1$, by epidermal keratinocytes, antigen-presenting dendritic cells, tumour cells and fibroblasts. In fact, virtually every cell type produces molecules with IL-1-type activity (Oppenheim et al. 1986).

IL-2, (formerly known as T cell growth factor, TCGF), allows helper and suppressor T cells and natural killer (NK) cells to grow in vitro (Miedema and Melief 1985). It shows no homology to known oncogene products or other haematopoietic regulators. DNA which codes for IL-2 has been cloned and the protein sequence has been derived from it. It has 133 amino acids. It is produced by most activated CD4+ and some CD8+ T cells. The mouse EL-4 lymphoma is a commonly used source of IL-2.

IL-2 plays at least two roles in B cell immune responses. Secretion of IL-2 by activated T cells induces proliferation of other T cells, which release IL-2 and BCGFs. IL-2 also acts directly on B cells. Both resting B and T cells have a few hundred IL-2 receptors per cell, the number increasing many times on activation, so that activated lymphocytes can be stimulated by IL-2. IL-2 stimulates colony formation by chronic lymphocytic leukaemia (CLL) B cells (Touw and Lowenberg 1985).

BCGF I, a weakly hydrophobic glycoprotein of 15–18 Kd under reducing conditions, 50–60 kD under non-reducing conditions, induces MHC class II expression and primes murine B cells for proliferation. Sources are murine T lymphocytes and the EL-4 T murine cell line. Similar lymphokines are produced by the Jurkat human T cell lymphoma and human T cell hybridomas. *BCGF II* appears to be the same as BCGF I.

Complement, in the form of cross-linked C3d, is reported to replace macrophage-derived α factors acting late in G_1, allowing entry into the S phase. Soluble C3d inhibits the action of α factors (Melchers et al. 1985). Complement deficiencies have long been associated with impairment of antibody responses.

Type C Factors (BCDFs)

Type C factors were originally called T cell replacing factors (TRFs). Many have been described, e.g. BCSF, BCDF I, BCDF II, BCDFμ, BIF and BRMF. It is not known whether some or all of them are the same, or substantially the same.

BCDF is obtained from activated T lymphocytes and a T cell hybridoma. BCDF from EL-4 T cell line is a hydrophobic glycoprotein of 30–40 kD with similar actions. BCDFs inducing a specific isotype, e.g. IgA or IgG1, have also been described.

Findings with factors like BMF (Sidman et al. 1984), which has been reported to act on both resting and activated B cells, make it hard to sustain the neat distinction between factors which act on resting B cells and those which act only on activated B cells.

Transferrin

Transferrin is a permissive factor which is absolutely required by normal and malignant lymphoid cells for proliferation, but does not induce further differentiation. The transferrin receptor is induced by specific growth factors binding to their respective receptors earlier in G_1 (Neckers 1984). When cells are exposed to interferon-α the expression of transferrin receptors is inhibited. This is considered to be one of the mechanisms by which interferon inhibits growth (Besancon et al. 1985). Expression of transferrin receptors in transformed malignant B cell lines (Raji, Daudi) is not dependent on cell cycle (i.e. they are expressed constitutively). These cells have no extrinsic requirement for growth factors, but are dependent on transferrin.

Interferon

Interferons are a group of proteins produced by a wide range of cells. Interferons are synthesised in response to infection by a virus, thus conferring resistance to a second viral infection.

There are three major types of interferon; IFN_α, IFN_β and IFN_γ. IFN_α used to be called leucocyte IFN. IFN_β was known as fibroblast interferon and the two together were named type I interferon. Type II interferon, produced by stimulated lymphocytes, is now known as IFN_γ. IFN_α and IFN_β are 166 amino acids long. IFN_γ has 146 amino acids. There are 10 or more fairly homologous genes for IFN_α on chromosome 9, having 80%–90% homology of their base sequences. One gene for IFN_β has been assigned to chromosome 9, which has 40%–50% homology with the IFN_α genes. However, there are many species of mRNA for IFN_β, suggesting that there is also a multigene β family. IFN_γ is not homologous with α and β interferons. There are slight differences between the products from cells and those produced by recombinant DNA technology. IFN_α and IFN_β share a common receptor, which is distinct from the receptor for IFN_γ. The effects of the three types on cells are the same, in general.

Macrophages produce IFN_α and IFN_β, as do cells from many other tissues, and T cells produce IFN_γ. Cycling T cell lines can produce IFN_γ without macrophages, whereas T cells from peripheral blood require, as well as a stimulus, the presence of macrophages. PHA, other mitogens and the mixed lymphocyte reaction (MLR) stimulate T cells to produce IFN_γ. 12-O-tetradecanoylphorbol-13-acetate (TPA) is also a powerful inducer and is strongly synergistic with phytohaemagglutinin (PHA). Various viruses and bacteria, double-stranded RNA, polyinosinic: polycytidylic acid (poly:IC) and bacterial products as well as certain simpler chemicals, induce interferon production. IFN_α and IFN_β production are induced within 4–6 h of viral stimulation, whereas IFN_γ is produced within 2–3 days.

Interferons act on cells and change biochemical functions in a way that makes virus replication no longer possible. A number of enzymes are induced, including one that generates oligoadenylates from ATP and a protein kinase that inhibits viral protein synthesis. However, there are many points of action. Interferons generally exert an antiproliferative effect; they inhibit mitogen-induced T cell proliferation and inhibit the plaque-forming response in vitro of B lymphocytes to antigens; they prolong all phases of the cell cycle. In addition, they may modify the phenotype of malignant cells, for example in melanoma cells by reducing the expression of melanoma antigens. IFN_α induces proliferation and differentiation of CLL B cells (Robèrt et al. 1985). Regression of tumours in some experimental tumours in vivo has aroused considerable interest in the therapeutic potential of interferon.

All interferons activate NK cells and macrophages. They cause enhanced expression of a variety of cell surface molecules, including β_2-microglobulin, MHC classes I and II products and Fc receptors. Pure interferons alone do not activate resting lymphocytes, but appear either to inhibit or enhance the activation of resting B cells, although the conditions for enhancement and inhibition have not been defined. Interferons are well reviewed by Kirchner (1984).

Other Factors

Lymphokines have been described which cannot easily be fitted, at this stage, into an ordered schema of lymphocyte differentiation. These include soluble immune response suppressor (SIRS), allogeneic effector factor (AEF) and various lymphotoxins. SIRS, a product of suppressor T cells, non-specifically inhibits B cell proliferation and antibody responses by an action on macrophages. Many other T lymphocyte factors may influence B cell activation by their effect on macrophage function, such as migration inhibition factor (MIF) and macrophage activation factor (MAF), which is possibly the same as IFN_γ. Leucocyte inhibitory factor (LIF), produced by both T and B lymphocytes, inhibits the random migration of polymorphonuclear leucocytes and enhances their phagocytic activity. Tumour necrosis factor (TNF) is discussed in Chapter 20 (see p. 353). Other lymphokines induce macrophages to release monokines that appear to suppress all kinds of immune responses. Lymphotoxins are produced by activated T and B cells. They lyse susceptible target cell lines. A lymphokine, named variously B-cell-derived enhancing factor (BEF), interleukin B or interleukin B4, has recently been described (reviewed by del Guercio et al. 1986). This factor, which is produced by B cells, enhances antibody responses in vitro and in vivo. It is proposed to act by preventing the differentiation of suppressor T cells.

Cellular Events in B Lymphocyte Activation

The biochemical processes involved in lymphocyte activation have been studied intensively in recent years (Wedner 1984; Cambier et al. 1985). A knowledge of these processes could be used to control malignant lymphocytes by enhancing immune responses against them or inhibiting their growth. Activation processes in lymphocytes have many features in common with those initiated in other cells by phorbol esters and growth factors.

Upon receipt of the first activation signal the phosphatidylinositol (PI) cycle is activated (Coggeshall and Cambier 1985) and protein kinases, particularly PKC but also cyclic-nucleotide-dependent protein kinases, are activated. Intracellular Ca^{2+} rises and there is a rise in intracellular pH. Ion channels are affected, resulting in a net efflux of H^+ ions and an influx of Ca^{2+}. The changes in T cells are similar (Imboden and Stobo 1985). Some polyclonal activators and phorbol esters activate protein kinase C but do not cause a rise in intracellular Ca^{2+}. The latter responses are inhibited by cyclosporin (Klaus and Chisholm 1986). The magnesium-stimulated, Na^+- and K^+-dependent adenosine triphosphatase (ATPase) and other ATPases of the plasma membrane generate and maintain the membrane gradients for K^+ and Na^+. The transport of glucose and amino acids is enhanced.

Some biochemical changes have been described that occur early in the membrane in response to an activating signal. The enzyme acetyl-coA:lysolecithin acyl-transferase (Resch and Ferber 1977) exchanges saturated for more unsaturated fatty acyl side chains of membrane phospholipids. Conversion of phosphatidylethanolamine to phosphatidylcholine by transmethylases I and II in the membrane results in phospholipids of the inner membrane translocating to the outer leaflet. BCDF induces phospholipid methylation and activation of serine esterase (Kishi et al. 1983).

Depolarisation, i.e. decrease of membrane potential, analogous to neuronal depolarisation, starts within minutes of an activating stimulus such as TPA and lasts 2–3 h (Monroe and Cambier 1983a). Repolarisation occurs over the next 7 h and is followed by a hyperpolarisation phase lasting 25–58 h. Depolarisation is monitored by decreased uptake of a carbocyanin dye $DiOC_5$ (discussed in Cambier et al. 1985).

When multivalent ligands bind to surface molecules, cell motility is induced and the ligand-receptor complexes aggregate as "patches" and then polar "caps". Ultimately the complexes are shed or endocytosed, and subsequently new receptors appear. After activation by SAC or anti-μ, detectable increases in cell size occur within 8 h, RNA synthesis is enhanced within 8 h and 50%–80% of resting B cells enlarge during the first 36 h. Increased expression of MHC class II product is detectable within 6–8 h of stimulation. The receptor for BCGF is expressed within the first few hours (Cooper 1985). After 8 h, enhanced RNA synthesis is stimulated by BCGF. DNA synthesis begins after 36 h in human B cells stimulated by high dose SAC or anti-μ. The surface protein 4F2 (see Table 8.5, p. 96) and transferrin receptor are not present on resting B cells. 4F2 is expressed during blast transformation (G_0 to early G_1), after which the B cell is responsive to BCGF. The transferrin receptor is expressed after BCGF has interacted with the cell. Similarly, receptors for calcitriol (1,25 dihydroxyvitamin D_3) are absent from resting B and T cells. Activation of normal T and B cells by mitogens and EBV causes expression of calcitriol receptors. Such receptors are also present on malignant T and B lines (Provvedini et al. 1983).

IL-1, IL-2 and IFN_γ or IFN_α do not enhance expression of MHC class II molecules by human B cells until the B cells have received an inducing stimulus. The density of MHC class II antigen on the murine B cell membrane increases fourfold during transition from G_0 to G_1, and rapidly decreases in the S and G_2 phases (Monroe and Cambier 1983b).

Bacterial lipopolysaccharide (LPS) binds to lymphocytes in less than 2 h and lymphocyte responses are initiated in the next 2–10 h (Morrison and Rudbach 1981). The earliest time at which DNA synthesis or immunoglobulin secretion can be detected is 16–24 h. Surface immunoglobulin disappears within 20 min of LPS stimulation of B cells, and appears in markedly greater concentrations as the B lymphocyte begins to proliferate. The addition of mitogens to lymphocytes is followed by stimulation of protein synthesis, within a period too short to involve the transcription of new mRNA. A large pool of stable inactive mRNA exists in quiescent lymphocytes.

The part played by the cyclic nucleotides in lymphocyte activation is still not clear. cAMP inhibits the proliferation of a variety of cells, including human lymphocytes. Elevation of cGMP levels, or an increase in cGMP:cAMP ratio may lead to, or favour cell proliferation.

The cytoskeleton is involved in the movement of surface receptors and in cell–cell interactions. Lattice microfilaments, composed of actin and myosin, are closely associated with the plasma membrane, forming a filamentous network. Stress microfilaments (actin cables) form a network of tight bundles running immediately beneath the inner surface of the plasma membrane. Microtubules, composed of tubulin, form a cytoplasmic network not directly connected to the plasma membrane. Cytochalasin B disrupts the lattice microfilaments, inhibiting lymphocyte movement. Cytochalasin B also inhibits blastic transformation. However, this may be an indirect effect, through inhibition of the function of ACs or suppressor T cells. Colchicine causes disaggregation of microtubules. It does not prevent the early metabolic response to antigen, but inhibits transition to the S phase.

The end result of transduction of an effective signal from an antigen or mitogen is regulation of the activity of genes, i.e. activation and inhibition of gene transcription. A number of oncogenes are among the genes activated by signals transmitted from the cell surface. Some of them encode proteins acting in the nucleus. Several changes in DNA and chromatin are associated with the activation of a gene. One is a change in the extent of methylation of cytosine bases in DNA. In general, the DNA of inactive genes is more heavily methylated than the DNA of active genes. The methylation pattern is passed on to daughter cells, so that genes that were active in the parent cell are active in its progeny. Certain proteins bind to active genes; these are named high motility group (HMG) proteins 14 and 17. Some chemical carcinogens are thought to inhibit the normal methylation process.

Phorbol esters have become potent tools in the research on normal and malignant lymphocytes, as they activate lymphocytes and induce differentiation, thereby helping to reveal the sequence of expression of phenotypic markers during differentiation. They also stimulate the secretion of lymphocyte products.

Normal peripheral blood and tonsil B lymphocytes, and leukaemic human B lymphocytes differentiate following TPA stimulation. The cytoplasm increases, becomes basic and vacuolated, and the nucleus becomes prominent. The cells resemble early plasma cells after 3 days, but fail to develop to fully mature plasmacytes, possibly because TPA inhibits microtubule formation.

After exposure to active phorbol esters, B lymphocytes undergo the maturation sequence MER+, R2+ →MER−, R2+ →MER− R2− (Forbes et al. 1982). Within 1 h the cells change to the MER−, R2+ phenotype and over the next 96 h there is a gradual conversion to the MER−, R2− stage. Cytoplasmic Ig appears at 12 h and steadily increases; sIg decreases (particularly sIgD). MHC class II antigens increase and persist at 96 h. B cells acquire receptors for complement (CR) in the process. Fc_γ receptors have mostly gone by 24 h while Fc_μ, CR and sIg are prominent at 24 h, but absent at 72–96 h. There is also a reduction or loss of the CD20 antigen and usually of CD21, when present. The phenotype which develops in response to TPA resembles that of hairy cell leukaemia. The sequence of events induced by PWM is different; Ig secretion begins only after the peak of DNA synthesis in PWM-stimulated B cells. It is unclear whether T cells are necessary for Ig production in TPA-stimulated cultures.

TPA induces expression of the the T cell antigen CD5 in normal and some malignant B lymphocytes (Miller and Gralow 1984). Whether this represents expression appropriate to a particular stage of differentiation, or "lineage infidelity", i.e. aberrant expression of a gene that is normally expressed by cells of a different lineage, is unknown. CD5 antigen is normally expressed by a small subset of B lymphocytes in lymph nodes and spleen. TPA is about 10% as mitogenic for human peripheral blood lymphocytes as optimal concentrations of Con A and is synergistic with the calcium ionophore A23187. TPA acts synergistically with PHA or Con A to induce proliferation of macrophage-depleted peripheral lymphocytes and enhances stimulation by CLL cells in the MLR, which is otherwise poor.

Pretreatment with TPA generally inhibits responses to lectins, LPS, anti-Ig and PBA. It is interesting that TPA inhibits mitosis of mouse lymphocytes, although it induces some changes, e.g. membrane depolarisation and increased class II MHC expression, associated with activation in these cell (Mond et al. 1981).

Phorbol esters may increase the cytotoxic activity of NK cells and antigen-specific cytotoxic lymphocytes (CTLs). They may either stimulate or inhibit the generation of CTLs in mixed lymphocyte culture. Phorbol esters increase phospholipid metabolism in lymphocytes and stimulate phosphorylation of the same protein substrates (p64 and p58 in B, p61 and p55 in T), as do other mitogens and anti-Ig, within 5 min of exposure (Earp et al. 1984). Many other enzymes are activated.

TPA induces, alone or synergistically with mitogens, production of various soluble mediators and lymphokines including IFN, IL-1 and IL-2. TPA is synergistic with PHA but cannot replace it as a stimulus for IL-2 production (Frank et al. 1981).

Low concentrations of TPA reversibly inhibit macrophage migration (Pick et al. 1982), an effect associated with an increase in the amount of tubulin present in polymeric form. This effect is prevented by colchicine. Other effects of TPA are production of plasminogen activator, prostaglandin release, enhancement of pinocytosis, induction of oxygen burst and increases in non-specific esterase and acid phosphatase. Macrophage-mediated tumour lysis may be inhibited by TPA (Baxter et al. 1982), although phagocytosis by macrophages may be stimulated. The addition of monocytes augments DNA synthesis by purified T cells stimulated by PHA (Sugawara and Ishizaka 1983).

TPA enhances the capping of various receptors and membrane molecules, including CD2 antigen and Con A receptor. The effect is dependent on energy and temperature, and requires functional microfilaments. It decreases membrane viscosity, an effect blocked by retinoic acid. It increases the uptake of deoxyglucose and aminoisobutyric acid (analogues of glucose and amino acids).

Conclusions

The term "activation" describes the process by which quiescent B cells are induced to proliferate and differentiate to mature plasma cells. The exquisite complexity of the cellular interactions involved in activation is evidently necessary to ensure the strictest control over a process that could, if uncontrolled, have dire consequences for the host. The capacity of cells to interact is governed by strict requirements for compatibility of expression of products of the MHC. The mechanism contains checks and balances that allow immune responses to be generated against foreign living matter while inhibiting responses against very similar molecules of the host's own tissues. The philosophical considerations are well reviewed by Forni (1985). This mechanism must also be controlled according to the persistence of the foreign invasion. Once the threat is over, the response must be turned off, but kept in a state of readiness for a subsequent quick response.

Activation of B cells takes place in two or more steps. The B cell must usually receive an antigen-driven first signal from a helper T cell. As a result of the first signal the B cell expresses receptors for factors which stimulate further steps in the process. ACs are generally necessary in the complex interactions between themselves and T and B lymphocytes. Identification of the cytokines which drive and inhibit B cell activation is leading to an understanding of disorders of lymphoid tissue and the development of new biological agents for the treatment of a wide range of human diseases.

As cellular processes involved in B cell activation are unravelled, a pattern is revealed that has much in common with events resulting from stimulation of target cells by hormones and growth factors. A stimulus that is successful in activating B cells leads to activation of the genome. The genes involved are members of the "competence" family, which contains the cellular oncogenes. The result is orderly expression of genes encoding proteins necessary for proliferation and differentiation.

References

Alpert SD, Jonsen ME, Broff MD, Schneeberger E, Geha RS (1981) Macrophage T-cell interaction in man: handling of tetanus toxoid antigen by human monocytes. J Clin Immunol 1: 21–29

Baxter CS, Fish L, Ferguson TA, Michael J, Bash J (1982) Effects of tumor-promoting agents on cells of the murine immune system: inhibition of antibody synthesis and of macrophage-mediated tumor cell cytotoxicity In: Hecker E et al. (eds) Carcinogenesis, vol 7. Raven, New York, pp 637–642

Bergstedt-Lindqvist S, Sideras P, MacDonald HR, Severinson E (1984) Regulation of Ig class secretion by soluble products of certain T-cell lines. Immunol Rev 78: 25–50

Besancon F, Bourgeade MF, Testa U (1985) Inhibition of transferrin receptor expression by interferon-alpha in human lymphoblastoid cells and mitogen-induced lymphocytes. J Biol Chem 260: 13074–13080

Biozzi G, Mouton D, Stiffel C, Bouthillier Y (1984) A major role of the macrophage in quantitative genetic regulation of immunoresponsiveness and antiinfectious immunity. Adv Immunol 36: 189–234

Brochier J, Bona C, Ciorbaru R, Revillard J-P, Chedid L (1976) A human T-independent B lymphocyte mitogen extracted from *Nocardia opaca*. J Immunol 117: 1434–1439

Brock JH, de Sousa M (1986) Immunoregulation by iron-binding proteins. Immunol Today 7: 30–31

Bruszewski WB, Bruszewski JA, Tonnu H, Ferezy SL, O'Brien RL, Parker JW (1984) Early mitogen-induced metabolic events essential to proliferation of human T lymphocytes: dependence of specific events on the influence of adherent accessory cells. J Immunol 132: 2837–2843

Cambier JC, Monroe JG, Coggeshall KM, Ransom JT (1985) The biochemical basis of transmembrane signalling by B lymphocyte surface immunoglobulin. Immunol Today 6: 218–222

Chen W-H, Munoz J, Fudenberg HH, Tung E, Virella G (1981) Polyclonal activation of human peripheral blood B lymphocytes by formaldehyde-fixed *Salmonella paratyphi* B. J Exp Med 153: 365–374

Clark EA, Shu G, Ledbetter JA (1985) Role of the Bp35 cell surface polypeptide on human B-cell activation. Proc Natl Acad Sci USA 82: 1766–1770

Clement LT, Tedder TF (1985) Antibodies reactive with class I antigens of the major histocompatibility complex (MHC) inhibit B cell activation. Fed Proc 44: 974

Coggeshall KM, Cambier JC (1985) B cell activation VI. Effects of exogenous diglyceride and modulators of phospholipid metabolism suggest a central role for diacylglycerol generation in transmembrane signalling by mIg. J Immunol 134: 101–107

Cooper MD (1985) In: Melchers F, Potter M (eds) Mechanisms of B cell neoplasia 1985. Editiones Roche, Basle, p 55

Cooper MD, Kearney JF, Gathings WE, Lawton AR (1980) Effects of anti-Ig antibodies on the development and differentiation of B cells. Immunol Rev 52: 29–53

Corbel C, Melchers F (1984) The synergism of accessory cells and of soluble alpha-factors derived from them in the activation of B cells to proliferation. Immunol Rev 78: 51–74

Coutinho A, Pobor G, Petterson S et al. (1984) T cell-dependent B cell activation. Immunol Rev 78: 211–224

DeFranco AL, Kung JT, Paul WE (1982) Regulation of growth and proliferation in B cell subpopulations. Immunol Rev 64: 161–182

del Guercio PD, Marcelletti JF, Katz DH (1986) B-cell lymphokines and activation of the immune system by internal structures. Immunol Today 7: 97–98

Earp HS, Austin KS, Buessow SC, Dy R, Gillespie GY (1984) Membranes from T and B lymphocytes have different patterns of tyrosine phosphorylation. Proc Natl Acad Sci USA 81: 2347–2351

Fauci AS (1983) Basic mechanisms of activation and immunoregulation of human B-lymphocyte responses. In: Fauci AS (moderator) Activation and regulation of human immune responses: implications in normal and disease states. Ann Intern Med 99: 61–75

Fauci AS, Ballieux RE (1982) Summary of workshop presentations and discussions. In: Fauci AS, Ballieux RE (eds) Human B-lymphocyte function: activation and immunoregulation. Raven, New York, pp 309–316

Forbes IJ, Zalewski PD, Valente L (1982) Human B-lymphocyte maturation sequence revealed by TPA-induced differentiation of leukaemic cells. Immunobiology 163: 1–6

Forni L (1985) From the point of view of the B cell: considerations on B-cell activation. Scand J Immunol 22: 235–243

Frank MB, Watson J, Mochizuki D, Gillis S (1981) Biochemical and biologic characterisation of lymphocyte regulatory molecules VIII Purification of interleukin 2 from a human T cell leukemia. J Immunol 127: 2361–2365

Helderman JH, Strom TB (1978) Specific insulin binding site on T and B lymphocytes as a marker of cell activation. Nature 274: 62–63

Howard M, Paul WE (1983) Regulation of B-cell growth and differentiation by soluble factors. Ann Rev Immunol 1: 307–333

Howard M, Nakanishi K, Paul WE (1984) B cell growth and differentiation factors. Immunol Rev 78: 185–210

Imboden JB, Stobo JD (1985) Transmembrane signalling by the T cell antigen receptor. Perturbation of the T3-antigen receptor complex generates inositol phosphates and releases calcium ion from intracellular stores. J Exp Med 161: 446–456

Kehrl JH, Fauci AS (1983) Identification, purification, and characterisation of antigen-activated and antigen-specific human B lymphocytes. J Exp Med 157: 1692–1697

Kirchner H (1984) Interferons: a group of multiple lymphokines. Semin Immunopathol 7: 347–374

Kishi H, Miki Y, Kikutani H, Yamamura Y, Kishimoto T (1983) Sequential induction of phospholipid methylation and serine esterase activation in a B cell differentiation factor (BCDF)-stimulated human B cell line. J Immunol 131: 1961–1965

Klaus GGB, Chisholm P (1986) Does cyclosporine act *in vivo* as it does *in vitro*? Immunol Today 7: 101–103

Lanzavecchia A (1985) Antigen-specific interaction between T and B cells. Nature 314: 537–539

Mayer LF, Thompson C, Fu SM, Kunkel HG (1984) T cell factors regulating B cell activation and differentiation. Curr Top Microbiol Immunol 113: 77–85

Melchers F, Erdei A, Schulz T, Dierich MP (1985) Growth control of activated synchronized murine B cells by the C3d fragment of human complement. Nature 317: 264–267

Miedema F, Melief CJM (1985) T-cell regulation of human B-cell activation. A reappraisal of the role of interleukin 2. Immunol Today 6: 258–259

Miller RA, Gralow J (1984) The induction of Leu-1 antigen expression in human malignant and normal B cells by phorbol myristic acetate (PMA). J Immunol 133: 3408–3414

Mond JJ, Seghal E, Kung J, Finkelman FD (1981) Increased expression of I- region-associated antigen (Ia) on B cells after cross-linking of surface immunoglobulin. J Immunol 127: 881–888

Monroe JG, Cambier JC (1983a) Level of mIa expression on mitogen-stimulated murine B lymphocytes is dependent on position in cell cycle. J Immunol 130: 626–631

Monroe JG, Cambier JC (1983b) B cell activation I. Anti-immunoglobulin-induced receptor cross-linking results in a decrease in the plasma membrane potential of murine B lymphocytes. J Exp Med 157: 2073–2086

Morrison DC, Rudbach JA (1981) Endotoxin-cell-membrane interactions leading to transmembrane signalling. In Inman FP (ed) Contemporary topics in molecular immunology, vol 8. Plenum, New York, pp 187–218

Muraguchi A, Kehrl JH, Butler JL, Fauci AS (1984) Regulation of human B-cell activation, proliferation and differentiation by soluble factors. J Clin Immunol 4: 337–347

Neckers LM (1984) Transferrin receptors regulate proliferation of normal and malignant B cells. Curr Top Microbiol Immunol 113: 62–68

Nossal GJV, Pike BL (1984) A reappraisal of "T-independent" antigens. II. Studies on single, hapten-specific B cells from neonatal CBA/H or CBA/N mice fail to support classification into TI-1 and TI-2 categories. J Immunol 132: 1696–1701

Opitz H-G, Opitz U, Lemke H, Hewlett G, Schreml W, Flad H-D (1977) The role of fetal calf serum in the primary immune response in vitro. J Exp Med 145: 1029–1038

Oppenheim JJ, Kovacs EJ, Matsushima K, Durum SK (1986) There is more than one interleukin 1. Immunol Today 7: 45–56

Persson UCI, Lennart LG, Hammarstrom LLG, Smith CIE (1977) Macrophages are required for the dextran-sulfate induced activation of B lymphocytes. J Immunol 119: 1138–1144

Persson UCI, Hammarstrom U, Moller G, Smith CIE (1978) The role of adherent cells in B and T lymphocyte activation. Immunol Rev 40: 79–101

Pick E, Keisari Y, Bromberg Y, Freund M, Yabukowski A (1982) Effect of tumor promoters in immunological systems — the macrophage as a target cell for the action of phorbol esters. In: Hecker E et al. (eds) Carcinogenesis, vol 7. Raven, New York, pp 625–634

Provvedini DM, Tsoukas CD, Deftos LJ, Manolagas SC (1983) 1,25-dihydroxyvitamin D_3 receptors in human leukocytes. Science 221: 1181–1183

Resch K, Ferber E (1977) Phospholipid metabolism of stimulated lymphocytes. Effects of phytohemagglutinin, concanavalin A and an anti-immunoglobulin serum. Eur J Biochem 27: 153–161

Robèrt K-H, Einhorn S, Juliusson G, Östlund L, Biberfeld P (1985) Interferon induces proliferation and differentiation in primary chronic lymphocytic leukaemia cells. Clin Exp Immunol 62: 530–534

Ròsen A, Gergely M, Jondal M, Klein G, Britton S (1977) Polyclonal Ig production after Epstein-Barr virus infection of human lymphocytes in vitro Nature 267: 52–54

Rosenberg SA, Lipsky PE (1981) The role of monocytes in pokeweed mitogen-stimulated human B cell activation: separate requirements for intact monocytes and a soluble monocyte factor. J Immunol 126: 1341–1345

Rosenberg SA, Lipsky PE (1982) The role of monocytes in human B-cell activation In: Fauci AS, Ballieux RE (eds) Human B-lymphocyte function: activation and immunoregulation. Raven, New York, pp 263–287

Scouros MA, Bohleber-Matza M, Murphy SG (1983) Kinetics of protein A activation of mononuclear cells from patients with chronic lymphocytic leukemia I. CLL B-cells are not intrinsically unresponsive to staphylococcal protein A. Leuk Res 7: 703–712

Sidman CL, Unanue ER (1978) Control of proliferation and differentiation in B lymphocytes by anti-Ig antibodies and a serum-derived cofactor. Proc Natl Acad Sci USA 75: 2401–2405

Sidman CL, Paige CJ, Schreier MH (1984) B cell maturation factor (BMF): a lymphokine or family of lymphokines promoting the maturation of B lymphocytes. J Immunol 132: 209–222

Sieckmann DG, Asofsky R, Mosier DE et al. (1978) Activation of mouse lymphocytes by anti-immunoglobulin. I. Parameters of the proliferative response. J Exp Med 147: 814–829

Sugawara I, Ishizaka S (1983) The degree of monocyte participation in human B- and T-cell activation by phorbol myristate acetate. Clin Immunol Immunopathol 26: 299–308

Touw I, Lowenberg B (1985) Interleukin 2 stimulates chronic lymphocytic leukemia colony formation in vitro. Blood 66: 237–240

Webb DR (1983) The biochemistry of antigen-specific T-cell factors. Ann Rev Immunol 1: 428–438

Wedner HJ (1984) Biochemical events associated with lymphocyte activation. Surv Immunol Res 3: 295–303

13 Immunoregulatory Mechanisms

Introduction

Much is known about the mechanisms for initiating immune responses, but less about how they are terminated. Once an immune response starts, it would never stop if there were no regulatory mechanisms. B cells from an immunised mouse which are injected into irradiated mice continue to multiply. In the normal vertebrate, the response to a single dose of antigen is very quickly reduced to a minimum. The primary antibody response to most antigens results in an exponential increase in the number of B lymphocytes secreting specific IgM antibody. This response is terminated 4–6 days after immunisation. Different antibody-secreting B cell subsets appear briefly at different times during this period (Brieva et al. 1984). Subsequent exposure to antigen leads to secondary immune responses which have distinct characteristics, occur more rapidly and are often more powerful. Complex organisation is necessary to control these responses.

Systems Controlling Immunological Function

The immune system can be viewed as being in a complex homeostasis. It can be argued that recognition of self, not non-self, is paramount; certainly the immune system normally responds against self, but keeps this autoimmune activity under control. Foreign antigen perturbs equilibrium, producing a regulatory shift leading ultimately to positive (immune) or negative (tolerance) responses. The response is geared to produce maximal destruction of foreign antigens, representing a potential pathogen, with minimal damage to self tissues.

Many systems of control are apparent:

1. Antibody exerts a negative feedback under some conditions. By combining with antigen, antibody competes with antigen receptors on the responding B cells. Feedback by specific antibody and idiotypic antibody is only effective if presented just before or at the time of immunisation. Infants can be protected against the damaging effects of rhesus antibodies by administration of the appropriate antibody to the mother. Inhibition of immune responses by passive administration of antibody requires whole IgG molecules. The $F(ab)_2$ fragment of antibody, lacking the Fc piece, is not effective. This suggests that the action of passively administered antibody action is through Fc receptors, on macrophages or B lymphocytes.

Antibody-antigen complexes, binding both through the specific antibody receptor and through the Fc receptor may exert an inhibitory effect on B cell differentiation. Antigen-antibody complexes can actually enhance immune responses, by binding to the surface of accessory cells (ACs) through Fc receptors. Complexes with a high ratio of antigen to antibody are effective in this way. They thereby enhance the effectiveness of antigen presentation. The free complement component C3d involved in antigen-antibody complexes exerts a negative influence, whereas cross-linked complement in antigen-antibody complexes is a positive factor in B cell activation (Melchers et al. 1985). T cells may also be involved in this mechanism. B cells are not affected by antigen-antibody complexes when the antigen and corresponding antibody in the complexes have a specificity differing from the specificity of the surface immunoglobulin receptor on the B cells, as the cross-linking must involve the B cell receptor for antigen.

2. The concentration of antigen is a major factor driving an immune response. Antigen may be neutralised by antibody and its concentration is reduced by catabolic processes in which macrophages are particularly important. B cells are inhibited in the production of antibody if they cannot attain an antigen-poor environment. Increases or decreases in the ratio of macrophages to lymphocytes may lead to an increase in suppressor cell activity. Activation of macrophages by T cell products has the same effect. Lymphokines from suppressor T cells may inhibit the presentation of antigen to B cells.

3. There are inherent genetic limitations. These genetic limitations are exerted both through the major histocompatibility complex (MHC) and through distinct genetic mechanisms. Inherited immune response (Ir) genes have been shown to determine responsiveness in mice to single antigenic specificities (epitopes). Mice can be bred for high and low antibody responses. Up to a dozen genetic loci may be involved, and some of these affect macrophage function.

In addition to these genes affecting immune responsiveness, the capacity to produce specific antibodies can, in some experiments, be shown to be linked to immunoglobulin genes. The basis of such a linkage is the inheritance of a certain repertoire for variable genes. There is an inherited capacity to produce an idiotype (a "public", inherited or cross-reacting idiotype, discussed later in this chapter; see p. 164) that is common to the range of antibodies formed against some antigens. In this case the gene for the variable region of the antibody occurs on the same chromosome as that carrying the genes for the constant region.

4. Interactions of T and B cells, and ACs are major factors in the control of immune responses, with restrictions on cellular interactions imposed by the MHC.

Cell–cell interactions may be mediated by direct contact, or by cytokines, factors released by cells of one type affecting the activity of another. Most antigens elicit a complex set of interacting T cells that regulate B cells and each other. These include antigen-specific helper T cells, several types of suppressor T cells and cytotoxic T cells. Contrasuppressor T cells interfere with suppression in a manner which is distinct from T cell help (Green and Ptak 1986; Lehner 1986).

Highly complex regulatory T cell networks and circuits are described: contra-suppressive networks, interactions of one set of T cells with another through receptor/anti-receptor interactions, and helper T cells recognising B cell receptors. Natural killer (NK) cells probably also help to terminate an antibody response.

5. Anti-idiotypic interactions occur in virtually every immune response.

6. Regulation of the production of virgin B and T cells, about which little is known, could influence immune responsiveness.

Suppressor Mechanisms

Suppressor T cells are major factors in the control of immune responses, acting on B cells (Sinclair 1983), on other T cells and on macrophages. Inhibition of antibody responses by T cells may be both antigen specific and non-specific (Callard 1984; Clement et al. 1984). There is a complex system of different T cell subclasses interacting with B cells and ACs. T cells that specifically induce suppressor T cells ("suppressor-inducers") are proposed to activate the suppressor network by secreting a soluble factor (TSiF). This recruits suppressor effector T cells from precursors, which in turn produce a T cell inhibitory soluble factor (TSeF). Contrasuppressor cells are postulated which render helper T cells refractory to the influence of suppressor T cells. Relatively large amounts of a T cell suppressive factor preventing activation of B cells can be generated in large-scale cultures of pig lymphocytes stimulated by concanavalin A (Russmann et al. 1985). One postulated mechanism of action of suppressor factors is blockage of the binding of lymphokines to receptors.

Immunological immaturity at birth may be a consequence of high suppressor cell activity (Argyris 1984). Suppressor T cell activity is strong in late embryonic and early postnatal life and declines subsequently. It is present without antigenic stimulation (Droege 1984).

There is increasing evidence that NK cells exert a regulatory action on the antibody response (James and Ritchie 1984). Large granular lymphocytes stained by monoclonal CP03 (HNK-1, Leu-7) antibodies specific for NK cells are preferentially localised in the B cell areas of lymphoid tissue, particularly the follicular centres of lymph nodes (Si and Whiteside 1983; Ritchie et al. 1983). NK cells seem to be closely associated with neoplastic nodules in lymphomas of follicular centre origin, but not in nodes involved by T cell lymphomas (Banerjee and Thibert 1983).

B cells activate NK cells in vitro to suppress B cell differentiation and antibody production stimulated by pokeweed mitogen (PWM), and this inhibitory action can be enhanced further by interferon. Such activated NK cells will lyse the B cells used for activation. NK cells may be effective at lower ratios per B cell than suppressor T cells, but NK cells at very low ratios may enhance B cell responses.

There are two suggested mechanisms of the specific recognition of B cells by NK cells. One is through transferrin receptors as targets (Vodinelich et al. 1983). Another is that they terminate antibody responses by elimination of ACs that have been exposed to antigen (Abruzzo and Rowley 1983).

Not all examples of unresponsiveness can be explained by the mechanisms described so far. Non-responsiveness may be due to insufficient association between MHC product and antigen to create an immunogenic complex. Immunological unresponsiveness may also result from absence of appropriate T cells from the repertoire. A class of suppressor cells called "veto cells" has been described, which seem to inhibit autoreactive lymphocytes (Miller 1986). Histamine suppresses lymphocyte transformation induced by the mitogen concanavalin A by a direct action on T cells (Brostoff et al. 1980). Lymphocytes from atopic subjects are more sensitive to the suppressive effects of histamine than lymphocytes from normal subjects.

Idiotypes

Idiotypes are important, not only because they are involved in the control of normal lymphocytes, but also because the idiotype network is considered to be important in tumour immunity (Broder and Waldmann 1978; Schreiber 1984) The use of anti-idiotypic antibodies is being investigated as a treatment of lymphoid malignancies. Idiotype constitutes a tumour-specific antigen on malignant lymphocytes, offering a specific target for immunological attack.

When an antibody (A) is injected into another species, it may induce the production of another antibody (B), which reacts specifically with A only. Antibody B is an anti-idiotypic antibody. It reacts with part of the antibody-combining variable region of A. The antigenic part of the variable region of antibody A is its idiotype. Idiotypes are thus serological markers of variable regions of antibodies. An idiotype is made up of individual antigenic sites known as idiotopes. Most of the idiotopes, but not all, are within the antigen-binding site. Antigen blocks antibody directed against binding-site idiotopes, but does not block the binding of anti-idiotypes directed against idiotopes outside the antibody-combining site. Idiotopes and anti-idiotopes are, of course, encoded by V, D and J immunoglobulin genes. Both heavy and light chains are involved in forming an idiotype in most cases.

An idiotype is described as "private" if it is a unique determinant on the variable region of antibodies from a single clone. A private idiotype is usually the result of gene rearrangement. If the same sequence is found on antibodies with differing antibody-combining specificities, it is described as "public". The capacity to synthesise such idiotypes is inherited. Public idiotypes are markers of germline V and possibly D genes. Such public or cross-reacting idiotypes are found in the sera of patients with autoimmune disease (Cunningham-Rundles and Cheung 1985).

Anti-idiotypic antibodies binding to combining sites of antibodies can substitute for antigen; they mimic antigen. They should be able to exert the same effect on a surface immunoglobulin receptor molecule as antigen, either stimulatory or inhibitory. These anti-idiotypic antibodies are said to provide an "internal image" of the antigen. According to this definition an internal image is a short amino acid sequence on the anti-idiotypic antibody presenting the same configuration as an epitope on an antigen. In the same way, an amino acid sequence on an immunoglobulin molecule may mimic a hormone or a growth factor by binding to the specific receptor, with consequences for the growth of non-lymphoid cells.

Idiotypes on T Cells

There is no fundamental difference between the combining sites on T and B cell receptors. T cells therefore have idiotypes. An anti-idiotypic antiserum may cross-react with, and be used as a probe for a T cell receptor. Anti-idiotypic antisera can activate T cells. Conversely, T cells can recognise idiotypes on antibody molecules.

Idiotypic Regulatory Network

Jerne (see review in Jerne 1984) proposed that the interaction between antibodies and anti-antibodies formed a regulatory network. In addition to antibody, lymphocytes with anti-idiotypic receptors can recognise the idiotypes on other lymphocytes. The idiotype network encompasses both T and B cell divisions of the lymphoid system. Suppressor T cells corresponding to B cell idiotypes can be induced in animals.

Production of anti-idiotypic antibodies is a normal component of the immune response, a physiological autoimmune response, but the extent of the control which the idiotypic network exerts on immune function remains to be determined. In the view of some, an equilibrium of idiotypes and anti-idiotypes exists, and disturbances of this equilibrium result in changes which constitute immune responses. Anti-idiotype induces an anti-anti-idiotype and so on. Possibilities exist for enormous complexity. Anti-idiotypic antibodies can both suppress and enhance idiotype expression, depending on the experimental conditions. By binding to T cell receptors for antigen, they may influence T cell function. Anti-idiotypic antibodies may enhance, if injected into mice in nanogram quantities, or suppress target idiotope expression, if injected in microgram amounts. Long-lasting suppression of specific antibody results from giving newborn animals corresponding anti-idiotypic antibodies intravenously or in milk. Preimmunisation with anti-idiotype will stimulate or inhibit a response limited to a particular idiotype.

Disturbances of the idiotype network have been invoked as causes of autoimmunity. Anti-idiotypic antibodies reacting with anti-DNA antibodies are present in patients with systemic lupus erythematosus, and may reflect disease activity.

Jerne has questioned the classic notion of "antibody-combining site". He asks, "Must we consider which one 'recognises' the other?" It is much simpler if the distinction between recognising and being recognised is avoided. The idiotypic network may depend on no more than the immunoglobulin molecules having sticky ends that adhere with varying affinities to protuberances on other molecules.

Introductory essays on the subject of idiotypes may be found in a Lancet Annotation (1984), Cooke et al. (1984) and Roitt et al. (1985).

Immunological Tolerance

Tolerance is impairment of the capacity to respond to an antigen, resulting from previous exposure to it. It has often been speculated that tolerance may be the reason for the failure of immunological surveillance of tumours. Immunological tolerance was clearly perceived by Owen (1945), who found that most bovine twins had a mixture of each other's erythrocytes and recognised that erythrocyte precursors from each twin fetus had become established in the other and had conferred on their new host a "tolerance" towards these "foreign" cells that lasted throughout life.

In general, tolerance to antigens is not inherited, although genetic unresponsiveness to protein antigens can be demonstrated in certain inbred strains of animals. Offspring can react to parental MHC antigens except those they have inherited. Reactions to antigens except MHC products occur naturally and are obviously under control in the healthy person. Autoantibodies are normally present in all healthy subjects, but usually in such low amounts that they may require sensitive tests to demonstrate them. The incidence of such autoantibodies increases with age. Mechanisms must exist to regulate B cells producing these autoantibodies. This immune reactivity directed at self-antigens probably involves 10%–20% of the lymphoid cell population (del Guercio et al. 1986).

Transplantation tolerance can be induced by injecting neonatal mice of one inbred strain (A) with haematopoietic cells from another inbred strain (B). The A strain can then accept skin grafts from the B strain. Tolerance can also be induced to inanimate soluble antigens. To induce tolerance in the adult, either large doses of antigen or repeated very low doses are needed. Induction of high dose ("high-zone") tolerance is enhanced by immunosuppressive drugs. 'Low-zone" tolerance, induced by very small doses of antigen, usually over a long time, results in paralysis or elimination of specific T cells, whereas in "high-zone" tolerance both T and B cells are made unresponsive. Tolerance can be induced for delayed hypersensitivity, a T cell function, in the absence of B cell tolerance.

The state of the antigen is important to the outcome of an antigenic challenge. Aggregated or particulate antigen is immunogenic; soluble antigen is weakly antigenic or tolerogenic in repeated low doses. A monovalent antigen does not induce unresponsiveness in vitro of the clones of T and B cells reacting specifically to that antigen. Thymus-independent (TI) antigens are relatively tolerogenic, possibly because of their polymeric nature and long persistence in the body. High doses of many TI antigens induce specific B cell tolerance, possibly through cross-linking of B cell receptors. As well as the epitope of the antigen (hapten), its carrier plays an as yet unclarified part in the mechanism of tolerance. Hapten-specific tolerance may be induced by haptens conjugated to TI antigens.

Tolerance is more easily induced in young than old cells. B cells from newborns are more susceptible than those from adults, but the age of the animal is less important than the age of the cells. Nevertheless, it is possible to induce tolerance in populations of mature cells (including memory B cells). Activated B cells synthesising antibody can still be switched off by antigen in high concentration.

There is no complete or unified view to account for tolerance to self in the presence of reactivity to similar non-self molecules. There is clearly a balance between the maintenance of tolerance to self antigens and the mounting of an immune response against foreign antigens, particularly when the foreign antigens resemble self components closely.

Tolerance results from a number of mechanisms:

1. *Clonal abortion.* Immature clones of T and B cells may be tolerised by low concentrations of multivalent antigen. The normal maturation of the cells in response to antigen is inhibited, so that they are not able to respond to subsequent antigenic challenge. B cells encountering antigen as they differentiate from pre-B cells, when they first develop sIgM receptors, are highly sensitive to such inhibition (Nossal 1983). Antigen leads to capping of the sIg on immature B cells, which is endocytosed and not resynthesised. Mature B cells do resynthesise Ig after capping.

2. *Clonal exhaustion.* By repeated challenge with TI antigens, all the B cells capable of responding to antigen may be stimulated to differentiate into short-lived antibody-producing cells, leaving no cells capable of responding to subsequent challenge.

3. *Suppression.* Suppressor T cells actively suppress T or B cell clones.

4. *Functional deletion of mature clones.* B cells which encounter thymus-dependent (TD) antigen without helper T cells being present or which are exposed to TI antigens in excess are inhibited. Helper T cells may also be deleted by antigen presented repeatedly or in excess. Low molecular weight forms of some antigens are tolerogenic. T cells must have IL-2 for proliferation. It has recently been suggested that exposure of T cells to antigen in the absence of IL-2 may paralyse helper T cells or activate suppressor T cells (Malkovsky and Medawar 1984). This may occur in the induction of neonatal tolerance, because there may be a relative inefficiency in the production of IL-2.

5. *Blockade of antibody-forming cells.* Excess of thymus-independent antigen interferes with secretion of antibody by B cells.

6. *Inhibition by anti-idiotypic antibodies and anti-idiotypic T cells.*

Maintenance of tolerance requires persistence of antigen, either in the form of living cells, as in the chimaeric state exemplified by Owen's bovine twins (Owen 1945), or repeated injection of foreign antigen. T cell tolerance in mice to soluble antigen can be induced in 2 days and lasts for 150 days. Induction of B cell tolerance takes a week and lasts 50 days. Recovery from tolerance is probably due to emergence of new clones.

Presentation of the hapten of a tolerogenic antigen on a new carrier will break tolerance. This probably occurs through the stimulation of new helper T cells which recognise the new carrier. Autoimmunity could arise if an autoantigen is presented on an unnatural carrier molecule of an infectious micro-organism. Examples are rheumatic fever after infection with certain streptococci, Chagas' disease from *Treponema cruzi* infection, both resulting from cross-reaction between antigens on the micro-organisms and heart muscle, and encephalomyelitis after immunisation against rabies with foreign brain tissue. Viruses may insert new proteins into cell membranes which act as new carriers for membrane epitopes.

Polyclonal B cell activators can break tolerance. Bacterial lipopolysaccharide can induce antibodies to DNA in mice. Epstein–Barr virus induces synthesis of IgM rheumatoid anti-immunoglobulin by a proportion of human B lymphocytes.

Reviews of tolerance may be found in Nossal (1983), Evans and Engelman (1985) and Feldman et al. (1985).

Regulatory Mechanisms in B Cell Malignancies

The possibility that malignant lymphocytes are susceptible to normal regulatory influences, particularly of specific helper and suppressor B cells, has been investigated extensively in experimental systems (Abbas and Klaus 1978; Lynch et al. 1979, 1980; Bankert and Abbas 1980; Abbas 1982). Helper and suppressor cells specific for the hapten trinitrophenol, (TNP) are present in mice bearing the TNP-binding myeloma MOPC 315. The helper T cells can enhance the number of myeloma cells secreting anti-TNP, and the suppressors markedly inhibit myeloma growth.

These myeloma cells can be modulated by defined antigens and anti-idiotypic antibodies (Bona 1980). Incompletely differentiated plasmablasts which retain antigen receptors may be influenced by antigen, whereas terminally differentiated cells, having lost their receptors, are refractory to antigen. The antibody specificity of myeloma proteins, where it has been determined, has been for autoantigens and idiotypes; antibody specificity for foreign antigens is rare. Growth requirements and mechanisms controlling the growth of human myeloma cells have been studied recently. Myeloma cells in vitro are influenced by lymphokines and MHC-bearing macrophages (Durie 1986).

The obvious questions are whether patients are completely tolerant of their lymphoid tumours, or whether there is ever a controlling mechanism affecting the malignant clone, even at the beginning. If an immunological control mechanism exists, could it possibly be activated as a means of treatment? Another question concerns the stimulus which induces differentiation of lymphoid neoplasms. Since antigen is considered necessary for the differentiation of normal resting lymphocytes, does antigen drive the differentiation of malignant clones? One possibility is that all malignant lymphocytes have immunological specificity for autoantigens. Alternatively, they must circumvent the requirement of normal lymphocytes for antigen to induce differentiation.

It is important to question whether anti-idiotypic antibodies are present in patients with lymphoid tumours, and, if not, what the reason for their absence may be. In experimental models anti-idiotype may influence immune responses positively or negatively, and it is hard to predict which way. It is possible that immunisation with anti-idiotype may influence malignant lymphocytes. Anti-idiotypic immunotoxin may have a role.

References

Abbas AK (1982) Immunologic regulation of lymphoid tumor cells: model systems for lymphocyte function. Adv Immunol 32: 301–368

Abbas AK, Klaus GGB (1978) Antigen-antibody complexes suppress antibody production by mouse plasmacytoma cells in vitro. Eur J Immunol 8: 217–220

Abruzzo LV, Rowley DA (1983) Homeostasis of the antibody response: immunoregulation by NK cells. Science 222: 581–585

Argyris BF (1984) The interaction between macrophages and suppressor cells in immunological maturation in mice. Immunol Today 5: 34–36

Banerjee D, Thibert RF (1983) Natural killer-like cells found in B-cell compartments of human lymphoid tissues. Nature 304: 270–272

Bankert RB, Abbas AK (1980) Myelomas as models to study activation and suppression of normal lymphocytes. In: Potter M (ed) Progress in myeloma. Biology of myeloma. Elsevier/North Holland, New York, pp 109–128

Bona C (1980) Regulation of the growth of myeloma tumor cells and non-neoplastic B cell clones by anti-idiotypic antibodies. In: Potter M (ed) Progress in myeloma. Biology of myeloma. Elsevier/North Holland, New York, pp 209–221

Brieva JA, Targan S, Stevens RH (1984) NK and T cell subsets regulate antibody production by human in vivo antigen-induced lymphoblastoid B cells. J Immunol 132: 611–615

Broder S, Waldmann TA (1978) The suppressor-cell network in cancer. N Engl J Med 299: 1281–1284, 1335–1341

Brostoff J, Pack S, Lydyard PM (1980) Histamine suppression of lymphocyte activation. Clin Exp Immunol 39: 739–745

Callard RE (1984) T-cell suppression of human antibody responses: specific or non-specific? Immunol Today 5: 258–261

Clement LT, Grossi CE, Gartland GL (1984) Morphologic and phenotypic features of the subpopulation of LEU-2+ cells that suppresses B cell differentiation. J Immunol 133: 2461–2468

Cooke A, Lydyard PM, Roitt IM (1984) Autoimmunity and idiotypes. Lancet II: 723–725

Cunningham-Rundles C, Cheung MKL (1985) Cross-reacting idiotypes in human sera. Immunol Today 6: 14–16

del Guercio P, Marcelletti JF, Katz DH (1986) B-cell lymphokines and the activation of the immune system by internal structures. Immunol Today 7: 97–98

Droege W (1984) Suppressor cells in immunological maturation. Immunol Today 5: 161

Durie BGM (1986) The immunology of multiple myeloma. Proceedings of the XXI congress of the International Society of Hematology, Sydney, May 1986, p 203 (abstract)

Evans RL, Engelman EG (1985) Progress toward understanding self-tolerance. Semin Hematol 22: 68–80

Feldman M, Zanders ED, Lamb JR (1985) Tolerance in T-cell clones. Immunol Today 6: 58–62

Green DR, Ptak W (1986) Contrasuppression in the mouse. Immunol Today 7: 81–86

James K, Ritchie AWS (1984) Do natural killer cells regulate B-cell activity? Immunol Today 5: 193–194

Jerne NK (1984) Idiotypic networks and other preconceived ideas. Immunol Reviews 70: 5–24

Lancet Annotation (1984) Anti-idiotypes for the clinician. Lancet II: 440–441

Lehner T (1986) Antigen presenting, contrasuppressor human T cells. Immunol Today 7: 87–92

Lynch RG, Rohrer JW, Odermatt B, Gebel HM, Autry UR, Hoover RG (1979) Immunoregulation of murine myeloma cell growth and differentiation: a monoclonal model of B cell differentiation. Immunol Rev 48: 45–80

Lynch RG, Rohrer JW, Gebel HM, Odermatt B (1980) Regulation of murine myeloma cell growth and differentiation: cellular and molecular mechanism and therapeutic implications In: Potter M (ed) Progress in myeloma. Biology of myeloma. Elsevier/North Holland, New York, pp 129–150

Malkovsky M, Medawar PB (1984) Is immunological tolerance (non-responsiveness) a consequence of interleukin 2 deficit during the recognition of antigen? Immunol Today 5: 340–343

Melchers F, Erdei A, Schulz T, Dierich MP (1985) Growth control of activated, synchronised murine B cells by the C3d fragment of human complement. Nature 317: 264–267

Miller RG (1986) The veto phenomenon and T-cell recognition. Immunol Today 7: 112–114

Nossal GJV (1983) Cellular mechanisms of immunologic tolerance. Annu Rev Immunol 1: 33–62

Owen RD (1945) Immunogenetic consequences of vascular anastomoses between bovine twins. Science 102: 400–401

Ritchie AWS, James K, Micklem HS (1983) The distribution and possible significance of cells identified in human lymphoid tissue by the monoclonal antibody HNK-1. Clin Exp Immunol 51: 439–447

Roitt IM, Thanavala YM, Male DK, Hay FC (1985) Anti-idiotypes as surrogate antigens: structural considerations. Immunol Today 6: 265–267

Russmann E, Kramer MD, Wissler JH, Schirrmacher V (1985) Biotechnical production and functional characterisation of leukocytic cytokine(s) with cytotoxic effect on resting but not activated thymocytes. Immunobiology 169: 389–402

Schreiber H (1984) Idiotype network interactions in tumour immunity. Adv Cancer Res 41: 291–321

Si L, Whiteside TL (1983) Tissue distribution of human NK cells studied with anti-Leu-7 monoclonal antibody. J Immunol 130: 2149–2155

Sinclair NRStC (1983) The influence of T lymphocytes on antibody-induced B-cell suppression. Immunol Today 4: 35–36
Vodinelich L, Sutherland R, Schneider C, Newman R, Greaves M (1983) Receptor for transferrin may be a "target" structure for natural killer cells. Proc Natl Acad Sci USA 80: 835–839

14 Technology of Investigation and Diagnosis

Introduction

Better understanding of the lymphoid malignancies results largely from the introduction of increasingly precise and sophisticated methods of investigation. Because populations of neoplastic lymphocytes have a very homogeneous marker profile and function, the study of immunological markers has not only provided essential information for the distinction of reactive and neoplastic lymphoid proliferations and the subtyping of lymphocytic leukaemias and non-Hodgkin's lymphomas, but has also taught us much about lymphoid differentiation.

The purpose of this chapter is to present the principles underlying the more recently developed techniques used in specialised laboratories, to provide source references to the details of the techniques, and to outline the principles underlying hybridoma technology and gene technology, which already have made enormous contributions and promise even more.

Hybridoma Technology and Monoclonal Antibodies

In 1975, Köhler and Milstein reported the fusion of normal murine splenic B lymphocytes with murine myeloma cells to produce a hybridoma cell line capable of secreting antibody of selected specificity. This started a revolution in immunological research, with a particularly significant impact on research into lymphoid malignancies. Using the machinery of the myeloma cell and the specificity of the antibody-producing splenic B cell with which it is fused, the hybridoma line can produce virtually unlimited amounts of monoclonal antibodies of extraordinary specificity, because each molecule, being the same, is directed against a single antigenic determinant. An ever-increasing battery of reagents can thus be produced to identify the antigenic determinants of lymphoreticular cells. These reagents offer, for the first time, standard antibodies for world-wide use.

Principles of Hybridoma Technology

Cultured, immortal myeloma cells are fused with normal, short-lived antibody-producing B cells to form immortal, antibody-secreting hybrids that have been called "hybridomas". The fusion of mouse myeloma cells with normal mouse splenic B cells results in nuclei containing chromosomes from the myeloma cells and the normal antibody-producing cells. Myeloma cells, lacking the enzyme hypoxanthine phosphoribosyl transferase, which is essential for growth in HAT (hypoxanthine, aminopterin, thymidine) medium do not survive, whereas hybrids grow because the normal B cells contribute the gene for this enzyme. The mouse spleen cells have a short life span in culture. The culture system, therefore, results only in growth of hybrid cells. Hybrids can also be generated from human antibody-forming cells with cultured myeloma cells.

Each viable hybrid is an individual and a potential founder of a clone, with the capacity to produce its unique antibody because it bears the rearranged immunoglobulin genes contributed by a normal splenic B cell. A crucial step is the selection of the few cells producing antibody of the required specificity from the millions arising at each fusion. To do this, the cells are diluted out so that approximately one is allotted to each culture well. After the clones have grown up, a sensitive procedure, such as an enzyme-linked immunoassay, is used to demonstrate those producing the required antibody. The desired clones so obtained can be grown in vitro or in vivo by injection into the peritoneal cavity of mice. The principles used to produce B hybridomas may also be utilised to produce T hybridomas that synthesise T lymphokines. Mouse T lymphoma cells have also been fused with human malignant T cells for the purpose of analysing chromosomal abnormalities in the malignant cells (Erikson et al. 1985).

The monoclonal antibodies useful in the diagnosis and classification of lymphoid malignancies are discussed in Chapter 8. They have almost replaced polyclonal antibodies produced in domestic animals for routine work such as the determination of T and B cell subsets and detection of monotypic malignant B cell populations. An antigen on normal lymphoid and reticular cells as well as cells of bone marrow origin, called the leucocyte common antigen (LCA), is recognised by several monoclonal antibodies. These antibodies are useful in differentiation of lymphoid neoplasms from carcinomas and sarcomas. Eight antibody clusters react selectively with cells of the T cell lineage. CD2, CD3 and CD5 antibodies react with nearly all peripheral blood T lymphocytes. The E (sheep erythrocyte) receptor is detected by CD2 antibodies. T cells express either CD4 or CD8 and a small percentage expresses both. Many monoclonal antibodies are available for characterisation of B cells. Monoclonal antibodies to constant regions of κ and λ immunoglobulin light chains detect B cells over a wide range of their differentiation pathways. CD20 antibodies bind to nearly all B lymphocytes from blood and lymphoid organs except plasma cells. Antibodies of the clusters CD19, CD21 and CD22 are differentiation stage-dependent B cell markers. Other monoclonal reagents including CD23 detect antigens expressed during activation. CD10 detects the common acute lymphocytic leukaemia antigen (CALLA) on primitive B cells. Large granular lymphocytes express an antigen recognised by antibodies of the CP03 cluster. Most monoclonal antibodies which react with monocytes and macrophages, such as M01 and Leu-M1 (CD11), also react with cells of the granulocyte series.

Gene Cloning

The use of recombinant DNA technology has made possible, in principle, the production of proteins encoded by virtually any structural gene. We can therefore look forward to having any desired protein hormone or growth factor for treatment of human disease. Interferon-α (IFN$_a$), now being used for the treatment of hairy cell leukaemia, and insulin, both produced by recombinant gene technology, are already in clinical use. This technology involves insertion of an isolated gene into a bacterial or mammalian cell which multiplies rapidly in vitro. The new clone of cells synthesises the product of the introduced gene. Many proteins are glycosylated in the natural state, but not in the bacterial recombinant product. Because of this and the difficulty of making host bacteria secrete the product of some engrafted genes, efforts are now being directed to the use of mammalian cell lines for the production of complete gene products.

There are three ways to obtain genes for insertion into producer cells. A gene may be taken from a cell known to contain it and inserted into a bacterium (Fig. 14.1). As explained below, this involves random insertion of genes into bacteria, creation of a large number of new clones of bacteria and identification of the clone containing the required gene. A gene may also be produced biochemically if the messenger RNA can be obtained, by the use of the enzyme reverse transcriptase. A third possibility is the chemical synthesis of a DNA sequence, if the sequence is known.

The principles of identification and production of a gene by cloning it in bacteria can be listed quite simply; the technical details are not so simple. The steps are:

1. *Fragmentation of a genome by restriction enzymes.* This involves cutting the DNA of a cell which has the gene into small segments with restriction enzymes (bacterial endonucleases) that break DNA molecules at precisely defined base sequences. A restriction enzyme cuts the human genome into approximately one million fragments.

2. *Introduction of genes into plasmids.* Plasmids are small circular chromosomes possessed by many bacteria, unlinked to the main chromosome. A DNA fragment can be inserted into the circular genome of a plasmid by opening its DNA ring with an enzymatic incision, joining the fragment to one end and closing the ring by the use of other enzymes. When a pool of diverse fragments is used, a heterogeneous population of hybrid plasmids is created.

3. *The hybrid plasmids are introduced into plasmid-free bacteria.*

4. *The plasmid-containing bacteria are dispersed on solid medium and allowed to form individual colonies.* A complete collection of cloned random fragments from a single organism is known as a "genomic library".

5. *The colonies containing the required gene must be identified.* The clone carrying the desired gene can be detected either by recognition of the gene, i.e. by gene probing, or of its products, using a sensitive assay.

6. *When a clone has been obtained which contains the required gene, it is grown up in large quantities.*

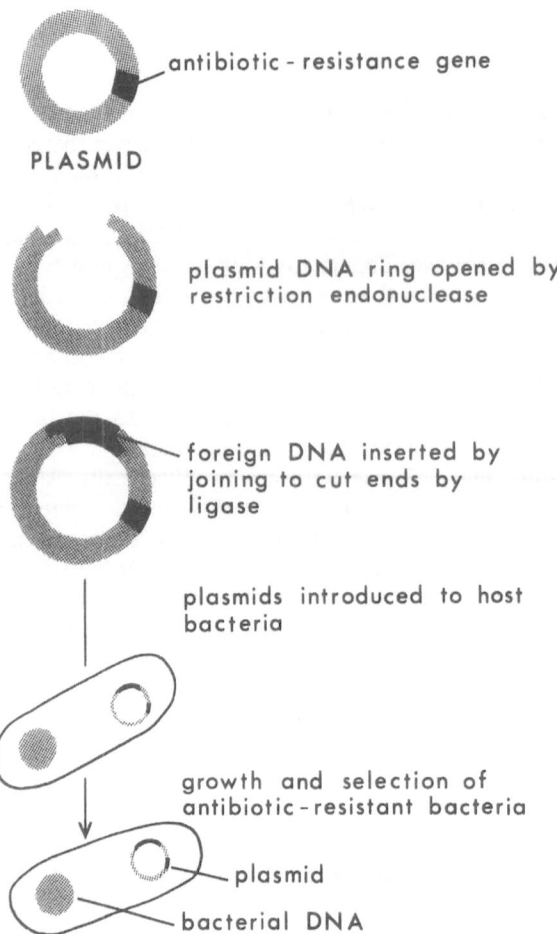

antibiotic - resistance gene

PLASMID

plasmid DNA ring opened by
restriction endonuclease

foreign DNA inserted by
joining to cut ends by
ligase

plasmids introduced to host
bacteria

growth and selection of
antibiotic - resistant bacteria

plasmid

bacterial DNA

Fig. 14.1. Gene cloning. Foreign DNA containing the desired gene is inserted into plasmids by enzymatically opening the DNA rings and joining the ends of the foreign segment to the ends of the plasmid DNA strand. The plasmid DNA also contains genes for antibiotic resistance. The bacteria are treated to allow ingress of recombinant DNA molecules. From the millions of bacteria arising in the culture only those with the antibiotic resistance gene grow in the presence of antibiotic. The clones containing the required gene must be identified by detection of either the unique DNA or its product.

Gene Probing

Molecular hybridisation permits the detection and identification of specific genes. Molecular hybridisation of specific sequences of DNA and RNA depends on the specific matching shown by the bases in nucleic acid. In this technique, a unique single-stranded gene sequence is labelled and used to detect complementary nucleic acid sequences derived from cell samples. Binding of homologous (comple-

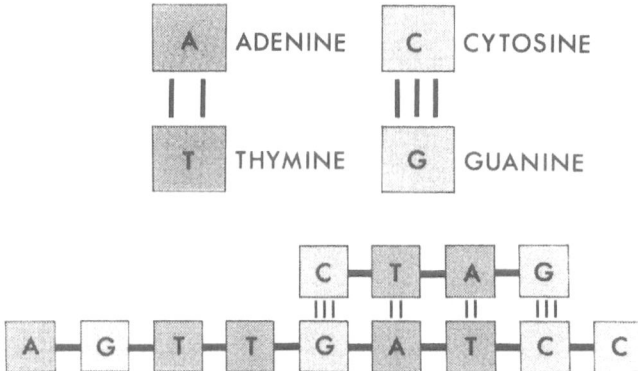

Fig. 14.2. Gene probing. Illustration of the principle of the specific matching of nucleic acid bases. Adenine pairs specifically with thymine and cytosine with guanine. If short sequences are tagged with a label, usually radioactive, a longer length of DNA can be "probed" to determine whether or not it contains complementary sequences following the base pair rules.

mentary) DNA molecules is highly specific and highly sensitive. The building blocks of nucleic acid are the nucleotides, each containing a base, a phosphate residue and a sugar (ribose in RNA or a desoxyribose in DNA). DNA contains only the four bases — thymine (T), adenine (A), cytosine (C) and guanine (G). The principle underlying hybridisation of DNA is that thymine pairs only with adenine and guanine only with cytosine (Fig. 14.2). In RNA, uracil takes the place of thymine.

Specific DNA sequences may be recognised by hybridisation of purified DNA in electrophoretic gels. The two strands of DNA must be separated (denatured) for hybridisation. Electrophoresed DNA is denatured by reacting the gel with alkali and the pattern is transferred to a sheet of nitrocellulose paper. The electrophoresed fragment enmeshed in nitrocellulose, containing a particular gene, is identified by allowing a short sequence of radioactive DNA, known as the probe, to hybridise with it. "Southern blotting" is the term used for DNA hybridisation with DNA deposited on nitrocellulose membranes, and "Northern blotting" for hybridisation with RNA. The DNA sequence to be used as a probe is synthesised or grown up in bacteria and labelled to high specific activity.

Gene probing may also be used to show that a gene is present in different positions in the genome in different individuals. If the DNA from a given individual is digested completely by a single restriction enzyme, a characteristic set of fragments is produced from every cell. Positions of many restriction sites may vary from one individual to another. Thus not all fragments produced by digestion of DNA from one individual will be of exactly the same length as those from another when the same restriction enzyme is used. The fragment containing a particular gene may be of different length in different individuals. This is called restriction fragment length polymorphism (RFLP). In practice the determination of the length of the fragments is made by electrophoresis in gel. The band labelled by the radioactive probe is found in a different position on the gel (Fig. 14.3). This indicates that the gene is present on a fragment of different length.

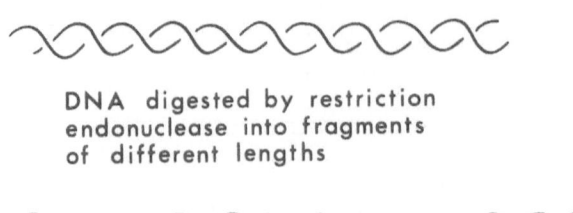

DNA digested by restriction
endonuclease into fragments
of different lengths

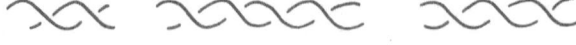

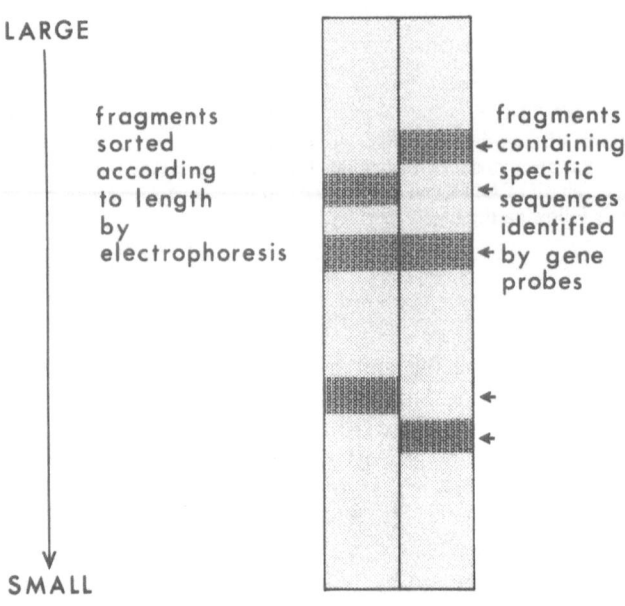

Fig. 14.3. Southern blotting of electrophoresed DNA fragments. When DNA is fragmented by a bacterial endonuclease it is cut wherever the specific sequence occurs in the DNA strand, resulting in a large number of fragments of varying sizes. The fragments are sorted by electrophoresis according to size into a smear along the length of the gel. A radioactive gene probe is allowed to react with an imprint of the gel on nitrocellulose. The fragments which contain the complementary sequence are recognised by autoradiography.

A lucid exposition of the basic procedures in gene technology may be read in Steel (1984), and a very readable account of the history of gene cloning has been written by Watson and Tooze (1981).

Immunodiagnostic Methods

Lymphoid cells from peripheral blood, bone marrow, fluids and effusions, as well as from lymphoid tissues, can be examined in suspensions or in sections. They may be examined fixed or unfixed, may be stained with labelled antibodies or histochemical reagents and may be studied by light or electron microscopy.

Collection of Specimens

In our laboratory, all biopsy material is obtained fresh and divided into three portions for the following procedures:

Portion 1: For morphological examination.
   a) A sliver is shaved off, fixed in 2.5% glutaraldehyde and stored for electron microscopic examination.
   b) Imprints are prepared from freshly cut surfaces of the remaining tissue, which is sliced thinly and fixed in buffered formalin or B5 solution for routine processing and embedding in paraffin.
Portion 2: For cell suspension studies. This portion is placed in RPMI 1640 and cell suspensions prepared for fluorescein-labelled monoclonal antibody studies.
Portion 3: For cryostat sections and cytocentrifuge preparations. One half of this remaining portion is covered in OCT embedding medium (Miles Laboratories) and snap frozen in liquid nitrogen, wrapped in aluminium foil and stored at $-70°$ C for subsequent cryostat section immunoperoxidase staining. The remaining tissue is placed in RPMI 1640 for preparation of cytocentrifuge smears (250 r/min for 5 min in a Shandon Cytospin II) for morphological examination and immunoperoxidase staining.

It is possible to examine lymphocytes from peripheral blood, bone marrow, cerebrospinal fluid, effusions and tissue biopsies after dispersion. Contemporary monographs describing details of collection techniques and preserving medium are available (Janossy 1981; Stevenson et al. 1983; Hamblin and Smith 1984).
   Cells collected in Hanks' phosphate-buffered saline (PBS), or heparin (20 units/ml) should be processed within a few hours of collection. If delays of more than 12 h are anticipated, samples should be taken into an equal volume of culture medium such as RPMI 1640 or Medium 199 or Minimum Essential Medium (MEM).
   Lymphocyte-rich suspensions are prepared by centrifugation of the heparinised blood or fluid through a Ficoll gradient. The cell layer at the interface is collected, washed in PBS and resuspended in a mixture of bovine serum albumin and culture medium (such as RPMI 1640).

Immunological Methods

Antibodies labelled with fluorochrome (fluorescein or rhodamine) may be used to stain living cells in suspension by direct or indirect immunofluorescence. In the direct method, cell membrane antigens are stained by a fluorochrome-labelled antibody, whereas, in indirect immunofluorescence staining, the unlabelled antibody first attaches to the cell and its presence is shown by staining with labelled anti-immunoglobulin. The indirect method offers greater sensitivity and the convenience of one indicator antibody to detect a range of unlabelled primary antibodies. Fluorescein is the most commonly used labelling agent but antibodies can also be labelled with rhodamine. Double labelling can be performed, i.e. simultaneous staining by one antibody labelled with fluorescein and another labelled with rhodamine. Localisation of each antibody is visualised by using different sets of optical filters, permitting simultaneous excitation of the green fluorescence of fluorescein and the orange fluorescence of rhodamine.

By counting 200 lymphocytes after applying different antibodies directed against immunoglobulin heavy and light chains, the percentages of lymphocytes bearing each chain can be obtained. Although polyclonal antibodies are satisfactory for this study, monoclonal antibodies are preferred as they offer greater reproducibility.

Surface antibody staining patterns will vary both in strength and distribution over the cell. Capping is commonly observed if the cells are not kept at 4° C or if azide has not been added to the suspension medium. Positive staining may assume several patterns of surface fluorescence: ringed, representing equatorial focusing on a cell having fluorescent antibody distributed uniformly over its surface; speckled or patched, with some gathering of surface antigen-antibody complexes into bright aggregates; and capped, the antigen-antibody complexes having accumulated at one pole of the cell. Non-viable cells which show artefactual diffuse homogeneous staining are excluded from the count. The intensity of fluorescence is recorded as dim, moderately bright and very bright. Dim and moderately bright fluorescence is displayed by cells of B-chronic lymphocytic leukaemia (B-CLL), whereas the cells of follicular centre cell lymphomas display bright fluorescence.

In the examination for intracellular markers it is necessary to fix the cells, thereby damaging the membrane so that the indicator reagents have access to cytoplasmic or nuclear material. For example, fixation in cold methanol or formalin can be used for the demonstration of the nuclear enzyme terminal deoxynucleotidyl transferase (TdT).

The examination for surface and cytoplasmic immunoglobulin serves as a powerful tool not only to identify B lymphocytes but also to recognise clonal, neoplastic growths. A reactive lymphocyte population will contain cells bearing the spectrum of heavy and light chains representing a polyclonal population, whereas a monoclonal population of B lymphocytes can be identified when the

Table 14.1. Surface marker analysis in three cases of B cell malignancy with cutaneous infiltration (Leong and Forbes 1982)

Histology	Tissue	E	PV	G	A	M	κ	λ	MRbc	Clonality
LH-N	Skin	9	86	0	0	88	91	0	3	Mκ
	Node	27	ND	0	0	72	70	0	6	Mκ
PDLL-D	Skin	13	80	ND	ND	72	21	64	ND	
	Node	30	70	5	0	75	12	50	2	Mλ
CLL	Skin	10	80	0	0	60	50	10	ND	Mκ
	Blood	3	85	21	4	70	80	7	45	Mκ

Note: Values given as percentage.
E, E-rosette; PV, polyvalent surface immunoglobulin; G, sIgG; A, sIgA; M, sIgM; κ, $sIg_κ$; λ, $sIg_λ$; MRbc, mouse rosette; LH-N, lymphocytic-histiocytic lymphoma nodular; PDLL-D, poorly differentiated lymphocytic lymphoma diffuse; CLL, chronic lymphocytic leukaemia; ND, not done.

vast majority of cells in the sample are homogeneous, particularly with respect to the light chain determinants. Observations that the neoplastic lymphocytes may bear two heavy chains are compatible with a sequential switch in the production of heavy chains, controlled at the gene level. Examples of reactive lymphoid hyperplasia with single class surface immunoglobulin have rarely been reported (Palutke et al. 1982; Levy et al. 1983). The significance of such examples of an increase of B lymphocytes with single class surface immunoglobulins is not clear and the possibility that such surface immunoglobulin patterns are a harbinger of neoplastic disease has been suggested (Levy et al. 1983).

The lymphocyte surface markers of three examples of B lymphoproliferative disorders with cutaneous infiltration in which monoclonality could be identified are shown in Table 14.1.

Rosette Formation

Indicator erythrocytes will form spontaneous rosettes by adhering to the surface of a lymphoid cell which possesses a receptor for molecules occurring on the erythrocytes. The receptors for the naturally occurring molecules were discovered fortuitously. The sheep erythrocyte (E) receptor is on the molecule identified by CD2 antibodies; its function may be related to T cell activation, but little is known of it.

T lymphocytes spontaneously form rosettes with unsensitised sheep erythrocytes. The E-rosette technique is still the most widely used test for the identification of T lymphocytes. The rosettes formed with unsensitised sheep red blood cells, however, are tenuous and readily disrupted. Pretreatment of sheep erythrocytes with either neuraminidase or 2-5-amino-ethylisothiouronium bromide (AET) enhances the binding and increases the stability of the rosettes. A variety of experimental manipulations have been reported which affect E-rosette scores and interpretation. Such methodological modifications over the past several years have resulted in increasing E-rosette percentages for normal human blood lymphocytes as reported from different laboratories, ranging from 5%–15% in 1970 to 50%–80% in 1973 (Stein 1978). Several factors including the physiological state of the individual, inhibitory serum factors in patients with neoplasms and Hodgkin's disease, radiotherapy and chemotherapy may produce an overall lowering of values, whereas other drugs such as levamisole enhance E-rosette scores (Parker 1980). E-rosette forming cells constitute 95%–100% in postnatal thymus, 50%–80% in peripheral blood and 20%–70% in lymph nodes (Stein 1978; Black et al. 1980).

Mouse erythrocytes form spontaneous rosettes with a subpopulation of B lymphocytes. These appear to be resting, early B lymphocytes, because peripheral blood lymphocytes lose their ability to form mouse erythrocyte rosettes following activation by any stimulus. The percentages of mouse erythrocyte rosetting-lymphocytes vary slightly according to the strain of mouse erythrocytes used in the assay (McGraw et al. 1981). We have shown the usefulness of this marker to distinguish CLL from lymphosarcoma cell leukaemia (Forbes et al. 1978) and this has been confirmed by others (Sugden and Lilleman 1982). Mouse rosette formation has rarely been observed in other conditions such as plasmacytoma, Waldenström's macroglobulinaemia and a proportion of patients with hairy cell leukaemia (HCL) (Gupta et al. 1976).

Immunofluorescence on Cryostat Sections

The detection of surface immunoglobulin has been adapted to cryostat sections of lymphoid tissue (Levy et al. 1977). It can be applied to both unfixed cryostat sections or to sections fixed lightly in acetone; however, it is virtually impossible to distinguish extracellular or interstitial immunoglobulin from membrane-bound immunoglobulin by this technique.

Immunohistochemical Methods

The wide acceptance of the immunofluorescence method in the study of lymphoid neoplasms paradoxically engendered the need for an alternative technique that avoided some of the disadvantages inherent in the use of fluorescein-conjugated antibodies. Immunofluorescent staining of lymphocytes in suspension has the major disadvantages of the impermanence of immunofluorescent preparations, the need for a special microscope system utilising ultraviolet light, and the poor morphological detail of immunofluorescence preparations. In addition, the use of lymphocyte suspensions has the inherent risk of selective enrichment or loss of a certain cell subset, because some cells can be suspended more easily than others and, because of the homogenisation process, focal abnormalities in lymphoid tissues cannot be appreciated. These handicaps are largely overcome by the application of immunohistochemical techniques to tissue sections.

The search for other light microscopical labels resulted in the use of enzyme systems, particularly peroxidase and, more recently, glucose oxidase and alkaline phosphatase. Enzyme labels are developed histochemically at the end of the antigen-antibody reaction and yield intensely coloured end-products which can be viewed in an ordinary light microscope. These permanent preparations offer the additional advantage that the reactions can be adapted to the electron microscope by using suitably prepared material and making the end-product electron dense, usually by osmication.

In an attempt to obtain amplification and greater sensitivity, various bridge techniques have been developed for the unlabelled antibody-enzyme method. The most widely used of these is the peroxidase-antiperoxidase (PAP) method of Sternberger. In our laboratory, we use the more recently introduced avidin-biotin peroxidase complex (ABC) technique of Hsu et al. (1981), because of its greater sensitivity.

The tissue antigens useful in the study of neoplasms can be broadly divided into two categories. The first consists of cytoplasmic antigens which can be demonstrated in routinely fixed paraffin-embedded tissue and the second comprises the membrane antigens which are largely destroyed by fixation and paraffin-embedding and are therefore best demonstrated in frozen sections.

Paraffin Sections

The immunoperoxidase method is particularly useful in the detection of cytoplasmic immunoglobulin in paraffin sections (Fig. 14.4), but small lymphocytes with

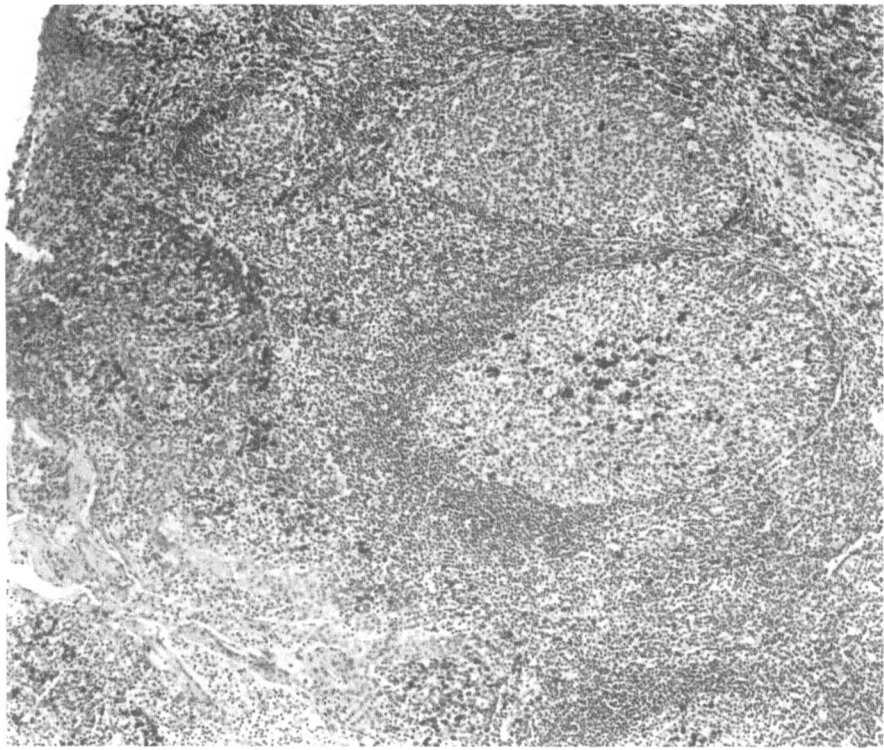

Fig. 14.4. Immunoperoxidase staining for cIg in formalin-fixed paraffin-embedded tonsil. Positive staining is seen in some cells of the germinal centres and in plasma cell in the subepithelial areas. (Anti-IgG, ABC technique, × 60)

easily detectable surface immunoglobulin show little cytoplasmic immunoglobulin (Melchers and Andersson 1974). Many tumours which can be identified in suspension as being of B cell origin by the presence of surface immunoglobulin do not stain for immunoglobulin by the immunoperoxidase technique in paraffin-embedded tissue (Callihan et al. 1979). Although this technique has the major advantage of being applicable to archived material with excellent preservation of morphological details (Fig. 14.5), immunoperoxidase studies on paraffin-embedded tissue have revealed lymphoma cells with a monotypic immunoglobulin staining pattern in only 42%–68% of cases (Curran and Jones 1979; Isaacson et al. 1980). A larger series of 89 cases of non-Hodgkin's lymphoma (NHL) showed monotypic cytoplasmic immunoglobulin in 16% of cases of nodular poorly differentiated lymphocytic lymphoma (Fig. 14.6), in 14% of diffuse poorly differentiated lymphocytic lymphoma and in only 30% of diffuse histiocytic lymphoma (DHL) (Pangalis et al. 1981).

In an attempt to improve the preservation of lymphocyte antigens in paraffin-embedded tissues, many different methods of fixation have been used. Formol sublimate, B5, Bouin's, Zenker's and cold ethanol solutions (Mason and Biberfeld 1980), fixation by microwave irradiation (Leong and Milios 1986) and the use of various proteolytic enzymes to unmask tissue antigens (Mason and Biberfeld

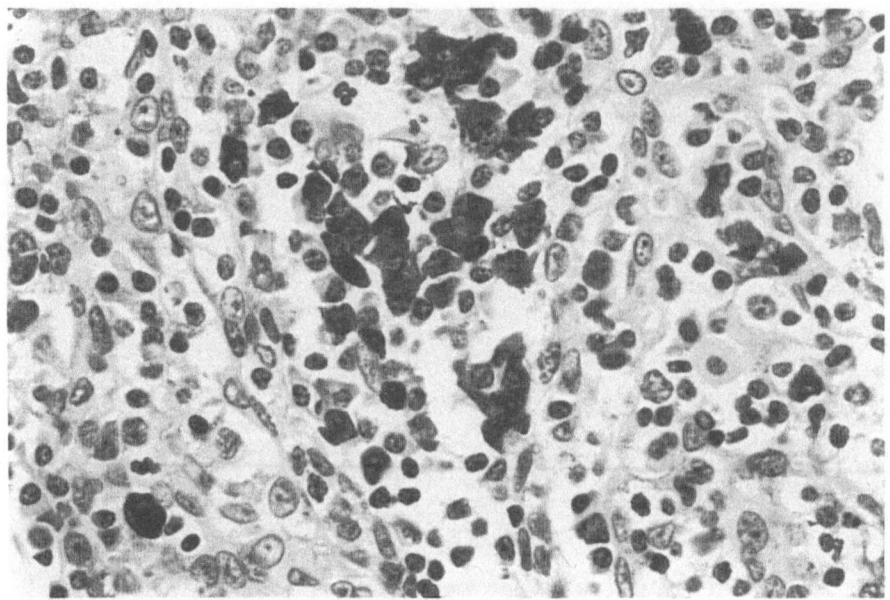

Fig. 14.5. Plasma cells in the sinuses of the tonsil stain distinctly for cIg_κ in paraffin section. Cellular morphology is distinct and the clock-face pattern of the plasma cell nuclei is discernible. (Anti-Ig_κ, ABC technique, × 500)

1980) all enhance the demonstration of cytoplasmic immunoglobulin but do not appear to improve the detection of lymphocyte surface antigens. Tissues fixed in cold acetone, embedded in low melting point paraffin wax and treated with hyaluronidase can be stained for lymphocyte surface antigens with monoclonal antibodies (Tanaka et al. 1984), but tissue sections obtained in this way are difficult to cut and morphological preservation is poor. A detailed study by Stein et al. (1985) indicates that antigenic denaturation during conventional tissue processing appears to occur during exposure to aldehyde-containing fixatives and to alcohol but not as a result of heating or exposure to melted paraffin wax. They showed that freeze-dried tissues embedded directly in paraffin wax retain surface antigens which can be displayed with an intensity equal to or greater than that observed on frozen sections.

Surface membrane Ig can be stained by the immunogold-silver method (Holgate et al. 1983a) in formol sublimate-fixed paraffin sections of NHL (Holgate et al. 1983b). This indirect immunohistochemical method employs immunoglobulin adsorbed to colloidal gold as the secondary antiserum. The gold particles introduced to antigenic sites are then revealed by a silver precipitation reaction. The technique is much more sensitive (reportedly up to 200-fold) than standard immunoperoxidase and immunogold staining methods.

Cryostat Sections

Currently, one of the most effective immunohistochemical methods of studying benign and malignant lymphoid tissues is the application of immunoperoxidase

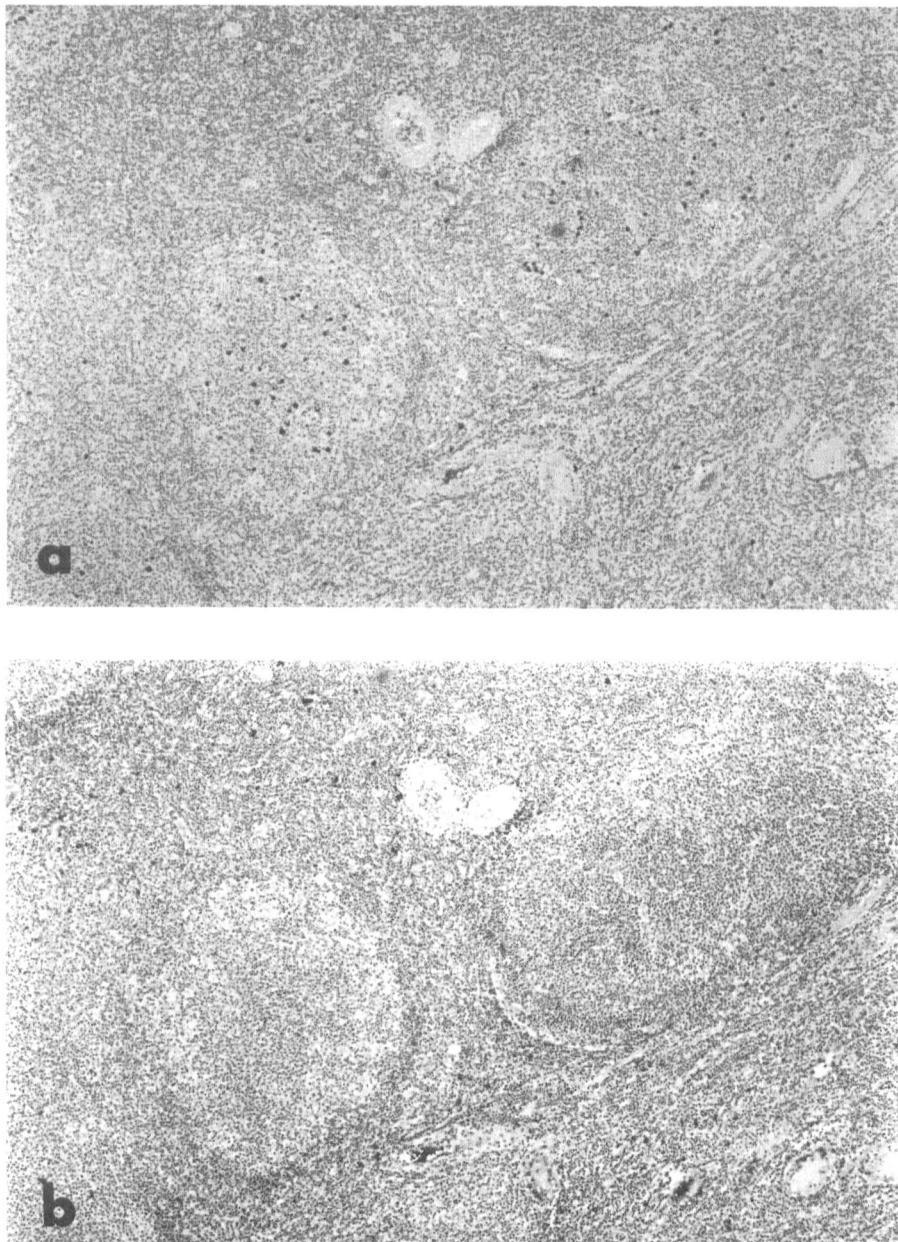

Fig. 14.6a,b. Consecutive paraffin sections of Bouin's-fixed lymph node with a follicle centre cell lymphoma, mixed cell type (centroblastic-centrocytic). **a** Scattered cells in the neoplastic follicles stain for cIg$_\kappa$. **b** Only extrafollicular cells stain for cIg$_\lambda$. (Avidin-biotin peroxidase, hemotoxylin counterstain, ×50)

techniques to frozen sections (Stein et al. 1980; Tubbs et al. 1981). The capacity to demonstrate surface membrane antigens in frozen sections eliminates many of the drawbacks of suspension studies already discussed and allows the anatomical pathologist to work with a permanent preparation and a medium with which he is familiar (Fig. 14.7). The technique involves the application of any of the indirect immunoperoxidase methods to frozen sections briefly fixed in cold acetone. Peroxidase-catalysed colour reaction is commonly carried out with 3, 3-diamino-benzidine tetra-hydrochloride (DAB) or with 3-amino-9-ethylcarbazole (AEC) or 4-chloro-1-naphthol, the latter two chromogens having the disadvantage of requiring aqueous mounting. DAB staining can be further enhanced with a variety of agents such as copper sulphate, nickel chloride, amidazole at alkaline pH or thioglycolic acid-silver nitrate.

Alkaline phosphatase is becoming increasingly popular in immunohistology as an alternative enzymatic system to immunoperoxidase, particularly in double-staining schemes along with peroxidase. In principle, it may be substituted for peroxidase in any system and has been employed in a method analogous to the PAP procedure (Mason et al. 1983). Alkaline phosphatase may be useful as a substitute for peroxidase in staining tissues which contain large amounts of endogenous peroxidase, such as in Hodgkin's disease. Glucose oxidase may be substituted for peroxidase in a manner analogous to the PAP method (Clark et al. 1982), because it has not been shown to exist in mammalian tissues. Glucose oxidase may be attractive in certain situations in which other enzymes generate high background. It is localised using a substrate of nitro-blue tetrazolium.

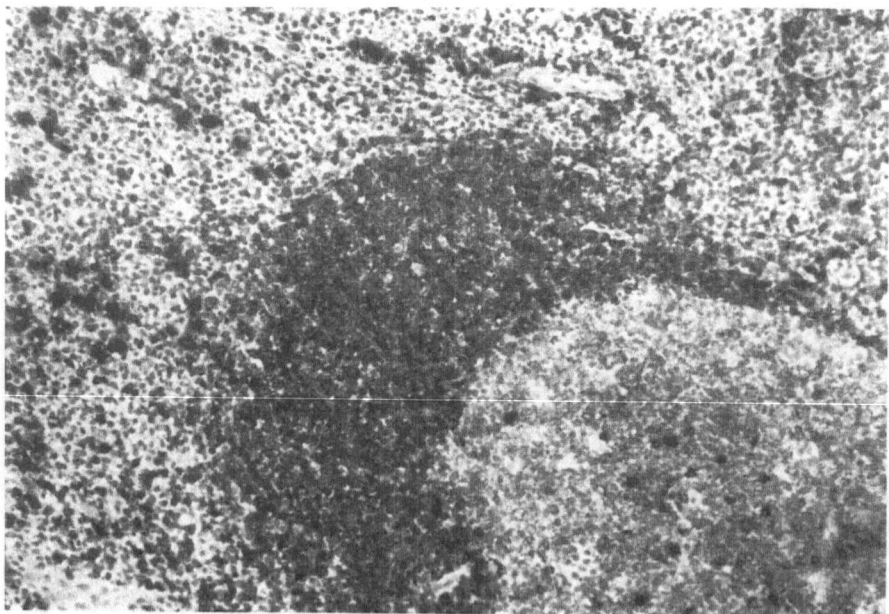

Fig. 14.7. Frozen section of tonsil showing marked membranous staining of mantle zone lymphocytes for sIgD. (Anti-IgD, modified ABC technique, × 125)

Nearly all of the techniques that have been discussed may be used in combination to detect two different antigens simultaneously in the same tissue section. Such double-staining techniques allow an accurate assessment of the topographic inter-relationships of two cell types, which may be useful in detecting neoplastic cells, for example malignant foci in lymph nodes. Double staining may also shed light on the histogenesis of proliferative patterns in identical or adjacent tissue sites which are histologically dissimilar, and on cellular interactions in inflammatory infiltrates.

Recently, microwave irradiation was introduced into the procedure of immunoperoxidase staining of lymphocyte membrane antigens (Leong and Milios 1986). Irradiation of the frozen section for a matter of a few seconds produces rapid drying and fixation of the tissue sections, and the subsequent exposure to a short burst of irradiation rapidly accelerates the reaction of the primary antibody and the cell surface antigen.

Falini et al. (1984) have applied the immunoalkaline phosphatase method to frozen sections of undecalcified bone marrow biopsies, successfully phenotyping acute leukaemias and labelling lymphocytes and their subsets in reactive and neoplastic conditions.

Imprints and Cytocentrifuge Preparations

The impermanence of fluorescent preparations and their poor morphological detail has led to the application of immunoperoxidase staining to cell smears, imprints and cytocentrifuge preparations. Air-dried smears and imprints prepared from peripheral blood and lymphoid tissues can be stained with the indirect immunoperoxidase technique following fixation in acetone at 4°C for 5–10 min (Banks et al. 1983; Giorno 1983) or with the immunoalkaline phosphatase method following 30 s of fixation in formol acetone (Erber et al. 1984). These techniques are very sensitive, permitting the use of high dilutions of monoclonal antibodies. They have the major advantages of permitting the simultaneous assessment of single cell morphology and immunological phenotype, an exercise not possible in immunofluorescent cell suspensions or in immunoperoxidase-stained frozen sections. Cytocentrifuge preparations can be made from buffy-coat cells isolated from peripheral blood in EDTA or from disaggregated lymphocytes obtained by passing minced fragments of biopsied lymphoid tissue through a wire mesh. The cells obtained are resuspended at 5×10^5 cells/ml in PBS with 30% horse serum albumin. Cytocentrifuge smears are prepared by spinning 0.2 ml aliquots (1×10^5 cells) of the suspension at 250 r/min for 5 min in a Cytospin II (Shandon Instruments, London, England).

Enumeration of lymphocyte subpopulations on cytocentrifuge smears of peripheral blood stained with an indirect ABC procedure is reliable and reproducible. When compared to flow cytometry employing direct immunofluorescence, the ABC procedure was not only a valid method of assessment but also appeared to detect a greater proportion of immunostained lymphocytes for all subsets tested than did flow cytometry (Paradis et al. 1984). This method of enumeration of lymphocyte subsets should prove to be increasingly popular as it possesses several important advantages over analysis by flow cytometry. It is more widely adaptable and less expensive than flow cytometer analysis since it utilises standard, commercially available reagents and simple laboratory equipment rather than the expensive and technologically complicated fluorescence-activated cell sorter. Furthermore, the ABC analysis produces a permanent record, as do all immuno-peroxidase techniques, whereas flow cytometry analysis employs a suspension of live cells that have a limited life span. Lastly, ABC analysis utilises one-tenth as many cells as does flow cytometry analysis. This is particularly useful in instances where only small numbers of lymphocytes are available for analysis, such as in bronchoalveolar lavage specimens or in small infants or patients receiving chemotherapy. In our laboratory, the enumeration of ABC-stained lymphocyte subsets on cytocentrifuge smears prepared from biopsy specimens is replacing immunofluorescence suspension surface marker analysis and is an important adjuvant to frozen section immunoperoxidase examination (Fig. 14.8).

Immunogold reagents are another effective labelling system for lymphocyte immunotyping in both light (Crockard and Catovsky 1983; DeWaele et al. 1983; Wybran et al. 1985) and electron microscopy (Geoghegan et al. 1978; Matutes and Catovsky 1982). The amplification of immunogold staining by a silver precipitation reaction has been demonstrated to be a sensitive method for revealing lymphocyte surface immunoglobulin in paraffin-embedded tissues (Holgate et al. 1983b). The recent adaptation of this staining technique to smears and cytocentrifuge preparations, which can be subsequently counterstained with standard panoptic Wright or May–Grunwald Giemsa stain, produces excellent morphological detail (Romasco et al. 1985).

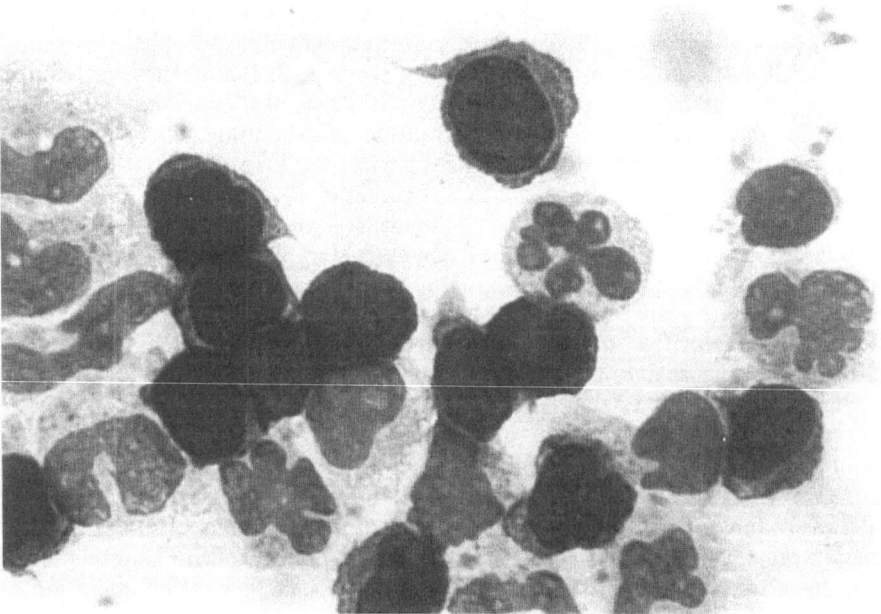

Fig. 14.8. Cytospin preparation of peripheral blood stained for T lymphocytes (CD3/Leu-4, modified ABC technique, × 1250)

Unfixed buffy-coat cells from blood or lymphoid tissues are incubated with the primary monoclonal antibody and washed in PBS before incubation with colloidal gold-labelled secondary goat anti-mouse antibodies. Buffy-coat smears or Cytospin preparations are then fixed in 1% glutaraldehyde in absolute ethanol before silver staining. In the presence of a reducing agent (hydroquinone), colloidal gold particles catalyse the reduction of silver ions (silver lactate). The progressive deposition of metallic silver encapsulates the gold probes producing a dense black silver shell, a label clearly visible in the light microscope. This new procedure is simple and rapid, being performed in less than 3 h. It is more sensitive than immunofluorescence and immunogold staining, and morphological examination and cell identification are greatly facilitated by the panoptic counterstains which can be used with this technique (Fig. 14.9).

The importance of correlating cytomorphological features with immunological markers cannot be overemphasised, especially in distinguishing T cell lymphoma from hyperplasia. Resting and reactive peripheral T cell populations are normally composed of mixtures of CD4 + helper T cells and CD8 + suppressor T cells, all of which express the pan T antigens such as CD2, CD3 and CD5. T cell lymphomas lack one or more of these pan T antigens and express either a pure helper or suppressor phenotype (Grogen et al. 1985; Weiss et al. 1985). However, the antigens of helper and suppressor T cells are not clonal markers and it is essential to confirm that the cytologically atypical lymphocytes are indeed T cells. This can be done by examining the morphology of E-rosetting lymphocytes (Leong et al. 1981) or Cytospin preparations or imprints of the cells marked by pan T antibodies using any of the immunoperoxidase techniques or the immuno-

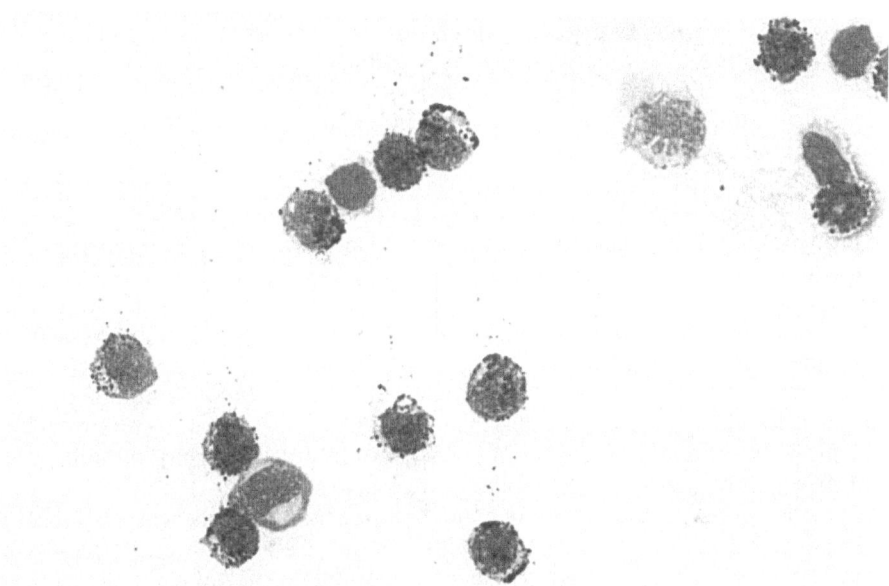

Fig. 14.9. Cytospin preparation of peripheral blood stained for T lymphocytes. Positive cells are covered by black silver particles. (CD3/Leu-4, immunogold silver, × 500)

gold-silver procedure described previously. A monoclonal T cell population can be demonstrated definitively by determination of the rearrangement of genes for the chains of the T cell receptor.

Histochemical Stains

Standard cytochemical techniques are available for the detection of intracellular substrates or the indirect demonstration of enzymes. Some 20 enzymes in lymphoid cells have been documented, although relatively few of these reactions have been studied in any great detail (Crockard 1984). Comprehensive accounts of the various cytochemical procedures are available (Hayhoe et al. 1980; Schwarze 1980) and recently these techniques have been standardised by an international committee (Shibata et al. 1985).

Periodic-acid Schiff

Periodic-acid Schiff (PAS) staining has limited application in the lymphoprolifera-tive disorders. Lymphocytes of CLL have increased glycogen content, making them PAS positive, and a positive PAS reaction has been reported in cells of B prolymphocytic leukaemia (Catovsky et al. 1974) and less commonly in T prolymphocytic leukaemia. The PAS reaction in lymphoproliferative disorders shows a great variability, greatly diminishing its diagnostic or prognostic value. Diastase-resistant PAS-positive globules represent immunoglobulin and charac-terise a lymphoma as a B cell neoplasm containing cytoplasmic immunoglobulin such as seen in lymphoplasmacytic/lymphoplasmacytoid lymphoma, follicle centre cell lymphomas and B immunoblastic lymphoma.

Non-specific Esterase

The esterases are a group of enzymes capable of hydrolysing a variety of aliphatic or aromatic esters in an acid or neutral pH. The term "non-specific esterase" refers to esterases with a preference for short-chain esters such as acetate or butyrate and distinguishes them from the specific esterase activity of granulocytes and mast cells using naphthol AS-D chloroacetate as a substrate. Non-specific esterase activity has been employed principally as a marker for mononuclear phagocytes, although it may be identified in a variety of other cell types including megakaryocytes, plasma cells and even epithelial cells. The presence of non-specific esterase activity which can be inhibited by sodium fluoride is useful for distinguishing monocytes and their precursors from cells of the granulocyte series.

For the identification of monocytic and megakaryocytic cells, α-naphthyl butyrate and α-naphthyl acetate are preferable substrates (Li et al. 1975). The α-naphthyl acetate esterase (ANAE) reaction is of diagnostic value for the recogni-tion of acute myelomonocytic leukaemia, immature histiocytic neoplasias, and other non-lymphoid tumours which must be considered in the differential diagnosis of certain types of NHL.

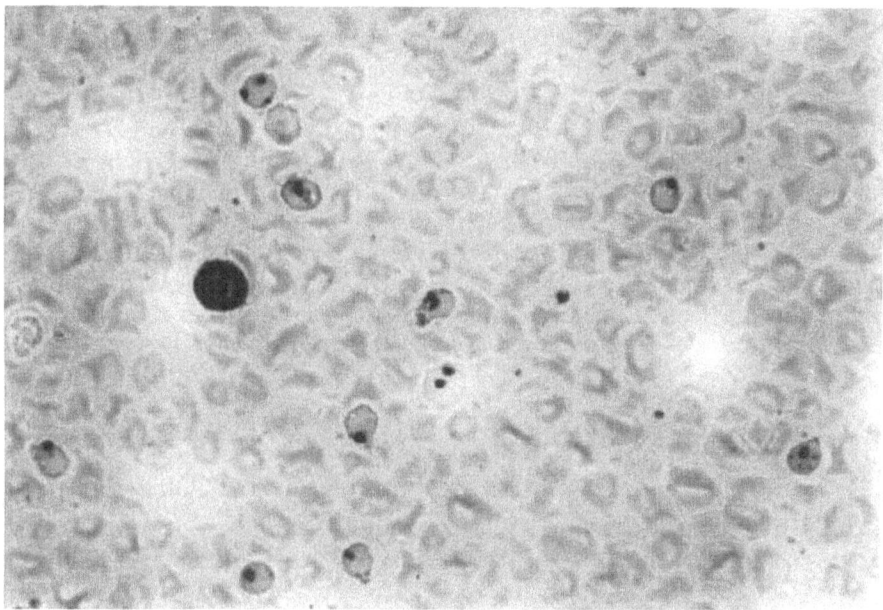

Fig. 14.10. α-naphthylacetate esterase staining of peripheral blood in a case of T-CLL. Dot-like staining is seen in the T lymphocytes while a larger monocyte shows diffuse positivity. (ANAE, × 500)

ANAE at pH 5.0 identifies the acid esterase of T lymphocytes. T lymphocytes contain one or occasionally two distinct spot-like granules or several smaller granules accumulated in a focal area of the cytoplasm distinct from the diffuse staining seen in monocytes and histiocytes (Fig. 14.10). Grossi et al. (1978) first reported that the characteristic dot-like ANAE reaction was associated almost entirely with T helper cells, T suppressor cells being unreactive. Subsequent work using a modified technique confirmed the spot-like ANAE reaction in T helper cells but also showed a paranuclear distribution of reaction product in T suppressor cells. It appears that the respective reaction patterns are not exclusively associated with either subset of T lymphocytes (Ferrarini et al. 1980; Basso et al. 1981; Van der Loo et al. 1981; Crockard et al. 1982). Although a higher proportion of T helper lymphocytes than T suppressor lymphocytes displays spot-like ANAE staining, the overlap precludes using ANAE reactivity as a means of distinguishing these respective T cell subsets (Armitage et al. 1982; Bernard and Dufer 1983; Crockard and Catovsky 1983; DeWaele et al. 1983). ANAE staining is applicable to frozen sections and to fresh tissue optimally fixed in Baker's fixative in cacodylate buffer at pH 7.4. Both techniques show distinctive dot-like positivity in T lymphocytes. Approximately 40%–50% of MHC class II-positive B lymphocytes in the peripheral blood are ANAE positive, although the vast majority display a diffuse staining (Bernard and Dufer 1983; Crockard and Catovsky 1983).

ANAE staining is quite variable in T cell malignancies. For example, granular ANAE reactivity has been observed in pre-T-ALL cells (Huhn et al. 1981), whereas in T-ALL cells weak or negative ANAE reactions have been reported

(McKenna et al. 1979; Veerman et al. 1983). Granular ANAE positivity or negative reactions have been recorded in T lymphoblastic lymphoma (Navas-Palacios et al. 1981), and the cells of T prolymphocytic leukaemia are said to show localised ANAE positivity (Crockard et al. 1982). ANAE staining is weak and diffuse in T-CLL, while Sézary cells are rich in hydrolytic enzymes including ANAE (Crockard et al. 1982). ANAE staining is variable in the peripheral T cell malignancies. We have found positive dot-like staining in node-based T cell lymphomas (Leong et al. 1981) in keeping with the mature post-thymic phenotype of the malignant T cells. A dot-like ANAE positivity has been observed in the cells of human B cell lymphoma cell lines and in cells of biopsy specimens from patients with multiple myeloma. However, none of the ANAE-positive B cell lymphomas have so far expressed a pronounced dot-like pattern (Schwarze 1980).

Acid Phosphatase

Acid phosphatases are a group of enzymes capable of hydrolysing phosphate ester in acid pH. They are located in lysosomes and have been considered the marker enzymes of these organelles. Positive activities are found in the cytoplasm of most nucleated haemic cells. The acid phosphatase reaction has two important applications in clinical haematology: the diagnosis of HCL and the discrimination between lymphoproliferative disorders of T and non-T cell type. A predominantly focal, often tightly packed accumulation of granules or one or more small dot-like granules makes up the reaction pattern of lymphoblastic lymphoma; it is also seen in T-ALL. Strong focal acid phosphatase reactivity is indeed characteristic of T lymphoblasts and may be regarded as a definite indication of the T cell nature of a lymphoblastic lymphoma or ALL in cases showing the constellation of male preponderance, a high blast count and a mediastinal mass in childhood. Acid phosphatase positivity is also seen in some B lymphocytes such as lymphoplasma-cytoid cells and plasma cells and their corresponding tumours. However, the pattern of staining in these instances is different, in that a semicircular or crescentic distribution is observed.

Tartrate-resistant Acid Phosphatase

Most cases of HCL and some cases of B and T prolymphocytic leukaemia show tartrate-resistant acid phosphatase (TRAP) positivity. This staining reaction is of high diagnostic value, even though a few cases of various other NHLs, such as B immunoblastic lymphoma, may be TRAP positive. TRAP has also been detected in Gaucher's cells, osteoblasts and macrophages of the thyroid gland. More recently, it has been shown to be an inducible differentiation marker for transformation of human blood monocytes into a specific subset of macrophages (Radzun et al. 1983).

Alkaline Phosphatase

Predominantly membrane-bound alkaline phosphatase activity is a characteristic feature of B cells in lymphoid follicles and of malignant lymphomas that are composed of or derived from germinal centres, particularly the mantle zones (Nanba et al. 1977; Weisenburger et al. 1981).

Other Enzyme Reactions

Naphthol-AS-D-chloroacetate esterase and peroxidase reactions are important stains in that they are consistently negative in lymphocytes and other lymphoid cells. These reactions are also of diagnostic value in the identification of granulocytes and their precursors, myelomonocytic cells and tissue mast cells, the peroxidase reaction being generally the more sensitive of the two. The naphthol-AS-D-chloroacetate esterase stain for tissue sections (Leder stain) is particularly useful for the identification of granulocytic sarcoma, an entity often difficult to separate from large cell lymphoma in tissue sections.

TdT is a DNA polymerase which has proved to be a useful intracellular marker because of its restricted distribution in cells of lymphoid tissues. This enzyme is present in blastic or immature cells of either T or pre-B cell type, mature lymphocytes and mitogen-stimulated lymphocytes showing no detectable TdT activity. TdT-positive cells are the major population in ALL and frequently appear as part of the leukaemic population during the "blast crisis" of chronic myelogenous leukaemia (CML), in acute non-lymphocytic leukaemia, and on exceedingly rare occasions in acute myelogenous or acute myelomonocytic leukaemia (Bollum 1979). The enzyme is frequently present in lymphoblastic lymphoma and on occasions has been reported in T-CLL and Sézary syndrome (Braziel et al. 1983). TdT can be effectively stained by antibodies with any immunofluorescence or immunoperoxidase procedure (Braziel et al. 1983; Tavares de Castro et al. 1984; Lanham et al. 1985).

Two other enzymes which may have a role to play in the distinction of B and T lymphocytes are the hydrolases β-glucuronidase and N-acetyl-β-glucosaminidase. β-Glucuronidase-positive cells in the peripheral blood appear to coincide in numbers with E-rosetting lymphocytes but glucosaminidase-reactive cells exceed E-rosetting cells in most instances (Crockard et al. 1983).

Table 14.2 shows the cytochemical profiles of various acute and chronic lymphoid leukaemias.

Flow Cytometry

Rapid advances in computing and electronics in the field of electronic cell counting led to the development of what was probably the first "clinically applicable" flow cytometer made by Bonner and associates in 1972 (Bonner et al. 1972). For comprehensive reviews of flow cytometric technology see papers by Shapiro (1983) and Lovett et al. (1984). The fluorescence-activated cell sorter (FACS) makes possible the rapid analysis of a monodispersed suspension of cells tagged by fluorochrome-labelled probes. This method of cell analysis by FACS has wide applications in the investigation of the lymphoid neoplasms, especially the leukaemias. Its application to the diagnosis of lymphomas and to the differential diagnosis between lymphomas and pseudolymphomatous lesions is

Table 14.2. Cytochemical profile of lymphoid leukaemias (after Crockard 1984)

Leukaemia type	Acid phosphatase	ANAE	β-glucuronidase	N-acetyl-β-glucosaminidase
Acute lymphoblastic leukaemia (ALL)				
T lineage:				
Pre-T-ALL	+/+ +[a]	±	+	+
T-ALL	+/+ +[a]	±	+	+
T-LbLy	+/+ +[a]	±/+	+	+
B lineage:				
Pre-B-ALL cALL	±/+	−/+	±/+	+/+ +
B-ALL	−/±	−/+	−	+
Chronic lymphocytic leukaemia (CLL)				
T lineage:				
T-PLL	+	+ +	+ +	+ +
T-CLL$_\gamma$	+ +	±	+ +	+ +
Sézary	+ +	+ +	+ +	+ +
ATL	±/+	±/+	±/+	+ +
B lineage:				
B-CLL	−/±	−/±	−/±	−
B-PLL	−/±	−/±	−/±	−
HCL	+ +[a]	−/±	−/±	−
MM	+ +	+ +	+ +	+ +

MM, Multiple myeloma; T-LbLy, T-lymphoblastic lymphoma
Strength of reaction: + +, strong; +, moderate; ±, weak; −, negative;
[a]Tartrate resistant.

somewhat more complex than for the diagnosis of lymphoid leukaemias. The reason for this greater complexity lies in the fact that heterogeneous populations of lymphocytes are usually found in lymph nodes, despite the presence of a lymphomatous infiltrate.

The partial involvement of a lymph node by the lymphoma and the presence of residual non-neoplastic lymphocytes in a suspension of cells made from the lymph node may render it difficult to establish the presence of a clear-cut monoclonal proliferation by cell surface phenotype analysis in the FACS. In such cases, either single parameter DNA analysis or multiparameter analysis using the Braylan technique may prove to be useful (Braylan et al. 1982). Loss of the architectural relationship in the homogenised lymphoid tissue is a handicap of this system of analysis. Because pathologists use tissue architecture in addition to individual cell morphology to diagnose disease, an attractive compromise is to combine the quantitative precise analytical capabilities of flow cytometry with qualitative immunohistochemical analysis. Other limitations of FACS are the difficulty of disaggregating certain tumours and tissues such as skin, and the expense currently involved. The instruments are expensive to acquire and to maintain, and highly qualified technical personnel are needed for correct operation. However, cytofluorometric analysis holds promise of exciting possibilities in the investigation of lymphoid neoplasms. To date, sophisticated refinements like the "kappa-lambda test" (Weinberg et al. 1984) indicate that the FACS is potentially capable of detecting small numbers of monoclonal B lymphocytes, providing a powerful tool for establishing lymphomatous involvement in cases which are equivocal by standard immunological methods. In the absence of applicable monoclonal markers for T lymphocytes, it is still not possible to detect "clonal excess" of T lymphocytes by this technology.

Ultrastructural Analysis

Electron microscopy is useful for studying lymphoid neoplasms. In general, the ultrastructural characteristics of human lymphocyte leukaemias and lymphomas conform to the light microscopic features. The presence of identifying characteristics such as specific granules, melanosomes, cell junctions and other organelles may be useful in distinguishing lymphomas from other anaplastic round cell tumours. The value of ultrastructural examination in lymphomas has been increased by the use of immunocytochemical techniques with labels such as peroxidase, ferritin or immunogold, by enzyme cytochemistry using electron-dense reaction products, and by rosette methods, particularly since the same techniques are useful for light microscopy.

Sampling is a major problem encountered in the electron microscopy of human lymphomas. The degree of involvement of a lymphoid organ by a lymphomatous process may be minimal or extensive, focal or diffuse. If diffuse, adequate sampling for electron microscopy presents little difficulty, however, if a node is only partially or focally involved, adequate sampling is essential. It is important therefore to confirm the presence of tumour involvement in thick plastic sections before examination is carried out by the electron microscope. The immunocytochemical demonstration of lymphocyte antigens by the electron microscope requires the use of labels with specific characteristics. These labels identify the sites of antigen-antibody reaction because they are inherently electron dense (metals), have a distinct configuration (ferritin, haemocyanin, tobacco mosaic virus, microspheres, etc.), or because they can produce an electron dense reaction product (enzymes). Horseradish peroxidase, an example of the last type, has proved to have a broad application, because it can be used for both light as well as electron microscopy. Other enzymes such as phosphatases can also be used, but the peroxidase label in conjunction with a chromogenic substrate such as diaminobenzidine, which is rendered electron opaque by treatment with osmium tetroxide, provides an excellent marker.

Cells in suspension stained by the immunogold-silver method described above are ideally suited to electron microscopic examination. Pre-embedding immunoperoxidase staining may also be applied to thick frozen sections of fixed tissue prior to post-fixation, embedding and ultra-thin sectioning. With this method, penetration into the thick sections is a limiting factor due to the large molecular size of the antibody or antibody-peroxidase conjugate, but the use of $F(ab')_2$ and peroxidase fragments helps to resolve the problem (Kraehenbuhl and Jamieson 1974; Nakane 1975). Post-embedding staining involves staining antigens at the surface of ultra-thin sections of resin-embedded tissue. Since the antigen is at the surface, penetration may not be a problem, but the effect of dehydrating agents and embedding resins on different antigens is unpredictable. In the case of lymphomas where the majority of the antigens of interest are on the cell membrane, penetration is not a problem, but the cells must be stained in suspension for the detection of surface determinants (Reyes et al. 1975).

Application of enzyme cytochemistry to the ultrastructural study of lymphoid neoplasms has been relatively limited. The principles governing reaction conditions and enzyme specificity are in general the same for electron microscopy as for light microscopy with the exception that the reaction product must be electron dense. The limitation of the light microscope in the accurate localisation of enzyme activity within the cell is avoided by the electron microscope, with which the exact location of an enzyme within an organelle is possible. A wide spectrum of enzymes including phosphatases (Poore et al. 1981), esterases (Boesen 1984), dehyrogenases, glycosidases and transaminases can be demonstrated if the reaction conditions and fixation are appropriate for the preservation of both enzyme activity and fine structure (Hayat 1973). Aldehydes generally preserve enzyme activity better than other fixatives and glutaraldehyde is the most widely used. Methods for detecting 5′-nucleotidase and ATPase ultrastructurally have been used in differentiating the different types of stromal cells in normal lymphoid tissue and lymphomas (Lennert and Niedorf 1969).

Conclusions

The development of an increasingly precise and sophisticated lymphocyte marker technology for the detailed characterisation of human lymphocyte subpopulations has already contributed significantly to the understanding of a number of disorders, particularly the immune deficiencies. It has also provided important insights into leucocyte differentiation and the cellular origin of leukaemias. The combination of traditional surface marker techniques with highly specific monoclonal antibodies and cytochemical staining has made it possible to define precisely the stages of human lymphocyte differentiation. Studies of human B cell-associated antigens on leukaemias and lymphomas indicate that tumours of B cell lineage can be related to B cell differentiation pathways (Anderson et al. 1984; Caligaris-Cappio and Janossy 1985). Such multiparameter studies have enabled the separation of ALL into five major clinical and prognostic subgroups (Foon et al. 1982). The immunological approach has established the heterogeneity of childhood ALL and has led to a change in the therapeutic approach to the ALL subtypes. Cells from patients with CLL, NHL and Sézary syndrome can also be classified by their reactivity with monoclonal antibodies (Foon et al. 1982).

While many of the current classifications of NHL are based purely on morphological criteria (Leong 1983), it is possible, using current immunological techniques, to classify NHLs according to their apparent cell of origin since lymphomas, like leukemias, may retain the markers and functions of the normal cell counterparts from which they arise. Careful correlation of morphology with markers may well allow recognition of morphological subtypes based on subtle, previously unrecognised histological features. Of even more importance, the antigenic phenotype of different lymphomas and leukaemias may be associated with distinctive clinical features and different responses to therapeutic regimens, as has already been well demonstrated in childhood ALL. In spite of the current confusion in classification, it is apparent that multiparameter studies and a functional approach will continue to enhance our understanding of the biology of the malignant lymphomas and lead to more rational evaluations of prognosis and selection of therapy.

References

Anderson KC, Bates MP, Slaughenhoupt BL, Pinkus GS, Schlossman SF, Nadler LM (1984) Expression of human B-cell-associated antigens on leukaemias and lymphomas: a model of human B-cell differentiation. Blood 63: 1424–1433

Armitage RJ, Linch DC, Worman CP, Cawley JC (1982) The morphology and cytochemistry of human T-cell populations defined by monoclonal antibodies and Fc receptors. Br J Haematol 51: 605–613

Banks PM, Caron BL, Morgan TW (1983) Use of imprints for monoclonal antibody studies: suitability of air-dried preparations from lymphoid tissues with an immunohistochemical method. Am J Clin Pathol 79: 438–442

Basso G, Semenzato G, Cocito MG, Pezzutto A, Agostini C, Zanesco L (1981) Cytochemical study in human lymphocyte subpopulations as defined by Fc receptors. Thymus 3: 195–201

Bernard J, Dufer J (1983) Cytochemical analysis of human peripheral blood lymphocyte subsets defined by monoclonal antibodies. Scand J Immunol 17: 89–93

Black RB, Leong AS-Y, Cowled PA, Forbes IJ (1980) Lymphocyte subpopulations in human lymph nodes: a normal range. Lymphology 13: 86–90

Boesen AM (1984) Ultrastructural localisation of acid alpha-naphthylacetate esterase in human normal and neoplastic lymphocytic and monocytic cells and in hairy cells. Scand J Haematol 32: 367–373

Bollum FJ (1979) Terminal deoxynucleotidyl transferase as a hematopoietic cell marker. Blood 54: 1203–1215

Bonner WA, Hulett HR, Sweet RG, Herzenberg LA (1972) Fluorescence activated cell sorting. Rev Sci Inst 43: 404–409

Braylan RC, Benson NA, Nourse V, Kruth HS (1982) Correlated analysis of cellular DNA, membrane antigens and light scatter of human lymphoid cells. Cytometry 2: 337–343

Braziel RM, Keneklis T, Donlon JA et al. (1983) Terminal deoxynucleotidyl transferase in non-Hodgkin's lymphoma. Am J Clin Pathol 80: 655–659

Caligaris-Cappio F, Janossy G (1985) Surface markers in chronic lymphoid leukemias of B-cell type. Semin Hematol 22: 1–12

Callihan TR, Braylan RC, Farnham R et al. (1979) Correlation between immunohistochemistry and cell surface markers in diffuse large cell ("histiocytic") lymphomas. Lab Invest 40: 244 (abstract)

Catovsky D, Galetto J, Okos A et al. (1974) Cytochemical profile of B and T leukaemic lymphocytes with special reference to acute lymphoblastic leukaemia. J Clin Pathol 27: 767–771

Clark CA, Downs EC, Primus FJ (1982) An unlabelled antibody method using glucose oxidase-antiglucose oxidase complexes (GAG): a sensitive alternative to immunoperoxidase for the detection of tissue antigens. J Histochem Cytochem 30: 27–34

Crockard A (1984) Cytochemistry of lymphoid cells: a review of findings in the normal and leukemic state. Histochem J 16: 1027–1050

Crockard A, Catovsky D (1983) Cytochemistry of normal lymphocyte subsets defined by monoclonal antibodies and immunocolloidal gold. Scand J Haematol 30: 433–443

Crockard A, Chalmers D, Matutes E, Catovsky D (1982) Cytochemistry of acid hydrolases in chronic B- and T-cell leukemias. Am J Clin Pathol 78: 437–444

Crockard AD, MacFarlane E, Jess H, Catovsky D (1983) Correlation of lymphocyte beta-glucuronidase and N-acetyl-beta-glucosaminidase with E-rosette formation. Histochem J 15: 179–183

Curran RC, Jones EL (1979) Non-Hodgkin's lymphomas: an immunohistochemical and histological study. J Pathol 129: 179–190

DeWaele M, DeMey J, Moeremans M et al. (1983) Immunogold staining method for the light microscopic detection of leukocyte cell surface antigens with monoclonal antibodies. J Histochem Cytochem 31: 376–381

Erber WN, Pinching AJ, Mason DY (1984) Immunocytochemical detection of T and B cell populations in routine blood smears. Lancet I: 1042–1046

Erikson J, Williams DL, Finan J, Nowell PC, Croce CM (1985) Locus of the *alpha*-chain of the T-cell receptor is split by chromosome translocation in T-cell leukemias. Science 229: 784–786

Falini B, Martelli MF, Tarallo F et al. (1984) Immunohistological analysis of human bone marrow trephine biopsies using monoclonal antibodies. Br J Haematol 56: 365–386

Ferrarini M, Cadoni A, Franzi AT et al. (1980) Ultrastructure and cytochemistry of human peripheral blood lymphocytes. Similarities between the cells of the third population and T gamma lymphocytes. Eur J Immunol 10: 562–570

Foon KA, Schroff RW, Gale RP (1982) Surface markers on leukemia and lymphoma cells: recent advances. Blood 60: 1–19

Forbes IJ, Zalewski PD, Leong AS-Y et al. (1978) B cell leukaemia distinguished from chronic lymphocytic leukaemia by surface markers. Aust NZ J Med 8: 532–538

Geoghegan WD, Scillian JJ, Ackerman GA (1978) The detection of human B lymphocytes by both light and electron microscopy utilising colloidal gold labelled anti-immunoglobulin. Immunol Commun 7: 1–12

Giorno R (1983) Characterisation of mononuclear cells in cytocentrifuge and imprint preparations using monoclonal antibodies and an avidin-biotin immunoperoxidase staining system. J Histochem Cytochem 31: 1326–1328

Grogan TM, Fielder K, Rangel C et al. (1985) Peripheral T cell lymphoma: aggressive disease with heterogenous immunotypes. Am J Clin Pathol 83: 279–288

Grossi CE, Webb SR, Zicca A et al. (1978) Morphological and histochemical analyses of two human T-cell subpopulations bearing receptors for IgM or IgG. J Exp Med 147: 1405–1417

Gupta S, Good RA, Siegal FP (1976) Rosette formation with mouse erythrocytes. III. Studies in patients with primary immunodeficiency and lymphoproliferative disorders. Clin Exp Immunol 26: 204–213

Hamblin TJ, Smith JL (1984) Cell markers on lymphocytes in suspension. Association of Clinical Pathologists' Broadsheet 112, December 1984, pp 1–12

Hayat MA (1973) Electron microscopy of enzymes. Principles and methods, vol I. Von Nostrand Rheinhold, New York, pp 1–149

Hayhoe FGJ, Quaglino D, Doll R (1980) Cytology and cytochemistry of acute leukemias. MRC Special Report Series No 304. HMSO, London

Holgate CS, Jackson P, Cowen PN, Bird CC (1983a) Immunogold-silver staining: new method of immunostaining with enhanced sensitivity. J Histochem Cytochem 31: 938–944

Holgate CS, Jackson P, Lauder I et al. (1983b) Surface membrane staining of immunoglobulins in paraffin sections of non-Hodgkin's lymphomas using immunogold-silver staining technique. J Clin Pathol 36: 742–746

Hsu S-M, Raine L, Fanger H (1981) A comparative study of the peroxidase-antiperoxidase method and an avidin-biotin complex method for studying polypeptide hormones with radioimmunoassay antibodies. Am J Clin Pathol 75: 734–738

Huhn D, Thiel E, Rodt H, Andreewa P (1981) Cytochemistry and membrane markers in acute lymphatic leukemia (ALL). Scand J Haematol 26: 311–320

Isaacson P, Wright DH, Judd MA et al. (1980) The nature of immunoglobulin-containing cells in malignant lymphoma: an immunoperoxidase study. J Histochem Cytochem 28: 761–770

Janossy G (1981) Membrane markers in leukemia. In: Catovsky D (ed) Methods in haematology. The leukemic cell. Churchill Livingstone, Edinburgh, pp 129–184

Köhler G, Milstein C (1975) Continuous cultures of fused cells secreting antibody of predefined specificity. Nature 256: 495–497

Kraehenbuhl JP, Jamieson JP (1974) Localisation of intracellular antigens by immunoelectron microscopy. Int Rev Exp Pathol 13: 1–53

Lanham GR, Melvin SL, Stass SA (1985) Immunoperoxidase determination of terminal deoxynucleotidyl transferase in acute leukemia using PAP and ABC methods: experience in 102 cases. Am J Clin Pathol 83: 366–370

Lennert K, Niedorf HR (1969) Nachweis von desmosomal verknupften Reticulum-zellen in follikularen Lymphomen. Virchows Arch [Cell Pathol] 4: 148–150

Leong AS-Y (1983) A critique of some contemporary classifications of non-Hodgkin's lymphoma. Which one should we now use? Pathology 15: 437–442

Leong AS-Y, Forbes IJ (1982) Immunological and histochemical techniques in the study of the malignant lymphomas: a review. Pathology 14: 247–254

Leong AS-Y, Milios J (1986) Rapid immunoperoxidase staining of lymphocyte antigens using microwave irradiation. J Pathol 148: 183–187

Leong AS-Y, Dale BM, Liew S-H et al. (1981) Node-based T-cell lymphoma. The clinical, immunological and morphological spectrum. Pathology 13: 79–95

Levy N, Nelson J, Meyer P et al. (1983) Reactive lymphoid hyperplasia with single class (monoclonal) surface immunoglobulin. Am J Clin Pathol 80: 300–308

Levy R, Warnke R, Dorfman RF, Haimovich J (1977) The monoclonality of human B-cell lymphomas. J Exp Med 145: 1014–1028

Li C-Y, Lam KW, Yam LT (1973) Esterases in human leukocytes. J Histochem Cytochem 21: 1–12

Lovett EJ, Schnitzer B, Keren DF et al. (1984) Application of flow cytometry to diagnostic pathology. Lab Invest 50: 115–140

Mason DY, Biberfeld P (1980) Technical aspects of lymphoma immunohistology. J Histochem Cytochem 28: 731–745

Mason DY, Abdulaziz Z, Falini B, Stein H (1983) Double immunoenzymatic labelling. In: Polak JM, Van Noorden S (eds) Immunocytochemistry. Practical applications in pathology and biology. Wright, Bristol, pp 113–128

Matutes E, Catovsky D (1982) The fine structure of normal lymphocyte subpopulations — a study with monoclonal antibodies and the immunogold technique. Clin Exp Immunol 50: 416–425

McGraw DJ, Kurec AS, Davey FR (1981) Mouse erythrocyte formation. A marker for resting B lymphocytes. Am J Clin Pathol 76: 177–183

McKenna RW, Brynes RK, Nesbit ME et al. (1979) Cytochemical profiles in acute lymphoblastic leukemia. Am J Pediatr Haematol Oncol 1: 263–275

Melchers F, Andersson J (1974) IgM in bone marrow derived lymphocytes. Changes in synthesis turnover and secretion and in numbers of molecules on the surface of B cells after mitogenic stimulation. Eur J Immunol 4: 181–188

Nakane PK (1975) Recent progress in the peroxidase-labelled antibody method. Ann NY Acad Sci 254: 203–211

Nanba K, Jaffe ES, Braylan RC et al. (1977) Alkaline phosphatase-positive malignant lymphoma: a subtype of B-cell lymphomas. Am J Clin Pathol 68: 535–542

Navas Palacios JJ, Valdes MD, Montalban-Pallares MA et al. (1981) Lymphoblastic lymphoma/leukemia of T-cell origin: ultrastructural, cytochemical and immunologic features of ten cases. Cancer 48: 1982–1991

Palutke M, Schnitzer B, Mirchandani I et al. (1982) Increased numbers of lymphocytes with single class surface immunoglobulins in reactive hyperplasia of lymphoid tissue. Am J Clin Pathol 78: 316–323

Pangalis GA, Nathwani BN, Rappaport H (1981) An immunocytochemical study of non-Hodgkin's lymphomas. Cancer 48: 915–922

Paradis IL, Merrall EJ, Krell JM et al. (1984) Lymphocyte enumeration: a comparison between a modified avidin-biotin-immunoperoxidase system and flow cytometry. J Histochem Cytochem 32: 358–362

Parker JW (1980) Immunological approach to lymphoid neoplasms. In: Van den Tweel JG (ed) Malignant lymphoproliferative diseases. Martinus Nijhoff, The Hague, pp 85–110

Poore TE, Barrett SG, Kadin ME, Bainton DF (1981) Ultrastructural localization of acid phosphatase in rosetted T and B lymphocytes of normal human blood. Am J Pathol 102: 72–83

Radzun HJ, Kreipe H, Parwaresch MR (1983) Tartrate-resistant acid phosphatase as a differentiation marker for the human mononuclear phagocyte system. Hematol Oncol 1: 321–327

Reyes F, Lejonc JL, Gourdin MF et al. (1975) The surface morphology of human B lymphocytes as revealed by immunoelectron microscopy. J Exp Med 141: 392–410

Romasco F, Rosenberg J, Wybran J (1985) An immunogold-silver staining method for the light microscopic analysis of blood lymphocyte subsets with monoclonal antibodies. Am J Clin Pathol 84: 307–316

Schwarze EW (1980) Cytochemical methods. In: Van den Tweel JG (ed) Malignant lymphoproliferative deseases. Martinus Nijhoff, The Hague, pp 137–148

Shapiro HN (1983) Multistation multiparameter flow cytometry: a critical review and rationale. Cytometry 3: 227–232

Shibata A, Bennett JM, Castoldi GL et al. (1985) Recommended methods for cytological procedures in haematology. International Committee for Standardization in Haematology (ICSH). Clin Lab Haematol 7: 55–74

Steel CM (1984) DNA in medicine. The tools. Lancet II: 908–911, 966–968

Stein H (1978) The immunologic and immunochemical basis for the Kiel classification. In: Lennert K (ed) Malignant lymphomas other than Hodgkin's disease. Springer, Berlin Heidelberg New York, pp 529–657

Stein H, Bonk A, Tolksdorf G et al. (1980) Immunohistologic analysis of the organisation of normal lymphoid tissue and non-Hodgkin's lymphomas. J Histochem Cytochem 28: 746–760

Stein H, Gatter K, Asbahr H, Mason DY (1985) Use of freeze-dried paraffin-embedded sections for immunohistologic staining with monoclonal antibodies. Lab Invest 52: 676–683

Stevenson GT, Smith JL, Hamblin TJ (1983) Immunological investigation of lymphoid neoplasms. Churchill-Livingstone, Edinburgh

Sugden PJ, Lilleyman JS (1982) Mouse red cell rosette formation and the colchicine sensitivity test: relative usefulness in the differential diagnosis of chronic lymphocytic leukaemia and B lymphocytic lymphoma. J Clin Pathol 35: 376–379

Tanaka M, Tanaka H, Ishikawa E (1984) Immunohistochemical demonstration of surface antigen of human lymphocytes with monoclonal antibody in acetone-fixed paraffin-embedded sections. J Histochem Cytochem 32: 452–454

Tavares de Castro J, San Miguel JF, Soler J, Catovsky D (1984) Method for the simultaneous labelling of terminal deoxynucleotidyl transferase (TdT) and membrane antigens. J Clin Pathol 37: 628–632

Tubbs RR, Sheibani K, Weiss RA, Sebek BA (1981) Immunohistochemistry of fresh frozen lymphoid tissue with the direct immunoperoxidase technic. Am J Clin Pathol 75: 172–174

Van der Loo EM, Cnossen J, Meijer CJLM (1981) Morphological aspects of T cell subpopulations in human blood: characterisation of the cerebriform mononuclear cells in healthy individuals. Clin Exp Immunol 43: 506–516

Veerman AJP, Huismans DR, Van Zantwijk CH (1983) Immunological phenotype related to acid alpha-naphthyl acetate esterase and acid phosphatase in childhood acute lymphoblastic leukemia. Acta Haematol 69: 32–35

Watson JD, Tooze J (1981) The DNA story. A documentary history of gene cloning. WH Freeman, San Francisco

Weinberg DS, Pinkus GS, Ault KA (1984) Cytofluorometric detection of B cell clonal excess: a new approach to the diagnosis of B cell lymphoma. Blood 63: 1080–1087

Weisenburger DD, Nathwani BN, Diamond LW et al.(1981) Malignant lymphoma, intermediate lymphocytic type: a clinical and pathologic study of 42 cases. Cancer 48: 1415–1425

Weiss LM, Crabtree GS, Rouse RV, Warnke RA (1985) Morphologic and immunologic characterization of 50 peripheral T-cell lymphomas. Am J Pathol 118: 316–324

Wybran J, Rosenberg J, Romasco F (1985) Immunogold staining: an alternative method for lymphocyte subset enumeration. Comparison with immunofluorescence microscopy and flow cytometry. J Immunol Methods 76: 229–238

15 B Cell Neoplasia

Introduction

B cell malignancies are more common than the T cell malignancies and have been recognised for a longer time, although T cells are the initiators and regulators of immune responses. A description of B cell malignancies is needed that includes the most recent classification and relates, as far as possible, to newer insights into basic mechanisms of neoplasms and immunology. The classification of B cell neoplasms, which has been traditionally based on clinical and pathological criteria, is evolving through the use of the battery of monoclonal antibodies now available. The definition during the past decade of molecular markers characteristic of differentiation stages and pathways in normal B cell ontogeny has facilitated a more precise classification.

However, the current classification of B cell leukaemias by surface markers has some inherent problems. It is impossible to know with certainty whether a particular malignant phenotype corresponds to a normal subclass and represents a stage in differentiation, or represents an anomalous pattern of gene expression peculiar to the malignant population. The term "lineage infidelity" refers to the concept that the malignant cells express genes not normally expressed by cells of the lineage to which they apparently belong (Greaves et al. 1986). As an example, lymphoid characteristics may be found in blast cells of patients with chronic myelogenous leukaemia (CML). As an alternative to lineage infidelity, Greaves et al. have proposed the term "lineage promiscuity" for the concept of transient expression by progenitor cells of a number of genes not normally expressed later in differentiation. Another problem is the likelihood that the majority of malignant cells, upon which we base our judgment of the differentiation stage of a particular tumour, are not the stem cells of the neoplasm. The phenotype of the recognisable malignant cells is largely determined by mechanisms described as "differentiation arrest", which probably affect all differentiation steps, including early stages having the capacity to proliferate. Some cells of a tumour must retain "self-renewal" capacity. This can only result from asymmetrical division, the production on one hand of a replica of the stem cell and on the other hand of a cell which proceeds both to division and to differentiation. It is probably the stem cells which must be eradicated if a patient is to be cured of his tumour.

As chromosomal abnormalities associated with B malignancies are being defined more precisely, it is becoming possible to include such information in the description of some leukaemias and lymphomas. With the rapid progress in mapping chromosomal locations of genes encoding specific lymphocyte structures and genes involved in growth and function of lymphocytes, chromosomal abnormalities are beginning to shed light on the mechanisms leading to malignancy. Perhaps the best example is Burkitt's lymphoma (BL), where reciprocal translocation brings the c-*myc* oncogene within the region of the immunoglobulin genes on chromosomes 2, 14 or 22. The translocation most commonly involves the distal regions of the long arms of chromosomes 8 and 14, bringing the c-*myc* oncogene to 14q32, within the region of the genes for the heavy chain of immunoglobulin, Ig_H. The activation of the c-*myc* oncogene results in increased synthesis of its product, a protein which binds to specific segments of DNA. This protein may, through its role as a regulator of mitosis, induce malignant transformation of the cell.

It would be very valuable if the description of the B cell neoplasms were to include details of abnormal expression of growth factor receptors or abnormal responsiveness to control mechanisms. When most human lymphoid tumour cells are placed in culture they do not proliferate and usually die by 7–10 days. This strongly suggests that growth factors which are operative in vivo are missing from the culture medium. The question of growth requirements may be better answered if the cells which are acting as stem cells for the cancers could be identified. In multiple myeloma, for example, there is disagreement as to whether a primitive stem cell exists. Studies with anti-idiotypic antibodies have demonstrated the neoplastic idiotype in pre-plasma cells of marrow and blood, but it is not certain that all myelomas grow from such early cells. Normal haematopoietic stem cells have requirements for growth different from those of their more differentiated progeny, and the growth requirements of the stem cells of a lymphoid neoplasm may also differ from those of the more mature cells of the lineage.

At present only a few aetiological factors associated with B cell malignancies are known. The Epstein–Barr virus (EBV) is virtually always associated with the endemic African BL, but a non-African, sporadic form occurs in its absence. Similarly, the HTLV-I virus is regularly associated with adult T cell lymphoma/leukaemia (ATL) in endemic areas, but the same T cell neoplasms occur in uninfected subjects. It would also be most useful if tumour-specific antigens could be found; a human malignancy-associated nucleolar antigen on T and B cell non-Hodgkin's lymphoma (NHL) as well as various types of lymphocytic leukaemia has been described recently, but its specificity is yet to be proven (Ford et al. 1984).

Immunological Abnormalities in Lymphoid Malignancies

Loss of humoral immune function is a characteristic of B cell malignancies. This is manifested first by failure to respond by antibody production to standard challenges such as tetanus toxoid and *Salmonella typhi* antigens. Most patients with low-grade follicular cell lymphomas have normal Ig levels, and symptomatic patients with bulky high-grade NHL are more likely to have hypogammaglobulinaemia. A few have a polyclonal hypergammaglobulinaemia. In some cases of differentiated B cell lymphomas hypergammaglobulinaemia is due to monoclonal immunoglobulin.

Lymphopenia is often found in patients with NHL, the frequency increasing with grade and stage of disease. About a third of patients with diffuse histiocytic lymphoma have severe lymphopenia of less than 1.0×10^9/litre (Jones et al. 1977). Similarly, the relatively few published studies of NHL have shown loss of delayed hypersensitivity in a proportion of advanced cases (Anderson et al. 1981). The lymphocyte response to mitogens has been studied fairly extensively in NHL, but the results have been inconsistent because of variation in technique; most studies do not take into account the individual subpopulations of lymphocytes in the test samples. The circulating lymphocytes are a very select population which does not necessarily reflect the disease in the lymphoid tissue. There are few studies of helper and suppressor T cell function in non-Hodgkin's lymphoma. Increased helper T function has been reported in one study (Gaijl-Peczalska et al. 1982). Whether a primary immunological abnormality precedes the development of the lymphoma and whether such an abnormality is involved in its pathogenesis are questions which cannot be answered at present.

Advancing disease is accompanied by advancing global immunological failure, with susceptibility to opportunistic micro-organisms. This is much greater if there is neutropenia. The description of immunological abnormalities in lymphomas is still in a relatively early stage. The availability of new tools, such as monoclonal antibodies to receptors of growth factors, will lead to new sophistication in the description of the abnormal immune function in patients with lymphoid neoplasms.

Chromosomal Abnormalities in B Cell Malignancies

Characteristic chromosomal abnormalities are frequently associated with B cell neoplasms (Table 15.1), although there has been doubt that they represent a primary manifestation or are related to the causation of the malignancy. The presence of an abnormal karyotype is significantly correlated with advanced clinical stage and shortened survival in chronic lymphocytic leukaemia (CLL). It is now claimed that chromosomal translocations are involved in more than 80% of human B cell neoplasms (Croce 1986) and that the neoplastic phenotype is the consequence of reciprocal chromosomal translocations involving the loci for immunoglobulin chains and proto-oncogenes or putative oncogenes. By juxtaposing proto-oncogenes with immunoglobulin gene loci, the transcription of the proto-oncogenes may be deregulated. Promoter genes in the immunoglobulin loci can activate transcription of genes at a distance on the same chromosome. Croce also suggests that the reciprocal translocations in B cell neoplasia are catalysed by the same enzymes that are involved in physiological gene rearrangements. However, not all of the reported chromosomal abnormalities involve chromosomes 2, 14 and 22, the sites of the genes encoding κ, heavy chain and λ chains, respectively.

In both acute lymphoblastic leukaemia (ALL) and acute myeloblastic leukaemia (AML), trisomy 21 is the most common chromosomal abnormality.

Table 15.1. Reported chromosomal abnormalities in B cell malignancies[a]

Neoplasm	Type of aberration
A. Chromosomal abnormalities in the B cell neoplasms	
ALL pre-B	t(1;14)(q23;p13.3)
ALL (not proven B ALL)	Trisomy 21
	del (9)(p21)
	t(9;22)(q34;q11)
	t(11;14)(q23;q32)
	t(11;19)(q23;p13)
	Translocations involving 6q14-q27
BL (ALL-L3)	t(2;8)(p12;q24)
	t(8;14)(q24.1;-32.3)
	t(8;22)(q24;q11)
B-CLL	Trisomy 12
	t(2;14)(p13;q32)
	Deletions and translocations involving 5p15-p13
	t(11;14)(q13;q32)
	t(13;14)(q22;q32)
	del (14)(q22-q24)
	t(14;17)(q32;q23)
	inv (17)(p11-q11)
B-PLL	Translocations involving 14q32
	del(3)(p13)
	t(6;12)(q15;q13)
	t(6;14)(q21;q24)
	t(11;14)(q13;q32)
HCL	del(14)(q22-q32)
Malignant lymphoma	t(1;14)(q21–25;q32)
	t(3;14)(p21;q32)
	t(11;14)(q13.3;q32.3)
	t(14;18)(q32.3;q21.3)
	t(14;19)(q32;q13)
	Other translocations involving 14q32
Multiple myeloma and plasma cell leukaemia	Trisomy 3, 5, 7, 9, 11
	t(11;14)(q13.3;q32.3)
	Other translocations involving 14q32
B. Chromosomes involved in rearrangements in B cell neoplasia	
Pre-B-ALL	1, 19
ALL	4, 6, 9, 11, 12, 14, 19, 21, 22
BL (ALL-L3)	2, 8, 14, 22
B-CLL	2, 5, 11, 12, 13, 14, 17, 19
HCL	14
PLL	3, 5, 6, 12, 14
Malignant lymphoma	1, 3, 11, 14, 18, 19
Multiple myeloma and plasma cell leukaemia	3, 5, 7, 9, 11, 14

[a]Data from report of Human Gene Mapping 8 (1985).

Trisomy 21 is also found in Down's syndrome, which is associated with an increased incidence of ALL. The translocation 14;18 is found in a number of cases of ALL and is also found in follicular lymphoma (Tsujimoto et al. 1984a) and diffuse large cell lymphoma (Juneja et al. 1986).

Because CLL cells are rarely seen in spontaneous mitosis and respond poorly to mitogens in vitro under ordinary conditions, it has been difficult to ascertain the karyotype of CLL cells. Phytohaemagglutinin (PHA) primarily stimulates T cells and usually reveals normal karyotypes. Chromosome analyses are possible in less than half of the cases of CLL when PHA is used as mitogen. The commonest abnormalities found are trisomy 12 and translocations involving chromosome 14 (Gale 1986). Trisomy 12 occurs in up to 25% of cases in which analyses are successful and the same abnormality is found in lymphocytic lymphoma of small cell type, which is regarded as a closely related disease. Trisomy 12 is usually the only abnormality in patients with early disease. Other patients may have clonal chromosomal abnormalities without involvement of chromosome 12.

The second most frequent chromosomal abnormality in CLL is translocation from one of several chromosomes to the long arm of chromosome 14 ($14q^+$); the usual breakpoint on chromosome 14 is q32. Abnormality of karyotype in CLL is correlated with advanced clinical stage, active disease and shortened survival but not with sex or age of the patient, duration of disease, treatment status, or the immunoglobulin heavy or light chain phenotype of the leukaemic cells. The yield of mitotic cells for karyotyping is better with the use of 12-O-tetradecanoylphorbol-13-acetate (TPA). TPA revealed chromosomal abnormalities (including trisomy 12 and deletion of chromosome 11 at band q22) in five of six cases of B-CLL (Callen and Ford 1983).

A translocation between chromosomes 18 and 14 with breakpoints at 18q21.3 and 14q32.3 is characteristic of follicular lymphoma (Tsujimoto et al. 1984a). The translocation involves a gene on chromosome 18 at band q21 that comes into apposition with the heavy chain gene locus on chromosome 14 (Tsujimoto et al. 1984b). This gene may be involved in the pathogenesis of the lymphoma. Translocation between chromosomes 11 and 14 with breakpoints at 14q32.3 and 11q13 occurs in small cell lymphocytic and large cell lymphomas. The breakpoint in these cases also occurs in the region carrying the heavy chain locus. A gene located in band q13 of chromosome 11 is translocated to the heavy chain gene region on chromosome 14 (Tsujimoto et al. 1984b, 1985). The gene involved is unrelated to any of the known retrovirus oncogenes. The potentially oncogenic DNA sequences at breakpoints of some translocations are now being cloned. The cloned gene in the breakpoint on chromosome 14 involved in the 11;14 translocation has been named *bcl-1*. It can be used as a probe to identify and characterise the gene involved in this translocation.

Three types of chromosome translocation are repeatedly observed in BL: t(8;14), t(8;22) and t(2;8), regardless of the geographic origin of the patient and evidence of EBV infection. A part of chromosome 8 is transferred to chromosomes 14, 2 or 22, most commonly to 14. The *myc* gene is frequently translocated very close to the region carrying heavy chain genes on chromosome 14. However, the sites of translocation relative to *myc* are variable; translocation can occur in or near the *myc* locus or at a distance from it. The sites of translocation relative to the antibody genes are also variable. Usually the heavy or light chain constant regions are involved, but examples of translocation to the middle of the V_H or V_L gene are also known. Translocations of c-*myc* into the immunoglobulin loci result in a general increase in c-*myc* mRNA, although this increase is variable. This increase depends more on a reduction in turnover of c-*myc* mRNA than on increased activation of the gene (Blanchard et al. 1985). The product of c-*myc* regulates gene activity by binding specifically to DNA, and excessive production of this regulator of mitosis may induce malignancy. The cause of these specific translocations is unknown. EBV does not appear to play a direct role in causing the translocations associated with BL, but may increase the number of B cells at risk of developing chromosome translocations during immunoglobulin gene rearrangements (Croce 1986). A resumé of the subject of immunoglobulin gene rearrangements and involvement of the c-*myc* oncogene may be read in Waldmann et al. (1985).

The chromosomal translocations and involvement of the *myc* gene in mouse plasmacytoma are remarkably similar to the changes in BL. In mouse plasmacytomas, chromosome 12 — the chromosome analogous to human chromosome 8 — is involved. The similarities in these two diseases confirm the importance of abnormalities of regulation of *myc* in malignant disease of the lymphoid tissues. However, what determines the plasma cell phenotype in one and the early B cell phenotype in the other is still unknown.

In summary, translocations involving human chromosome 14 and different donor chromosomes are relatively commonly found in B cell neoplasms, particularly of adults. The t(11;14)(q13;32) chromosome translocation is observed in CLL, diffuse B cell lymphoma and multiple myeloma (Yunis 1983) and the t(14;18)(q32;21) translocation is observed in follicular lymphomas. The chromosomal breakpoints on chromosome 14 directly involve the heavy chain locus. Specific loci on chromosomes 11 and 18 may be involved in the oncogenic process in malignant B cells carrying these translocations. Certain gene segments, such as that named bcl-1, when involved in translocations, may function as oncogenes in the causation of B cell neoplasms of man.

Oncogene Activation in B Cell Neoplasia

The carcinogenic mechanism of avian leukosis viruses, which do not introduce an oncogene, is by activation of the c-*myc* oncogene through integration of the viral promoter next to the proto-oncogene. It was therefore thought that the same proto-oncogene may be activated in human lymphocyte cancers.

The results obtained so far of analysis of c-*myc* RNA, representing expression of the oncogene, are not easy to interpret. c-*myc* mRNA has a very short half-life; an increase in detectable specific RNA could be due to reduced turnover or increased synthesis, or, conversely, a small increase could indicate a large rise in synthesis. Very variable levels of expression of c-*myc* were observed in ALL (Ferrari et al. 1985). Modest increases were found in nodular, poorly differentiated lymphocytic lymphoma, diffuse histiocytic lymphoma (DHL) and in some cases of CLL, but not in T cell lymphomas examined in one study (Zeller et al. 1984). c-*myc* sequences seem to be present in normal number and without rearrangement in most cases of CLL (Ferrari et al. 1985). c-*myb* may be differentially expressed in AML and ALL, but not CLL or CML.

Immunoglobulin Gene Rearrangements

A malignant lymphocyte must arise after the process of receptor gene rearrangement has begun. The evidence for this comes from the observation that all progeny of the original malignant cell bear the same individual gene rearrangement. Without these gene rearrangements, a malignant cell cannot be recognised as a lymphocyte. The definitive indicator of a monoclonal malignant lymphocyte population is therefore a unique, uniform rearrangement of the immunoglobulin or T receptor genes. Each B cell malignancy has a single, unique detectable Ig gene rearrangement. This rearrangement is a sensitive and specific tumour marker. A monoclonal expansion of B cells is distinguishable from a polyclonal expansion because, in the latter, no single immunoglobulin gene rearrangement is detectable. The Ig gene rearrangement of a leukaemic B cell clone is detectable when its DNA constitutes 5% or even less of an admixture with polyclonal lymphocyte DNA. Identification of uniform Ig gene rearrangements is particularly useful in the detection of B cell lymphomas in which a predominant infiltration of T cells may hide a small monoclonal B cell neoplasm.

It is possible to classify B cell neoplasms according to the extent of rearrangement of these genes, as the heavy chain genes are normally rearranged first, then the κ light chain genes, and subsequently the λ chain genes. This maturation sequence of immunoglobulin gene rearrangements, heavy chain→κ light chain→λ light chain, can be observed in B cell malignancies. Mature B cell leukaemias have rearrangements of both heavy and light chain genes. B cell malignancies that reflect the initial stages of B cell development express only the most proximally located constant regions producing IgM or simultaneous IgM or IgD.

"Non-T-, non-B-" ALL cells lack surface Ig, fail to rosette with sheep erythrocytes and do not react with monoclonal antibodies specific for T cell antigens. They are clonal expansions of B cell precursors, having complete or incomplete rearrangements of J_H segments of their heavy chain genes, and surface antigens associated with early development (Korsmeyer et al. 1981; Waldmann et al. 1985). These precursor B cell leukaemias can be classified according to the sequence: rearrangement of the D_H segment to the J_H segment→addition of a V_H segment→κ rearrangement→λ rearrangement. MHC class II expression and heavy chain gene rearrangements precede the presence of CD10 and the antigens recognised by the monoclonal antibodies CD19, CD20 and CD24. CD20 may be found on the more mature B cell precursor leukaemias.

Many of these cases of non-B-, non-T-ALL fail to produce cytoplasmic μ chain, representing incomplete D_H-J_H intermediate rearrangement or ineffective, aberrant V_H-D_H-J_H rearrangements. Light chain rearrangements are found in half of these cases, with patterns indicating that κ rearrangement precedes λ rearrangement. Some cases fail to express immunoglobulin, despite having apparently complete gene rearrangements. Some mature further when cultured in the presence of TPA, and express cIg or sIg.

Almost 10% of T cell lymphomas have partially rearranged Ig heavy chain genes. Also, occasional myeloid cells with heavy chain rearrangements have been observed (Rovigatti et al. 1984). Light chain genes are rarely rearranged in malignant T cells. Rearrangement of Ig heavy chain genes has also been reported in T cell lines (Rovigatti et al. 1984). Conversely, rare cases of B-CLL and of B cell immunoblastic lymphoma show rearrangement of both Ig heavy chain and the β

chain of the Ti receptor. Because of the rearrangement of Ig heavy chain genes in some T cell neoplasms, it is theoretically not safe to rely only on detection of a common rearrangement of heavy chain genes for the diagnosis of B cell neoplasia. Demonstration of both heavy and light chain gene rearrangements within a tumour is unequivocal evidence of the B cell lineage of a neoplasm, as rearrangement of immunoglobulin light chain genes is rarely found in T cell neoplasms.

Most blast cells in CML blast crisis belong to the B cell precursor series. Rearrangement of heavy chain genes is demonstrable in most, and of light chain genes in less than half of these cases (Bakhshi et al. 1983). In one reported case, different stages of genetic maturation were shown during the course of the disease (Bakhshi et al. 1983). The heavy chain rearrangements were identical, but in one crisis the light chain genes were in the germline status. Occasionally, the lymphoblasts in such cases have demonstrable cytoplasmic Ig and express CD20 and CD24.

Since monoclonal populations are normally generated in immune responses, detection of the clonal rearrangement of immunoglobulin genes is not absolute evidence of neoplasia, at least theoretically. Oligoclonal tumours arising in patients receiving immunosuppressive therapy for organ transplantation may not all be malignant, as some regress if therapy is withheld.

References

Anderson TC, Jones SE, Soehnlen BJ, Moon TE, Griffith K, Stanley P (1981) Immunocompetence and malignant lymphoma: immunologic status before therapy. Cancer 48: 2702–2709

Bakhshi A, Minowada J, Arnold A et al. (1983) Lymphoid blast crises of chronic myelogenous leukaemia represent stages in the development of B-cell precursors. N Engl J Med 309: 826–831

Blanchard J-M, Piechaczyk M, Dani C et al. (1985) c-myc gene is transcribed at high rate in Go-arrested fibroblasts and is post-transcriptionally regulated in response to growth factors. Nature 317: 443–445

Callen DF, Ford JH (1983) Chromosome abnormalities in chronic lymphocytic leukemia revealed by TPA as a mitogen. Cancer Genet Cytogenet 10: 87–93

Croce CM (1986) Molecular mechanisms involved in human B and T neoplasia. Proceedings of the XXI Congress of the International Society of Hematology, Sydney, May 1986, p 3 (abstract)

Ferrari S, Torelli U, Selleri L et al. (1985) Study of the levels of expression of two oncogenes, c-myc and c-myb, in acute and chronic leukaemias of both lymphoid and myeloid lineage. Leuk Res 9: 833–842

Ford RJ, Cramer M, Davis F (1984) Identification of human lymphoma cells by antisera to malignancy associated nucleolar antigens. Blood 63: 599–565

Gaijl-Peczalska KJ, Chartrand SL, Bloomfield CD (1982) Abnormal immunoregulation in patients with non-Hodgkin's malignant lymphomas. I. Increased helper function of peripheral T lymphocytes. Clin Immunol Immunopathol 23: 366–378

Gale RP (1986) Chromosomes, oncogenes and retroviruses in chronic leukemias. In: Champlin R (moderator) Chronic leukaemias: oncogenes, chromosomes, and advances in therapy. Ann Intern Med 104: 671–677

Greaves MF, Chan LC, Furley AWJ, Watt SM, Molgaard HV (1986) Lineage promiscuity in haemopoietic differentiation and leukemia. Blood 67: 1–11

Human Gene Mapping 8 (1985) Eighth international workshop on human gene mapping, Helsinki, Finland, 4–10 August, 1985. Cytogenet Cell Genet 40 (1–4): 567–788

Jones SE, Griffith K, Dombrowski P, Gaines JA (1977) Immunodeficiency in patients with non-Hodgkin's lymphomas. Blood 49: 335–344

Juneja S, Cooper I, Hodgson G et al. (1986) Cytokinetic, immunologic and cytogenetic heterogeneity of diffuse large cell lymphoma (DLCL) Proceedings of the XXI congress of the International Society of Hematology, Sydney, May 1986, p 330 (abstract)

Korsmeyer SJ, Hieter PA, Ravetch JV, Poplack DG, Waldmann TA, Leder P (1981) Developmental hierarchy of immunoglobulin gene rearrangements in human leukaemic pre-B cells. Proc Natl Acad Sci USA 78: 7096–7100

Rovigatti U, Mirro J, Kitchingman G et al. (1984) Heavy chain immunoglobulin rearrangements in acute nonlymphocytic leukemia. Blood 63: 1023–1027

Tsujimoto Y, Yunis J, Onorato-Showe L et al. (1984a) Molecular cloning of the chromosomal breakpoint of B-cell lymphomas and leukemias with the t(11;14) chromosome translocation. Science 224: 1403–1406

Tsujimoto Y, Finger LR, Yunis J, Nowell PC, Croce CM (1984b) Cloning of the chromosome breakpoint of neoplastic B cells with the t(14;18) chromosome translocation. Science 226: 1097–1099

Tsujimoto Y, Jaffe E, Cossman J et al. (1985) Clustering of breakpoints on chromosome 11 in human B-cell neoplasms with the t(11;14) chromosome translocation. Nature 315: 340–343

Waldmann TA, Korsmeyer SJ, Bakhshi AJ, Arnold A, Kirsch IR (1985) Molecular genetic analysis of human lymphoid neoplasms. Immunoglobulin genes and the c-*myc* oncogene. Ann Intern Med 102: 497–510

Yunis J (1983) The chromosomal basis of human neoplasia. Science 221: 227–236

Zeller N, Cossman J, Jaffe ES, Tsichlis P (1984) Expression of c-*myc* sequences in human lymphomas In: Magrath IT, O'Connor GT, Ramot B (eds) Pathogenesis of leukemias and lymphomas. Raven, New York, pp 363–371

16 B Cell Leukaemias

Introduction

The classification of B cell leukaemias has traditionally been based on clinical and pathological criteria. Monoclonal antibody technology now allows these neoplasms to be classified according to the differentiation stage of the corresponding normal lymphocyte, although, as discussed previously (see Chap. 15, p. 199), such a classification does not take into account the likelihood that the stem cells of the leukaemias may not be at that stage of differentiation. As the properties and molecular markers of these different stages of B cell maturation continue to be defined with increasing precision, so will the classification of B cell leukaemias continue to evolve.

Both leukaemias and lymphomas apparently involve B cells at different stages and pathways of maturation or differentiation (Salmon and Seligmann 1974), and formal proof of the monoclonal nature of B cell lymphomas has long been established (Brouet and Seligmann 1977; Habeshaw et al. 1979). The differentiation stages of normal B cells to which the B cell leukaemias correspond are set out in Table 16.1.

Lymphomas and leukaemias are usually reported as different entities, but there is, without doubt, an overlap in their evolution. Lymphomas are distributed irregularly in lymphoid tissues throughout the body, whereas "leukaemia" implies a systemic distribution of abnormal cellular proliferations, always involving the bone marrow and usually characterised by abnormal cells circulating in the peripheral blood. Some lymphomas, as it will become apparent, are notorious for their systemic involvement of the bone marrow, peripheral blood and cerebrospinal fluid, besides being present as tumour masses in various lymphoid tissues and viscera. Such examples make the conceptual distinction of the terms "leukaemia" and "lymphoma" difficult. In the case of lymphomas of small round lymphocytes or well-differentiated lymphocytic lymphoma, which are clearly related to the leukaemic proliferation called chronic lymphocytic leukaemia (CLL), the term "leukaemia/lymphoma" may seem more reasonable than either "leukaemia" or "lymphoma".

Table 16.1. B cell differentiation and corresponding neoplasms

Normal B cell phenotype	Corresponding malignant subtype	Marker
Pre-pre-B	Acute lymphoblastic leukaemia (ALL)	MHC class II + CD19 + CD20 ± CD22 + (cytoplasm) CD24 ± TdT + CD10 ±
Pre-B	Pre-B-ALL	cμ + MHC class II + CD10 + CD19 ± CD20 + CD22 + (cytoplasm) CD24 + (MER +)
Early B	B-ALL	sIgM MHC class II + CD10 ± CD19 + CD20 + CD21 + CD22 + (cytoplasm) CD23 + CD24 + MER +
Intermediate B	Chronic lymphocytic leukaemia (CLL) Diffuse well-differentiated lymphocytic lymphoma	sIgM +, D ± MHC class II + CD10 ± CD19 + CD20 + CD21 + CD22 + (cytoplasm and surface) CD23 + CD24 + MER + Y29/55 +
Mature B	Hairy cell leukaemia (HCL) Diffuse poorly differentiated lymphoma Nodular lymphoma	sIg + + MHC class II + CD19 + CD20 + CD21 + CD22 + (cytoplasm and surface) CD23 + CD24 + MER ± Y29/55 +
Activated B cell	HCL B lymphomas	T10 + MER- CD23 + sIg +/+ + MHC class II + CD19 + CD20 + CD24 +

Table 16.1. (*continued*)

Early plasma cell	Waldenstrom's macroglobulinaemia	sIg+ MHC class II+ CD19± CD20+ CD24+ T10+ PCA-1+ PC-1+ cIg+ cIg+
Terminally differentiated	Multiple myeloma	PCA-1+ PC-1+ MHC class II± CD10±

Acute Lymphoblastic Leukaemia

Acute leukaemia is the most common malignancy in childhood, making up three quarters of the cases and having a peak incidence between 2 and 6 years of age. In adults, acute lymphoblastic leukaemia (ALL) occurs mostly in the third and fourth decades.

ALL has provided important insights into the aetiology of lymphoid malignancy; an increased incidence of ALL was seen in children exposed to atomic blasts. Therapeutic and diagnostic irradiation, toxic chemicals, particularly cytotoxic drugs, and genetic abnormalities are recognised causative factors associated with ALL. Down's syndrome, Fanconi's anaemia, Bloom's syndrome, Klinefelter's syndrome, ataxia-telangiectasia, Wiskott–Aldrich syndrome and other congenital immunodeficiencies are aetiologic associations which have been discussed previously (see Chap. 2, p. 16–17; Chap. 5, p. 41).

ALL is a heterogeneous disease as defined by clinical, morphological, cytochemical and immunological criteria. The wide range of clinical responses to therapy has also suggested its heterogeneity.

Using morphological, biochemical and enzymatic parameters, and with the aid of phenotype analysis, ALL can be divided into major prognostic groups. Immunological phenotyping of blast cells from peripheral blood (from the bone marrow, should the leucocyte count be less than 10×10^9/litre), clearly identifies five subcategories of childhood ALL: (1) non-B, non-T, (2) pre-B, (3) B, (4) pre-T and (5) T cell types. About 75% of ALL patients have blast cells that are negative for conventional B and T markers. This group of non-B-, non-T-ALL is largely made up of cases bearing the common ALL antigen (CALLA) recognised by antibodies of CD10, the remainder being of the unclassified cell type (Chessells et al. 1977; Miller 1980; Foucar 1981).

The leukaemia primarily involves the bone marrow and the peripheral blood. Enlargement of lymph nodes and the spleen is common and the leukaemic cells may disseminate to almost any site of the body, producing signs and symptoms related to the site of involvement. These widely disseminated sites, particularly the meninges and gonads, constitute reservoirs for recurrences after treatment. The major clinical manifestations are related to the deficiency of normal haematopoietic cells resulting from bone marrow infiltration. Patients may present with anaemia, or with bleeding resulting from a deficiency of platelets, or with infection resulting from granulocytopenia and immunodeficiency.

The diagnosis is made on the presence of circulating blast cells, which are also present in bone marrow. Very early in the disease, infiltration of the bone marrow may be only focal, resulting in little alteration to the peripheral blood picture.

The appearance of ALL cells varies considerably. Until immunological and genetic markers became available, the classification of ALL was based on morphological features. The French-American-British (FAB) classification (Bennett et al. 1976) proposed three categories of ALL, based on morphological criteria, such as the amount of cytoplasm, prominence of nucleoli, basophilia of cytoplasm and other features. L1 represents the type of acute leukaemia common in childhood. L2, which is less common in children, sometimes requires differentiation from myeloblastic leukaemia without maturation and is sometimes designated "undifferentiated leukaemia", whereas L3 includes Burkitt's lymphoma (BL).

Phenotype of ALL Cells

The earliest identifiable B cell precursors (designated "pre-pre-B cells" in Table 16.1) may lack detectable B cell antigens and sIg but have a clear genetic commitment to the B cell lineage, as shown by rearrangement of immunoglobulin genes. The first set of pre-B cells identified were large cells which contained small amounts of cytoplasmic µ heavy chain, but undetectable sIg. These pre-B cells give rise, either by direct transition or by dividing once, to small non-dividing lymphocytes which express surface membrane immunoglobulin of IgM type and are regarded as the earliest form of immunologically competent peripheral small B lymphocytes. Pre-B cells containing cytoplasmic µ chain but lacking sIg can be first seen within human fetal liver at 9–10 weeks and in bone marrow by about the 15th week (see Table 10.1, p. 116). The term "pre-B cell leukaemia" includes cases with all of these early forms of B cell which precede those expressing sIg. The clinical and laboratory characteristics of pre-B cell leukaemia in childhood have been summarised by Cristo et al. (1979).

Of the non-B, non-T forms of ALL, approximately 20% have been shown to have blasts which contain cytoplasmic µ chain (Vogler et al. 1978; Brouet et al. 1979; LeBien et al. 1982) so that this subset is felt to be a pre-B-ALL instead of non-B-, non-T-ALL. Of the remaining non-B-, non-T-ALL cases, many have been demonstrated to show heavy chain gene rearrangements, providing strong evidence that as a group they belong to the early B cell lineage. Furthermore, approximately 60% of such leukaemias display only heavy chain gene rearrangements, with their light chain genes being retained in the germline configuration (Korsmeyer et al. 1981, 1983a).

This group of ALL may also be categorised accurately by the use of a battery of monoclonal antibodies (Flug et al. 1985). The earliest antigen displayed appears to be CD19, followed by CD24, CD20, cytoplasmic CD22, CD10 and cytoplasmic µ chains. The developmental hierarchy established by the use of these monoclonal antibodies on leukaemic cells is confirmed by the sequence in early ALL cells treated with 12-O-tetradecanoylphorbol-13-acetate (TPA). Terminal deoxy-nucleotidyl-transferase (TdT) is found in early B-ALL but its expression is variable. Common and pre-B-ALL cells also express receptors for interleukin 2 (IL-2) (Touw et al. 1985).

B cell ALL constitutes about 2% of all ALL cases. This group of ALL is identified by the presence of membrane-bound immunoglobulin molecules. The leukaemic cells usually synthesise monoclonal sIgM with little or no sIgD, in contrast to the presence of both IgM and IgD at the surface of non-neoplastic B-derived cells. Class II major histocompatibility complex (MHC) products seem invariably to be expressed on the surface of the neoplastic blasts, which inconsistently display Fc and complement receptors. B cell ALL as a group has a very poor prognosis, even poorer than T-ALL (Wolff et al. 1976; Maheu et al. 1981).

It has been proposed that non-T-ALL can be subdivided into phenotypically defined subgroups on the basis of MHC class II, CD10, CD19, CD20 and cIgM (Anderson et al. 1984). The observation that all non-T-ALL strongly express MHC class II antigen indicates that this antigen develops very early in B cell precursors. CD19 is also strongly expressed on the non-T-ALL and with decreased intensity on more mature neoplasms. CD10 is expressed on slightly fewer non-T-ALL than CD19. It appears to follow CD19 in B cell ontogeny. The CD20 antigen appears at about the same time as CD10 (see Table 11.2, p. 130; Fig. 11.1, p. 131) and is found on only 50% of non-T-ALL.

CML is a clonal haematopoietic malignancy that arises from a remarkable pluripotent cell which also gives rise to all of the non-malignant lineages of blood cells. Because of the multipotential capacity and differentiative ability, considerable uncertainty has surrounded the nature of the blast crisis which can occur during the terminal phase of this disease.

Morphological, cytochemical, biochemical and immunological studies have indicated that this increasing portion of blast cells in the bone marrow and peripheral blood is heterogeneous. In addition to the classic myeloblastic or myelofibrotic proliferation, lymphoblastic, promyelocytic, megakaryoblastic, and erythroblastic transformations have been described. The lymphoid blast cells in Philadelphia chromosome-positive CML are identical antigenically and enzymatically to the typical non-B-, non-T-ALL cells seen in children, being TdT +, MHC class II +, CD9 +, CD10 + and CD24 +. cIgM has also been found in the blast cells, and heavy-chain as well as light-chain rearrangements have been demonstrated, indicating that cells in most episodes of lymphoid crisis in CML are genetically committed B cell precursors (Bakhshi et al. 1983; Ford et al. 1983).

Prognosis in ALL

The prognosis in this group of leukaemias is largely determined by the type and the clinical extent of the disease. Up to 80% 2-year survivals have been reported for childhood ALL. "Cures", i.e. 5- and 10-year disease-free intervals are not rare and remissions have also been obtained in adults. The presence of CD10 represents a favourable prognostic factor for children with ALL (Bowman et al. 1979; Morgan and Hsu 1979). Its absence may increase the likelihood of a poor response to therapy, whether or not high-risk clinical features are present.

The non-B, non-T cell ALL seen in adults differs clinically and morphologically from the more common childhood type. The cells in adults are usually L2 in the FAB classification. The remission rate in adults is lower than in children. There is earlier relapse, and the median survival is much shorter. Childhood common ALL tends to present with a low blood white cell count and to attain a high remission rate and a longer duration of the first complete remission in contrast to B and T cell ALL. Non-B, non-T cell leukaemia has the best prognosis of the three major groups (Brouet and Seligmann 1978).

B-Chronic Lymphocytic Leukaemia

CLL has a special place in the history of the malignant lymphocyte as the first recognised lymphocyte malignancy. It continues to offer much for the study of the oncology of the lymphocyte because of the ready availability of the malignant cells and their normal counterparts. The first description of leukaemia is attributed to Virchow in 1845, although in 1827 Velpeau described a case with very large liver and spleen and thick blood like gruel and in 1845 Bennett in Scotland had also recognised leukaemia. The two main varieties of chronic leukaemia were first recognised in 1857 by Friedreich. Kundrat introduced the term "lymphosarcoma" in 1893 to describe a related disease affecting lymph nodes but without leukaemia. Türk used the term "lymphomatoses" in 1903 to indicate similarities between lymphosarcoma and CLL. Minot and Isaacs (1924) reported the results of radiotherapy in a sizeable series of leukaemic patients. Treatment with ^{32}P was introduced in 1936 and with nitrogen mustard in 1949. Adrenocorticotrophic hormone and adrenal steroids were used after 1950. In 1971, CLL lymphocytes were shown to be of B cell lineage (Wilson and Nossal 1971). A review of the history of CLL and the historical references may be found in Rundles (1977).

The evidence of the monoclonality of B-CLL is as follows:

1. Only κ or λ light chains are expressed by a malignant population.
2. A specific cytogenetic abnormality may be expressed by all cells.
3. Only one and the same idiotype of immunoglobulin is expressed on all leukaemic cells of the patient.
4. A single glucose-6-phosphate dehydrogenase (G6PD) enzyme isotype is expressed in females with CLL who are heterozygous for the X-linked marker G6PD.
5. The cells have a uniform immunoglobulin gene rearrangement.

Granulocytes, erythrocytes, platelets, and T lymphocytes from patients with B-CLL display both enzyme isotypes of G6PD in proportions similar to those found in skin (Fialkow et al. 1977), whereas only one isotype is found in the CLL cells, indicating that the progenitor cells of CLL express only B lymphocyte differentiation (Fialkow et al. 1978). This contrasts with the multipotential haematopoietic stem cell which is involved in CML, myeloid metaplasia and polycythaemia vera. The blast crisis of CML may involve myeloblasts, promyelocytes, megakaryoblasts, erythroblasts or lymphoblasts. When blastic transformation occurs in CLL, the blast cells express the same idiotype as the B-CLL cells, indicating derivation from the original malignant clone and not from the recruitment of hitherto normal lymphoid cells (Brouet et al. 1977; Delsol et al. 1981).

CLL accounts for 25% of all leukaemias in the western world. About 95% of all cases of CLL are of B cell type, most of the remainder being malignant T cell proliferations. The annual incidence in the State of South Australia over the years 1977–1981 was 3.5 and 2.6 per 100 000 for males and females respectively (population 654 274 males, 664 603 females in 1981; Central Cancer Registry Unit, South Australia 1985). Two-thirds of those affected are over 60 years of age, and 90% are over 50 years. CLL is an age-related disease and actually never occurs before the third decade of life (Lennert 1978). B-CLL is extremely rare in Japan and is less common in the Chinese and Japanese living in America than in the Caucasian population.

Lymphocytosis, generally $20-600 \times 10^9$/litre, enlarged lymph nodes and spleno-megaly are found in most patients, but in at least one-quarter of cases the diagnosis is made incidentally in asymptomatic patients. Other lymphoid tissues which may be enlarged include the tonsils and adenoids, and the retroperitoneal and mesenteric lymph nodes. The lymphocytes accumulate in various organs, mostly without apparent disturbance of function. The commonest symptom is fatigue. Fever is very uncommon in the absence of infection. Anaemia, granulocytopenia and thrombocytopenia result from the infiltration of the bone marrow. Anaemia may also result from reduced red cell survival associated with splenome-galy, autoimmune haemolytic anaemia (AIHA) in 5%–10% of cases (the Coombs' test for red cell-associated Ig is positive in up to 20% of patients with CLL) and the activity of T_γ cells which suppress erythroid precursors. The pathogenesis of AIHA has not been explained.

Between 10% and 15% of all patients live for up to 15 years requiring little or no treatment for their disease; 15% or more die within a year from aggressive disease. Although uncommon, spontaneous remission from CLL has been reported from time to time. The leukaemic cell mass usually increases at a steady rate and lymphocytosis often reaches a plateau which may persist for months or years. There is slowly progressive infiltration of the bone marrow. In the majority of cases, discrete lymph node enlargement occurs in an apparently random manner, and enlargement of the spleen or liver follows after months or years, especially if the disease is not treated. In a minority of cases, splenic enlargement occurs without lymph node enlargement. The blood lymphocyte count correlates poorly with the degree and extent of tissue infiltration.

CLL terminates either in infection associated with immunodeficiency or in other complications such as AIHA. Herpes zoster infection occurs at some time in the course of the disease in 10% of all cases. Impaired resistance to infection in CLL is related to depression of immunological function and to treatment with alkylating agents and corticosteroids. Neutropenia is a potent cause of susceptibility to infection. Both primary and secondary antibody responses are severely impaired. T cell mediated natural killer (NK) and antibody-mediated cytotoxicity seem to be impaired in most patients.

Several systems of staging CLL have been described. The staging system of Rai et al. (1975) uses five groups:

Stage 0: when lymphocytosis is 15×10^9/litre or higher, with lymphocytes amounting to 40% or more of the nucleated cells in the bone marrow, no enlargement of lymph nodes, spleen or liver, haemoglobin concentration of 11 g/dl or greater and a platelet count of at least 100×10^9/litre

Stage I: as in Stage 0 plus lymphadenomegaly

Stage II: as in stage 0 plus splenomegaly, hepatomegaly, or both

Stage III: as in Stage 0 plus anaemia (haemoglobin less than 11 g/dl)

Stage IV: as in Stage 0 plus thrombocytopenia (platelets less than 100×10^9/litre).

This clinical staging system has been widely accepted and verified; however, some attempts to improve this classification have been carried out. An International Workshop on CLL (1981) has recommended a modified system for CLL staging in which patients are classified according to the presence or absence of anaemia and/or thrombocytopenia (Group C) and the number of "lymphoid" areas enlarged (Groups A and B). This International Workshop has particularly encouraged the investigation of methods to predict, within each of the A, B and C groups, subsets of patients who develop a progressive or aggressive clinical course as compared with patients whose clinical course is benign or stable. It is not considered a final system of staging but provides advantages in planning treatment and in research because clinical stages are limited to three.

The prognostic value of bone marrow histological patterns in CLL has been evaluated by some authors. In a study of 115 patients, cases with diffuse bone marrow infiltration had a poor prognosis as compared with cases presenting with a nodular or mixed (nodular and diffuse) pattern (Gray et al. 1974). More recently, a multivariate survival analysis of 329 cases showed that bone marrow histological pattern appears to be a better single prognostic parameter than any one of the variables employed in current clinical staging systems (Rozman et al. 1984). Dividing bone marrow involvement into four patterns — interstitial, nodular, mixed and diffuse patterns — they showed that patients with interstitial and nodular bone marrow involvement had a longer survival than those with mixed and diffuse patterns. In the interstitial pattern of involvement there is some degree of replacement of normal haematopoietic tissue by mature lymphocytes but there is preservation of fat cells and bone marrow structure. The nodular pattern comprises nodules of mature lymphocytes, the nodules being larger than normal lymphoid follicles and lacking germinal centre differentiation. Fat cells are preserved and there is no interstitial infiltration. The mixed pattern is defined as a combination of interstitial and nodular patterns. Lastly, the pattern of diffuse lymphoid infiltration shows massive replacement of normal haematopoietic tissue as well as fat cells. In this study high peripheral lymphocyte counts correlated with the diffuse type of bone marrow involvement rather than the extent of involvement. The same group of workers had previously demonstrated a certain degree of correlation between bone marrow patterns and clinical stages, although it is far from being absolute (Rozman et al. 1981; Montserrat and Rozman for the Spanish Cooperative Group for CLL Study 1983). In some cases it may be extremely difficult to categorise the pattern of bone marrow infiltration.

Serum immunoglobulin levels are commonly normal in early CLL. With progression of the disease, the serum immunoglobulin levels fall, although this does not appear to correlate with the Rai staging of the disease. A decrease of all classes of serum immunoglobulin is found in 40% of patients (Slungaard and Smith 1981), and a reduction of one or more Ig classes is found in more than 70% of patients (Schwarzmeier et al. 1981). The decrease in Ig levels tends to correspond with the extent of bone marrow involvement. Abnormal levels of gamma globulin are found sporadically in family members of patients with CLL (Gunz et al. 1975), and a familial incidence of CLL is recognised, although the pattern of inheritance has not been established.

Although Lennert (1978) stated that "... a case of 'CLL' with paraproteinemia is in all probability an 'immunocytoma'. Paraproteinemia does not occur in CLL", somewhat less than 10% of cases of CLL have easily detectable levels of monoclonal protein in the blood, the most common being an IgM monoclonal gammopathy. Monoclonal light chains are found in the urine of three-quarters of the patients and these light chains are similar to those expressed on the leukaemic cells. Antibodies prepared against monoclonal-free light chains from the urine of CLL patients will react with the patient's leukaemic cells (Tutt et al. 1983). More than half of these proteins are pentameric IgM.

A "pure splenomegalic" form of B-CLL has been described (Dighiero et al. 1979). Progressive enlargement of the spleen without significant enlargement of peripheral lymph nodes as the salient presenting feature is seen in about 5% of CLL. This condition is distinct from prolymphocytic leukaemia because the morphology and the phenotype of the lymphocytes are those of B-CLL and the highest lymphocyte counts rarely overlap with those at the lower end of the range for prolymphocytic leukaemia. The prognosis of the pure splenomegalic form of CLL is said to be considerably better than average. In particular, when the spleen is very large, hypersplenism leads to anaemia and thrombocytopenia, and the patients are inappropriately staged as III or IV in the Rai system or C according to the International Workshop system. Successful treatment of hypersplenism with radiotherapy, chemotherapy or splenectomy produces excellent results. It has been suggested that this distinct clinical pattern may reflect the behaviour of a non-circulating B cell of splenic marginal zones (Kumararatne and MacLennan 1981; Kumararatne et al. 1981) with splenic homing properties (Galton and MacLennan 1982).

Second neoplasms occur in an estimated 10%–15% of cases of CLL. The occurrence of many of the tumours is largely attributable to the age of the patients. Excluding basal cell carcinomas, the most common tumours are squamous cell carcinomas of the skin. Other tumours seen in patients with CLL include squamous and glandular tumours of the lung and carcinoma of the colon. Treatment with ^{32}P or prolonged treatment with alkylating agents definitely increase the risk of occurrence of myelomonocytic leukaemia. Sézary syndrome has also developed after prolonged treatment with chlorambucil (Ferme et al. 1981).

In 3%–10% of patients with CLL, the disease evolves into a diffuse "histio-cytic" lymphoma (Richter 1928). The malignant cells are not true histiocytes but represent large lymphoid cells, which have been shown in some cases to derive from the same clone of B cells, sharing the same sIg phenotype (Brouet et al. 1977; Delsol et al. 1981). The transformation is announced by the appearance of a sudden and striking deterioration of the general condition with weight loss, fever and massive enlargement of lymph nodes. In some cases lymphocytosis decreases and a monoclonal immunoglobulin may appear in the serum (Long and Aisenberg 1975). This transformation of CLL to a large cell lymphoma is postulated to occur only in CLL of memory cells. This "memory cell CLL" is considered to be due to an increased proliferation of immunoblasts capable of differentiating to memory lymphocytes. A block in this differentiaton would eventuate in immunoblastic proliferation without maturation and a large cell lymphoma would ensue (Ezdinli and Nanus 1983). Richter's syndrome, according to this postulate, can occur only with memory CLL. "Virgin" CLL could also conceivably undergo aggressive transformation, but, in this instance, the proliferative precursor cell would be the pre-B cell and the disease should convert into B-ALL as described by Brouet et al. (1973).

The morphological features and membrane phenotype of CLL B cells usually remain unchanged throughout the course of the disease. "Prolymphocytoid" transformation occurs in parallel with deteriorating clinical condition, increasing size of lymph nodes and the spleen, resistance to treatment, deterioration in bone marrow function and increasing immunodepression (Enno et al. 1979). In many cases the transformed cells have retained the phenotype of the population of smaller CLL cells, but cases in which the phenotype was that of prolymphocytic leukaemia cells have been reported (Kjeldsberg and Marty 1981). Terminal transformation into a "blastic" phase that is refractory to therapy is much less common in CLL than in chronic myeloid leukaemia. In such cases the disease is characterised by the appearance of increasing numbers of cells larger than the majority, with more cytoplasm, less condensed chromatin, sometimes irregular nuclear outlines and a distinct nucleolus.

A benign variant of CLL has recently been recognised. Twenty cases of Rai Stage 0 CLL showed a monoclonal B cell lymphocytosis and stable benign disease without progression for between 6.5 and 24 years (Han et al. 1984). Three patients had spontaneous regressions and all followed a prolonged asymptomatic or benign clinical course, with essentially normal humoral and cellular immunity and normal karyotype. Indices of good prognosis as found in these patients were: sIgM or sIgD phenotype or both; CD5+, RFA4+, FMC7+ (Caligaris-Cappio et al. 1984a); absence of chromosomal abnormalities; normal T-cell response to mitogens; and normal delayed hypersensitivity responses. The bone marrow in these cases may be normal or may show a nodular or interstitial pattern of infiltration. Immunoglobulin levels are generally normal and total T cell counts may be elevated. Such cases of benign monoclonal B cell lymphocytosis should be distinguished from those with persistent polyclonal lymphocytosis of B lymphocytes (Gordon et al. 1982), a rare, non-neoplastic condition possibly related to smoking (Carstairs et al. 1985).

Lymphocyte Kinetics

In CLL, there is an increase of the intravascular lymphocyte pool relative to the readily accessible extravascular compartment. Exchange of lymphocytes between lymph nodes and blood is partially intact, but recirculation between bone marrow and blood appears to be blocked. Moreover, the leukaemic cells also do not leave the tissues as readily as normal lymphocytes. This possible impairment of recirculation has been suggested to result from an abnormality of the lymphocyte surface (Vincent and Gunz 1970).

The disease results from a slow accumulation of relatively long-lived malignant B cells, rather than from rapid proliferation. The predominant cell in CLL is long-lived with a life span of 1–5 years and about 90% of the blood lymphocytes have a turnover time in excess of 1 year. The rest, both large and small lymphocytes, have

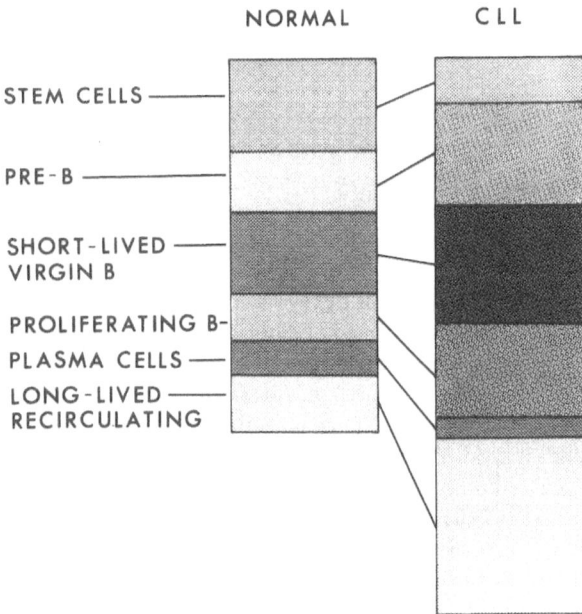

Fig. 16.1. Cell kinetics in chronic lymphocyte leukaemia (CLL). The unidentified precursor pool, from which the malignant clone arises, is presumably normal or reduced in size, as is the size of the pool of normal B cells responding to antigen. There is gross enlargement of the long-lived recirculating B cell pool. The pre-B cells, which normally do not divide more than once, are the putative stem cells but the virgin and proliferating B cell pool (stippled) can presumably contribute to the malignant population by proliferating. The number of cells maturing to plasma cells is reduced.

half lives of 3–8 days. Although the accumulation is due principally to the increased life span of the lymphocytes, more than normal numbers of lymphocytes are produced (up to 10 times more long-lived and up to 25 times more short-lived lymphocytes). The average life span of the short-lived lymphocytes is in the normal range. The number of B cells in S phase, i.e. taking up tritiated thymidine, is increased in cases with a higher lymphocyte count (Moayeri and Sokel 1979). Doubling times between 4 and 19 months have been measured in circulating lymphocytes (Theml et al. 1977). This is slow relative to non-Hodgkin's lymphomas (NHLs), which have a doubling time of 1 month. Even after treatment the cell numbers increase exponentially at about the same rate. These kinetics are represented schematically in Fig. 16.1.

Morphology

B-CLL cells are relatively uniform, often normal-looking small lymphocytes (8–10 μm) with a compact, round to oval nucleus and coarse chromatin. The cells may rupture easily during the preparation of smears, causing the appearance of "smudge cells". Some cells have slightly irregular or notched nuclei and the nucleoli are ring-like, small and central. The scanty cytoplasmic rim is slightly basophilic.

At the ultrastructural level, the cytoplasm contains few organelles, which include mitochondria, lysosomes, ribosomes and short endoplasmic reticulum. The cytoplasmic membrane is usually smooth or may show short blunt microvilli. Blast forms are usually infrequent.

The bone marrow and peripheral blood are said to be involved exclusively at an early stage in CLL. As previously described, the pattern of infiltration may be nodular, interstitial, diffuse or mixed. Infiltration, overgrowth and replacement of the bone marrow often develop slowly over a period of years. The phenotypes of the dominant lymphoid population within the bone marrow infiltrate and the blood are identical (Pizzolo et al. 1984).

The percentage of T cells in the bone marrow infiltrate of patients with B-CLL is often high and may be greater than that in the peripheral blood. The CD4+ inducer subset predominates in the marrow, in contrast to the peripheral blood where the CD8+ suppressor/cytotoxic phenotype predominates (Caligaris-Cappio and Janossy 1985; Markey et al. 1986). The accumulation of T helper cells in both the bone marrow and lymph nodes may have a role to play in the expansion of the neoplastic clone, whereas the T helper cell depletion and relative increase of T suppressor/cytotoxic cells in the blood and at other sites may contribute to the immunodeficiency of B-CLL patients. The reversal of the CD4:CD8 ratio does not correlate with the clinical stage and in many patients it is due to a low absolute number of CD4+ cells rather than an increase in numbers of CD8+ cells (Markey et al. 1986). Although the percentage of T cells in the peripheral blood is low, the absolute number of T cells is often increased. This contrasts with the relatively low blood T lymphocyte count in almost all patients with follicular lymphomas of the small cell type. Delayed hypersensitivity remains relatively normal in most patients. The T cells in CLL may not react with anti-CD3, although the antigen can be revealed by treatment with neuraminidase (Kay and Kaplan 1984).

Peripheral blood lymphocytosis may remain at a plateau during the expansion of the lymphoid mass in the marrow, nodes and spleen. Bone marrow function is maintained by the conversion of yellow to red marrow until there is overgrowth by the leukaemic infiltrate. Cytopenias develop when the lymphoid tissue comprises about half of the marrow.

There is a diffuse infiltration of the lymph nodes by the leukaemic cells producing a histological picture which is indistinguishable from diffuse well-differentiated lymphocytic lymphomas. The predominant cell in this disease, as in CLL, is considered to be earlier in the B cell differentiation pathway than lymphomas of the follicle cells and of the medulla. As in the marrow, the lymph nodes appear to attract and sequester T helper cells, which, it has been speculated, may play a role in the genesis of the neoplastic clone (Caligaris-Cappio and Janossy 1985). The histological appearances of lymph node involvement by CLL are discussed under well-differentiated lymphocytic lymphomas (see Chap. 17, p. 248).

Phenotype

Circulating B-CLL cells express membrane Ig which is usually of the IgM and IgD classes, but may also be IgG. Monoclonality is proven by the demonstration that the leukaemic cells from a patient all bear the same idiotype or the same rearrangement of immunoglobulin genes. These cells differ in some aspects from most normal B cells in the peripheral blood. While the total Ig content is comparable to that of normal B lymphocytes, cIgM is higher and sIg is one tenth as dense as that of normal B cells. Lymphocytes lacking sIg may be present in large numbers in occasional cases (Forbes et al. 1979), and the number of such "null" cells which bear mouse erythrocyte receptors (MER) may vary greatly during the course of the disease. Rarely, cases may express both B and T cell antigens (in addition to CD5), although such cases are clinically not classic examples of B-CLL (Brouet and Prieur 1974; Bona and Fauci 1980). These cases are reminiscent of the 10% of leukaemic T cell populations that can be shown to have Ig heavy chain rearrangement. Patients with biclonal proliferations of CLL have occasionally been reported, having one population with κ light chains and another with λ light chains.

B-CLL cells generally also express MER, C3d receptors (CD21 antigen), and receptors for Helix pomatia agglutinin but they wholly lack the CD10 (CALLA) cell surface antigen. The coexpression of MHC class II, CD19, CD20, CD21 and sIg defines the phenotype of most B-CLL. Of interest are the observations that the majority of patients with B-CLL (94%) also expresses the T cell-associated antigen, CD5, and that in the resting state the neoplastic cells which express MER and MHC Class II antigens express receptors for IL-2.

E-rosette formation is found in a small proportion of cases of B-CLL. In some, it is the consequence of monoclonal sIg with "Forssman-like" antibody activity. Forssman antibodies are naturally occurring heterophile antibodies that react with antigens on sheep erythrocytes.

In general, B-CLL cells are thought to correspond to immature B cells of the phenotype MHC Class II+, CD19+, CD20+, CD21+, sIg+ and CD5+ found in the mantle zones of fetal lymphoid follicles, and B-CLL could be the malignant counterpart of this population of lymphocytes. The neoplastic cells of a given patient with B-CLL, however, do not all belong to a single maturation stage and, furthermore, they often bear activation antigens such as Y29/55 and 9.4, giving rise to debate about the differentiation stage of the leukaemic cells.

Cellular Abnormalities in CLL

Leukaemic cells from patients with CLL have been studied extensively for functional and biochemical differences that might underlie the neoplastic change. Vast numbers of presumed biochemical abnormalities have been described, but unfortunately these results have been described from work mostly carried out on impure populations of cells, done before the existence of T and B lymphocytes was known and before other subsets were distinguished. A short synopsis is presented.

B-CLL lymphocytes have membrane abnormalities in the form of higher fluidity associated with a higher cholesterol content, reduced amino acid transport, lower 5′-nucleotidase and a lower but more uniform sIg which forms caps poorly.

Many enzymes such as adenosine deaminase, cAMP phosphodiesterase, lysosomal enzymes (except acid phosphatase) and adenylate cyclase, have lower activity in CLL cells. Neutral maltase is virtually absent, although this enzyme occurs in high levels in myeloma cells. Some other enzymes, such as fluoride-resistant α-naphthyl butyrate esterase and α-naphthyl acetate esterase (ANAE) are present in CLL cells but are not found in normal B cells.

The cytoskeleton of the neoplastic cells is also abnormal. The patterns of vimentin intermediate filaments, microtubules and microfilaments are abnormal and the actin content is reduced. These abnormalities may account for the easy smudging of CLL cells in smears and the enhanced susceptibility of the cells to drugs such as colchicine and vinca alkaloids which disrupt microtubules. CLL cells are killed by a 100 000-fold lower concentration of colchicine than are normal blood lymphocytes. This extraordinary sensitivity is reversed within minutes by exposure in vitro to TPA (O'Connor 1985).

Chromosomal abnormalities, rearrangements of immunoglobulin genes and abnormalities of oncogenes in CLL cells have been discussed previously. The neoplastic cells show a greater capacity to repair chromosomal damage caused by ultraviolet light or by X-irradiation when compared with normal B cells. This property has been attributed to the presence of a DNA-binding protein involved in repair which is not found in normal lymphocytes (Huang et al. 1975).

Functional abnormalities have also been recorded in CLL cells. CLL B cells stimulate poorly in the mixed lymphocyte reaction (MLR) despite the expression of MHC Class II products (Chiorazzi et al. 1979; Halper et al. 1979). The neoplastic lymphocytes also respond suboptimally to polyclonal activators such as bacterial lipopolysaccharide (LPS), and anti-β_2 microglobulin, possibly because of the dilution of T lymphocytes and changes in the ratios of T cell subpopulations. The neoplastic lymphocytes generally respond better to dextran sulphate, a stimulator of intermediate B cells, but the neoplastic cells synthesise little Ig. B-CLL cells are also poorly activated by Epstein–Barr virus (EBV), a process requiring the presence of T cells. Few antibody-forming cells result and few immortal cell lines have been established (Rickinson et al. 1982). Some CLL populations are inhibited by anti-Ig while others can be induced to synthesise Ig by polyclonal stimuli plus allogenic T cells or T cell supernatants. B-CLL cells appear to have an intrinsic defect which prevents full maturation to antibody-secreting cells.

Unstimulated CLL cells secrete intact IgM, IgD and free light chains in vitro. A significant proportion of the circulating IgM and IgD in CLL patients is synthesised by the leukaemic cells.

The response of CLL lymphocytes to T cell mitogens is generally poor, peaking at 5–7 days rather than at 72 h, as is the norm. However, isolated T lymphocytes from patients with CLL respond better and even normally in some cases and also function normally in a one-way mixed lymphocyte reaction (MLR). Studies on the functional capacity of T cells from patients with CLL have shown variable results. There is an indication in some studies that B-CLL cells are under the influence of suppressor T cells. T lymphocytes in B-CLL make normal amounts of IFN$_\gamma$ and IL-2 on stimulation with TPA or phytohaemagglutinin (PHA), but the IL-2 is directly absorbed by the malignant B cells. This finding has led to the interesting suggestion that the rapid removal of IL-2 contributes to abnormalities of T cell function (Foa et al. 1984). The reversal of the CD4+/CD8+ ratio found in the blood is not seen in the lymph nodes and in the bone marrow, where CD4+ cells exceed CD8+ cells.

There appears to be no evidence to suggest that the poor activation of the leukaemic B cells is due to poor function of the accessory cells (ACs). The capacity of monocytes from CLL patients to enhance T cell responses to mitogens is normal.

NK cells are numerically increased but functionally depressed in CLL (Foa et al. 1984). Furthermore, they cannot be stimulated to improved function by interferon. These important observations need to be examined further. The population of NK cells may be expanded but immature; active NK cells may, as in ordinary immune responses, be capable of exerting functional control on neoplastic B cells. It has also been suggested that defective NK cell function in CLL may play a part in the development of second malignancies.

Malignant Stem Cell

It is not yet possible to identify the stem cells in CLL. The ability to do so has more than theoretical implications. Cure of CLL by bone marrow purging, an approach currently under trial, is aimed at the elimination of the malignant stem cells. This method of treatment requires the identification of a marker that is expressed by all the cells which are capable of multiplying to maintain the malignant clone of B lymphocytes.

B Cell Prolymphocytic Leukaemia

Prolymphocytic leukaemia (PLL) was first described by Galton (Galton et al. 1974) as a subtype of CLL with lymphocytes which were morphologically different. The disease, which makes up about 10% of the chronic leukaemias, is characterised by a subacute course, and, unlike B-CLL, splenic enlargement appears early and is often massive at presentation. Lymph node enlargement is either absent or minimal except as a terminal development (Galton et al. 1974; Catovsky 1977). Peripheral lymphocyte counts are high, often exceeding 100×10^9/litre and lymphocyte morphology is characteristic and different from CLL cells. The majority of patients are men older than 60 years (range 46–77 years) and the main presenting symptoms are weight loss, weakness, fever, fatigue and abdominal discomfort because of massive splenomegaly. The liver is also enlarged and skin lesions occur occasionally, while anaemia is uncommon.

Alkylating agents and chemotherapy usually fail to produce a significant response, and splenic irradiation is of value in some cases (Oscier et al. 1981); the majority of patients die between 3 and 12 months after diagnosis.

Morphology and Phenotype

The prolymphocyte is larger than both a normal or a CLL lymphocyte. It has more cytoplasm, a prominent nucleolus, and, distinct from a blast cell, has relatively condensed nuclear chromatin. In a proportion of PLL patients, the morphology of the cell departs slightly from that typically seen and irregularity of nuclear membrane and clefting may occur. In others, the cell size may be no more than that in CLL.

By light microscopy, there do not appear to be major morphological differences between the B cell and T cell types of PLL. ANAE staining shows one or two distinct red dots in T cell PLL, and acid phosphatase may be demonstrated, whereas both these enzymes are negative or only weakly positive in B cell PLL. The cells in the majority of PLL patients have the membrane characteristics of B lymphocytes. Surface Ig shows a bright fluorescence when stained with fluorescein-conjugated anti-Ig reagents, in contrast to the faint or weak staining seen in the cells of B-CLL. In B cell PLL there is a slightly higher incidence of patients with IgG or IgA on the cell membrane as compared with B cell CLL. B-PLL cells are further distinguished from B-CLL cells in that they show reactivity with FMC7 monoclonal antibody and a low capacity for binding mouse red cells. Rearrangement of both heavy and light chain alleles have been demonstrated (Melo et al. 1985).

The unfortunate historical term "prolymphocyte" implies that it is a precursor lymphocyte, but there is no evidence for this. The high density of sIg, and the finding of more lymphocytes expressing sIgG and sIgA indicates that PLL cells are more mature than CLL cells. This is consistent with the lack of expression of MER. Furthermore, the presence of obvious monoclonal immunoglobulins in the serum is more commonly encountered in B-PLL. It appears that PLL cells and CLL cells are programmed for different traffic routes, but the cell determinants responsible for this are unknown. On the basis of the surface marker phenotype, it has been suggested that the counterpart of the PLL B cell is seen in the lymphocyte corona or mantle zone of lymph nodes (Gobbi et al. 1983).

Hairy Cell Leukaemia

Hairy cell leukaemia (HCL) or leukaemic reticuloendotheliosis constitutes less than 2% of all adult leukaemia. It is primarily a lymphoma of splenic B cells, although the normal counterpart of the highly characteristic hairy cell is not known.

The mean age at presentation is 55 years, and males predominate. Common presenting complaints are weakness, fatigue, infection, easy bruising and abdominal pain from splenomegaly. Early splenic enlargement is a characteristic feature and the most common finding is a pancytopenia of variable degree and the presence of hairy cells in the peripheral blood of 90% of patients (Golomb et al. 1978; Bouroncle 1979). A frank leukaemic picture with over 50% of hairy cells is seen in one-third of patients, but in only a minority is the total leucocyte count over 10×10^9/litre at diagnosis. Pancytopenia is due in varying degree to bone marrow failure and hypersplenism. Hepatomegaly may occur but lymph nodes and other lymphoid organs are not involved.

Two patients with massive splenomegaly were reported to achieve complete haematological and clinical remission after splenectomy, including clearance of the bone marrow (Bouroncle 1979; Slater et al. 1979), suggesting that a predominantly splenic form of HCL may exist. Rarely, patients with pancytopenia and circulating hairy cells but without splenic enlargement have been reported.

The prognosis of HCL is directly related to the degree of pancytopenia (Jansen and Hermans 1982). The overall median survival is between 40 and 60 months. In a comprehensive multicentre study, Jansen and Hermans (1982) showed a significantly prolonged survival for splenectomised patients (median survival of 90 months) as compared with non-splenectomised patients (median survival of less than 30 months). The benefit of splenectomy relates to the extent of improvement of the pancytopenia and to the size of the spleen, since patients with spleens of less than 4 cm below the costal margin may not benefit from splenectomy (Jansen and Hermans 1982). It has also been suggested that poor bone marrow function at presentation and absence of splenomegaly are associated with poor response to splenectomy and a shorter survival (Catovsky 1983). It also appears that about two-thirds of patients with HCL will require other therapeutic measures in addition to splenectomy. Good responses to alkylating agents, anthracycline antibiotics and intensive leukephoresis have been reported (Catovsky 1983).

HCL responds to treatment with IFN_α. Several clinical trials are currently in progress to assess the benefit, indications and methods of administration. The reasons for the responsiveness of HCL to IFN are not clear.

Cases of HCL expressing κ light chains have been reported to have a better prognosis than those with λ light chains. However, the various heavy chain classes of sIg did not correlate with survival time (Jansen et al. 1984).

Morphology and Phenotype

An essential element for the diagnosis of HCL is the presence of the characteristic mononuclear cell with irregular cytoplasmic outlines and, often, clearly identifiable long villous processes. These hair-like cytoplasmic projections are seen in the transmission electron microscope as a mixture of about equal numbers of slender, finger-like microvilli and broad-based, tongue-like pseudopods, corresponding to the microvilli and ruffles, respectively, seen in the scanning electron microscope (Fig. 16.2) (Katayama and Schneider 1977). The hairy cells display a characteristic ribosome-lamella complex consisting of a central space and an outer sheath of multiple parallel lamellae with rows of ribosomes evenly spaced between the lamellae (Fig. 16.3) (Katayama et al. 1972). While this structure is not specific to HCL and can be seen in cells of CLL and lymphosarcoma cell leukaemia, it occurs in a much higher frequency, being observed in as many as 90% of hairy cells, with each hairy cell containing one to several ribosome-lamella complexes (Katayama and Schneider 1977). Nuclear pockets, which are relatively frequent in lymphocytes of other haematological disorders, are rare in the cells of HCL. Normal sIgG + B cells may show cytoplasmic processes similar to those found on hairy cells, whereas most sIgM + lymphocytes have smooth surfaces, a difference which correlates with the higher incidence of sIgG expressed by hairy cells in comparison with other heavy chains.

The hairy cells contain an isoenzyme of acid phosphatase (isoenzyme 5) that is not inhibited by the presence of tartaric acid (Yam et al. 1971). The presence of tartrate-resistant acid phosphatase (TRAP) is the most characteristic cytochemical feature of hairy cells. The proportion of positive cells is variable, and, in a few patients, the TRAP reaction may be completely negative. On the other hand, rare cases of chronic T cell leukaemia also have TRAP and the isoenzyme has rarely been found in Sézary cells and cells of PLL and lymphomas. ANAE and α-naphthyl butyrate have been described as weakly or moderately positive in the hairy cells, sometimes producing a characteristic reaction in the form of fine to

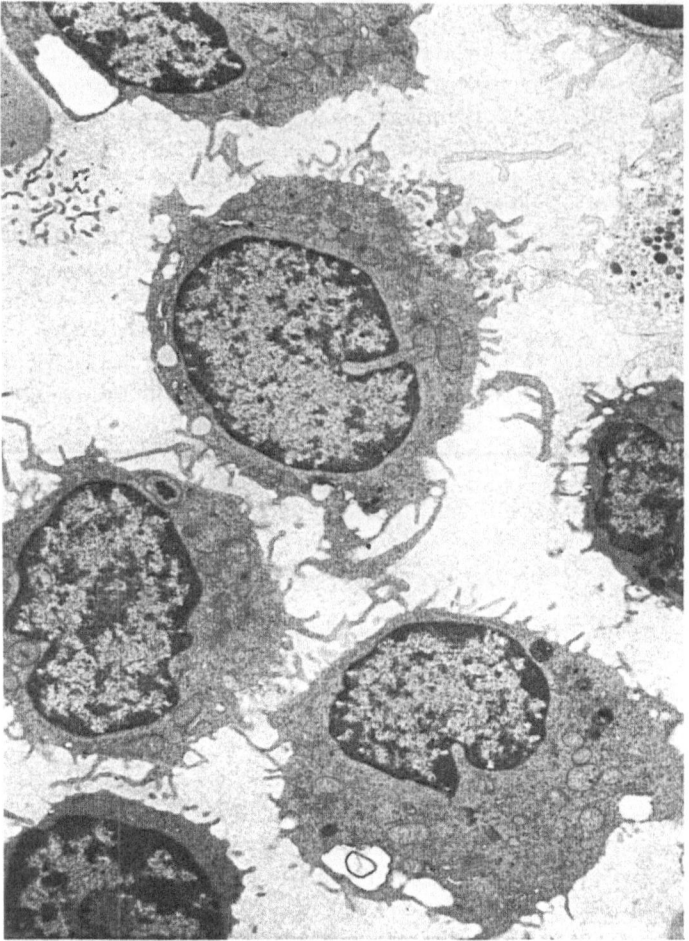

Fig. 16.2. HCL showing peripheral blood leukaemic cells with characteristic finger-like microvilli and broader tongue-like projections. (Uranyl acetate, lead citrate, × 6000)

coarse granules with a crescent configuration (Higgy et al. 1978). Hairy cells also have peroxidase activity in the nuclear envelope and in the strands of endoplasmic reticulum but not in the Golgi saccules or granules.

Early studies of the origin of HCL produced puzzling results. The hairy cells appeared to react with many kinds of anti-immunoglobulin antibodies and to ingest particles, suggesting a mixed B lymphocyte/monocyte phenotype. When precautions were taken to prevent the non-specific binding of anti-immunoglobulin reagents, the sIg in the hairy cells were demonstrated to be monoclonal with respect to light chains in almost every case studied (Golomb et al. 1982; Jansen et al. 1982). The hairy cells most commonly express sIgG and a high proportion carry multiple isotypes all with light chain restriction (Fig. 16.4). sIgMD is encountered in only a minority of cases. The results of monoclonal antibody studies confirm the B cell lineage of most cases of HCL and also show the presence

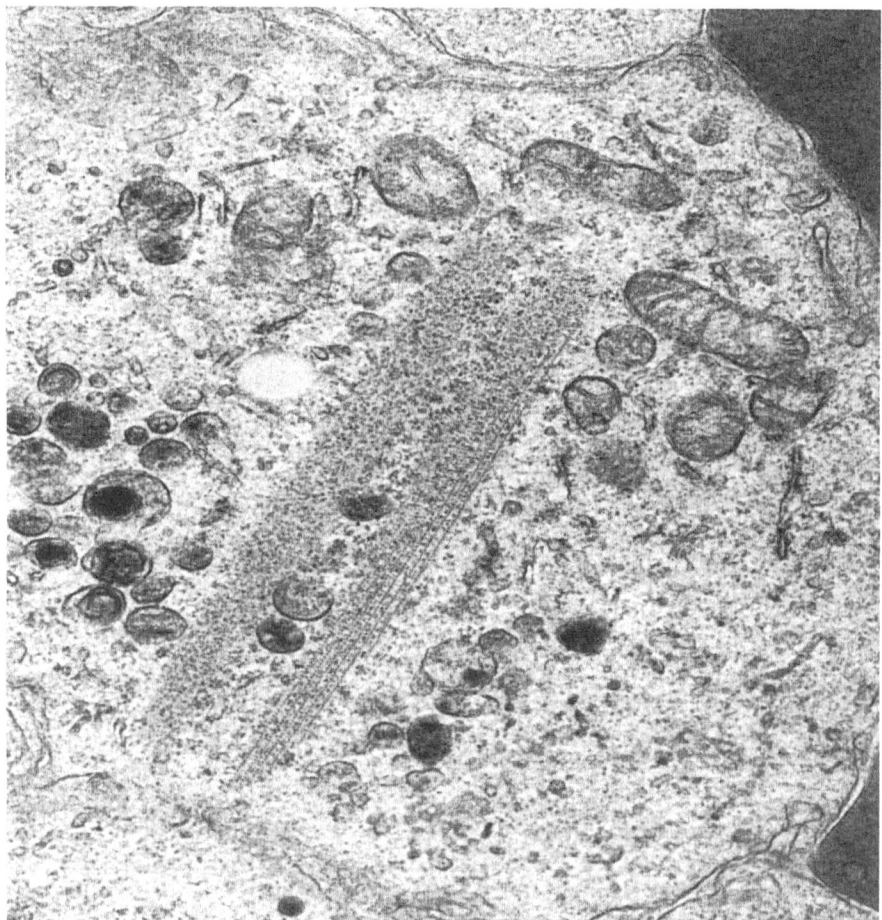

Fig. 16.3. Ribosome-lamella complex in a hairy cell. Parallel lamellae alternating with rows of evenly spaced ribosomes are arranged in a sheath around a central space. (Uranyl acetate, lead citrate, × 23 000)

of multiple phenotypes. Hairy cells bear the pan-B markers CD20, CD22, CD24 and Y29/55 (Jansen et al. 1982) and usually FMC7 and RFA4 (Caligaris-Cappio et al. 1984b), but not the T cell-associated antigens CD1, CD3, CD4, CD7 and CD8. Many have antigens reacting with OKM1 (CD11) antibody, which binds to certain myeloid cells as well as to monocytes. They are also unreactive with monoclonal antibodies against CD5, CD21, CD23 and Tü33 and also lack the meshwork of associated dendritic reticulum cells (Falini et al. 1985). Monoclonal antibodies HC1 and HC2 have been described as specific for HCL (Posnett et al. 1982; Falini et al. 1985). Hairy cells may be MER+ and may express CD1 and CD2 when in culture. They also have IL-2 receptors (CD25) but do not respond to IL-2 in culture (Korsmeyer et al. 1983b).

Autoradiograms of the hybridised DNA in 11 spleens involved by HCL have revealed rearrangements of a heavy chain gene and at least one light chain gene. In

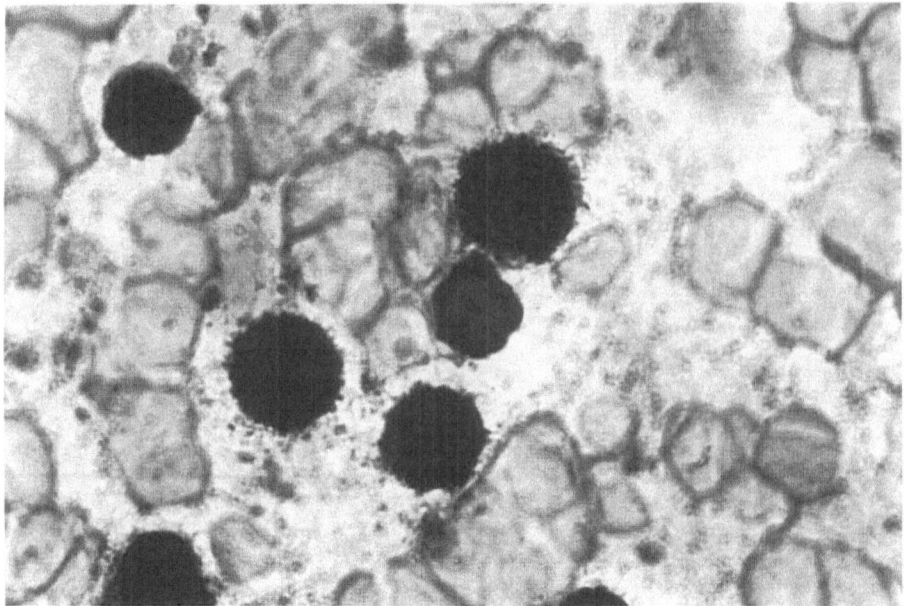

Fig. 16.4. HCL showing marked staining of leukaemic cells for cIg. Notice the staining of the "hairy" cytoplasmic projections. (Anti-Ig6-modified avidin-biotin peroxidase technique, × 1250)

addition, in all cases in which immunoglobulin could be detected within the cells, a rearrangement was present in the DNA of the corresponding immunoglobulin gene. In three cases in which no immunoglobulin was detected, rearrangements were found. These findings confirm the B lymphocyte character of the majority of cases of this leukaemia (Cleary et al. 1984).

The expression of IL-2 receptors suggests that the hairy cell is an activated B cell or an early plasma cell. When CLL B cells are incubated with TPA they express a phenotype resembling that of HCL cells. They become TRAP+, FMC7 and MER– and also develop membrane perturbations similar to those of HCL cells. However, the cells retain the CD5 antigen. The sIg staining in HCL is stronger than that seen in CLL; by using an electron immunoperoxidase technique Mori et al. (1984) have detected immunoglobulins in the perinuclear space and endoplasmic reticulum as well as at the surface of the hairy cells. Such results support the conclusion that hairy cells are commonly derived from immunoglobulin-producing B cells at an earlier stage of differentiation than plasma cells, and that HCL represents a maturation arrest somewhere in between CLL and multiple myeloma (Jansen et al. 1981).

Bone Marrow in HCL

Bone marrow aspirates are characteristically unsuccessful in HCL because of a combination of cellular infiltration and myelofibrosis. Bone marrow biopsy has

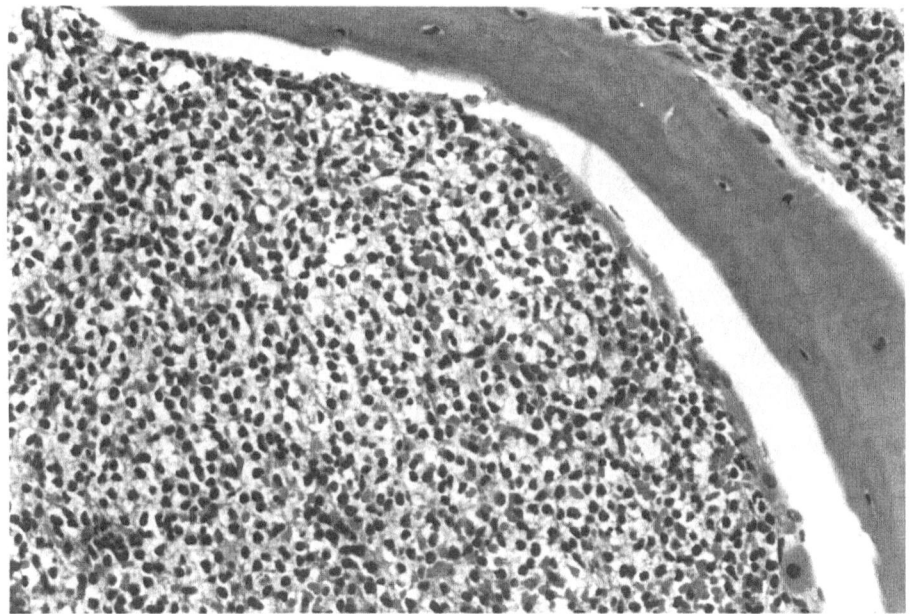

Fig. 16.5. Bone marrow infiltrated by sheets of neoplastic cells. Note the clear cytoplasm, which forms a halo around the rather uniform nuclei. (H & E, × 500)

been demonstrated to be a valuable diagnostic procedure, revealing diffuse involvement in the majority. Partial or focal involvement occurs in less than one third of cases.

The bone marrow shows an infiltration by bland, uniform, mononuclear cells with well-defined nuclei and distinct cytoplasmic borders. Mitotic figures are rare. The infiltrating cells have abundant amounts of water-clear or finely reticulated cytoplasm which imparts a halo around their finely stippled nuclei (Fig. 16.5). Nucleoli are inconspicuous, and there is often folding of the nuclear membrane, producing a coffee-bean appearance in the nucleus. Reticulin stains invariably show an increase in reticulin fibres around individual neoplastic cells. The reticulin stain is also useful in demonstrating focal and patchy involvement of the bone marrow. Subtle infiltration of mononuclear cells can appear to be so innocuous that on low-power examination the most immediate impression is that of a vague expansion of haematopoietic islands (Burke 1978).

Recent reports have drawn attention to the occurrence of osteolytic lesions in patients with HCL. Five patients in a series of 150 had bone lesions (Weh et al. 1979). The femur was the most frequent site of involvement. The bone lesions are described as resembling myeloma deposits (Rosenthal et al. 1979).

Spleen and Liver in HCL

Clinical splenomegaly occurs in over 90% of patients with HCL, and massive enlargements of over 6000 g have been reported (Bouroncle 1979). Isotope studies

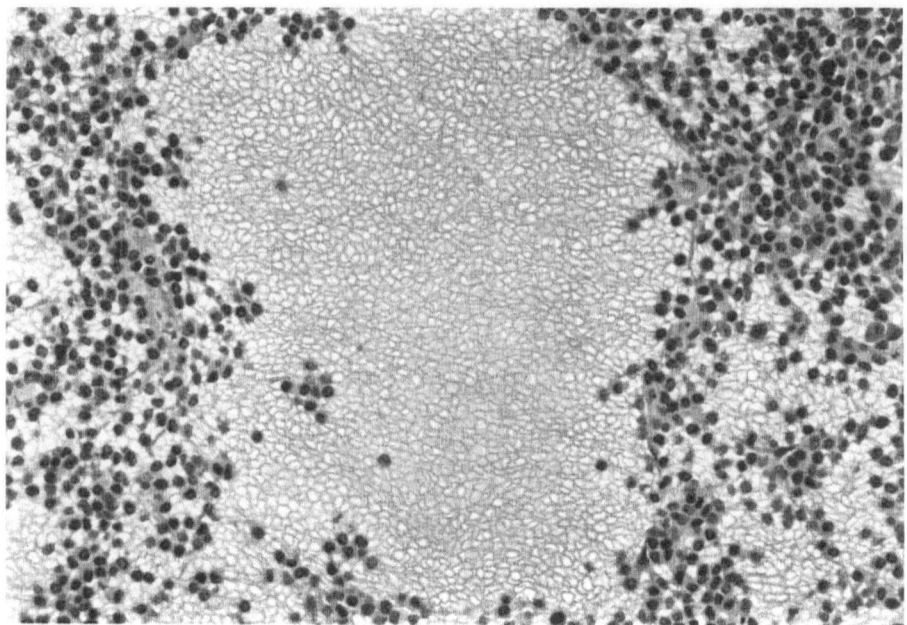

Fig. 16.6. 2500 g spleen in HCL. A "blood lake" is shown lined by hairy cells of uniform appearance. (H & E, × 500)

show that the splenic red blood cell pool is exceptionally large when compared with other disorders with the same degree of splenomegaly. The anatomical basis for this difference relates to the unique changes in the spleen in HCL. Variably prominent distended spaces filled with erythrocytes and resembling dilated sinuses are present. These large "blood lakes" (Fig. 16.6) within the splenic red pulp are lined by one or more layers of circumferentially arranged hairy cells and lack endothelial lining and the ring fibres which form the normal support of red pulp sinuses. This replacement of normal endothelial cells by hairy cells intimately adherent to the pre-existing reticulum network has been suggested to be responsible for the formation of the pseudosinuses and angiomatous lesions seen in the spleen (Nanba et al. 1977). Similar angiomatous lesions are seen in the liver, although up to 20% of livers from patients wtih HCL may not show infiltration by hairy cells at necropsy. Hairy cells appear to possess strong properties of adherence and have been shown in vitro to adhere to surfaces of glass, gelatin-cotton filters and plastic. They attach selectively to hepatic sinusoidal endothelial cells, their processes extending through endothelial pores or through the endothelial cell cytoplasm into the space of Disse. The cytoplasmic extensions bifurcate in the space of Disse to provide anchorage for the hairy cells.

Recently, a syndrome resembling periarteritis nodosa syndrome has been described in association with HCL. Hairy cells were demonstrated in the walls of medium-sized arteries involved by chronic inflammation (Krol et al. 1983).

Chronic Cold Agglutinin Disease

Cold agglutinins are antibodies that have the extraordinary property of combining with red cell antigen in the cold so that haemolysis leading to severe anaemia may result at the temperature of blood circulating through the extremities in cold weather. Chronic cold agglutinin disease (CCAD) is a monoclonal B lymphoproliferative disease which usually has limited proliferative potential. The clinical manifestations are the result of the secretion of monoclonal antibodies that combine in the cold with glycoconjugates bound to proteins and/or lipids of the membranes of erythrocytes and other cells of the body. These antigens are present on the lymphocytes themselves. The cold agglutinins are classified according to the sugar in the glycoconjugate and the protein or lipid to which it is attached. They are of considerable interest from the viewpoint of the genetics of the immune response because they show a strong relationship between antibody specificity and class of heavy chain. Most cold agglutinins are of the IgMκ type. Those of the IgG and IgA classes are almost invariably of cold agglutinin subtypes that react with different specific types of antigen.

Cold agglutinins are normally produced in very small quantities in health. Infection, particularly with EBV and *Mycoplasma pneumoniae*, sometimes induces transient development of high levels of cold agglutinin, and these autoantibodies are found infrequently in a wide range of other illnesses such as hepatic cirrhosis and systemic lupus erythematosus.

Persistent cold agglutinins may be found in association not only with most of the B lymphomas, but also Hodgkin's disease, angioblastic lymphadenopathy and even sinus histiocytosis, and a variety of benign and malignant neoplasms.

In addition to cases in which CCAD is associated with an obvious lymphoma, the disease may also exist without an obvious lymphoma. CCAD often follows a static course, and patients may survive for several decades with no obvious lymphoproliferative manifestations, although some may show lymphocytic infiltration of the bone marrow. About 15% of patients are said to die from a malignant lymphoma. In common with benign paraproteinaemia with non-pathogenic antibody, spontaneous regression may also occur. The cold agglutinins have been reviewed recently by Pruzanski and Katz (1984).

Lymphoplasmacytoid Lymphoma

Lymphoplasmacytoid lymphoma is a group of disorders with a range of clinical presentations. The term "Waldenström's macroglobulinaemia" is applied to the clinical syndrome when both a lymphoplasmacytic proliferation and a monoclonal increase in IgM can be demonstrated. Although some patients may be asymptomatic, an insidious onset of fatigue, weakness, weight loss and bleeding in the form of epistaxis, dependent purpura or gastrointestinal tract haemorrhage are common presenting symptoms. These are often accompanied by generalised lymphadenomegaly, neurological and retinal changes and hepatosplenomegaly. In addition to an almost invariably present Coombs' negative, normocytic, normochronic anaemia, there may be a cryoglobulinaemia, Bence Jones proteinuria and an increased serum viscosity. About one-half of the patients with Waldenström's macroglobulinaemia manifest symptoms which are related to specific physical and chemical properties of the IgM molecules. Their high intrinsic viscosity and ability to interact with other proteins such as clotting factors produce an increase in resistance to the flow of plasma. The resulting hyperviscosity syndrome is manifested in rouleau formation, retinal haemorrhages and exudates and visual impairment. The impaired circulation may produce deafness, headaches, dizziness, somnolence, stupor, paresis, seizures and peripheral neuropathy. Many of these neurological manifestations change frequently with time. Involvement of the bone marrow by the proliferating lymphoid cells, observed in 90% of cases, may result in marrow failure, but a leukaemic phase is rarely present until the terminal stages. The lymphocytosis which occurs may require differentiation from CLL; however, the cytology of the circulating cells is generally more pleomorphic and the cells may have varying degrees of plasmacytoid features.

The diagnosis of Waldenström's macroglobulinaemia is usually made on a biopsy of bone marrow or lymph node in conjunction with serum protein abnormalities. Lymphoplasmacytoid cells are found diffusely permeating through the lymph nodes, often with preservation of sinusoidal structures. The histological features are described in detail in the section on B cell lymphomas.

In lymphoplasmacytoid tumours it is not uncommon to find intracellular cytoplasmic inclusions of intact Ig. These accumulations of Ig in the cells can be quite large and are thought to be the result of a disturbance in secretion. Accordingly, the lymphoplasmacytoid lymphoma is a neoplasm of the secreting derivatives of B lymphocytes. This is an important distinction from CLL, the cells of which usually produce sIg but little secretory Ig.

A small percentage of patients with lymphoplasmacytoid lymphomas present with retrobulbar tumours and involvement of the conjunctiva and eyelids. The tumour sometimes proceeds from the orbit to the skin of the face or elsewhere. In addition, some patients have tumour only in the skull and skeletal muscles, especially in the extremities. These tumour infiltrates of lymphoplasmacytoid cells occur as nodules, either singly or widely spread over the body (Lennert 1978).

Plasma Cell Dyscrasias

Multiple Myeloma

Multiple myeloma is the most common form of malignant plasma cell neoplasm in man. It shows an increased incidence in first-degree relatives, and correlations with the HLA Cw5 complex and immunoglobulin allotypes have been demonstrated. Ionising radiation is an aetiological factor, and associations with chronic antigenic stimulation, rheumatoid arthritis, chronic osteomyelitis, hereditary spherocytosis and Gaucher's disease have been suggested. Plasmacytomas can be induced in high frequency in BALB/c mice by experimental manipulations such as the implantation of mineral oil, plastics or pristane. The relevance of this model to human lymphoid malignancies is strengthened by the occurrence of chromosomal translocations analogous to those seen in BL. Lastly, a viral aetiology has been postulated because of the natural occurrence of plasmacytosis in mink as a result of infection with Aleutian disease virus. The virus can be transmitted to humans but does not appear to cause disease.

Multiple myeloma is an autonomous and progressive proliferation of plasma cells, many of which are cytologically immature or atypical. Although the plasma cell is the marker for the disease, the stage of B cell differentiation at which malignant transformation occurs is not known with certainty. In multiple myeloma there is considerable individual variation in the nature and severity of the clinical manifestations. The diffuse plasma cell infiltration of the marrow results in osteolysis, producing spherical deposits of plasma cells which are confined firstly to areas of red bone marrow but are found eventually throughout the skeleton. Osteolytic lesions and osteoporosis may also be associated with diffuse bone marrow infiltration, thus supporting the accumulating evidence that osteolysis in this disease is probably due to a secondary osteoclast activation rather than to direct bone destruction by tumour cells. In the majority of cases the plasma cells secrete an intact monoclonal immunoglobulin plus excess of free light chains. In about 10%–15% of cases the paraprotein consists only of light chains (Bence Jones protein).

Impairment of renal function may result from the precipitation of light chains in renal tubules and glomeruli, hypercalciuria and hypercalcaemia, hyperuricosuria and hyperuricaemia, pyelonephritis, myelomatous cellular infiltration, amyloidosis, or from iatrogenic causes such as nephrotoxic antibiotics, and, rarely, certain urographic contrast materials. The so-called myeloma kidney is unique and consists of atrophy and degeneration of renal tubular lining cells and apparent destruction of tubules by laminated eosinophilic casts that are occasionally surrounded by multinucleated giant cells.

In the minority of cases small numbers of plasma cells circulate in the peripheral blood, the spleen may be palpably enlarged, and soft tissues of the face, orbit, chest wall or spinal cord may be infiltrated by direct extension from neighbouring bony deposits.

The median survival of patients with multiple myeloma is now about 2–3 years. Patients who respond to therapy have longer median survivals, ranging from 3 to 5 years. Cures have not been obtained. The majority of patients die of progressive disease with or without the superimposition of other contributing factors such as renal failure and/or bacterial sepsis. A small number of patients develop immunoblastic sarcomas, a not-infrequent phenomenon observed in other lymphoproliferative and immunoproliferative disorders.

Malignant Stem Cell

In multiple myeloma there are generally billions of myeloma cells, all secreting the same Ig, usually IgG, indicating that the disease is clonal. Its clonal origin has also been confirmed by G6PD studies. Usually the blood lymphocyte count is not increased, but the Ig idiotype found free in the serum is detected on the surface of many circulating B cells as well as their precursors, indicating that myeloma reflects the proliferation of a clone of lymphoid cells which ultimately differentiates into Ig-secreting plasmacytes. Opinions differ on whether the malignant stem cell in myeloma is primitive or moderately differentiated. Most of the malignant cells are produced in the marrow, although immature malignant cells may sometimes be detected in the blood and a relatively high proportion of circulating pre-B cells expressing CD24 has been found (Pilarski et al. 1985). These different levels of differentiation in myeloma are in contrast to CLL, in which most patients have a restriction in the maturation of the leukaemic clone. Indeed, myeloma has rarely been described in association with CLL, indicating two levels of differentiation in possibly the same malignant process (Fermand et al. 1985).

Plasma Cell Leukaemia

Plasma cell leukaemia is a rare disorder representing a late and often terminal presentation of disseminated plasmacellular neoplasms. The clinical and pathological features of this disease resemble those of an acute leukaemia rather than typical multiple myeloma. Plasma cell leukaemia has been defined as having greater than $0.5-2 \times 10^9$ circulating plasma cells per litre at the time of presentation (Kyle et al. 1974; Woodruff et al. 1978).

Patients with plasma cell leukaemia present with enlarged spleens and sometimes palpable lymph nodes. There is anaemia and thrombocytopenia with renal impairment, leukocytosis and leukoerythroblastosis from extensive bone marrow infiltration by plasma cells. Despite the extent of the infiltration lytic bone lesions are exceptional. Serum and urinary paraproteins are found as in myelomatosis. The disease runs a rapid course despite therapy, and survival beyond 1 year is exceptional.

Localised Plasmacytoma

Localised plasma cell neoplasms account for about 6%–10% of all plasma cellular tumours and may occur as solitary plasmacytoma of bone and extramedullary plasmacytoma. The relationship between such plasma cell neoplasms and multiple myeloma is not well understood. Some authors consider these lesions to be different clinical manifestations of a single neoplastic process, whereas others consider them to be discrete clinical entities with different prognoses (Callihan et al. 1983).

Solitary Plasmacytoma of Bone

Solitary plasmacytoma of bone is a rare tumour which arises as a lytic lesion in a single bone and is indistinguishable histologically from multiple myeloma and extramedullary plasmacytoma. The average age of onset of solitary plasmacytoma of bone is in the early sixth decade as compared with the seventh decade for multiple myeloma, suggesting that solitary plasmacytoma may be a pre-myelomatous condition. The axial skeleton is affected more frequently than the appendicular skeleton. The vertebral column, pelvis, and femur are the most common sites and pain is the usual presenting symptom. Intraosseous lesions may break through the cortex to form soft tissue masses and compress or invade the adjacent spinal cord or nerves resulting in neurological symptoms. Investigation fails to reveal involvement of any other site. After treatment by excision, radiotherapy, or both, the disease may recur locally or the patient may remain without recurrence for years. However, the disease is apt to recur even after periods of some 20 years in a form indistinguishable from myelomatosis.

Extramedullary Plasmacytoma

"Extramedullary plasmacytoma" refers to circumscribed masses of neoplastic plasma cells which present in a site remote from bone and bone marrow. Although histologically and cytologically indistinguishable from multiple myeloma they have a very different natural history. The tumours may arise in Waldeyer's ring, the submucosa of the upper respiratory tract and oral cavity, the gastrointestinal tract mucosa, the skin and subcutis, or any other site where antibody formation occurs. At the time of presentation, lymph nodes draining an extramedullary plasmacytoma are not infrequently involved. The more malignant forms may resemble immunoblastic sarcoma and metastasise to lymph nodes, skin and bone. In contrast to multiple myeloma, the bone metastases, though discrete and lytic, show no predilection for red bone marrow and may appear at sites rarely involved in multiple myeloma such as the small bones of the extremities. Diffuse infiltration of marrow does not occur, except secondarily by spread from lytic deposits.

With regard to immunological abnormalities, about one-quarter of patients have a monoclonal gammopathy and an even smaller percentage have Bence Jones proteinuria. Generally, patients with a few foci of involvement, either with or without regional node involvement, show unremarkable protein levels and normal immunoelectrophoresis.

For a truly localised plasmacytoma, local treatment represents adequate therapy. This takes the form of surgery to remove accessible tumour followed by high-dose radiation therapy. Patients with clinically disseminated disease should receive chemotherapy as for multiple myeloma.

Monoclonal Gammopathy of Undetermined Significance

The monoclonal gammopathies are a group of disorders characterised by proliferation of a single clone of plasma cells that produce a homogenous, monoclonal protein. The term "benign monoclonal gammopathy" has commonly been applied to the presence of the monoclonal protein in persons without evidence of multiple myeloma, macroglobulinaemia, or other related diseases. This term appears to be inadequate because it cannot be predicted whether a monoclonal protein will remain benign or will produce symptomatic myeloma or macroglobulinaemia. Kyle (1982) therefore proposed the term "monoclonal gammopathy of undetermined significance" to designate the monoclonal hyperglobulinaemia secreted by a relatively small benign clone of B cells. It has been estimated that the appearance of a recognisable paraprotein (equivalent to 5 g/litre) usually reflects a tumour mass of at least 5×10^9 cells. The immunoglobulin synthesised in excess may be of any class, but only M, D and A heavy chain classes are seen in clinical practice; IgD and IgE monoclonal proliferations are very rare.

Monoclonal immunoglobulin is present in the serum of apparently healthy people at a frequency which increases to about 3% in the population over the age of 70 years (Kyle and Bayrd 1976). The concentration of monoclonal immunoglobulin remains essentially unchanged during many years of observation, and may occasionally decline spontaneously to undetectable levels. Malignancy develops, however, in at least one-fifth of patients in whom the concentration of immuno-globulin rises and frank myelomatosis ensues. In monoclonal gammopathy of undetermined significance (MGUS) it is usual for the paraprotein concentration to remain below 25 g/litre, the polyclonal serum immunoglobulins to remain at concentrations within their normal ranges, and for monoclonal light chains to be undetectable in the urine. Occasionally, patients whose condition remains stable have shown serum paraprotein concentrations above 25 g/litre, subnormal levels of one or more of the polyclonal serum immunoglobulins, and bone marrow plasma cell counts of above 3%. The plasma cells may show monoclonality, and monoclonal light chains may be found in the urine (Bast et al. 1981). The distinction from early progressive myelomatosis or other antibody-secreting tumours can be made only by following the patients regularly. The absence of J chains in the marrow of some patients with MGUS, in contrast to myelomatosis, may help the diagnosis (Bast et al. 1981).

Heavy Chain Diseases

Heavy chain diseases (HCD) are immunoproliferative disorders characterised by the secretion of structurally abnormal monoclonal heavy chain proteins devoid of attached light chains. Because of genetic deletion, the incomplete heavy chain in these rare diseases cannot be coupled with the corresponding light chain. The disease synthesising the α heavy chain is the least uncommon of the group and those synthesising the γ and μ chains are excessively rare.

The clinical presentation of heavy chain disease is characteristic. The common form of α chain disease occurs in young adults in poor socioeconomic circumstances, most frequently in the Middle East. This disorder is characterised by a plasma cell proliferation that primarily involves the small intestine, and the term "immunoproliferative small intestinal disease (IPSID)" has been recommended for the condition. Symptoms of chronic diarrhoea, steatorrhea, abdominal pain and distension, nausea, vomiting and weight loss are common, and presenting signs include cachexia, clubbing, abdominal tenderness and abdominal masses. In contrast to γ and μ HCD, hepatosplenomegaly is absent.

The pathological features of IPSID have been described under a variety of names, most common of which are "Mediterranean abdominal lymphoma" or "primary intestinal lymphoma of the Mediterranean type". The lymphomas in the small intestine have been variably described as immunoblastic sarcomas, pleomor-phic lymphoma, mixed lymphocytic-histiocytic lymphomas and histiocytic lymphomas (Haghighi 1983). In the lamina propria and superficial submucosa of the small bowel uninvolved by malignant lymphoma, there is a dense, diffuse lymphoplasmacellular infiltrate (Callihan et al. 1983; Isaacson et al. 1983). It has been suggested that this infiltrate represents a premalignant or pretumoural stage which transforms, in the small bowel and/or mesenteric lymph nodes, to a large cell malignant lymphoma (Callihan et al. 1983). The actual frequency of transfor-mation to a malignant lymphoma of the large cell type is unknown. It occurred in 36% of patients with α HCD in Selzer's series (Selzer 1979), whereas a third of Lewin's patients developed large cell lymphomas (Lewin 1976). The lymphoma cells, which presumably arise from the ancestral progenitors of the plasma cell-secreting α chain, also synthesise only α chains.

In some cases of IPSID, prolonged antibiotic treatment prior to the onset of lymphomatous transformation has resulted in resolution. In an uncommon variant, the lungs are the major organs affected.

HCD with synthesis of γ chains is more variable; it can occur at any age and may present in benign or malignant forms as lymphoma. Associated fever, malaise and erythema and oedema of the soft palate and uvula have been described. HCD synthesising μ chain afflicts older patients who have a CLL-like condition with characteristic large vacuolated plasma cells.

Lymphosarcoma Cell Leukaemia

Flashman and Leopold (1929) were perhaps the first to observe that a leukaemic phase may develop late in the course of a lymphosarcoma. It was later observed that a lymphosarcoma cell leukaemia (LSCL) with distinctive circulating malignant cells could be the presenting manifestation of lymphosarcoma. The distinctive cells with "notched nuclei" were morphologically similar to the malignant cells seen in the lymphosarcomatous nodes. Applying the classification of Gall and Rappaport, Schnitzer et al. (1970) concluded that LSCL was the leukaemic phase of poorly differentiated lymphocytic lymphoma, but subsequent reports have established that a leukaemic phase may occur in the other subtypes of NHL (Schnitzer and Kass 1973; Nathwani et al. 1976) of both B and T cell lineages.

Come et al. (1980) found that a leukaemic phase occurred in 14% of 214 patients with NHL. They also reported that in the patients with nodular poorly differentiated lymphotic lymphoma in whom the peripheral blood was involved at the time of presentation or later, the rate and extent of response to treatment and the survival approached those in patients with similar disease but who were not leukaemic. These findings confirm the prevalent view that neither bone marrow nor peripheral blood involvement at diagnosis correlates with survival in nodular poorly differentiated lymphocytic lymphoma. In the case of diffuse large cell lymphoma, leukaemic conversion appeared to be a terminal event associated with unresponsive disease in multiple sites, again without appearing to exert an important independent effect on prognosis.

The cells of LSCL usually differ from the lymphocytes of CLL by the presence of a very narrow rim of cytoplasm and an irregular, angular, seldom round nucleus that often reveals indentation. These notched or cleaved nuclei are often distinctive, but, on occasion, separation from the cells of CLL on morphological grounds alone is difficult. The surface marker characteristics, however, allow accurate identification. LSCL cells show dense sIg compared with the faintly staining cells of CLL. Furthermore, they lack MERs, which are present in CLL cells (Forbes et al. 1978). LSCL cells when placed at 37° C show redistribution of surface immunoglobulin by the formation of bright caps, a property not shared by the cells of CLL.

More recently, cytofluorometric analysis including the sensitive "kappa-lambda test" has demonstrated the presence of circulating monoclonal lymphocytes in non-leukaemic patients with B cell lymphomas (Ligler et al. 1980; Weinberg et al. 1984). Such small numbers of malignant cells in the peripheral blood were previously not detectable by morphological observation and standard immunological techniques. Monoclonal lymphocytes can now also be detected by analysis for clonal rearrangements of Ig or Ti genes and the same rearrangement can be demonstrated in the tumour as in the circulating malignant cells (Hu et al. 1985). Detection of malignant lymphoma cells in blood may confirm a diagnosis of malignant lymphoproliferative disease when biopsy is not possible, for example when no tumour is evident. Clonal rearrangements have been found in blood cells in patients in clinical remission. The detection of circulating malignant cells raises a number of questions: Can the technique be used to assess (1) the efficacy of primary treatment, (2) the recurrence of tumour and (3) the need for further treatment before recurrence of the disease is otherwise detectable?

It appears, therefore, that the term "LSCL" will have less relevance as we accept that spill-over of malignant cells into the peripheral blood can occur in NHL of both B and T cell lineages and that a considerable overlap exists between lymphoma and leukaemia.

References

Anderson KC, Bates MP, Slaughenhoupt BL, Pinkus GS, Schlossman SF, Nadler LM (1984) Expression of human B-cell-associated antigens on leukaemias and lymphomas: a model of human B-cell differentiation. Blood 63: 1424–1432

Bakhshi A, Minowada J, Arnold A et al. (1983) Lymphoid blast crises of chronic myelogenous leukemia represent stages in the development of B-cell precursors. N Engl J Med 309: 826–831

Bast EJEG, VanCamp B, Boom SE et al. (1981) Differentiation between benign and malignant monoclonal gammopathy by the presence of the J chain. Clin Exp Immunol 44: 375–382

Bennet JM, Catovsky D, Daniel MT et al. (1976) Cooperative Group Proposals for the classification of acute leukaemia. Br J Haematol 33: 351–358

Bona CA, Fauci AS (1980) In vitro idiotypic suppression of chronic lymphocytic leukemia lympho- cytes secreting monoclonal immunoglobulin M anti-sheep erythrocyte antibody. J Clin Invest 65: 761–767

Bouroncle BA (1979) Leukemic reticuloendotheliosis (hairy cell leukemia). Blood 53: 412–436

Bowman WP, Melvin SL, Aur RJ et al. (1979) Patterns of cell membrane markers and clinical prognostic features in acute lymphocytic leukemia (ALL) of childhood. Proc Am Assoc Cancer Res 20: 156–161

Brouet JC, Prieur A (1974) Membrane markers on chronic lymphocytic lymphoma cells. A B cell leukemia with rosettes due to antisheep erythrocyte antibody activity of the membrane bound IgM and a T cell leukemia with surface immunoglobulin. Clin Immunol Immunopathol 2: 481–486

Brouet JC, Seligmann M (1977) Chronic lymphocytic leukaemia as an immunoproliferative disorder. Clin Haematol 6: 169–184

Brouet JC, Seligmann M (1978) The immunological classification of acute lymphoblastic leukemias. Cancer 42: 817–827

Brouet JC, Preud'homme J-L, Seligmann M et al. (1973) Blast cells with monoclonal surface immunoglobulin in two cases of acute blast crisis supervening on chronic lymphocytic leukaemia. Br Med J 4: 23–24

Brouet JC, Preud'homme JL, Flandrin G et al. (1977) Membrane markers in "histiocytic" lymphomas (reticulum cell sarcomas). J Natl Cancer Inst 56: 631–633

Brouet JC, Preud'homme JL, Penit C, Valensi F, Rouget P, Seligmann M (1979) Acute lymphoblastic leukemia with pre-B-cell characteristics. Blood 54: 269–273

Burke JS (1978) The value of bone-marrow biopsy in the diagnosis of hairy cell leukemia. Am J Clin Pathol 70: 876–884

Caligaris-Cappio F, Janossy G (1985) Surface markers in chronic lymphoid leukemias of B cell type. Semin Hematol 22: 1–12

Caligaris-Cappio F, Gobbi M, Campana D et al. (1984a) B-chronic lymphocytic leukaemia patients with stable benign disease showing a distinctive membrane phenotype. Br J Haematol 56: 655–660

Caligaris-Cappio F, Janossy G, Campana D et al. (1984b) Lineage relationship of chronic lymphocytic leukemia and hairy cell leukemia: studies with TPA. Leuk Res 8: 567–578

Callihan TR, Holbert JM, Berard CW (1983) Neoplasms of terminal B-cell differentiation: the morphologic basis of functional diversity. In: Sommers Sc, Rosen PP (eds) Malignant lymphoma. A Pathology Annual Monograph. Appleton Century Crofts, Norwalk, Connecticut, pp 169–268

Carstairs KC, Francombe WH, Scott JG, Gelfand EW (1985) Persistent polyclonal lymphocytosis of B lymphocytes induced by cigarette smoking? Lancet I: 1094 (letter)

Catovsky D (1977) Hairy-cell leukemia and prolymphocytic leukemia. Clin Haematol 6: 245–268

Catovsky D (1983) Prolymphocytic and hairy cell leukemias. In: Gunz FW, Henderson ES (eds) Leukemia. Grune and Stratton, New York, pp 759–781

Central Cancer Registry Unit, South Australia (1985) Cancer in South Australia 1977–1983 South Australian Health Commission, Lutheran Publishing House, South Australia

Chessells JM, Hardisty RM, Rapson NT, Greaves MF (1977) Acute lymphoblastic leukaemia in children: classification and prognosis. Lancet II: 1307–1309

Chiorazzi N, Fu SM, Montazeri G et al. (1979) T cell helper defect in patients with chronic lymphocytic leukemia. J Immunol 122: 1087–1090

Cleary ML, Wood GS, Warnke R, Chao J, Sklar J (1984) Immunoglobulin gene rearrangements in hairy cell leukemia. Blood 64: 99–104

Come SE, Jaffe ES, Andersen JC et al. (1980) Non-Hodgkins's lymphomas in leukemic phase: clinicopathologic correlations. Am J Med 69: 667–674

Cristo W, Vogler L, Sarrif et al. (1979) Clinical and laboratory characterisation of pre-B-cell leukemia in children. Blood 54 (Suppl 1):183a (abstract)

Delsol G, Laurent G, Kuhlein E et al. (1981) Richter's syndrome. Evidence for the clonal origin of the two proliferations. Am J Clin Pathol 76: 308–315

Dighiero G, Charron D, Debre P et al. (1979) Identification of a pure splenic form of chronic lymphocytic leukaemia. Br J Haematol 14: 169–174

Enno A, Catovsky D, O'Brien M, Cherchi M, Kumaran TO, Galton DA (1979) "Prolymphocytoid" transformation of chronic lymphocytic leukemia. Br J Haematol 41: 9–18

Ezdinli EZ, Nanus DM (1983) B-lymphoproliferative disorders: a proposed unified pathogenetic pathway. Hematol Oncol 1: 297–319

Falini B, Schwarting R, Erber W et al. (1985) The differential diagnosis of hairy cell leukemia with a panel of monoclonal antibodies. Am J Clin Pathol 83: 289–300

Fermand JP, James JM, Herait P, Brouet JC (1985) Associated chronic lymphotic leukemia and multiple myeloma: origin from a single clone. Blood 66: 291–293

Ferme JM, Andrien G, Flandrin G, Bernard J (1981) Sézary syndrome occurring ten years after monoclonal gammopathy treated for four years by chlorambucil. Leuk Res 5: 168–171

Fialkow PJ, Jacobson RJ, Papayannopoulou T (1977) Chronic myelocytic leukemia: clonal origin in a stem cell common to the granulocyte, erythrocyte platelet and monocyte/macrophage. Am J Med. 63: 125–129

Fialkow PJ, Najfeld V, Reddy AL, Singer J, Steinmann L (1978) Chronic lymphocytic leukemia: clonal origin in a committed B-lymphocyte progenitor Lancet II: 444–446

Flashman DH, Leopold SS (1929) Leukosarcoma: with report of a case beginning with a primary retroperitoneal lymphosarcoma and terminating with leukemia. Am J Med Sci 177: 651–656

Flug F, Dodson L, Wolff J (1985) B-lymphocyte associated differentiation antigen expression by 'non-B, non-T' acute lymphoblastic leukemia. Leuk Res 9: 1051–1058

Foa R, Lauria F, Lusso P et al. (1984) Discrepancy between phenotypic and functional features of natural killer T-lymphocytes in B-cell chronic lymphocytic leukaemia. Br J Haematol 58: 509–516

Forbes IJ, Zalewski PD, Leong AS-Y et al. (1978) B cell leukaemia distinguished from chronic lymphocytic leukaemia by surface markers. Aust NZ J Med 8: 532–538

Forbes IJ, Zalewski PD, Cowled PA, Sage RE (1979) Maturation in B lymphocytic leukaemia. J Clin Lab Immunol 1: 329–331

Ford AM, Molgaard HV, Greaves MF, Gould HJ (1983) Immunoglobulin gene organisation and expression in haemopoietic stem cell leukemia. EMBO J 2: 997–1001

Foucar K (1981) Acute leukemias I: acute lymphoblastic leukemia. Lab Med 12: 404–410

Galton DAG, MacLennan ICM (1982) Clinical patterns in B lymphoid malignancy. Clin Haematol 11: 561–587

Galton DAG, Goldman JM, Wiltshaw E et al. (1974) Prolymphocytic leukemia. Br J Haematol 27: 7–11

Gobbi M, Caligaris-Cappio F, Janossy G (1983) Normal equivalent cells of B cell malignancies: Analysis with monoclonal antibodies. Br J Haematol 54: 393–403

Golomb HM, Catovsky D, Golde DW (1978) Hairy cell leukemia A clinical review based on 71 cases. Ann Intern Med 89: 677–683

Golomb HM, Davis S, Wilson C, Vardiman J (1982) Surface immunoglobulins of hairy cells of 55 patients with hairy cell leukemia. Am J Haematol 12: 397–401

Gordon DS, Jones BM, Browning SW et al. (1982) Persistent polyclonal lymphocytosis of B lymphocytes. N Engl J Med 307: 232–236

Gray JL, Jacobs A, Block M (1974) Bone marrow and peripheral blood lymphocytosis in the prognosis of chronic lymphocytic leukemia. Cancer 33: 1169–1178

Gunz FW, Gunz JP, Veale AMO, Chapman CJ, Houston IB (1975) Familial leukemia: a study of 909 families. Scand J Haematol 15: 117–131

Habeshaw JA, Catley PF, Stansfeld AG, Brearley RL (1979) Surface phenotyping, histology and the nature of non-Hodgkin's lymphoma in 157 patients. Br J Cancer 40: 11–34

Haghighi P (1983) Primary small intestinal lymphoma and immunoproliferative small intestinal disease: an update. In: Sommers SC, Rosen PP (eds) Malignant lymphoma. A Pathology Annual Monograph. Appleton Century Crofts, Norwalk, Connecticut, pp 269–295

Halper JP, Fu S-M, Gottlieb AB, Winchester RJ, Kunkel HG (1979) Poor mixed lymphocyte reaction stimulatory capacity of leukaemic B cells of chronic lymphocytic leukemia patients despite the presence of Ia antigens. J Clin Invest 64: 1141–1148

Han T, Ozer H, Gavigan M (1984) Benign monoclonal B-cell lymphocytosis — a benign variant of CLL: clinical, immunologic, phenotypic and cytogenetic studies in 20 patients. Blood 64: 244–252

Higgy KE, Burns GF, Hayhoe FGJ (1978) Identification of the hairy cells of leukaemic reticuloendotheliosis by an esterase method. Br J Haematol 38: 99–106

Hu E, Trela M, Thompson J et al. (1985) Detection of B-cell lymphoma in peripheral blood by DNA hybridisation. Lancet II: 1092–1095

Huang ATF, Riddle MM, Coons LS (1975) Some properties of a DNA-unwinding protein unique to lymphocytes from chronic lymphocytic leukemia. Cancer Res 35: 981–986

International Workshop on CLL (1981) Chronic lymphocytic leukaemia: proposals for a revised prognostic staging system. Br J Haematol 48: 365–367

Isaacson P, Al-Dewachi HS, Mason DY (1983) Middle Eastern intestinal lymphoma: a morphological and immunohistochemical study. J Clin Pathol 36: 489–498

Jansen J, Hermans J (1982) Clinical staging system for hairy cell leukemia. Blood 60: 571–577

Jansen J, Schuit HRE, Meijer CJLF et al. (1981) Cell markers in hairy cell leukemia. In: Kanapp W (ed) Leukemic markers. Academic, New York, pp 179–193

Jansen J, Schuit HRE, Meijer CJLF, van Niewkoop JA, Hÿmans W (1982) Cell markers in hairy cell leukemia studied in cells from 51 patients. Blood 59: 52–60

Jansen J, Schuit HRE, Hermans J, Hijmans W (1984) Prognostic significance of immunologic phenotype in hairy cell leukemia. Blood 63: 1241–1244

Katayama I, Schneider GB (1977) Further ultrastructural characterization of hairy cells of leukemic reticuloendotheliosis. Am J Pathol 86: 163–182

Katayama I, Li CY, Yam LT (1972) Ultrastructural characteristics of the "hairy cells" of leukemic reticuloendotheliosis. Am J Pathol 67: 361–370

Kay NE, Kaplan ME (1984) Defective expression of T cell antigens in chronic lymphocytic leukaemia: relationship to T-cell dysfunction. Br J Haematol 57: 105–111

Kjelsberg CR, Marty J (1981) Prolymphocytic transformation of chronic lymphocytic leukemia. Cancer 48: 2447–2451

Korsmeyer SJ, Hieter PA, Ravetch JV et al. (1981) Developmental hierarchy of immunoglobulin gene rearrangements in human leukemic pre-B cells. Proc Natl Acad Sci USA 78: 7096–7100

Korsmeyer SJ, Arnold A, Bakhshi A et al. (1983a) Immunoglobulin gene rearrangement and cell surface antigen expression in acute lymphocytic leukemias of T cell and B cell precursor origins. J Clin Invest 71: 301–313

Korsmeyer SJ, Greene WC, Cossman J et al. (1983b) Rearrangement and expression of immunoglobulin genes and expression of Tac antigen in hairy cell leukemia. Proc Natl Acad Sci USA 80: 4522–4526

Krol T, Robinson J, Bekeris L, Messmore H (1983) Hairy cell leukaemia and a fatal periarteritis nodosa-like syndrome. Arch Pathol Lab Med 107: 583–585

Kumararatne DS, MacLennan ICM (1981) Cells of the marginal zone of the spleen are lymphocytes derived from recirculating precursors. Eur J Immunol 11: 865–879

Kumararatne DS, Bazin H, MacLennan ICM (1981) Marginal zones: the major B cell compartment of rat spleens. Eur J Immunol 11: 858–864

Kyle RA (1982) Monoclonal gammopathy of undetermined significance (MGUS): a review. Clin Haematol 11: 123–150

Kyle RA, Bayrd ED (1976) The monoclonal gammopathies, multiple myeloma and related plasma cell disorders. American Lecture Series. Thomas, Springfield Ill

Kyle RA, Maldonado JE, Bayrd ED (1974) Plasma cell leukemia. Arch Intern Med 133: 813–818

LeBien TW, Bollum FJ, Yasmineh WG, Kersey JH (1982) Phorbol ester-induced differentiation of a non-T, non-B leukemic cell line: model for human lymphoid progenitor cell development. J Immunol 128: 1316–1320

Lennert K (1978) Malignant lymphomas other than Hodgkin's disease. Springer, Berlin Heidelberg New York, p 119

Lewin KJ, Kahn LB, Novis BH (1976) Primary intestinal lymphoma of "Western" and "Mediterranean" type α chain disease and massive plasma cell infiltration. A comparative study of 37 cases. Cancer 38: 2511–2528

Ligler FS, Smith RG, Kettman JR et al. (1980) Detection of tumor cells in the peripheral blood of nonleukemic patients with B-cell lymphoma: analysis of "clonal excess". Blood 55: 792–801

Long JC, Aisenberg AC (1975) Richter's syndrome. A terminal complication of chronic lymphocytic leukaemia with distinct clinico-pathologic features. Am J Clin Pathol 63: 786–795

Maheu M, Baker MA, Falk JA, Taub RN (1981) Immunologic diagnosis and monitoring of human acute leukemias. Am J Pathol 103: 139–158

Markey G, Alexander HD, Agnew AND et al. (1986) Enumeration of absolute numbers of T lymphocyte subsets in B-chronic lymphocytic leukaemia using an immunoperoxidase technique: relation to clinical stage. Br J Haematol 62: 257–273

Melo JV, Foroni L, Brito Bapapulle VB et al. (1985) Prolymphocytic leukemia of B cell type: rearranged immunoglobulin (Ig) genes with defective Ig production. Blood 66: 391–398

Miller DL (1980) Acute lymphoblastic leukemia. Pediatr Clin North Am 27: 269–274

Minot GB, Isaacs R (1924) Lymphatic leukaemia; age incidence, duration, and benefit derived from irradiation. Boston Med Surg J 191: 1–9

Moayeri H, Sokal J (1979) In vitro leukocyte thymidine uptake and prognosis in chronic lymphocytic leukemia. Am J Med 66: 773–778

Montserrat E and Rozman C for the Spanish Cooperative Group for CLL Study (1983) Bone marrow biopsy in chronic lymphocytic leukemia: a study of 208 cases. Haematologia 16: 73–83

Morgan E, Hsu CCS (1979) Prognostic implications of a leukemia-associated antigen in children with null cell acute lymphocytic leukemia. Blood 54 (Suppl 1): 198a (abstract)

Mori N, Tsunodar R, Kojima M et al. (1984) Ultrastructural localisation of immunoglobulins in hairy cell leukemia. Hum Pathol 15: 1042–1047

Nanba K, Soban EJ, Bowling MC, Berard CW (1977) Splenic pseudosinuses and hepatic angiomatous lesions. Distinctive features of hairy cell leukemia. Am J Clin Pathol 67: 415–426

Nathwani BN, Kim H, Rappaport H (1976) Malignant lymphoma, lymphoblastic. Cancer 38: 964–983

O'Connor TWE (1985) Phorbol ester-induced loss of colchicine ultrasensitivity in chronic lymphocytic leukemia lymphocytes. Leuk Res 9: 885–895

Oscier DG, Catovsky D, Errington RD, Goolden AW, Roberts PD, Galton DA (1981) Splenic irradiation in B-prolymphocytic leukaemia. Br J Haematol 48: 577–584

Pilarski LM, Mant MJ, Reuther BA (1985) Pre-B cells in peripheral blood of multiple myeloma patients. Blood 66: 416–422

Pizzolo G, Ambrosetti A, Semezato G et al. (1984) B cells in chronic lymphocytic leukemia. Comparative analysis of blood and bone marrow. Blut 49: 69–73

Posnett DN, Chiorazzi N, Kunkel HG (1982) Monoclonal antibodies with specificity for hairy cell leukemia cells. J Clin Invest 70: 254–261

Pruzanski W, Katz A (1984) Cold agglutinins — antibodies with biological diversity. Clin Immunol Rev 3: 131–168

Rai KR, Sawitsky A, Cronkite EP, Chanana AD, Levy RN, Pasternak BS (1975) Clinical staging of chronic lymphocytic leukemia. Blood 46: 219–234

Richter NN (1928) Generalised reticular cell sarcoma of lymph nodes associated with lymphatic leukemia. Am J Pathol 4: 285–299

Rickinson AB, Finerty S, Epstein MA (1982) Interaction of Epstein-Barr virus with leukaemic B cells in vitro. I. Abortive infection and rare cell line establishment from chronic lymphocytic leukaemic cells. Clin Exp Immunol 50: 347–354

Rosenthal RL, Steiner GC, Golub BS (1979) Hairy cell leukemia: historical aspects and bone involvement. Mt Sinai J Med (NY) 46: 237–242

Rozman C, Hernandez-Nieto L, Montserrat E, Brugues R (1981) Prognostic significance of bone marrow patterns in chronic lymphocytic leukaemia. Br J Haematol 47: 529–537

Rozman C, Montserrat E, Rodriguez-Fernandez JM et al. (1984) Bone marrow histologic pattern — the best single prognostic parameter in chronic lymphocytic leukemia: a multivariate survival analysis of 329 cases. Blood 64: 642–648

Rundles RW (1977) Chronic lymphocytic leukemia. In: Williams WJ, Beutler E, Erslev AJ, Rundles RW (eds) Hematology. McGraw-Hill, New York, pp 1002–1020

Salmon SE, Seligmann M (1974) B-cell neoplasia in man. Lancet II: 1230–1233

Schnitzer B, Kass L (1973) Leukemic phase of reticulum cell sarcoma (histiocytic lymphoma). A clinical and ultrastructural study. Cancer 31: 547–559

Schnitzer B, Loesel LS, Reed RE (1970) Lymphosarcoma cell leukemia: a clinicopathologic study. Cancer 26: 1082–1096

Schwarzmeier JD, Radaskiewicz T, Graminger W et al. (1981) Chronisch lymphatisch Leukaemie vom B-Zellen Typ: Klinisch und morphologische Untersuchungen zur diagnostischen Abgrenzung. Klin Wochenschr 59: 1313–1318

Selzer G, Sherman G, Callihan TR, Schwartz Y (1979) Primary small intestinal lymphomas and α-heavy-chain disease. A study of 43 cases from a pathology department in Israel. Isr J Med Sci 15: 111–123

Slater NG, Barkhan P, Williams HJH (1979) Hairy cell leukemia — apparent cure with reversal of marrow fibrosis. Clin Lab Haematol 1: 65–68

Slungaard A, Smith MJ (1981) Serum immunoglobulin in chronic lymphocytic leukemia. Scand J Haematol 12: 112–120

Theml H, Love R, Begemann H (1977) Factors in the pathomechanism of chronic lymphocytic leukemia. Annu Rev Med 28: 131–141

Touw I, Delwel R, Bolhuis R, van Zanen G, Lowenberg B (1985) Common and pre-B acute lymphoblastic leukemia cells express interleukin 2 receptors and interleukin 2 stimulates in vitro colony formation. Blood 66: 556–561

Tutt AL, Stevenson FK, Smith JL, Stevenson GT (1983) Antibodies against urinary light chain idiotypes as agents for detection and destruction of human neoplastic B lymphocytes. J Immunol 131: 3058–3063

Vincent PC, Gunz FW (1970) Control of lymphocyte level in the blood. Lancet II: 342–344

Vogler LB, Crist WB, Bockman DE et al. (1978) Pre-B cell leukemia: a new phenotype of childhood lymphoblastic leukemia. N Engl J Med 298: 872–878

Weh HJ, Katz M, Bray B, Rodat O, Degos L, Flandrin G (1979) Lesions osseuses au cours des leucemies a tricholeucocytes. Nouv Presse Med 8: 2253–2254

Weinberg DS, Pinkus GS, Ault KA (1984) Cytofluorometric detection of B cell clonal excess: a new approach to the diagnosis of B cell lymphoma. Blood 63: 1080–1087

Wilson JD, Nossal GJV (1971) Identification of human T and B lymphocytes in normal peripheral blood and in chronic lymphocytic leukemia Lancet II: 788–791

Wolff LJ, Richardson ST, Neiburger JB et al. (1976) Poor prognosis of children with acute lymphocytic leukemia and increased B-cell markers. J Pediatr 89: 956–958

Woodruff RK, Malpas JS, Paxton AM, Lister TA (1978) Plasma cell leukemia (PCL): a report on 15 patients. Blood 52: 839–845

Yam LT, Li CY, Lam KW (1971) Tartrate-resistant acid phosphatase isoenzyme in the reticulum cells of leukemic reticuloendotheliosis. N Engl J Med 284: 357–360

17 B Cell Lymphomas

Introduction

The classification of malignant lymphoma has always been a controversial subject, well-reflected in Rupert Willis' statement, "nowhere in pathology has a chaos of names so clouded clear concepts as in the subject of lymphoid tumours" (Willis 1948). Despite the fact that non-Hodgkin's lymphoma is at least twice as common as Hodgkin's disease, it is interesting that this larger group of lymphoid neoplasms has not been given a name of its own but has come to be identified as so-called NOT or non-Hodgkin's lymphomas. Terms like "reticulosis" and "reticulosarcoma" reflected prevailing concepts of the times and it was only in 1956 that the modern era of non-Hodgkin's lymphoma (NHL) classifications began, with the publication of Rappaport's classification (Rappaport et al. 1956). The Rappaport classification, based purely on morphological criteria, found favour among pathologists and clinicians alike for its relative simplicity and ease of application. General usage soon established the clinical relevance of this morphological classification. However, in the past two decades, developments in cellular immunology have led to radical changes in our concepts of the function and morphology of the lymphoid system. The accumulating information on the biology of lymphocytes resulted in objections to the validity of Rappaport's terminologies and the concepts inherent in his classification. Within a short period some five major classifications for NHL were proposed. While three of these were based purely on morphological grounds (Bennett et al. 1974; Dorfman, 1974; Mathe et al. 1976), the classifications of Lukes and Collins (1974) and of Lennert (Gerard-Merchant et al. 1974; Lennert et al. 1975) were based on a functional or immunological approach. Although the latter classifications involved different terminology and some variation in concept of the various cell origins, both Lukes and Lennert recognised that lymphomas did indeed reflect, very closely, the normal cellular components of lymphoid tissue. Conceived initially on a morphological basis, these classifications are strongly supported by immunological parameters.

In an attempt to curb the confusing proliferation of classifications, the National Cancer Institute in Bethesda, Maryland, commissioned an international multi-institutional clinicopathological study into the five major classifications including that of Rappaport (The Non-Hodgkin's Lymphoma Classification Project 1982). This study found that all these classifications were clinically relevant and useful for prognostication. The study also recommended a Working Formulation in which NHLs were divided by morphological criteria into three prognostic groups, and more importantly, this formulation provided a means of translation among the major contemporary systems of classification. The adoption of what is essentially a morphologically based classification has received strong criticisms from several authorities (reviewed by Leong 1983). Accumulated immunological data indicate that lymphocytic leukaemias and malignant lymphomas are composed of neoplastic lymphocytes and their morphological and behavioural characteristics are reflections of the morphology and biology of the normal lymphoid progenitor cells. If one conforms to the modern principle of classifying tumours by ontogeny, that is, according to their cell of origin or according to the normal cell which the tumour most closely resembles morphologically and phenotypically, then the classification of malignant lymphomas should reflect an immunological or functional basis and take into account the biology of the normal lymphocyte. It would appear, therefore, that we are not yet at the stage of achieving a classification which is both scientifically and clinically acceptable. The Working Formulation may fulfil the role of a clinically oriented system and will have to bridge the gap until the ultimate classification of NHL evolves.

In this chapter, in keeping with the approach also adopted for T cell malignancies, the B cell lymphomas will be grouped by anatomical compartments. B cell lymphomas occur in lymph nodes and less commonly in extranodal sites. It is appropriate to recapitulate the anatomical compartments of lymph nodes and the classification of the cells within these compartments (see Chap. 8). It is possible to divide the lymph node into different anatomical compartments (Fossum and Ford 1985) and to classifiy the cells within these compartments according to functional and morphological criteria and current concepts of their ontogeny. B lymphocytes can be found in the following lymph node compartments:

1. The deep cortex, containing recirculating small lymphocytes and immunoblasts within the cortical sinuses
2. The superficial cortex, containing follicle centre cells within primary and secondary follicles and mantle zone lymphocytes in perifollicular mantle zones
3. The medulla, containing plasma cells within the medullary sinuses.

Several hypothetical schemes have been proposed for antigen-dependent B lymphocyte maturation. These schemes recognise essentially similar stages of differentiation and progression. The mature B lymphocytes of the deep cortical sinuses of the lymph node can, in response to antigen, differentiate along one of two parallel pathways (Thorbecke et al. 1974; Lennert 1978; Weissman et al. 1978; Coico et al. 1983) which are depicted in Fig. 17.1. In the primary immune response, small sIgM +, sIgD + lymphocytes are transformed directly into immunoblasts and then into IgM-producing plasmacytoid lymphocytes and plasma cells (Harris and Bhan 1985). In the late primary and secondary immune response, the B lymphocytes undergo a transformational sequence within the follicle centres. Lukes and Collins (1974), from their studies on the normal follicle centre and its relationship to the classification of malignant lymphoma, conceived

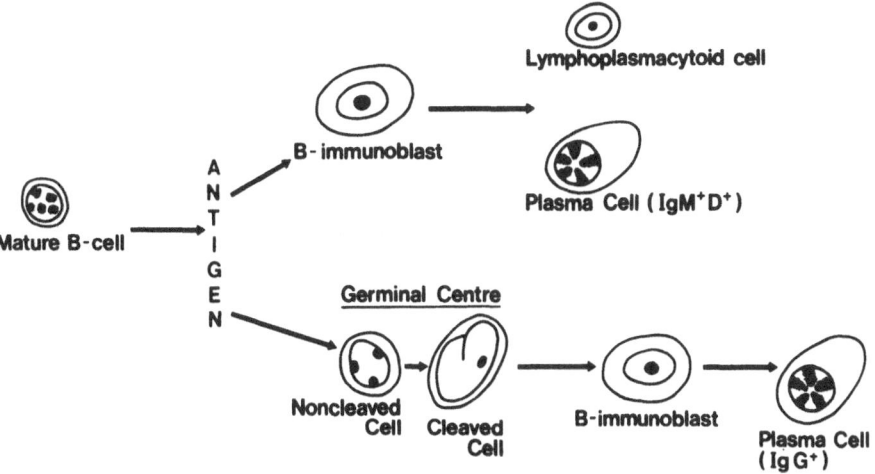

Fig. 17.1. Proposed maturation pathways of B lymphocytes in the lymph node.

the sequence of maturation as progressing from the small mature lymphocyte to cleaved cell to non-cleaved cell. Lennert (1978), however, depicted the reverse, with progression from the non-cleaved cell (centroblast) to cleaved cell (centrocyte). This latter pattern of B cell maturation is supported by the studies of Isaacson et al. (1980), which showed that only small amounts of immunoglobulin were detected in both benign and malignant large non-cleaved cells in contrast to increased amounts in cleaved cells. In vitro studies employing uptake of tritiated thymidine confirm this sequence of maturation from non-cleaved cells to cleaved cells of the germinal centre. The greatest incorporation of labelled thymidine, indicating a high rate of proliferation, was found in non-cleaved cells of the basal zone of the follicle centres. These labelled cells were later found to migrate to the upper or light zone, which contain mainly cleaved cells and only a few non-cleaved cells in the compartmentalised follicle centres (Hanna 1964; Koburg 1967). More recent morphometric studies of the nuclear morphology of transformed B lymphocytes in follicle centres provide additional support for this sequence of maturation (Dardick et al. 1983a). The transformed B lymphocytes are presumed to exit from the germinal centres as large B immunoblasts. These are believed to continue their replication cycle as they move to the medullary cords of the lymph node where they differentiate into the IgG-or IgA producing plasma cells of the secondary immune response and into small memory B lymphocytes which may re-enter the transformational sequence if again appropriately stimulated by the same antigen. The lymph node compartments and their corresponding B cells and tumours are listed in Table 17.1.

It is felt that this approach will allow a correlation of cell function with morphology and ontogeny and yet retain many of the histological features and terminologies which are important pointers to prognosis. The terminology of Lukes and Collins (1974) is used for the B cell lymphomas, with the exception of "intermediate cell lymphoma", a neoplasm derived from cells of the mantle zone. This term was introduced by Braylan et al. (1975) but has not been included as a separate entity in the major classifications of NHL.

Table 17.1. Lymph node compartments, B cell types and corresponding tumours

Anatomical compartment	B cell type	Neoplasm	Cell size	Pattern	Grade
Deep cortex:					
Cortical sinuses	Small lymphocytes	Small lymphocytic	Small	Diffuse	Low
		Plasmacytoid-lymphocytic lymphoma	Small	Diffuse	Low
	Immunoblasts	Immunoblastic sarcoma	Large	Diffuse	High
Superficial cortex:					
Primary and secondary follicles	Follicle centre cells	Follicle centre cell lymphoma	Small or large or mixed	Follicular or diffuse	Low or intermediate
Mantle zone	Mantle zone or intermediate cells	Mantle zone or intermediate cell lymphoma	Small	Diffuse with vague nodules	Low
Medulla:					
Medullary sinuses	Plasma cells	Plasmacytoma	Small	Diffuse	Low

In our approach to the classification of B cell lymphomas, it is appropriate to discuss the two major histological features which have been shown to be of prognostic relevance. The Working Formulation is largely based on these two factors — tumour growth pattern and tumour cell size. The course of a lymphoma and choice of treatment regimen is closely related to the pattern of tumour growth within the lymph node.

Rappaport et al. (1956) felt that there was no proven relationship between the nodules of nodular lymphoma and normal follicles or germinal centres. However, subsequent immunological studies have provided evidence that all lymphomas with a nodular growth pattern, regardless of cytological subtype, are derived from cells with the characteristics of follicle centre cells and are therefore of B cell lineage (Lennert 1973; Jaffe et al. 1974; Leech et al. 1975). Thus, follicular centre cell lymphomas fall into two major categories, "follicular" lymphoma and "diffuse" lymphoma. Follicular lymphomas are associated with a "favourable" prognosis or generally "low grade" disease (with the exception of malignant lymphoma, follicular, predominantly large cell type), whereas, diffuse lymphomas have an "unfavourable" prognosis or represent "intermediate" or "high-grade" disease in the Working Formulation (Table 17.2).

The question arises as to whether the extent of follicular involvement influences prognosis, that is, does complete involvement of a node with closely packed tumour nodules imply a better course for the patient than one which is involved largely by a diffuse pattern of infiltration with only focal or partial nodularity? Earlier data indicated that any degree of follicularity imparted a favourable prognosis compared with lymphomas with a diffuse pattern (Warnke et al. 1977; Lennert 1981; Herrmann et al. 1982). More recent data have suggested that the degree of follicularity may, in fact, relate to differences in the length of the course

Table 17.2. Working Formulation of the non-Hodgkin's
lymphomas for clinical usage

Low grade
  ML, small lymphocytic
  ML, follicular, predominantly small cleaved cell
  ML, follicular, mixed small cleaved and large cell

Intermediate grade
  ML, follicular, predominantly large cell
  ML, diffuse small cleaved cell
  ML, diffuse, mixed small and large cell
  ML, diffuse large cell

High grade
  ML, large cell immunoblastic
  ML, lymphoblastic
  ML, small non-cleaved cell

Miscellaneous
  Composite
  Mycosis fungoides
  Histiocytic
  Extramedullary plasmacytoma
  Unclassifiable

ML, malignant lymphoma.

of the disease and that patients with lesions having a greater degree of follicularity have had more prolonged courses than those showing fewer follicles.

Cell size is the other important morphological parameter. Small cell size is equated with lesions of low aggressiveness, and large cells generally represent lesions with more rapid tumour growth, causing symptoms such as fever and weight loss and a shorter clinical course. Large "blast" forms represent the actively proliferating cells in the maturation pathway of B lymphocytes, whereas the small lymphocytes represent either memory lymphocytes or early mature cells, the end-stage cells associated with slow turnover rates. Lymphomas of small lymphocytes therefore display less mitotic activity and less phagocytic activity than lymphomas of large cells. Similarly, plasma cells and plasmacytoid cells which are end-stage cells have slow turnover rates and are less aggressive tumours.

The follicular pattern seen in lymph node sections can be replicated in extranodal tissues. Closely packed nodules in extranodal sites indicate an origin of the lymphoma in follicular centres; however, follicularity in such locations should be interpreted with caution as an apparent "nodular" pattern can result from compartmentalisation of tumour imposed by the intrinsic structures of the extranodal tissue or by reactive fibrosis. In the bone marrow, aggregates of lymphocytes or lymphoid nodules may not reflect true follicle formation as seen in lymphoid nodules in the bowel, skin and other extranodal sites. In the spleen a nodular pattern may be produced by expansion of the splenic white pulp which is not truly representative of malignant follicles. The reverse is also true in that a diffuse lymphoma may appear as localised aggregates of nodules in the bone marrow or as prominent nodules in the sites of Malpighian corpuscles in the spleen.

B Cell Lymphomas of the Deep Cortex

B lymphocytes occur in the deep cortex of lymph nodes as recirculating small lymphocytes and as immunoblasts, all contained within the cortical sinuses.

Well-differentiated Lymphocytic Lymphoma

Malignant small (round) B lymphocytes of the deep cortical sinuses give rise to diffuse proliferations of well-differentiated lymphocytes which permeate through the lymph node producing effacement of normal architecture but sometimes resulting only in minimal disturbance of the basic vascular and lymphatic structures (Fig. 17.2). Follicular structures are not found in the monotonous infiltrate of small round lymphocytes with inconspicuous nucleoli, clumped chromatin, scanty cytoplasm and rare or absent mitoses (Fig. 17.3). However, not infrequently, admixed with these normal-appearing lymphocytes are seen scattered large cells with round vesicular nuclei and one or two prominent nucleoli. These "blast" cells may occur in clusters and show occasional mitoses. They have been referred to as pseudofollicular "growth centres" (Pangalis et al. 1977) and their significance is not clear (Fig. 17.4).

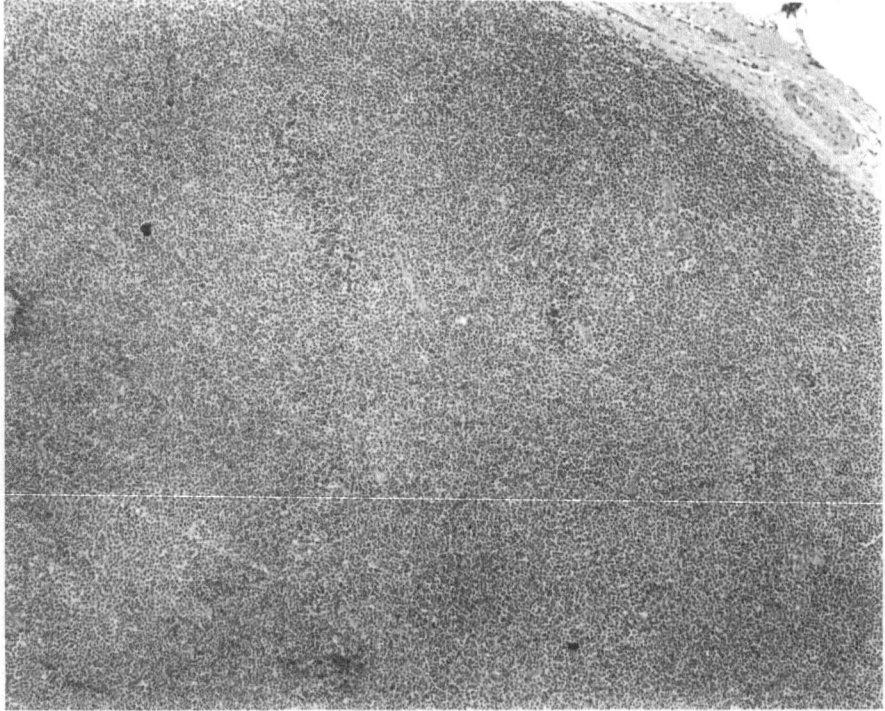

Fig. 17.2. Well-differentiated lymphocytic lymphoma (WDLL) with diffuse effacement of lymph node architecture by a monotonous infiltrate of small lymphocytes. (H & E, × 50)

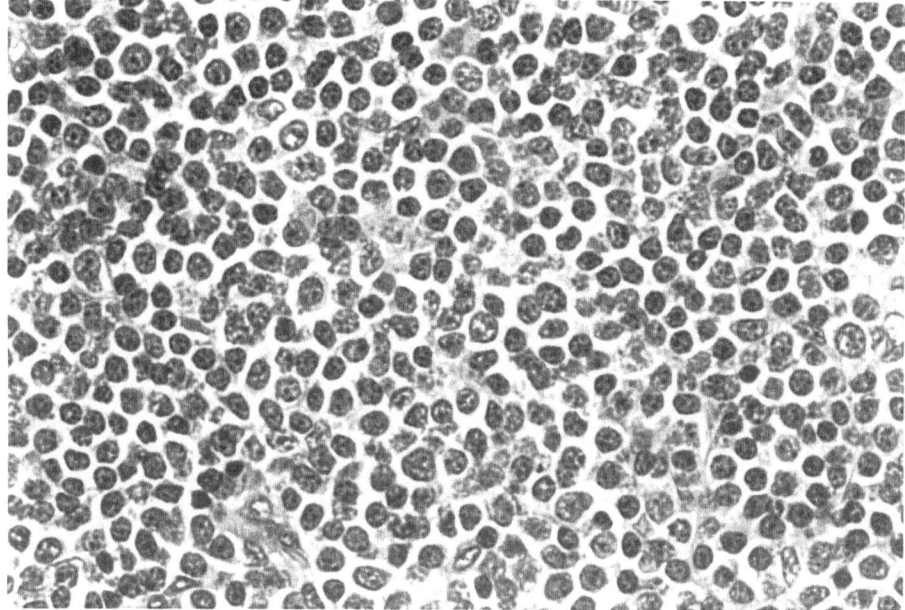

Fig. 17.3. The uniform small lymphocytes of WDLL. Note the mature "well-differentiated" morphology. (H & E, × 500)

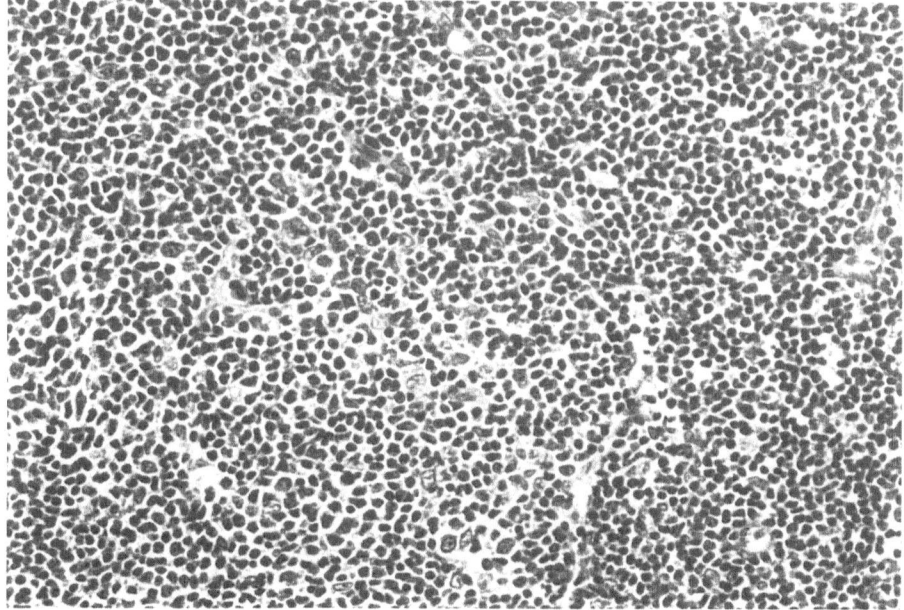

Fig. 17.4. Pseudofollicular "growth centre" in WDLL. A collection of larger cells with round vesicular nuclei and one or two nucleoli are present. (H & E, × 125)

The term "well-differentiated" applied to this group of small lymphocytic lymphoma is used in the morphological sense. From a functional standpoint the term may not be appropriate as these small lymphocytes are more fittingly called resting or mature lymphocytes and do not represent the well-differentiated stage of a lymphocyte. Well-differentiated lymphocytic lymphoma (WDLL) is a disease of the middle and older age groups. It is commonly so indolent that patients have minimum symptomatology, and the diagnosis is often made in individuals during a routine medical examination or work-up for other medical problems. Despite the frequent presence of wide dissemination at diagnosis, WDLL shows an indolent clinical course with prolonged survival, with or without evidence of persistent disease (Jones et al. 1973). There may be localised or generalised lymphadenomegatly with involvement of the bone marrow and leukaemia; however, neither morphological features (Rappaport 1966; Pangalis et al. 1977) nor surface marker studies (Aisenberg et al. 1973; Braylan et al. 1976) of the involved tissue appear to predict the presence or absence of peripheral blood involvement. It is believed that WDLL and B cell chronic lymphocytic leukaemia (B-CLL) represent different phases of the same disease; however, in many patients, leukaemia never develops even when the bone marrow is involved (Pangalis et al. 1977). Lennert (1978) considers all diffuse lymphomas of small lymphocytes to represent CLL and classifies the non-leukaemic forms of the disease as lympho-plasmacytoid lymphomas (immunocytomas). Although the common presentation includes bone marrow and peripheral blood lymphocytosis together with mild, if discernible, lymphadenomegaly and splenomegaly, patients may occasionally present with extranodal tumours of small B lymphocytes (Evans 1982), and leukaemia may or may not develop in such patients.

WDLLs demonstrate a predominance of lymphocytes with complement receptors, Fc receptors, receptors to mouse erythrocytes, and a monoclonal pattern of sIg (faint to intermediate brightness), sometimes showing both IgM and IgD heavy chains and a single light chain on the neoplastic cells (Pinkus and Said 1978; Leong et al. 1979; Aisenberg et al. 1983). In an attempt to establish if B-CLL, WDLL and extranodal WDLL represent proliferations of B cells at the same stage of differentiation or if they are immunologically distinct entities, Harris and Bhan (1985) recently studied a small series of cases with the B cell differentiation antibodies B1 (CD20), B2 (CD21), major histocompatibility complex (MHC) class II, T1 (CD5) and CD10 (CALLA) as well as with antibodies to immunoglobulin heavy and light chains. Their findings suggested that WDLL with leukaemia and WDLL without leukaemia may represent B cells at slightly different stages of differentiation. CD5-positivity was seen only in tumours associated with leukaemia and was present in 80% of cases. Of these, 90% were nodal and 50% expressed IgD as well as IgM. None contained IgG or IgA. In contrast, non-leukaemic cases were predominantly extranodal, CD5-negative, and lacked IgD.

Ultrastructural examination reveals that a great majority of the lymphocytes in this tumour have round nuclei with coarsely clumped chromatin (Mori and Lennert 1969; Cawley and Hayhoe 1973). There are no indentations of the nuclear membrane; however, occasional nuclear pockets are found. Nucleoli are inconspicuous and frequently have a characteristic ring-shaped pattern. The cytoplasm is rather scanty and contains a small or moderate number of mitochondria, numerous free ribosomes, a small Golgi apparatus, and a few rough endoplasmic reticulum cisternae. Cytoplasmic microfilaments may be present in some cells. The growth centres are composed of prolymphocytes which have a roughly oval

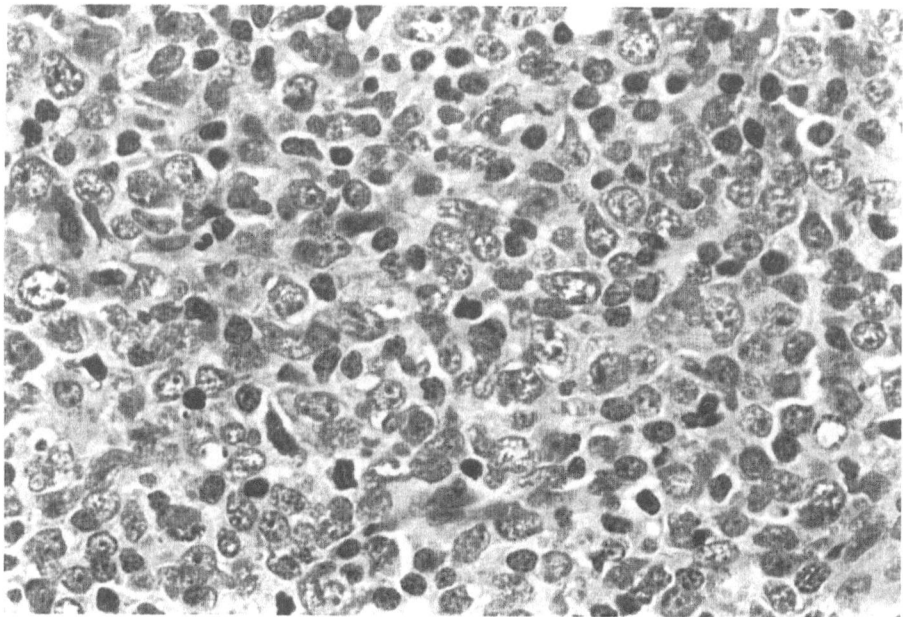

Fig. 17.5. Richter's syndrome occurring in a 78-year-old man with a 3-year history of WDLL. Note the conversion to a diffuse lymphoma of large cell type. (H & E, × 500)

nucleus and a well-developed nucleolus, less-clumped nuclear chromatin and more abundant cytoplasm.

Although WDLLs have an indolent course, they may occasionally undergo progression to an aggressive tumour with an accelerated clinical course composed of large blast cells or "histiocytes" (Fig. 17.5). This conversion to a "histiocytic" lymphoma has been commonly referred to as "Richter's syndrome" (Richter 1928; Long and Aisenberg 1975).

Information from three separate series suggests a 3%–10% incidence of diffuse "histiocytic" lymphomas (DHLs) in patients with WDLL/CLL (Trump et al. 1980). DHLs occurred within a median interval of 24 months (range, less than 1 month to 156 months) from the diagnosis of WDLL/CLL. Clinically this aggressive phase is heralded by the sudden onset of fever, asymmetrical lymphadenomegaly, hepatosplenomegaly and visceral involvement (Enno et al. 1979; Kjeldsberg and Marty 1981), but there were no features to predict its development. The exact mechanism of this conversion is not known but it probably represents development of a subclone of the pre-existing WDLL/CLL in which differentiation is more severely arrested. Most studies have shown the immunoglobulin idiotype on the large cell lymphoma to be identical to that on the small lymphocytes of the pre-existing WDLL/CLL (Brouet et al. 1973, 1977; Enno et al. 1979; Harousseau et al. 1981; Kjeldsberg and Marty 1981), indicating that the large cell lymphoma arises as a clonal progression of WDLL/CLL. One case of Richter's syndrome has been reported in which the WDLL cells and large cell lymphoma cells had monoclonal surface immunoglobulin of different light chain classes (Splinter et al. 1978).

Plasmacytoid Lymphocytic Lymphoma

The term "plasmacytoid lymphocytic lymphoma" describes a group of lymphomas with a range of clinical presentations. They have been called well-differentiated lymphocytic lymphoma with plasmacytoid features (Rappaport), plasmacytoid lymphocytic lymphoma (Lukes–Collins) and lymphoplasmacytic/lymphoplasmacytoid (LP immunocytoma; Kiel). Although the proposed place of these lymphomas in the scheme of the functional classification has been at the opposite end of the spectrum from WDLLs, they are tumours of small cells with a slow rate of turnover and a clinically indolent course generally similar to that of WDLL/CLL. Essentially, these lymphomas of small B lymphocytes show varying degrees of differentiation towards plasma cells. Plasmacytoid lymphocytic lymphomas mostly affect patients in the sixth and seventh decades who may present with a variety of symptoms which include fever, night sweats, lethargy, anorexia, loss of weight and arthralgia and often show a paraprotein in the blood and urine. Coombs' positive haemolytic anaemia occurred in 13.5% of cases in one series (Lennert 1981). Many of the tumours produce IgM heavy chains and are associated with the physical and laboratory findings of Waldenström's macroglobulinaemia. However, the tumour may produce other heavy chains but may not secrete these immunoglobulins. Many patients display a lymphocytosis in the peripheral blood of more than 4×10^9/litre with an appearance similar to that of CLL, although the circulating cells are said to show greater cytoplasmic basophilia (Lennert 1981). The bone marrow is almost always involved with tumour at the

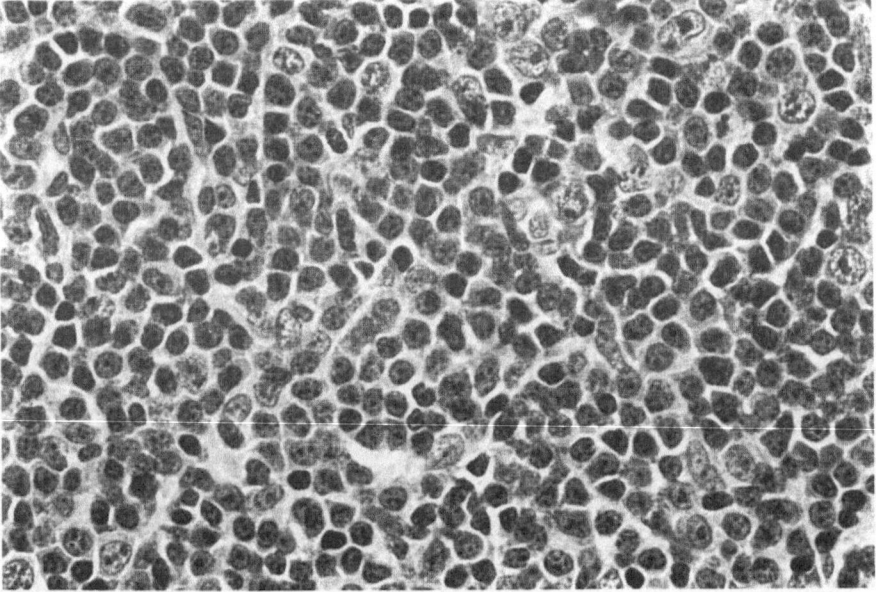

Fig. 17.6. Plasmacytoid lymphocytic lymphoma in a patient with Waldenström's macroglobulinemia. The lymph node contains a diffuse infiltrate of plasmacytoid lymphocytes with small round nuclei and the coarse chromatin pattern of lymphocytes, but, more often, eccentric dense cytoplasm. (H & E, $\times 500$)

time of diagnosis, and lymphadenomegaly and organomegaly are not generally remarkable.

Histologically, these tumours differ from WDLLs in their obvious plasma cell and plasmacytoid cell component (Heinz et al. 1981). The tumour cells have nuclei which are similar in appearance to those of small round lymphocytes, being of similar size and of similar chromatin distribution (Fig. 17.6). However, they are often eccentrically located as in plasma cells and the cells are larger by virtue of more characteristically dense cytoplasm. The frequent presence of globular intracytoplasmic and intranuclear inclusions of PAS-positive immunoglobulins is a useful cytological feature to distinguish plasmacytoid lymphocytic lymphomas from proliferations of small lymphocytes. The tumour cells may form solid infiltrating masses but in lymph nodes they characteristically infiltrate the medullary cords and paracortex leaving the sinuses intact (Fig. 17.7).

Electron microscopic examination shows large numbers of lymphocytes mixed with a much smaller number of plasma cells, plasmacytoid lymphocytes and immunoblasts. Plasmacytoid lymphocytes have abundant heterochromatin and an inconspicuous nucleolus, resembling the nucleus of the small lymphocyte. The cytoplasm contains abundant long cisternae of rough endoplasmic reticulum which are arranged around the nucleus (Lennert and Müller-Hermelink 1975). Appearances range from such cells to mature plasma cells with intermediate forms showing peripherally clumped nuclear chromatin, large Golgi apparatus and numerous polyribosomes. Intranuclear inclusions of granular or fibrillar material corresponding to the PAS-positive Dutcher bodies may be observed in plasmacy-

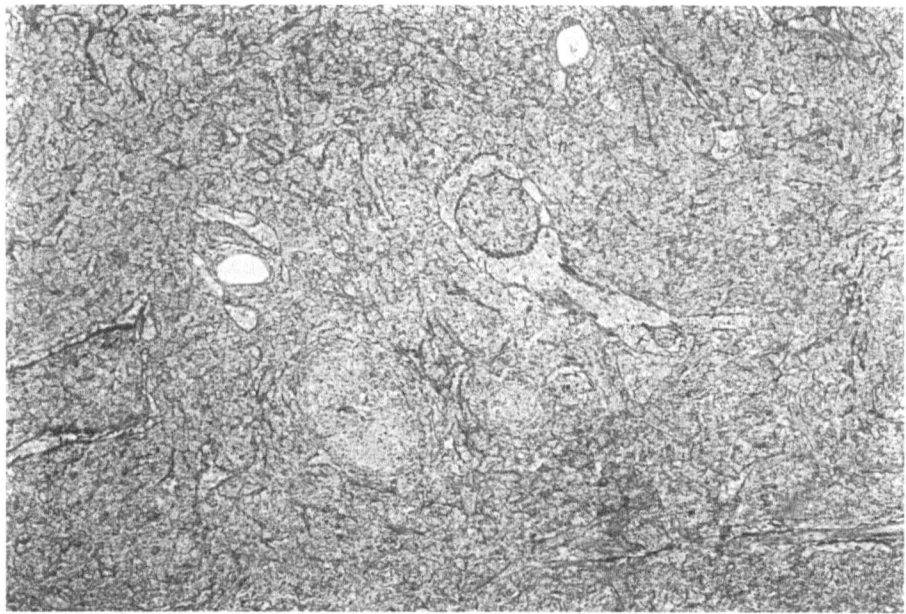

Fig. 17.7. Plasmacytoid lymphocytic lymphoma. A reticulin stain shows the preservation of lymph node sinuses in the diffuse infiltrate. (Reticulin stain, × 50)

toid lymphocytes as well as plasma cells, and Russell bodies and crystalline inclusions occur in the rough endoplasmic reticulum (Kuhn 1967; Mori and Lennert 1969; Cawley and Hayhoe 1973; Kaiserling 1977).

B Immunoblastic Sarcoma

The B immunoblastic sarcoma is a high-grade lymphoma, composed of uniformly large pleomorphic immunoblasts. Unfortunately, the variation in the reported incidence of this tumour suggests that the criteria employed for diagnosis are not universally uniform (Nathwani 1979). Immunoblasts should be clearly separated from the large non-cleaved cells of the follicular centre. B immunoblastic sarcomas often reflect plasma cell characteristics with moderate to abundant amounts of well-defined, dense, pyroninophilic cytoplasm containing immunoglobulin as discrete cytoplasmic inclusions or as nuclear inclusions. The cells have round or oval nuclei with a single prominent central nucleolus. Some workers accept considerable morphological variation in this group of tumours with a spectrum of transformed plasmacytoid cells and variable numbers of large cells, ranging from a few in some lesions to those lesions in which the large cells predominate (Fig. 17.8) (Schneider et al. 1985). Other workers suggest that the term "immunoblastic sarcoma" should be used only when immunoblasts predominate and produce a fairly monotonous tumour (Wright and Isaacson 1983). Occasional pleomorphic forms with large and multiple nucleoli and giant bizarre tumour cells may be seen. Large non-cleaved lymphomas of follicular centre origin, in contrast, show few plasmacytic cells and have two to three nucleoli that are frequently apposed to the nuclear membrane and a narrow rim of amphophilic cytoplasm which is moderately pyroninophilic. The distinction of immunoblastic sarcoma from diffuse large non-cleaved cell lymphoma is important, as the former is classified as a high-grade lymphoma in the Working Formulation while the latter falls into the intermediate grade group. The two entities, however, appear to be part of a spectrum, and the exact point of separation of large non-cleaved cell lymphomas from immunoblastic sarcomas can sometimes be difficult. Furthermore, immunoblastic sarcoma sometimes develops in patients with CLL, lymphoplasmacytoid lymphomas and follicular centre cell lymphomas (Spiro et al. 1975). Currently, it may be difficult to separate B immunoblastic sarcoma from T immunoblastic sarcoma on histological criteria without the aid of immunohistochemical techniques. Schneider et al. (1985) suggested, on the basis of a light microscopic study of 47 immunologically defined cases of immunoblastic sarcoma, that plasmacytoid differentiation, seen most consistently as amphophilic staining of the cytoplasm, generally characterised immunoblastic sarcoma of B cells (Fig. 17.8).

These tumours can arise as primary tumours in gut, lymph nodes, Waldeyer's ring, bone marrow, spleen or any other tissue where immunoblasts may be found physiologically. When the tumour is focal, such as within the gut, complete cures can sometimes be achieved by surgical resection alone. Spread appears to be by infiltration and metastases rather than by physiological migration (Galton et al. 1978). Serum and urine from patients with immunoblastic sarcoma should be examined for the presence of paraprotein. Bone marrow trephine may reveal focal marrow infiltration, but involvement of the peripheral blood is unusual.

Ultrastructurally, the tumour cells have large, round or oval nuclei with dispersed chromatin and one or two striking, large nucleoli, usually placed

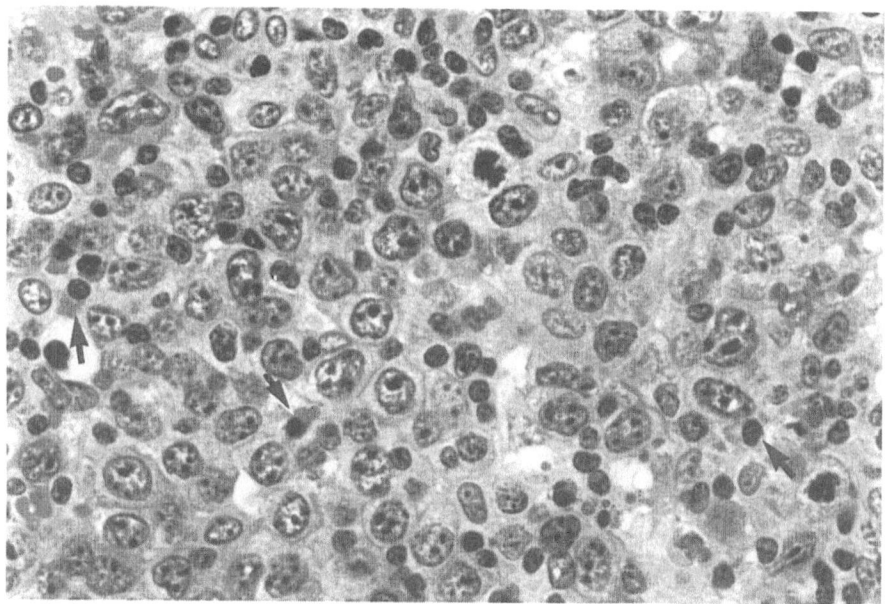

Fig. 17.8. Immunoblastic sarcoma of B cell type composed of a diffuse infiltrate of mostly large cells with moderate to abundant amounts of dense, well-defined cytoplasm and nuclei which contain large, centrally located nucleoli. Scattered, smaller plasmacytoid cells are present (*arrows*). (H & E, × 500)

centrally. Rough endoplasmic reticulum is generally scanty but numerous ribosomes and polyribosomes are present. A well-developed Golgi complex and a few mitochondria are seen. Cytoplasmic PAS-positive inclusions correspond to immunoglobulin accumulated in the perinuclear spaces and cisternae of the rough endoplasmic reticulum. The occasional plasmacytoid cells which are present show many rough endoplasmic reticulum cisternae.

B Cell Lymphomas of the Superficial Cortex

In the superficial cortex of the lymph node, the B lymphocytes form discrete follicles composed of a follicle or germinal centre surrounded by a mantle of small lymphoyctes which is broadest over the pole of the follicle centre closest to the lymph node capsule, or to the epithelium in the case of the tonsil. The follicle centre cells are B lymphocytes, the majority of which are cleaved cells or centrocytes with irregular, indented nuclei, varying in size up to twice that of a small lymphocyte. Small centrally located nucleoli may be present and the cytoplasm is pale and indistinct. Non-cleaved cells or centroblasts usually occur in smaller numbers and have round, pale-staining vesicular nuclei with one to three nucleoli often apposed to the nuclear membrane. The cytoplasm is usually sparse and intensely basophilic. Follicle centres show a spectrum of changes varying with the duration of antigenic stimulation. Masses of large non-cleaved cells appear a few days after antigenic exposure. These cells soon show active mitosis and are followed by the appearance of cleaved cells which mostly accumulate beneath the "cap" of mantle zone cells producing the familiar light or upper zone of the follicle centre. The pale staining of this zone is due to a lower cell density and to the weak basophilia of the cleaved cells. The light zone also contains a moderate number of small lymphocytes, some immunoblasts and occasional plasma cells. The non-cleaved cells are concentrated in the dark or basal zone of the follicle centre (Fig. 17.9). Large pale histiocytes with apoptotic bodies or tingible body macrophages and dendritic reticulum cells are other important components of the follicle centres.

Immunostaining reveals that the vast majority of cells in the primary lymphoid follicles are B lymphocytes with surface IgM and IgD. Few cells are sIgA-positive,

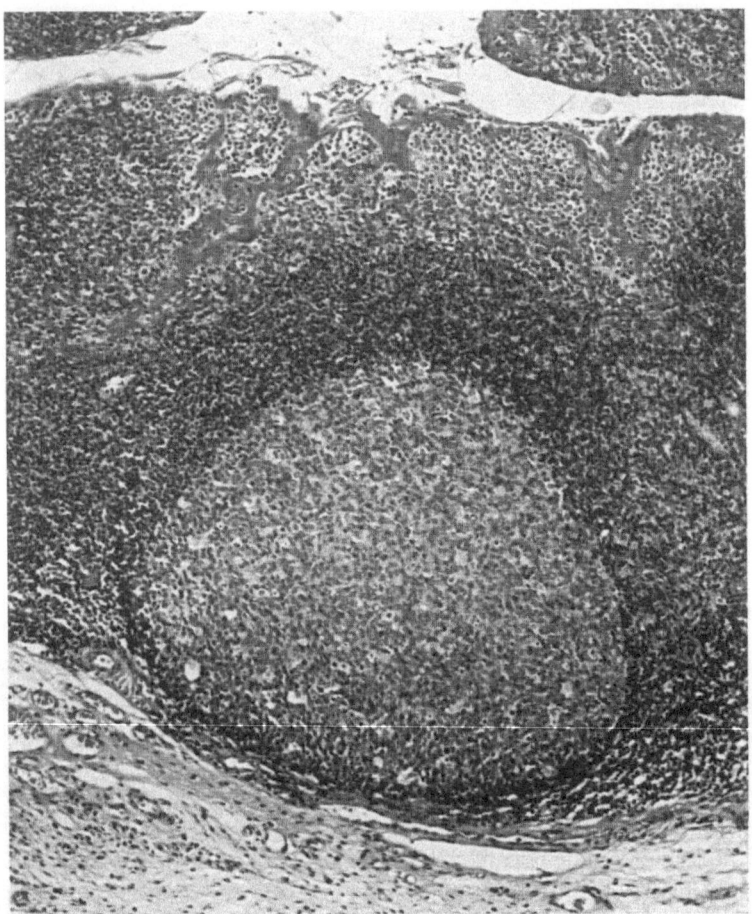

Fig. 17.9. Germinal centre in a tonsil showing the "cap" of mantle zone cells closest to the epithelial surface. A light zone of paler staining cleaved cells is present beneath the mantle zone and a basal dark zone composed of more densely packed non-cleaved cells is discernible. (H & E, × 75)

but sIgG-positive B cells are not detectable. B cells in primary follicles express κ and λ light chains in a mosaic-like pattern, and cytoplasmic Ig is not detected. Very few CD4- or CD8-positive T lymphocytes are interspersed among the B cells.

In the secondary follicles, non-cleaved cells or centroblasts which accumulate mostly in the basal or dark zones, are decorated by pan-B antibody and stain only weakly or not at all for surface IgM, G or A (Stein H. et al. 1980). The cleaved cells or centrocytes present in the upper light zones, on the other hand, always appear to express IgM and the pan-B antigen. Staining of entrapped immunoglobulins by the dendritic processes of the dendritic reticulum cells in the follicle centres makes it difficult to evaluate membrane Ig staining of follicle centre cells. Cytoplasmic immunoglobulin is only rarely found in non-cleaved cells, but up to 30% of cleaved cells contain cIgM, cIgG or cIgA (Stein et al. 1982). Both light chain types occur, indicating that the population of cIg-producing cells is polyclonal (Curran and Jones 1978a). The number of cIg-positive cleaved cells and the preponderance of the cIg class varies from follicle centre to follicle centre depending on the duration of antigen stimulation (Hsu and Jaffe 1984a,b). Both non-cleaved and cleaved cells are generally reported not to display IgD, CD10 (CALLA) or MHC class II (HLA-DR) antigens, although Hsu and Jaffe (1984b) believe that sIgD can be demonstrated in early follicle centre cells.

Plasma cells containing cytoplasmic immunoglobulin occur only in small numbers within the follicle centres. Large numbers of plasma cells are often seen overlying the mantle zone cap of small lymphocytes.

The follicular mantle zone cells which surround the germinal centre have the same phenotype as cells of the primary follicle and appear identical, being sIgM- and sIgD-positive as well as showing C3R and HLA-DR antigens (Stein et al. 1980, 1982).

T lymphocytes recognised by CD4 and the pan-T CD3 antibodies are found in the follicular mantle zone as well as in the light zone of the follicle centres. T cell subset analysis reveals that nearly all the T cells in the light zones are of the helper subset staining with OKT4 and Leu-3a (CD4) (Fig. 17.10), whereas in the follicular mantle as well as in primary follicles both helper and suppressor T cells occur in small numbers.

Follicular Centre Cell Lymphoma

Malignant lymphocytes of follicular lymphomas have characteristics of B cells of the follicular centres. Their morphology reflects that of the follicular cleaved and non-cleaved cells and they may grow in a follicular or in a diffuse pattern or show a mixture of these two patterns of growth. As discussed previously (see p. 246–7), both morphology and tumour cell size have prognostic implications. It is also important to recognise the follicular growth pattern for prognostic reasons, and its recognition identifies the tumour as being of follicular centre cell origin and therefore a B cell lymphoma. While earlier classifications separated NHLs into lymphocytic, mixed and histiocytic groups (Rappaport et al. 1956), it has now been established that many such lymphomas arise from follicle centres and show varying admixtures of cleaved and non-cleaved follicular centre cells of different sizes. Rappaport's "histiocytes" represent stimulated follicular centre cells, and true histiocytic lymphomas are now recognised to be very uncommon.

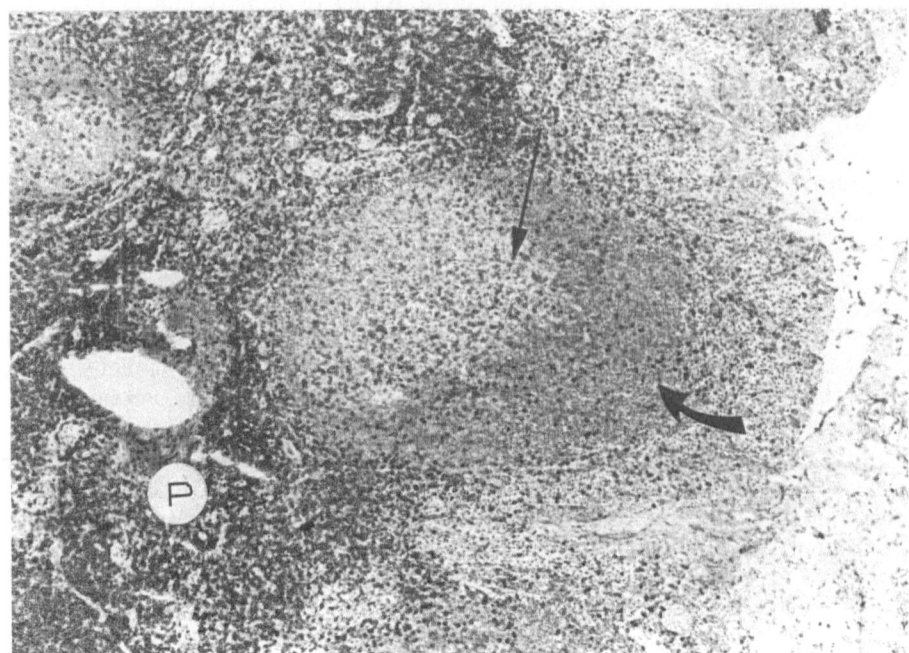

Fig. 17.10. CD4-positive T helper cells are present, mainly in the mantle zone (*curved arrow*) and light zone (*straight arrow*) of the germinal centre. Paracortical T cells also stain strongly positive (*P*). (Leu-3a, modified avidin-biotin peroxidase technique, × 50)

Small Follicular Centre Cell Proliferations

Follicular centre cell lymphoma of small cleaved lymphocytes occurs mainly in middle-aged and older individuals. There is no striking sex preponderance. The small cleaved lymphocytes typically grow as closely placed lymphomatous follicles with distinct margins but lacking the well-formed mantle of small lymphocytes which is characteristic of reactive follicle centres. The lymph node architecture is effaced by these neoplastic follicles (Fig. 17.11), which may also form in the perinodal connective tissue as well as in the hilar adipose tissue of the lymph node.

Within the neoplastic follicles, the cells are heterogeneous and, as is the case with most malignant lymphomas, the full spectrum of follicle centre cells may be represented. The majority of the cells, however, are small cleaved cells or "poorly differentiated lymphocytes" or centrocytes which are slightly larger than normal lymphocytes and display scanty cytoplasm, irregular and often indented nuclear outlines and a more open chromatin pattern than that of normal lymphocytes. There may also be one to three small inconspicuous nucleoli (Fig. 17.12). A small number of non-cleaved cells may be found, some of which may be larger with basophilic cytoplasm. Mitotic figures are usually infrequent. The small cleaved cells may infiltrate the tissue between follicles and may extend into the lymph node capsule and perinodal tissues. Sclerosis in the form of fine compartmentalisation of the node by collagen bundles or as coarse sclerosis or hyalinisation of the

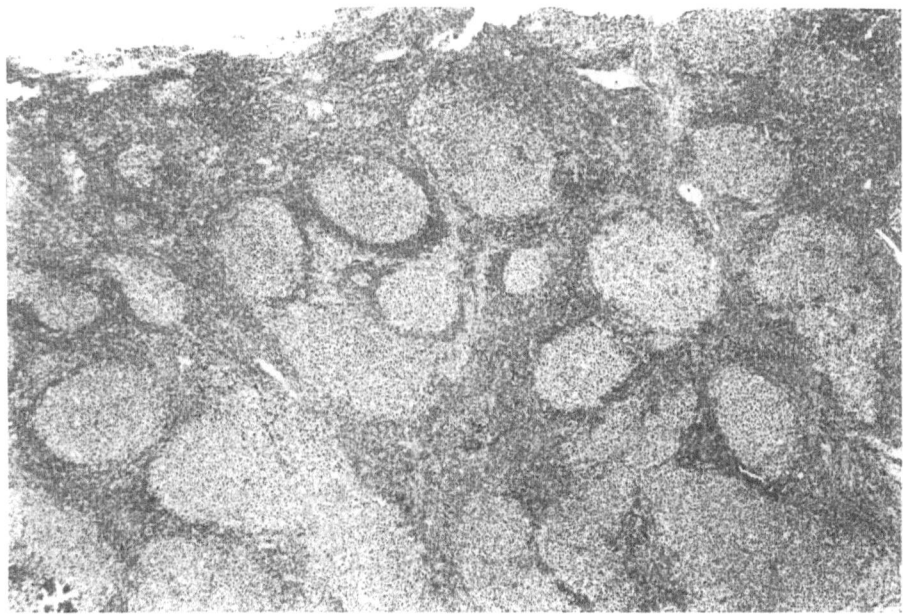

Fig. 17.11. Distinct follicular pattern of a follicular centre cell lymphoma, small cleaved type (centroblastic/centrocytic). (H & E, × 25)

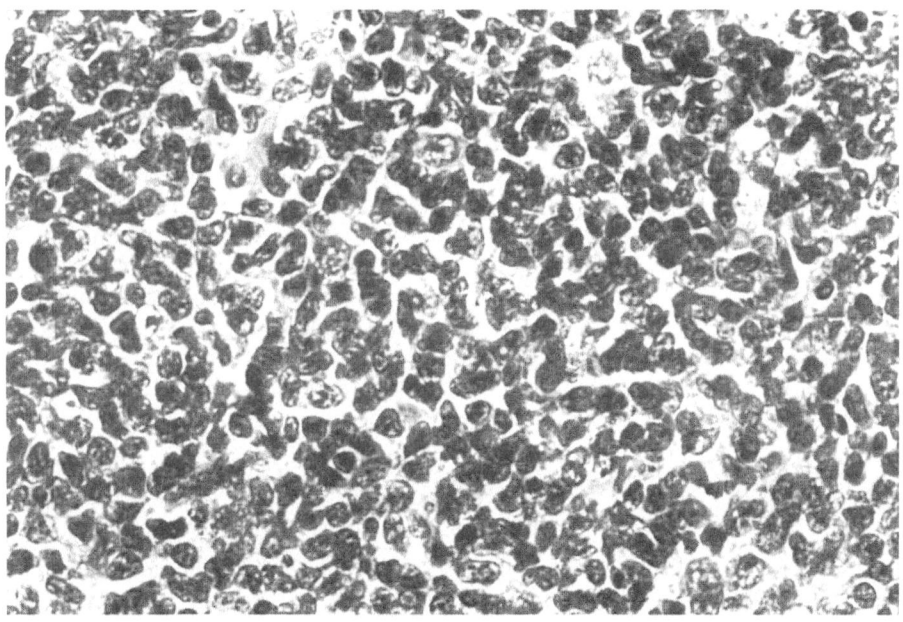

Fig. 17.12. Small cleaved cell within the follicles of a follicular centre cell lymphoma (centroblastic/centrocytic). The neoplastic cells are small and show irregular nuclear outlines and scanty cytoplasm (H & E, × 500)

neoplastic follicles has been shown to be a feature of favourable prognostic significance (Bennett 1975).

Follicular small cleaved cell lymphomas are indolent tumours, despite the fact that approximately two-thirds of the patients are in stage III or IV at the time of presentation (Jones et al. 1973; Lennert 1981; Herrmann et al. 1982). Despite this wide dissemination of the lymphoma the patients may not have systemic symptoms. Leukaemia has been reported in up to 15% of patients (Lennert 1981), the leukaemic cells being differentiated from CLL by the presence of nuclear clefting. One of the most important clinical characteristics of follicular centre cell lymphoma is its biphasic nature. During its indolent phase it is responsive to most therapeutic manoeuvres; however, when it eventually becomes aggressive and invasive, it is usually impossible to gain more than transient ascendency over the neoplasm. In a large number of cases there is a histological transition from follicular to the diffuse type, frequently accompanied by a shift of predominance from small to large lymphoid cells and a transition to an aggressive clinical behaviour. Cullen et al. (1979) reported cytological transformation in 4 of 21 patients with follicular small cleaved cell lymphomas in relapse. Risdall et al. (1979) and Lennert (1981) noted that up to 40% of patients with follicular small cleaved cell lymphomas had converted to a high-grade, diffuse, large non-cleaved centroblastic lymphoma at necropsy; York et al. (1984) estimated a transformation incidence of 17%. Despite aggressive chemotherapy, average survival after transformation was only 7 months (range, 1–23 months; York et al. 1984).

Ultrastructurally, cleaved cells differ from small lymphocytes mainly in their nuclear morphology. They have deeply cleaved nuclear membranes and the heterochromatin is less dense than that of normal small lymphocytes. Their scanty cytoplasm contains a few small mitochondria and rough endoplasmic reticulum cisternae, a small Golgi apparatus and numerous monoribosomes. Small microfilament bundles, lipid droplets, centrioles and lysosome-like dense granules are observed in some cells (Rilke et al. 1978). Large cleaved cells have similar indented nuclei which are larger and show more signs of morphological activation. The chromatin is more dispersed, the nucleoli, Golgi apparatus and rough endoplasmic reticulum are more prominent, and polyribosomes and mitochondria are more abundant that in the small cleaved cells. Non-cleaved cells, which are present in smaller numbers, have large oval or oblong nuclei, dispersed chromatin and one or more prominent nucleoli with a well-developed nuclear membrane. Nucleoli are apposed against the nuclear membrane. Polyribosomes are much more abundant and larger than in the cleaved cells, while monoribosomes are rarely present in the cytoplasm. Well-developed Golgi apparatus, electron-lucent mitochondria, small amounts of granular and agranular endoplasmic reticulum and a few lysosomes are found in the cytoplasm.

Mixed Follicular Centre Cell Proliferations

Because of variation in the composition of the neoplastic follicles, a follicular, mixed small cleaved and large cell lymphoma is recognised in the Working Formulation. This mixed cell category is designated to encompass cases of follicular lymphoma in which there is no clear preponderance of one cell type (small or large) over the other. The large cells, which may have cleaved or non-cleaved nuclei, are frequently two to three times the diameter of normal small lymphocytes and have vesicular nuclei with one to three nucleoli which are apposed to the nuclear membrane.

Large Follicular Centre Cell Proliferations

When the majority of the cells in the lymphomatous proliferation are large follicular centre cells, the grade of malignancy is higher and the prognosis worsens correspondingly. Large cell proliferations of the follicle centre include large cleaved follicular centre cell lymphoma and large non-cleaved follicular centre cell lymphoma. A follicular growth pattern of these lesions reflects their origin in the follicle centre. However, while discrete follicular patterns are occasionally observed in either large cleaved cell or large non-cleaved cell types, partial follicularity, with diffuse effacement of architecture elsewhere, is more often encountered. Large follicular centre cell lymphomas occur mainly in individuals after the second decade. These lymphomas have also been reported occasionally in children and they show no sex predisposition.

Large follicular centre cell lymphomas may be composed of cells having a range of sizes and morphology, but the majority of cells should have nuclei which are larger than those of macrophages in the same tissue section. It is possible to classify large follicular centre cell lymphomas into large cleaved cell type or large non-cleaved cell type depending on the predominating cell. A population of small lymphocytes with cleaved or indented nuclei may also be present but it will clearly be in the minority. If the process is focally dominated by non-cleaved cells, it is regarded as representing the non-cleaved cell type. Although nuclear cleavage is an important distinguishing factor between the two cell types, they also differ in other aspects such as in the amount of cytoplasm and the prominence and location of nucleoli. Large cleaved cells have irregular, indented nuclei and have minimal cytoplasm and inconspicuous nucleoli (Fig. 17.13). Large non-cleaved cells show oval, vesicular nuclei and usually possess a narrow rim of cytoplasm which may be amphophilic or basophilic and pyroninophilic. One or more prominent and distinctive nucleoli are typically situated apposed to the nuclear membrane on the short axis of the nucleus (Fig. 17.14). Large non-cleaved lymphomas tend often to be almost monomorphous and are rapidly growing tumours associated with abundant mitoses and many macrophages. Sclerosis, particularly of the fine trabecular type, may be prominent in association with both large cleaved or non-cleaved lymphomas, resulting in compartmentalisation of cells simulating an epithelial neoplasm.

The ultrastructural appearances of large cell lymphomas are basically similar to those of normal transformed lymphocytes (Gillespie 1978; Osborne et al. 1980; Azar et al. 1982). The nuclei are of moderate size, with smooth profiles where cleavage or nuclear blebs are not present. The chromatin is fine and evenly dispersed, and the nucleoli are prominent in many of the cells. Many free ribosomes and polyribosomes are found in the moderate to abundant cytoplasm, and sparse cisternae of endoplasmic reticulum may be seen in the large non-cleaved cells and occasional immunoblastic cells. Mitochondria are generally sparse and a few lipid droplets may be present.

While it has been recognised that large cell lymphoma cells may show some ruffling of their cytoplasmic borders, the presence of numerous microvillus-like cytoplasmic projections has been recognised only recently as a presentation of

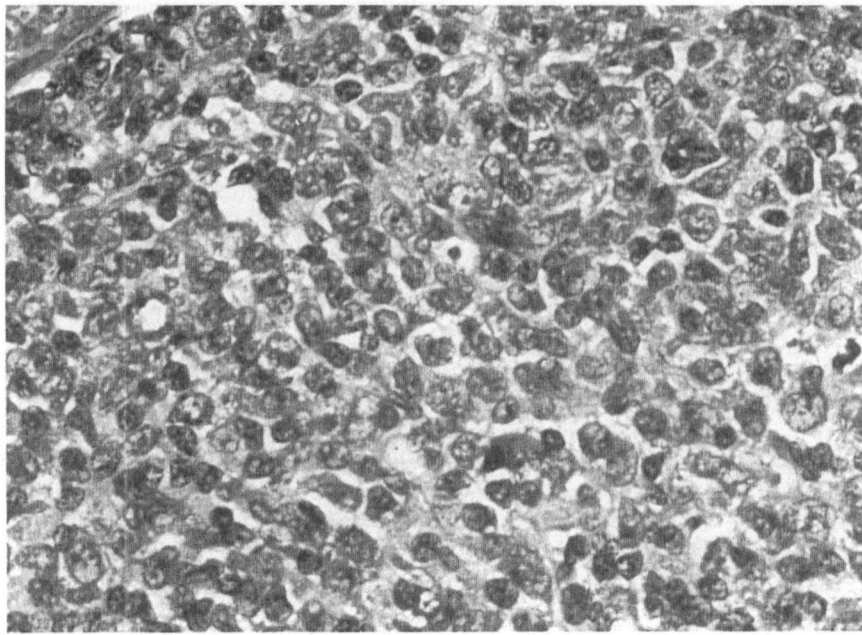

Fig. 17.13. Large cleaved cell lymphoma (centroblastic/centrocytic) with tumour cells showing marked nuclear folds and irregularities, inconspicuous nucleoli and scanty cytoplasm. (H & E, × 500)

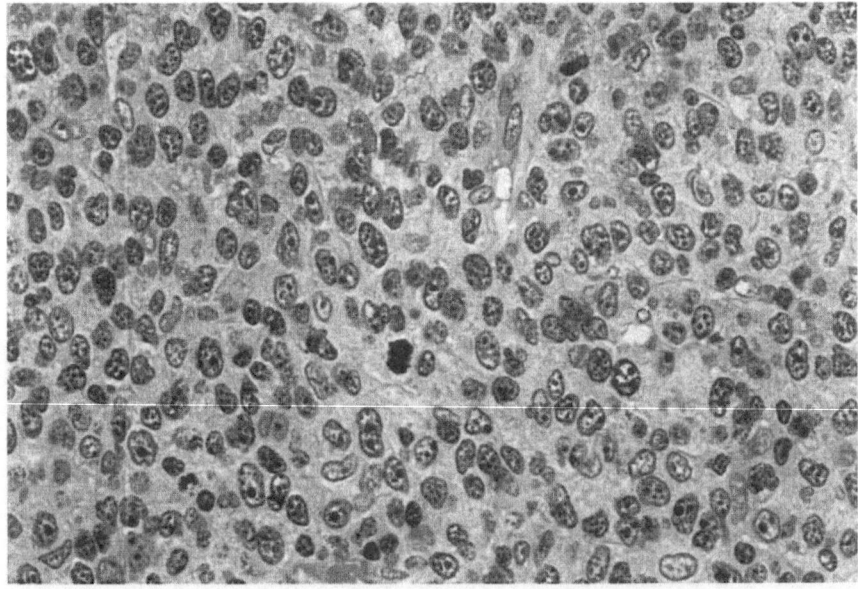

Fig. 17.14. Large non-cleaved follicular centre cell lymphoma (centroblastic) consisting of a monomorphous infiltrate of large cells with moderate amounts of cytoplasm and vesicular nuclei which contain one or more distinctive nucleoli, often apposed to the nuclear membrane. Mitotic figures are frequent. (H & E, × 500)

some uncommon cases of large cell lymphoma (Osborne et al. 1983). This striking ultrastructural appearance has prompted some authors to name the lymphoma "anemone cell tumour" (Sibley et al. 1980). This unusual appearance of a large cell lymphoma requires careful differentiation from carcinomas and mesotheliomas which it may simulate.

Signet-ring Cell Lymphoma

On occasion, follicular centre cell lymphoma cells may show a prominent cytoplasmic vacuole which indents and displaces a crescent-shaped nucleus, giving a "signet-ring" appearance to the tumour cells (Fig. 17.15). Most of the reported cases of signet-ring cell lymphoma have been examples of follicular, small cleaved or mixed lymphomas (Kim et al. 1978; Moir 1980; Harris et al. 1981; Silberman et al. 1984) and in a few instances have been large cell lymphomas (van den Tweel et al. 1978; Dardick et al. 1983b). In the majority of cases studied, the signet-ring formation is reported to result from abnormal accumulation of immunoglobulin within the cytoplasm of the tumour cells (Fig. 17.16) (Kim et al. 1978; Harris et al. 1981; Silberman et al. 1984). However, two recent reports identified three cases of signet-ring, diffuse, large cell lymphomas to be of T lymphocyte lineage (Grogan et al. 1985; Weiss et al. 1985a). Ultrastructural examination of the B cell-lineage neoplasms has shown the presence of striking cytoplasmic vacuoles, usually filled with microvesicles which have been assumed to be related to aberrant immunoglobulin synthesis (Iossifides et al. 1980; Navas-Palacios et al. 1983; Dardick et al.

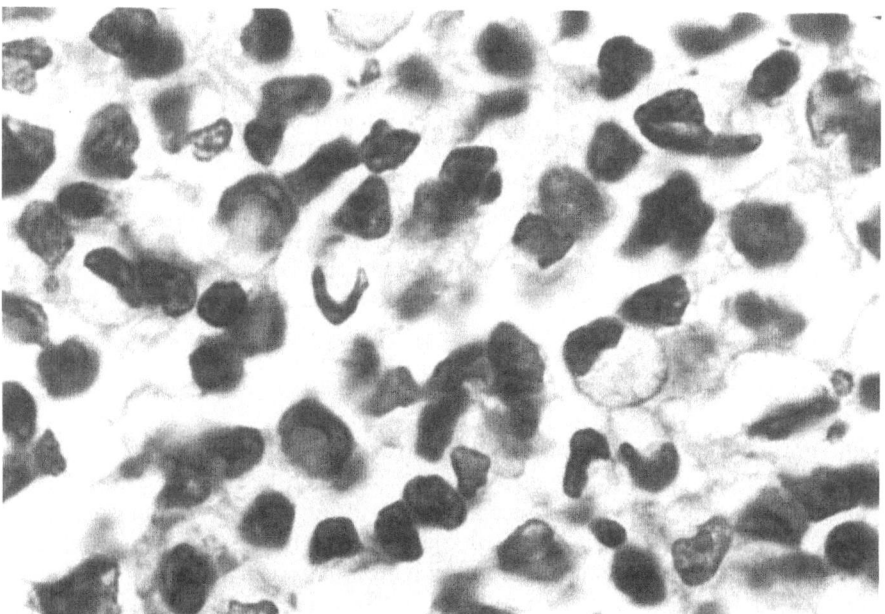

Fig. 17.15. Signet-ring cell lymphoma. Cytoplasmic vacuoles displace and indent the nuclei to produce the signet-ring appearance. (H & E, × 1250)

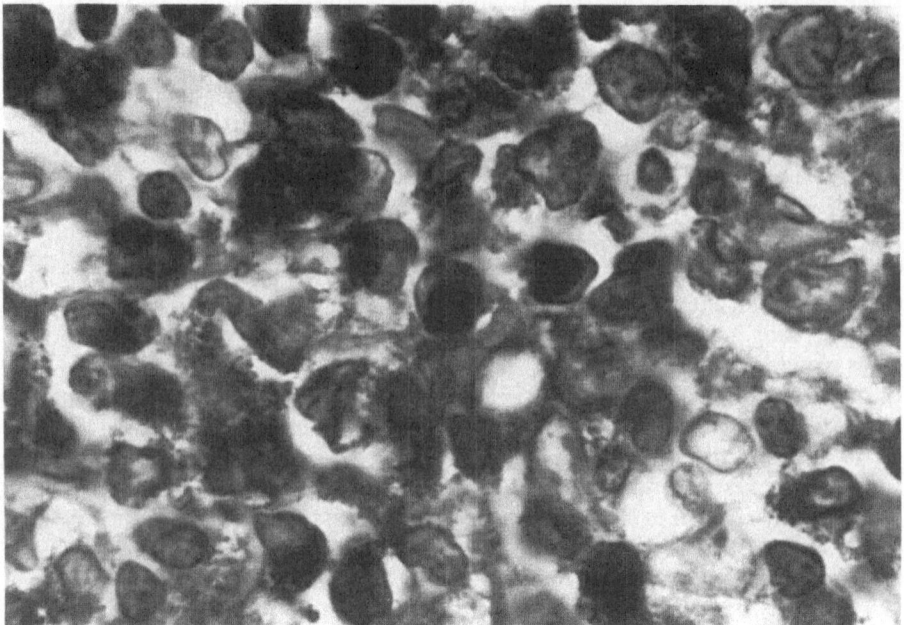

Fig. 17.16. Signet-ring cell lymphoma. The cytoplasmic vacuoles stain strongly for cIgG. Staining for cIgK was also positive, while cIgλ positivity was found in only occasional normal-appearing lymphoid cells. (anti-IgG, avidin-biotin peroxidase, × 1250)

1983b). The presence of similar microspherules within lucent spaces in T cell-derived signet-ring cell lymphomas makes it unlikely that they represent immunoglobulin. An origin from lysosomal or microvesicular bodies has been postulated by Harris et al. (1981). Grogan et al. (1985) feel that these giant vacuoles may result from the internalisation of surface T cell antigens or from sequestration of T cell antigen-containing Golgi-derived vesicles.

It appears that the recognition of signet-ring cells is only of histological and biological interest and at present imparts no special prognostic or clinical implication to the lymphoma.

Phenotype of Follicular Centre Cell Lymphomas

Initial immunocytochemical studies on follicular centre cell lymphomas employed fluorescence staining of lymphocytes in suspension, but, because of their inherent disadvantages, suspension techniques are slowly being replaced by immunohistochemical staining of cryostat sections and accompanying tissue imprints and cytospin preparations. Follicular centre cell lymphomas have receptors for C3 and Fc portion of IgG, MHC class II antigen and one light chain type (Fig. 17.17). Previous studies have usually shown a single heavy chain, most frequently IgM, although examples of multiple heavy chain expression have been occasionally encountered (van Heerde et al. 1980; Stein RS et al. 1980; Harris et al. 1982;

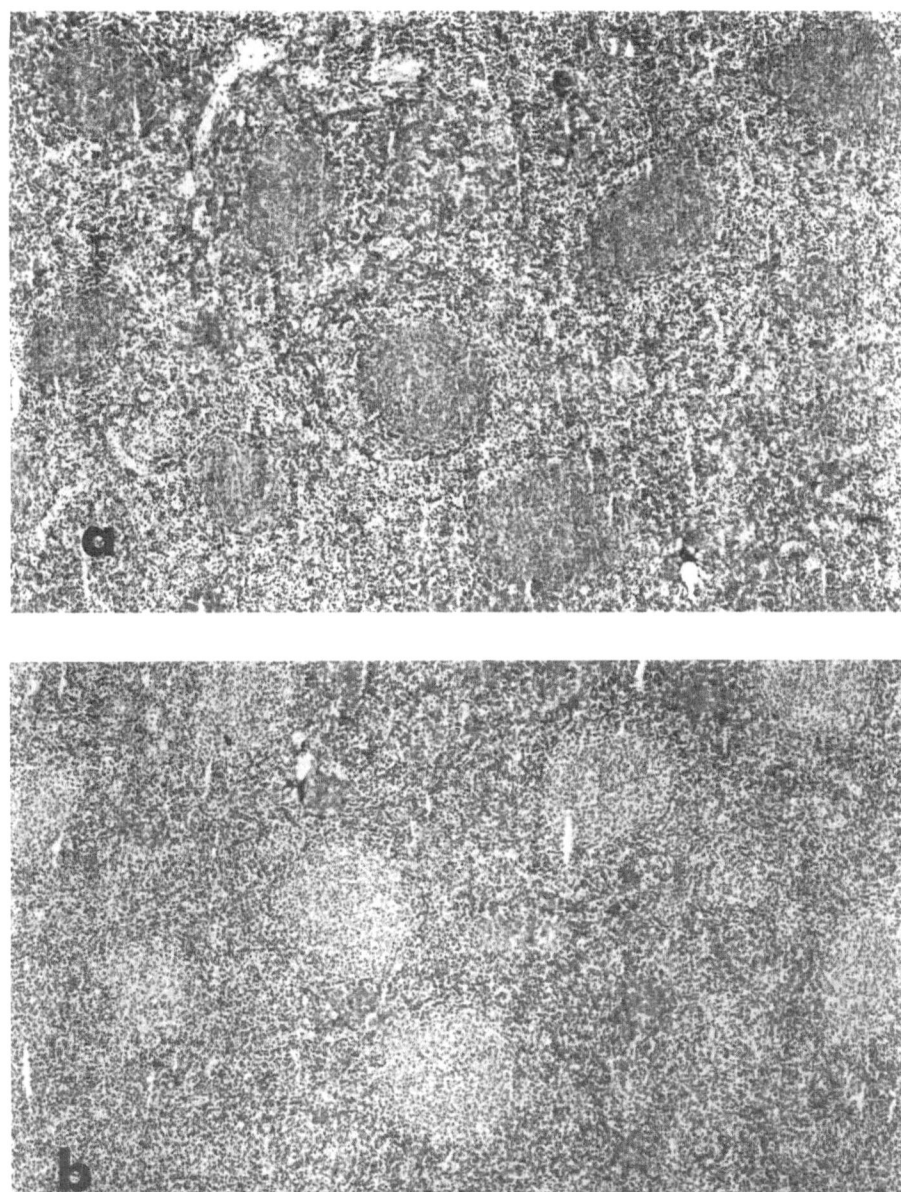

Fig. 17.17a,b. Immediate consecutive frozen sections of a follicular centre cell lymphoma, small cleaved cell type (centroblastic/centrocytic) showing the same field. Positive staining for sIg_κ is seen in the neoplastic follicles in **a**, whereas only benign interfollicular cells stain for $sIg\lambda$ in **b**. (Avidin-biotin peroxidase, haematoxylin counterstain, × 50)

Rudders et al. 1983). IgM may occur in combination with either IgD or IgG, although IgD combined with IgG and IgG or IgM alone has also been found (Lauder et al. 1985). It has been asserted that a double heavy chain phenotype is associated with a more slowly progressive clinical course (Rudders et al. 1983); however, this has not been confirmed. Generally, the prognosis has not been shown to correlate with specific heavy or light chain expression (Stein et al. 1979). One study reported a higher incidence of bone marrow involvement in patients whose lymphoma cells expressed λ light chain as compared with κ light chain (Filippa et al. 1978) Another study, while being unable to confirm this finding, suggested that bone marrow involvement appeared to occur more frequently in follicular centre cell lymphomas with sIgM than those with sIgG (Cousar et al. 1979). It has been claimed that lymphomas with a follicular pattern more commonly express κ light chain than diffuse lymphomas, where λ light chain expression is more common (Leech et al. 1975). Recently, Lauder et al. (1985), in an immunohistochemical study of 57 cases of B cell lymphoma followed for a minimum period of 1 year, indicated that tumours expressing λ light chain tumours had a tendency to be associated with poorer treatment response. It is interesting that large non-cleaved follicular centre cell (centroblastic) tumours more commonly express λ light chain (Stein H et al. 1980), and CLL (Mellstedt et al. 1978), multiple myeloma (Jancelewicz et al. 1975) and light chain disease (Shustik et al. 1976) with λ phenotype have a worse prognosis.

In rare cases, light chain staining of follicular lymphomas may pose a problem. Some workers (Stein et al. 1982; Swerdlow et al. 1985) have reported that neoplastic follicles occasionally bind both anti-κ and anti-λ antisera. The explanation of this observation remains uncertain. Immunoglobulin may not be demonstrable within the neoplastic follicles (Lukes et al. 1978; Warnke and Levy, 1978; Aisenberg et al. 1983; Harris and Bhan 1983), possibly because the cells are proliferations of surface immunoglobulin-negative follicular centre B cells which can normally be found in follicle centres (Hsu et al. 1983; Hsu and Jaffe 1984b). Two recent studies using combined immunophenotypic, functional and genotypic analysis made it possible to assign almost every case of sIg-negative, E-rosette-negative NHL to the B or T cell lineage, the majority being B lineage neoplasms (Knowles et al. 1985; Cleary et al. 1985). Such multiparametric immunophenotypic analyses demonstrate that truly "null-cell" NHL is probably very rare.

Other monoclonal antibodies have been applied to follicular centre cell lymphomas. Tubbs et al. (1981) and Swerdlow et al. (1985) reported that CD20 (B1) frequently stained the neoplastic follicles. In cases of extensive interfollicular lymphoma, numerous interfollicular CD20+ cells were identified. CD21 (B2) always identified the follicles, but even in the presence of interfollicular lymphoma, only occasional interfollicular cells stained with the antibody (Swerdlow et al. 1985). CD21 also decorated dendritic reticulum cells within the follicles. CD24 (BA1) was usually definitely positive in the follicles but it was weak or even negative in some cases of follicular centre cell lymphomas. Lastly, CD9 (BA2) usually stained the lymphomatous follicles diffusely, although rarely it was weak and even negative in 2 out of 24 cases (Swerdlow et al. 1985).

CD5+ B cells may occasionally be observed in follicular lymphomas (Burns et al. 1983; Knowles et al. 1983). This antibody also stains WDLL and B-CLL (Aisenberg et al. 1983). It has been suggested that CD5+ follicular lymphomas are not of follicular centre cell type but may represent intermediate or mantle zone lymphomas (centrocytic) (Cossman et al. 1984; Harris et al. 1984).

Immunohistochemical staining of the mantle-like structures surrounding neoplastic follicles of follicular centre cell lymphomas has revealed that at least some of the small lymphocytes are IgM +, IgD + polyclonal B cells similar both morphologically and immunologically to the mantle zone cells of reactive lymphoid follicles (Stein H et al. 1980; Harris and Data 1982; Lauder et al. 1985). The origin of these polyclonal mantle-zone lymphocytes is not apparent. It has been proposed that they represent residual marginal zones of primary follicles that have been invaded and displaced by "homing" tumour cells. They could represent B lymphocytes mounting an immunological reaction against the tumour, or both the polyclonal mantle-zone cells and the dendritic reticulum cells found within the lymphomatous follicles may be normal host cells which have in some way been induced to participate as "innocent bystanders" in the formation of neoplastic structures.

Normal reactive follicles contain T cells, predominantly of the T helper phenotype, in the light zone immediately beneath the follicular mantle (Poppema et al. 1981b; Stein et al. 1982). Neoplastic follicles also invariably contain T cells (Fig. 17.18) and their presence has given rise to much speculation. T cells are known to be involved in normal follicle formation (Jacobson et al. 1975) and it has been suggested that they may also participate in the formation of neoplastic follicles (Harris and Bhan 1983). Although they are generally considered reactive until the clonality of the T cells can be determined, the possibility remains that they may be part of the neoplasm. There may be differences in subset distributions within follicular lymphomas as compared with physiological hyperplasia (Dvoretsky et al. 1982; Harris and Bhan 1983). Approximately one-third of intrafollicular

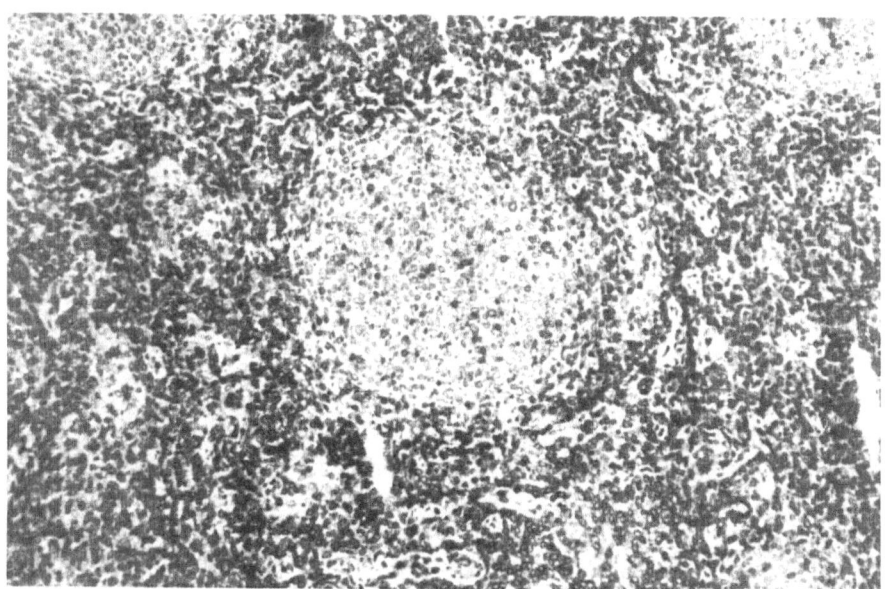

Fig. 17.18. Scattered T lymphocytes are seen in a neoplastic follicle in a follicular centre cell lymphoma, small cleaved cell type (centroblastic/centrocytic). Numerous T cells are present in the interfollicular areas. (Leu-4, modified avidin-biotin peroxidase, × 125)

T lymphocytes are CD8 +, in contrast to non-neoplastic follicles in which very few CD8+ lymphocytes are present. Natural killer (NK) and other large granular lymphocytes staining with CP03 (Leu-7) may also be very numerous within neoplastic follicles (Swerdlow and Murray 1984). T cells of helper phenotype have been reported to form perifollicular rims in about one-quarter of the cases studied (Swerdlow et al. 1985). These CD8+ rims are probably similar to the B cell-negative rims previously described (Tubbs et al. 1981). It has been proposed that these represent hyperplasia of the normal accentuation of T helper cells at the mantle–germinal centre interface in reactive nodes (Swerdlow et al. 1985).

T cells are usually even more numerous in interfollicular areas (Fig. 17.18) (Dvoretsky et al. 1982; Harris and Data 1982; Habeshaw et al. 1983). Their function is also uncertain. In all probability they represent remnants of pre-existing node or passive T cell traffic. There is both morphological as well as immunological evidence to suggest a T cell response. Large activated T cells may be observed in the interfollicular areas associated with prominent post-capillary venules (Papadimitriou and Papacharalampous 1979; Swerdlow et al. 1985). Although usually within the normal range, the T helper/T suppressor ratio may be very high or low (Habeshaw et al. 1983; Aisenberg et al. 1983). The T lymphocytes may also be CD25+ (Tac+) and MHC class II+, indicating their activated state. Recent cases of pleomorphic T cell malignant lymphomas have been reported in association with, or following, follicular B cell lymphomas (Jennette et al. 1982; York et al. 1985), fuelling further speculation that T cells may have a role in the formation of neoplastic follicles.

Intermediate and Mantle Zone Lymphomas

A variety of names has been given for this group of lymphomas. Nanba et al. (1977) described an alkaline phosphatase-positive B cell lymphoma which they later called "lymphocytic lymphoma of intermediate differentiation" (Mann et al. 1979). Rappaport's group described "malignant lymphoma, intermediate lympho-cytic type" (Weisenburger et al. 1981) and a follicular variant which they called "mantle zone lymphoma" (Weisenburger et al. 1982). It appears that these are a group of closely related tumours with minor variations in histological growth patterns. They are B cell lesions which appear to originate from the small lymphocytes of the mantle zones of the lymphoid follicles (Palutke et al. 1982). These relatively indolent tumours (not listed in the Working Formulation), tend to occur in middle-aged and older individuals and generally have clinical character-istics similar to those in patients with lymphomas of small cleaved follicular centre cells.

The lesions are characterised by widely expanded small lymphocyte mantles which surround large reactive follicle centres (Fig. 17.19). The small lymphocytes have slightly irregular nuclei with clumped chromatin and scanty cytoplasm (Fig. 17.20), cytological features apparently intermediate between the small round B cells of the more peripheral areas of the follicle mantle and the small cleaved cell within the follicle centre. This lymphoma may sometimes assume a diffuse growth pattern with a vague nodularity, but the cytological features of the infiltrating cells are similar in both patterns of growth. The diffuse proliferation with vague nodularity and the intermediate cytological features have made this tumour difficult to classify in the past. It has not been included as a separate entity in the

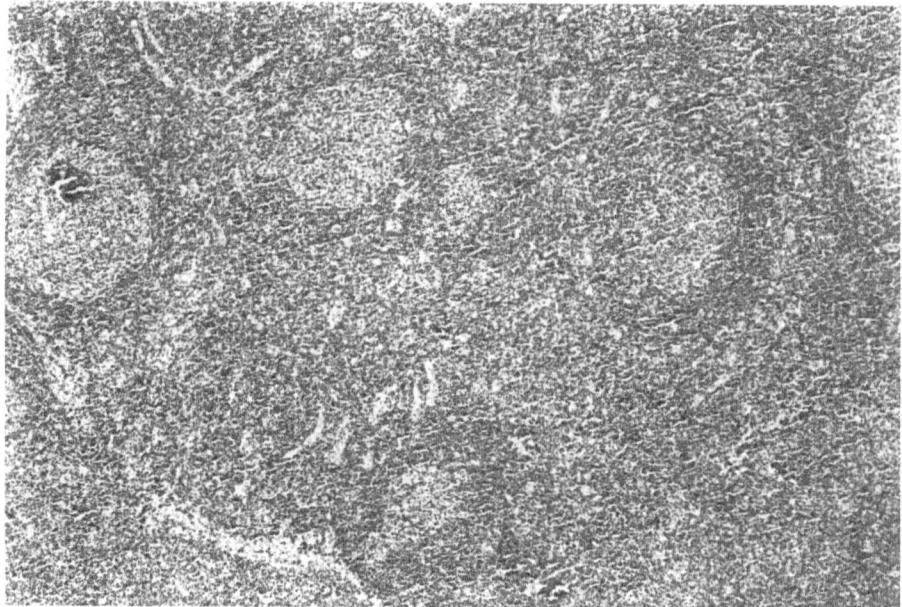

Fig. 17.19. Intermediate or mantle zone lymphoma with widely expanded mantle zones of small lymphocytes surrounding large reactive follicle centres. (H & E, × 50)

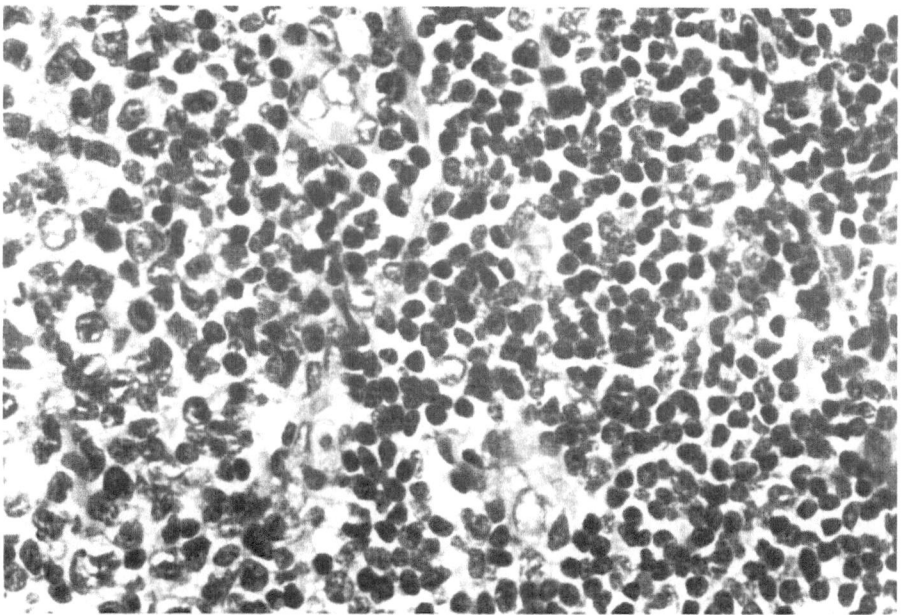

Fig. 17.20. The mantle zone cells are small with irregular nuclear outlines and the coarse chromatin pattern of small lymphocytes. They have an appearance intermediate between the small lymphocyte and the small cleaved cell of the follicle centre. (H & E, × 500)

major lymphoma classifications and has previously been placed with either WDLL or poorly differentiated lymphocytic lymphoma (small cleaved follicular centre cell lymphoma). More recently, Swerdlow et al. (1983) have suggested that many cases of mantle zone lymphomas probably represent a small subset of malignant lymphoma of the centrocytic type in the Kiel classification. Morphological and immunohistochemical studies performed on four cases of multiple lymphomatous polyposis, a distinctive type of primary gastrointestinal lymphoma, led Isaacson et al. (1984) to believe that it might represent a form of mantle zone lymphoma.

Immunological studies have revealed monoclonal B cell populations with sIg of intermediate density, usually of the IgM or IgMD type (Jaffe et al. 1977). Alkaline phosphatase activity was present in three out of six cases examined. This enzyme is normally found in cells of the mantle zone and primary follicles but has also been described in other B cell lymphomas (Nanba et al. 1977; Poppema et al. 1981a).

A recent study by Cossman et al. (1984) suggested that it is possible to distinguish the subclasses of low-grade B cell lymphomas by their expression of immunological determinants known to be developmentally regulated in normal B cells. WDLL (intermediate and mantle zone lymphomas) and follicular centre cell lymphomas all expressed monoclonal sIg, MHC class II, CD21 and CD9. Staining with other monoclonal antibodies revealed unique immunological phenotypes for each subclass of low-grade B cell lymphoma. WDLLs were CD5+, CD9−; mantle zone lymphomas were CD5+, CD9+; follicular centre cell lymphomas were CD5−, CD9−. CD9, CD20 and CD24 and sIg appeared to stain with different intensities among the three lymphoma subclasses. The relative fluorescence intensities of each of the three CD markers followed the same pattern: follicular centre cell lymphoma > mantle zone lymphoma > WDLL. The expression of these immunological determinants suggested that low-grade B cell lymphomas represent arrested, and possibly sequential, stages of B cell differentiation.

B Cell Lymphomas of the Medulla: Plasmacytoma

Localised plasma cell neoplasms may present as solitary lesions of bone or as extramedullary plasmacytomas. The relationship between the disseminated disease multiple myeloma and localised plasmacytoma is not well understood (Wiltshaw 1976; Corwin and Lindberg 1979). Some authors feel these lesions are different clinical manifestations of a single neoplastic process, whereas others consider them to be discrete entities with specific clinical features and prognostic characteristics (Callihan et al. 1983). Extramedullary plasmacytomas have been described in almost every organ, most frequently in the paranasal sinuses, nasopharynx, oropharynx and skin. Other locations include the salivary glands, breast, lung, thyroid and gonads. Primary lymph node plasmacytoma is rare, accounting for only 0.8% of NHL in the Kiel series (Lennert 1981). Extramedullary plasmacytomas can be multiple in up to 45% of patients, and draining lymph nodes may be involved in as many as 20% of patients (Wiltshaw 1976). Extramedullary plasmacytomas are most frequent after the age of 50 years, the majority being diagnosed in the 50- to 70-year age group.

Initial presentations may relate to the site of the tumour and include pain, epistaxis, dysphagia, dyspnoea or hoarseness. Although clinical response to surgery and/or low-dose radiation is good, local recurrence within 5 years of initial treatment has been reported in 30%–50% of cases. High-dose radiation of more than 50 Gy (5000 rads) is associated with a local recurrence rate of less than 10% (Bataille and Sany 1981). In approximately 40% of patients with extramedullary plasmacytoma, the disease may spread beyond the sites of presentation and to draining lymph nodes. About 25% of these patients develop multiple myeloma while others show skeletal or soft tissue involvement (Wiltshaw 1976).

Paraproteinaemia and paraproteinuria are less frequent in extramedullary plasmacytoma than multiple myeloma because of the smaller bulk of the tumour. About one-quarter of patients with extramedullary plasmacytoma have a monoclonal gammapathy, and even fewer show Bence Jones proteinurea.

The histopathology is usually straightforward. Regardless of the organ involved, the architecture is usually, but not invariably, distorted or destroyed by a monotonous proliferation of plasma cells with cytological features not dissimilar to that of multiple myeloma cells (Fig. 17.21). Varying degrees of pleomorphism may be seen, and less differentiated tumours with a more open chromatin pattern and single central nucleolus may be difficult to distinguish from B immunoblastic sarcoma. If submucosal tumours ulcerate, inflammatory cells may become mixed with the otherwise monomorphic neoplastic cells, especially in a superficial location near the ulcer. In lymph nodes primarily involved by plasmacytoma, the tumour often appears to start in the medullary region and spread to the cortex, producing entrapment of reactive lymphoid follicles among the sheets of plasma cells. Amorphous proteinaceous deposits of amyloid may be seen within the tumour, sometimes evoking a giant cell response.

The tumour cells are intensely pyroninophilic with a pale area adjacent to the nucleus corresponding to the Golgi apparatus. PAS-staining is diffuse or granular and intranuclear PAS-positive inclusions may be seen. Immunohistochemical staining is invaluable in demonstrating the monoclonality of the neoplastic cells (Fig. 17.21).

Undifferentiated B Cell Lymphomas

Undifferentiated B cell lymphomas are high-grade lymphomas which are called undifferentiated because of their size, the tumour cells approximating to the size of macrophage nuclei in the same tissue sections (Tindle 1984). This category encompasses not only Burkitt's lymphoma (BL) but also lymphomas which have previously been designated undifferentiated, non-Burkitt's type. "Undifferentiated" cells in these lymphomas correspond to the small non-cleaved cells of the follicle centres. The term "small non-cleaved cells" refers to their size relative to large non-cleaved cells, the nuclei of small non-cleaved cells being clearly larger than those of small lymphocytes. Cytologically, they appear as smaller counterparts to the large non-cleaved follicular centre cells in nuclear detail, but their cytoplasm is readily discernible as a dense perinuclear rim. These transformed lymphocytes have the characteristics of "blasts" with low nuclear/cytoplasmic ratio, fine chromatin, prominent nucleoli and dense and intensely pyroninophilic

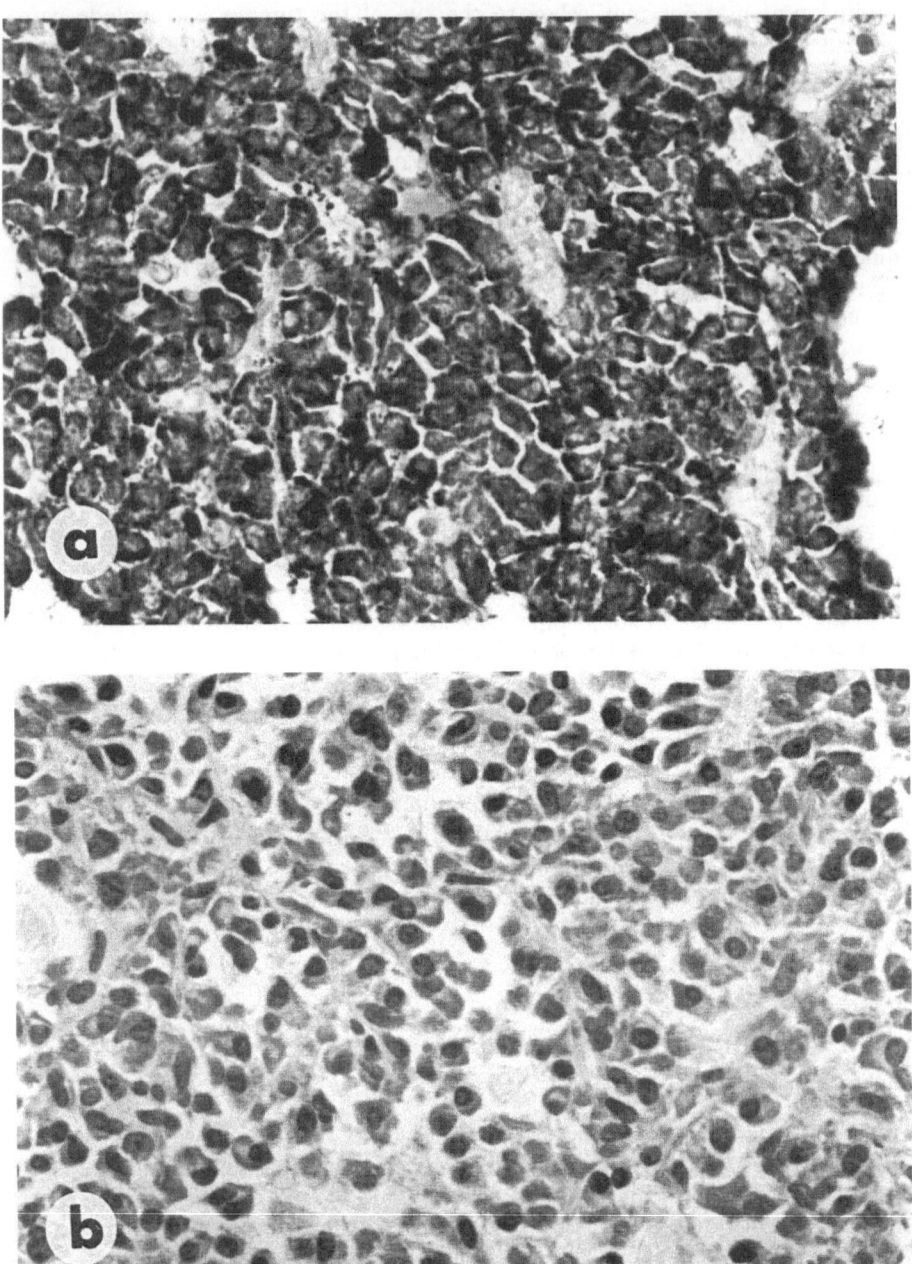

Fig. 17.21a,b. Plasmacytoma of nasopharynx showing positive staining for cIg$_\kappa$ in **a** and negative staining for cIgκ in **b**. The moderate pleomorphism of the tumour cells which are readily recognised as plasma cells, is discernible in **b**. (Avidin-biotin peroxidase, haematoxylin counterstain, × 500)

cytoplasm (Fig. 17.22). They show a very rapid cell turnover with a short doubling time, a high mitotic index and many tingible body macrophages mixed among the tumour cells. Small diffuse non-cleaved follicular centre cell lymphomas are rarely observed with a follicular pattern, probably because their high turnover rate results in a loss of propensity to retain a follicular structure.

The tumour, when expressed as an essentially monomorphous proliferation is classified as "Burkitt's type". Classic BL in Africa has a peak incidence in the first decade of life and comprises about 21% of NHL in childhood (Kjeldsberg et al. 1983). A typical presentation is with massive involvement of the jaws, commonly with involvement of kidneys and retroperitoneal tumour (Wright 1964). Neurological involvement, in the form of spinal cord compression and nerve palsies, may be a presenting feature but is more common in relapse (Magrath and Ziegler 1979). Massive bilateral ovarian involvement is common in girls, and the testes are involved in about 10% of the boys with BL. Infiltration of both breasts occurs during pregnancy and lactation. Involvement of other abdominal and thoracic viscera and of the endocrine glands is common in comparison with the low tumour bulk involving lymph nodes, spleen and lungs.

The nuclei of tumour cells in BL are uniform, approximating to those of macrophages. They are usually round but may occasionally be ovoid and show slight indentation of membranes. The nuclear membrane is prominent and the coarsely reticular chromatin is irregularly distributed and usually condensed at the nuclear membrane and around the nucleoli, of which there are three to four. Mitotic figures are numerous. The narrow rim of cytoplasm is amphophilic or basophilic and intensely pyroninophilic, except for a pale area at the nuclear hof.

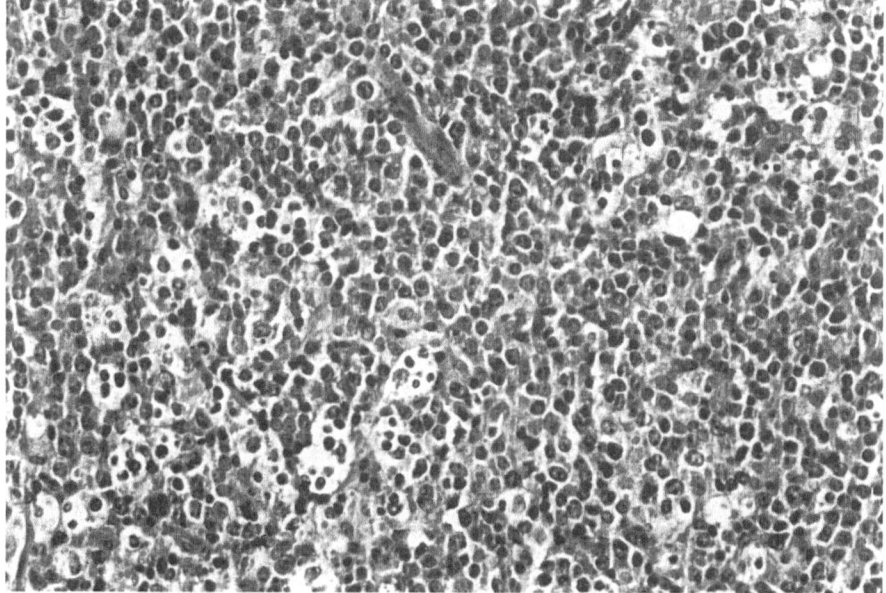

Fig. 17.22. Undifferentiated lymphoma, non-Burkitt's type. The tumour cells have non-cleaved nuclei which approximate to the size of macrophage nuclei seen in the section. Mitotic figures are numerous and tingible-body macrophages are plentiful. (H & E, × 300)

A variable number of cytoplasmic vacuoles is a characteristic, albeit, not constant feature. These vacuoles correspond to lipid droplets which are lost during fixation. The neoplastic cells may appear cohesive and "squared off" when the cytoplasm of one cell abuts that of another. A characteristic feature is the presence of scattered non-neoplastic macrophages having abundant clear or foamy cytoplasm containing pyknotic phagocytosed nuclear remnants among the tumour cells imparting a "starry-sky" appearance. Although the growth pattern of BL is classically diffuse, occasional lymphomatous follicles may be evident, implying a relationship to follicle centres.

The cells of BL not only resemble the small non-cleaved cells of follicle centres morphologically but also immunologically. Many cases of both African endemic and non-African sporadic BL have been shown to have high density monoclonal surface immunoglobulin on the malignant cells (Klein 1971; Flandrin et al. 1975; Mann et al. 1976). It has been demonstrated that tumour cells in culture synthesise immunoglobulin (van Furth et al. 1972), most commonly IgMκ (Mann et al. 1976).

American cases of BL have been reported in which the foci of tumour cells appear to be confined to single follicle centres of lymph nodes and Peyer's patches, suggesting an origin from, or homing to, such follicle centres (Mann et al. 1976). American cases of BL may differ from African cases in that they do not contain EBV DNA and do not express receptors for C3 and EBV (Magrath et al. 1980), suggesting that they may arise from a different clone of cells that do not express, or only weakly express, receptors for C3 and EBV. The chromosomal abnormalities which have been observed in most cases of BL, regardless of whether the EBV genome is present, do not appear to distinguish between endemic and non-endemic forms of the disease.

Electron microscopy shows rounded monomorphic nuclei which are pale and occasionally indented. Heterochromatin is sparse and peripherally located along the nuclear membrane (Epstein and Achong 1965; Berard et al. 1969; Flandrin et al. 1975). Nuclear pockets are characteristic but not diagnostic. Nucleoli are prominent. The cytoplasm is dark because of the presence of numerous polyribosomes and free ribosomes. Only short runs of rough endoplasmic reticulum are seen and mitochondria are few in number, often aggregated at one pole of the cell. Lipid droplets and clear vesicles are present. Annulate lamellae are observed in some cases (Epstein and Achong 1965).

Extranodal B Cell Lymphomas

The involvement of sites that are not primary organs of the lymphoreticular system may occur as part of a disseminated lymphomatous process, or may present as the primary tumour, remaining localised at these sites for varying periods of time. Wright and Isaacson (1983) believe that the involvement of extranodal sites in disseminated lymphoma rarely represents a random distribution but probably reflects the physiological circulation of the normal counterparts of the tumour cells. The characteristic involvement of the jaws by BL is an age-dependent phenomenon possibly related to dental development, and the striking involvement of the breasts during pregnancy and lactation may be the result of physiological migration of B lymphocytes to the breasts during these periods. Similarly, it is believed that B cell lymphomas may arise as primary tumours within physiological extranodal lymphoid tissues, as in the gastrointestinal tract, or in pathological collections of lymphocytes, as in Hashimoto's disease of the thyroid.

Extranodal tissues commonly involved by B cell lymphomas include the gastrointestinal tract, breast, thyroid, salivary gland, lung, skin, orbit, central nervous system, bone, ovary and testes. The differentiation of these extranodal lymphomas from reactive or inflammatory hyperplasia has been a major diagnostic problem, giving rise to the term "pseudolymphoma" to describe those tumour-like infiltrations which histologically are not clearly neoplastic and yet, on occasion, after variable periods of time, appear to evolve into lymphoma.

In many instances the diagnostic difficulty is compounded by the small size of the biopsy material available for examination. In an analysis of 22 gastric lymphoproliferative lesions in which biopsies and subsequent surgical specimens were available for examination, Saraga et al. (1981) noted that only 13 of the endoscopic biopsies were correctly diagnosed.

The histological features which have been generally applied to distinguish lymphomatous infiltrates from non-neoplastic processes include a monomorphous infiltrate of lymphoid cells, absence of follicle centres, destruction of the intrinsic architecture of the extranodal tissue, and isolation and destruction of the intrinsic epithelial structures such as colloid follicles in the thyroid and mucous glands in the gastrointestinal tract. However, it is often necessary to take multiple sections in order to establish the presence or absence of these diagnostic features. Appearances in a small biopsy sample from an otherwise polymorphous reactive process can mimic a monomorphous infiltrate, and plasmacytoid differentiation in a plasmacytoid lymphocytic lymphoma or superimposed inflammatory changes caused by tumour necrosis or ulceration may render the lymphoma misleadingly polymorphous.

Malignant lymphomas of the thyroid are mostly of B cell origin (Maurer et al. 1979) and have been frequently associated with lymphocytic thyroiditis (Lindsay and Dailey 1955; Burke et al. 1977; Compagno and Oertel 1980; Hamburger et al. 1983). Reactive follicles may be caught up in the lymphomatous infiltrate at the interface between the tumour and thyroiditis, their presence leading to the erroneous diagnosis of a benign process. An analogous situation may occur in other extranodal lymphomas which frequently arise in a background of inflammation or autoimmune diseases. Malignant B cell lymphoma of the salivary gland is frequently observed in Sjøgren's syndrome (Talal and Bunim 1964; Zulman et al. 1978; Schmid et al. 1982), and gastric lymphoma has been associated with atrophic gastritis (Vimadalal et al. 1983). Associations between achlorhydria and gastric ulcer with gastric lymphoma have been suggested (Hertzer and Hoerr 1976). Lymphoid hyperplasia adjacent to gastric lymphoma has been described (Lewin et al. 1978; Ranchod et al. 1978), and an instance of focal lymphoid hyperplasia preceding gastric lymphoma has been reported (Wolf and Spjut 1981).

In the lung, a few peribronchial reactive follicle centres and intralesional giant cell granulomas have been seen frequently in unequivocal lymphomas (Koss et al. 1983; Herbert et al. 1984). As a general rule, follicle centres should be absent or inconspicuous in extranodal lymphomas (Saltzstein 1963; Colby and Carrington 1983), but the associated conditions listed above may complicate the diagnostic appearance.

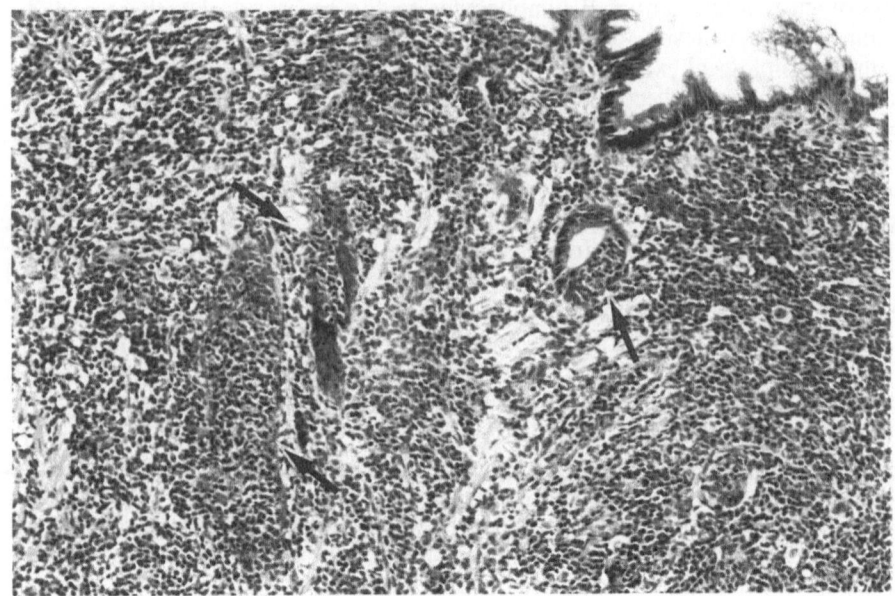

Fig. 17.23. A "lymphoepithelial lesion" is seen in a gastric lymphoma. Large cleaved cells are present infiltrating the gastric glandular epithelium (*arrows*). (H & E, × 50)

Involvement of lymph nodes adjacent to the extranodal tissue, when present, provides incontrovertible evidence of lymphoma. The finding of many cleaved follicular centre cells outside follicle centres is highly suggestive of a lymphomatous process. The invasion of individual glands in the gastrointestinal tract mucosa (Isaacson and Wright 1983) and of the colloid follicles in the thyroid (Compagno and Oertel 1980; Wright and Isaacson 1983; Anscombe and Wright 1985) by cleaved cells, either singly or in groups, when present, has been said to be pathognomonic of follicular centre cell lymphoma (Fig. 17.23). Wright and Isaacson (1983) considered the lymphoid infiltrates of the myoepithelial islands in salivary gland lymphomas as analogous to the glandular invasion seen in gastrointestinal tract and thyroid follicular centre cell lymphomas.

The problem of separation of lymphoma from pseudolymphoma is particularly accentuated in small biopsy specimens. Some authors have stated that the distinction in some sites, like the lung, is not possible on histological criteria alone (McNamara et al. 1969) and that all pseudolymphomas should be regarded as lymphomas (Gwynne-Jenkins and Salm 1971) or as pre-malignant lymphoma (Gibbs and Seal 1978). The introduction of immunocytochemical techniques that can identify monotypic (monoclonal) neoplastic proliferations from polytypic (polyclonal) reactive infiltrates has provided a method for resolving this problem (Knowles et al. 1982; Weiss et al. 1985b).

Immunoperoxidase studies on fixed tissues have shown that the majority of gastric lymphomas are of B cell type (Radaszkiewicz and Dragosis 1980; Yamanaka et al. 1980; Saraga et al. 1981; Vimadalal et al. 1983). Initial experience with immunological studies performed on frozen sections and cell suspensions from fresh tissue obtained at endoscopy or at the time of surgery has shown that this is an effective method of distinguishing between benign and malignant small cell lymphoid proliferations in the stomach (Vimadalal et al. 1983).

The classification of intestinal lymphomas, in particular those confined to the small intestine, has caused controversy for some time. Some authors believe them to be mainly of B cell type (Henry and Farrer-Brown 1977; Otto et al. 1981; Saraga et al. 1981; Haghighi 1983; Isaacson et al. 1983; Morgan et al. 1985) or to be "histiocytic" lymphomas by Rappaport's classification (Lewin et al. 1978; MacLennan et al. 1981). Isaacson and Wright (1978a, b) reported that immuno-histochemical studies revealed that the majority of small intestinal lymphomas in England were true histiocytic neoplasms. Furthermore, many of their cases of "malignant histiocytosis" were associated with proven coeliac disease. Recently, however, using both analysis for rearrangement of T cell receptor genes and immunocytochemical techniques on fresh frozen tissue, Isaacson et al. (1985) found four cases of so-called "malignant histiocytosis" to be of T cell origin.

In the past, there has been considerable controversy over the histological distinction between the benign lymphoepithelial lesion of the salivary gland, which is a characteristic feature of Sjøgren's syndrome, and malignant lymphoma. Many of these benign lymphoepithelial lesions have over the course of time, been associated with malignant lymphomas of B cell type (Azzopardi and Evans 1971; Hyman and Wolff 1976; Zulman et al. 1978). In an examination of 45 cases of benign lymphoepithelial lesion or "myoepithelial sialadenitis" (MESA), Schmid et al. (1982) were able to demonstrate confluent areas of monotypic lymphoplasmacytoid cells or immunoblasts in the salivary glands of 26 patients, 14 of whom developed extrasalivary gland malignant lymphoma of similar histological type. In 16 cases, the monotypic cells were focal within the salivary gland; nonetheless, 4 cases progressed to extrasalivary gland malignant lymphoma. It would appear, therefore, that many of these cases of so-called MESA are, in fact, malignant lymphoma localised to the salivary gland for variable periods (1.5–12 years in Schmid's series) before extrasalivary gland malignant lymphoma manifests.

The slow evolution characteristic of salivary gland malignant lymphomas is also often seen in some primary malignant lymphomas which occur in the gut, lung and thyroid. Mucosal B cells proliferate in response to antigenic stimulation and their progeny then circulate through the local lymph nodes, thoracic duct and bloodstream, eventually returning to the mucosa as plasma cells or B memory cells (McDermott and Bienenstock 1979) which are probably incapable of further proliferation. In a series of papers on malignant lymphomas of these mucosa-associated lymphoid tissues, Wright and colleagues (Isaccson and Wright 1983; Herbert et al. 1984; Moore and Wright 1984; Anscombe and Wright 1985) have postulated that the physiological circulation and homing patterns of these specific mucosa-associated lymphoid tissues may account for the long clinical courses of these diseases. Distinct circulatory pathways and homing patterns for the gut-associated lymphoid tissue (Bienenstock et al. 1973a, b) have been established. These physiological circulation patterns may account for the observation that mucosa-associated lymphomas often remain localised for long periods of time, in contrast to follicular centre cell lymphomas of peripheral lymphoid tissue which often present with bone marrow and peripheral blood involvement, representing stage III or IV disease. It is believed that when mucosa-associated lymphomas do metastasise, they spread to other sites of mucosa-associated lymphoid tissue (Herbert et al. 1984; Moore and Wright 1984).

The skin is another extranodal site of lymphoma where distinction from reactive proliferations poses a major diagnostic problem (Krishnan et al. 1983; Burg et al. 1984). Skin infiltration, which may occur during the course of almost any disseminated malignant lymphoma or leukaemia, accounts for approximately 20% of the extranodal manifestations of most B cell lymphomas (Lennert 1981). As a general rule, the criteria favouring a pseudolymphomatous infiltration over a follicular centre cell lymphoma are: (1) a solitary lesion on the head, (2) a wedge-shaped infiltrate forming follicles and sharply demarcated follicle centres and (3) the polymorphous nature of the infiltrate containing an admixture of large numbers of macrophages, plasma cells and eosinophils (Burg and Braun-Falco 1983; Burg et al. 1984).

Immunocytochemical staining is extremely useful in the identification of the neoplastic infiltrates (Kerl and Kresbach 1984). In contrast to cutaneous T cell lymphomas which are epidermotrophic (Leong et al. 1980), follicular centre cell lymphomas spare the papillary dermis and show a perivascular distribution, predominantly in the reticular dermis. The tumour often extends through the full thickness of the dermis into the subcutaneous fat with infiltration and destruction of blood vessels, nerves and skin appendages; these are additional features which are helpful in identifying malignant B cell infiltrates (Long et al. 1976). The difficulty in identifying primary lymphomas of the skin is accentuated by the fact that such lesions may remain localised for varying periods of time. Of the 25 primary lymphomas of the skin reported by Long et al. (1976), 22 developed extracutaneous lymphoma after periods ranging from 6 months to 5 years.

Small lymphocytic infiltrates of ocular structures, similar to those in other extranodal sites, may cause difficult diagnostic problems. Clinical features and routine histopathological techniques are often not sufficient for the separation of reactive from neoplastic lesions. In many instances immunohistochemical staining has proven to be especially useful in diagnosis (Knowles et al. 1979; Astarita et al. 1980; Jakobiec et al. 1982; Turner et al. 1984). Well-differentiated monoclonal lesions displayed no evidence of extraorbital disease, while a 50% incidence of extraorbital lymphoma occurred in the "less well-differentiated lymphomas" (Jakobiec et al. 1982).

The breast may be involved in disseminated malignant lymphoma, but primary lymphoma of the breast is rare, accounting for between 0.04% and 0.53% of all forms of malignancy in the breast (Mambo et al. 1977; Navas and Battifora 1977; Lin et al. 1980; Tateno et al. 1983). Lymphoma of the ovary is uncommon and tends to occur before the fifth decade (Chorlton et al. 1974; Paladuga et al. 1980), in contrast to malignant lymphoma of the testes which occurs after the fifth decade of life (Gowing 1976) usually as part of a disseminated disease (Turner et al. 1981).

Primary malignant lymphomas of bone are reported to be almost as common as those associated with disseminated lymphoma (Boston et al. 1974). The majority of cases appear to be of follicular centre cell origin (Mahoney and Alexander 1980).

Primary malignant lymphomas of the central nervous system are relatively rare. They account for 0.3%–1.5% of all intracranial neoplasms, occurring almost exclusively in the brain parenchyma (Allegranza et al. 1984). Advanced malignant lymphoma may secondarily involve the brain, large cell lymphomas tending to invade the substance of the brain, whereas small cell lymphomas show leptomeningeal seeding (Law et al. 1975; Venables et al. 1980). Central nervous system relapse is particularly high in lymphoblastic and diffuse undifferentiated lymphomas (Johnson et al. 1984). Immunohistochemical studies indicate that the majority of central nervous system lymphomas are of B cell lineage (Taylor et al. 1978; Allegranza et al. 1984), T cell variants representing a minority (Pinkus et al. 1979).

Hodgkin's Disease

Although notable advances have been made in the management of Hodgkin's disease (HD), the fundamental nature of the disease continues to be controversial. Despite many morphological and experimental studies of HD and Reed–Sternberg cells, the origin and identity of these cells continue to be the subject of debate. Among the leading candidates have been the reticulum cell (including reticular cell and stem cell), the histiocyte, the lymphoblast, the plasmablast, the megakaryocyte and myeloid cells (reviewed by Taylor 1983). Contemporary candidates have included the macrophage (Mori and Lennert 1969; Kaplan and Gartner 1977; Kadin et al. 1978), dendritic reticulum cells (Curran and Jones 1978b) and interdigitating reticulum cells (Poppema et al. 1982; Kadin 1982).

A T cell origin has been proposed, largely on the circumstantial evidence of decreased T cell immune function in HD. It was postulated that a virus-altered T cell could trigger a chronic graft versus host reaction resulting in malignant transformation of a bystander reticulum cell. Alternatively, a virus could transform the T cell directly into a Hodgkin tumour cell. Immunological studies, however, have not consistently shown Reed–Sternberg cells to possess markers of T lymphocytes, indicating that it is unlikely that Reed–Sternberg cells are closely related to T cells at either early or late stages of thymocyte differentiation.

The identification of immunoglobulin either within or on the surface of Reed–Sternberg cells has led to the suggestion that they are derived from B lymphocytes. In most cases the immunoglobulin was polyclonal or bitypic, associated with both κ and λ light chains. The failure to demonstrate J chain in the Reed–Sternberg cells suggested that they do not synthesise immunoglobulin but may have acquired exogenous immunoglobulin by internalisation of immune complexes circulating in the serum, or, alternatively, that the immunoglobulin could enter Reed–Sternberg cells by passive absorption through a leaky cell membrane, possibly damaged by tumour-directed antibodies.

While these observations apply to the most common forms of HD — mixed cellularity and nodular sclerosing types — it has been proposed that the unique Reed–Sternberg variant (L and H cell) in nodular lymphocyte-predominant HD is derived from an atypical B immunoblast which originates in progressively transformed germinal centres (Poppema et al. 1979).

In contrast to the other types of HD which initially involve the T zones of the node, lymphocyte-predominant HD appears to originate in the B cell areas. A single type of immunoglobulin light chain and J chains were found in the lymphocytic and histiocytic (L and H) variants, compatible with a B cell derivation.

Clinically, nodular lymphocyte-predominant HD also appears distinct; it is characterised by asymptomatic localised disease, which is usually cervical or axillary and frequently recurs at the same site, and is associated with an excellent prognosis even without therapy (Poppema et al. 1979). Some further support is given in the observation that the L and H variants do not stain for LeuM1 (CDw15) antigen, whereas Reed–Sternberg cells in other forms of HD were consistently strongly immunoreactive for this antigen (Pinkus and Said 1985). The studies by Stein et al. (1985) with Ki-1, a monoclonal antibody raised against a HD-derived cell line, suggest that Reed–Sternberg cells may represent malignant counterparts of lymphoid cells of either T or B cell origin that are in an activated state and hence only rarely encountered in normal lymphoid tissue. Ki-1 stains small mononuclear cells in the parafollicular zones of normal lymphoid tissue.

The identity of the malignant cell in HD is likely to be revealed by DNA hybridisation. An early study has yielded a surprising result. Cells from blood from a patient with HD in a leukaemic phase were morphologically like Reed–Sternberg cells and expressed sIgμ, CD19, CD20, MHC class II, CD10 (CALLA), Ki-1, but not sIgκ, sIgλ or T cell antigens. Immunoglobulin gene analysis showed rearrangement of the VDJ region of the heavy chain, a heavy chain allele in the germline configuration and rearrangement of the κ chain (Linch et al. 1985), indicating its B cell nature.

References

Aisenberg AC, Bloch KJ, Long JC (1973) Cell-surface immunoglobulins in chronic lymphocytic leukemia and allied disorders. Am J Med 55: 184–189

Aisenberg AC, Wilkes BM, Harris NL (1983) Monoclonal antibody studies in non-Hodgkin's lymphoma. Blood 61: 469–475

Allegranza A, Mariani C, Giardini R, Brambilla MC, Boeri R (1984) Primary malignant lymphomas of the central nervous system: a histological and immunohistological study of 12 cases. Histopathology 8: 781–791

Anscombe AM, Wright DH (1985) Primary malignant lymphoma of the thyroid — a tumor of mucosa-associated lymphoid tissue: review of 76 cases. Histopathology 9: 81–97

Astarita RW, Minckler D, Taylor CR et al. (1980) Orbital and adnexal lymphomas. A multiparameter approach. Am J Clin Pathol 73: 615–621

Azar HA, Espinoza CG, Richman AV, Saba SR, Wang T (1982) "Undifferentiated" large cell malignancies. An ultrastructural and immunocytochemical study. Hum Pathol 13: 323–333

Azzopardi JG, Evans DJ (1971) Malignant lymphoma of parotid associated with Mikulicz disease (benign lymphoepithelial lesion). J Clin Pathol 24: 744–752

Bataille R, Sany J (1981) Solitary myeloma: clinical and prognostic features of a review of 114 cases. Cancer 48: 845–851

Bennett MH (1975) Sclerosis in non-Hodgkin's lymphomata. Br J Cancer 31 (Suppl II): 44–52

Bennett MH, Farrer-Brown G, Henry K et al. (1974) Classification of non-Hodgkin's lymphomas. Lancet II: 405–406

Berard CW, O'Connor GT, Thomas LB, Torloni H (1969) Histopathological definition of Burkitt's tumor. Bull WHO 40: 601–607

Bienenstock J, Johnston N, Perey DYE (1973a) Bronchial lymphoid tissue. I. Morphologic characteristics. Lab Invest 28: 686–692

Bienenstock J, Johnston N, Perey DYE (1973b) Bronchial lymphoid tissue. II. Functional characteristics. Lab Invest 28: 693–698

Boston HC, Dahlin DC, Ivins JC, Cupps RE (1974) Malignant lymphoma (so-called reticulum cell sarcoma) of bone. Cancer 34: 1131–1137

Braylan RC, Jaffe ES, Berard CW (1975) Malignant lymphomas. Current classification and new observations. In: Sommers SC (ed) A Pathology Annual Monograph. Appleton Century Crofts, New York, pp 213–270

Braylan RC, Jaffe ES, Burbach JW, Frank MM, Johnson RE, Berard CW (1976) Similarities of surface characteristics of neoplastic well-differentiated lymphocytes from solid tissues and from peripheral blood. Cancer Res 36: 1619–1625

Brouet JC, Preud'homme JL, Seligmann M, Bernard J (1973) Blast cells with monoclonal surface immunoglobulin in two cases of acute blast crisis supervening on chronic lymphocytic leukemia. Br Med J 4: 23–24

Brouet J-C, Preud'homme JL, Flandrin G, Chelloul N, Seligmann M (1977) Membrane markers in "histiocytic" lymphomas (reticulum cell sarcomas). J Natl Cancer Inst 56: 631–633

Burg G, Braun-Falco O (1983) Cutaneous lymphomas, pseudolymphomas, and related disorders. Springer, Berlin Heidelberg New York

Burg G, Kerl H, Schmoeckel C (1984) Differentiation between malignant B-cell lymphomas and pseudolymphomas of the skin. J Dermatol Surg Oncol 10: 271–275

Burke JS, Butler JJ, Fuller LM (1977) Malignant lymphomas of the thyroid A clinical pathologic study of 35 patients including ultrastructural observations. Cancer 39: 1587–1602

Burns BF, Warnke RA, Doggett RS et al. (1983) Expression of a T-cell antigen (Leu-1) by B-cell lymphomas. Am J Pathol 113: 165–171

Callihan TR, Hobert JM Jr, Berard CW (1983) Neoplasms of terminal B-cell differentiation: the morphologic basis of functional diversity. In: Sommers SC, Rosen PP (eds) Malignant lymphoma. A Pathology Annual Monograph. Appleton Century Crofts, Norwalk, Connecticut, pp 169–268

Cawley JC, Hayhoe FGJ (1973) Ultrastructure of hemic cells: a cytological atlas of normal and leukemic blood and bone marrow. Saunders, Philadelphia

Chorlton I, Norris HJ, King FM (1974) Malignant reticuloendothelial disease involving the ovary as a primary manifestation. A series of 19 lymphomas and 1 granulocytic sarcoma. Cancer 34: 397–407

Cleary ML, Trela MJ, Weiss LM, Warnke R, Sklar J (1985) Most null large cell lymphomas are B lineage neoplasms. Lab Invest 53: 521–525

Coico RF, Bhogal BS, Thorbecke GJ (1983) Relationship of germinal centres in lymphoid tissue to immunologic memory. VI. Transfer of B-cell memory with lymph node cells fractionated according to their receptors for peanut agglutinin. J Immunol 131: 2254–2257

Colby TV, Carrington CB (1983) Lymphoreticular tumors and infiltrates of the lung. Pathol Annu 18(1): 27–70

Compagno J, Oertel JE (1980) Malignant lymphoma and other lymphoproliferative disorders of the thyroid gland. A clinico-pathologic study of 245 cases. Am J Clin Pathol 74: 1–11

Corwin J, Lindberg RD (1979) Solitary plasmacytoma of bone versus extramedullary plasmacytoma and their relationship to multiple myeloma. Cancer 43: 1007–1013

Cossman J, Neckers LM, Hsu S et al. (1984) Low-grade lymphomas. Expression of developmentally regulated B-cell antigens. Am J Pathol 115: 117–124

Cousar JB, Stein RS, Flexner JM et al. (1979) Pathologic and immunologic features of bone marrow and peripheral blood involvement in follicular centre cell lymphomas. Lab Invest 40: 14 (abstract)

Cullen MH, Lister TA, Brearley RL et al. (1979) Histological transformation of non-Hodgkin's lymphoma. A prospective study. Cancer 44: 645–651

Curran RC, Jones EL (1978a) The lymphoid follicles of the human palatine tonsil. Clin Exp Immunol 31: 251–259

Curran RC, Jones EL (1978b) Hodgkin's disease: an immunohistochemical and histological study. J Pathol 125: 39–51

Dardick I, Sinnott NM, Holl R et al. (1983a) Nuclear morphology and morphometry of B lymphocyte transformation. Implications for follicular centre cell lymphomas. Am J Pathol 111: 35–49

Dardick I, Srinivasan R, Al-Jabi M (1983b) Signet-ring cell variant of large cell lymphoma. Ultrastruct Pathol 5: 195–200

Dorfman RF (1974) Classification of non-Hodgkin's lymphoma. Lancet II: 961–962

Dvoretsky P, Wood GS, Levy R, Warnke RA (1982) T-lymphocyte subsets in follicular lymphomas compared with those in non-neoplastic lymph nodes and tonsils. Hum Pathol 13: 618–625

Enno A, Catovsky D, O'Brien M et al. (1979) "Prolymphocytoid" transformation of chronic lymphocytic leukemia. Br J Haematol 41: 9–18

Epstein MA, Achong BG (1965) Fine structural organisation of human lymphoblasts of a tissue culture strain (EBI) from Burkitt's lymphoma. J Natl Cancer Inst 34: 241–253

Evans HL (1982) Extranodal small lymphocytic proliferation: a clinico-pathologic and immunocyto-chemical study. Cancer 49: 84–96

Filippa DA, Lieberman PH, Erlandson RA et al. (1978) A study of malignant lymphomas using light and ultramicroscopic cytochemical and immunologic technices. Correlation with clinical features. Am J Med 64: 259–268

Flandrin G, Brouet JC, Daniel MT, Preud'homme JL (1975) Acute leukemia with Burkitt's tumor cells: a study of 6 cases with special reference to lymphocyte surface markers. Blood 45: 183–188

Fossum S, Ford WL (1985) The organisation of cell populations within lymph nodes: their origin, life history and functional relationships. Histopathology 9: 469–499

Galton DAG, Catovsky D, Wiltshaw E (1978) Clinical spectrum of lymphoproliferative diseases. Cancer 42: 901–910

Gerard-Merchant R, Hamlin I, Lennert K et al. (1974) Classification of non-Hodgkin's lymphomas. Lancet II: 406–408

Gibbs AR, Seal RME (1978) Primary lymphoproliferative conditions of lung. Thorax 33: 140–152

Gillespie JJ (1978) The ultrastructural diagnosis of diffuse large cell ("histiocytic") lymphoma. Fine structural study of 30 cases. Am J Surg Pathol 2: 9–20

Gowing NFC (1976) Malignant lymphoma of the testes. In: Pugh RCB (ed) Pathology of the testes. Blackwell Scientific, Oxford, pp 334–355

Grogan TM, Richter LC, Payne CM, Rangel CS (1985) Signet-ring cell lymphoma of T-cell origin. An immunocytochemical and ultrastructural study relating giant vacuole formation to cytoplasmic sequestration of surface membrane. Am J Surg Pathol 9: 684–692

Gwynne-Jenkins BA, Salm R (1971) Primary lymphosarcoma of lung. Br J Dis Chest 65: 225–230

Habeshaw JA, Bailey D, Stansfeld AG, Greaves MF (1983) The cellular content of non Hodgkin lymphomas: a comprehensive analysis using monoclonal antibodies and other surface marker techniques. Br J Cancer 47: 327–351

Haghighi P (1983) Primary small intestinal lymphoma and immunoproliferative small intestinal disease: an update. In: Sommers SC, Rosen PP (eds) Malignant lymphoma. A Pathology Annual Monograph. Appleton Century Crofts, Norwalk, Connecticut, pp 269–293

Hamburger JI, Miller JM, Kini SR (1983) Lymphoma of the thyroid. Ann Intern Med 99: 685–693

Hanna MG Jr (1964) An autoradiographic study of the germinal centre in the spleen white pulp during early intervals of the immune response. Lab Invest 13: 95–104

Harousseau JL, Flandrin G, Tricot G et al. (1981) Malignant lymphoma supervening in chronic lymphocytic leukemia and related disorders Richter's syndrome: a study of 25 cases. Cancer 48: 1302–1308

Harris M, Eyden B, Read G (1981) Signet ring cell lymphoma: a rare variant of follicular lymphoma. J Clin Pathol 34: 884–891

Harris NL, Bhan AK (1983) Distribution of T-cell subsets in follicular and diffuse lymphomas of B-cell type. Am J Pathol 113: 172–180

Harris NL, Bhan AK (1985) B-cell neoplasms of the lymphocytic, lymphoplasmacytoid, and plasma cell types: immunohistologic analysis and clinical correlation. Hum Pathol 16: 829–837

Harris NL, Data RE (1982) The distibution of neoplastic and normal B-lymphoid cells in nodular lymphomas: use of an immunoperoxidase technique on frozen sections. Hum Pathol 13: 610–617

Harris NL, Poppema S, Data RE (1982) Demonstration of immunoglobulin in malignant lymphomas. Use of an immunoperoxidase technic on frozen sections. Am J Clin Pathol 78: 14–21

Harris NL, Nadler LM, Bhan AK (1984) Immunohistologic characterization of two malignant lymphomas of germinal centre type (centroblastic/centrocytic and centrocytic) with monoclonal antibodies. Follicular and diffuse lymphomas of small-cleaved-cell type are related but distinct entities. Am J Pathol 117: 262–272

Heinz R, Stacher A, Pralle H et al. (1981) Lymphoplasmacytic/lymphoplasmacytoid lymphoma: a clinical entity distinct from chronic lymphocytic leukemia? Blut 43: 183–192

Henry K, Farrer-Brown G (1977) Primary lymphomas of the gastrointestinal tract. I. Plasma cell tumours. Histopathology 1: 53–76

Herbert A, Wright DH, Isaacson PG, Smith JL (1984) Primary malignant lymphoma of the lung: histopathologic and immunologic evaluation of nine cases. Hum Pathol 15: 415–422

Herrmann R, Barcos M, Stutzman L et al. (1982) The influence of histologic type on the incidence and duration of response in non-Hodgkin's lymphoma. Cancer 49: 314–322

Hertzer NR, Hoerr SO (1976) An interpretive review of lymphoma of the stomach. Surg Gynecol Obstet 143: 113–124

Hsu S, Jaffe ES (1984a) Phenotypic expression of B-lymphocytes. I. Identification with monoclonal antibodies in normal lymphoid tissues. Am J Pathol 114: 387–395

Hsu SM, Jaffe ES (1984b) Phenotypic expression of B-lymphocytes. II. Immunoglobulin expression of germinal centre cells. Am J Pathol 114: 396–402

Hsu SM, Cossman J, Jaffe ES (1983) Lymphocyte subsets in normal human lymphoid tissues. Am J Clin Pathol 80: 21–30

Hyman GA, Wolff M (1976) Malignant lymphomas of the salivary glands. Review of the literature and report of 33 new cases, including four cases associated with the lymphoepithelial lesion. Am J Clin Pathol 65: 421–438

Iossifides I, Mackay B, Butler JJ (1980) Signet-ring cell lymphoma. Ultrastruct Pathol 1: 511–517

Isaacson P, Wright DH (1978a) Intestinal lymphoma associated with malabsorption. Lancet I: 67–70

Isaacson P, Wright DH (1978b) Malignant histiocytosis of the intestine: its relationship to malabsorption and ulcerative jejunitis. Hum Pathol 9: 661–677

Isaacson P, Wright DH (1983) Malignant lymphoma of mucosa-associated lymphoid tissue, a distinctive type of B-cell lymphoma. Cancer 52: 1410–1416

Isaacson P, Wright DH, Judd MA et al. (1980) The nature of the immunoglobulin-containing cells in malignant lymphoma: an immunoperoxidase study. J Histochem Cytochem 28: 761–770

Isaacson P, Al-Dewachi HS, Mason DY (1983) Middle Eastern intestinal lymphoma: a morphological and immunohistochemical study. J Clin Pathol 36: 489–498

Isaacson PG, Maclennan KA, Subbuswamy SG (1984) Multiple lymphomatous polyposis of the gastrointestinal tract. Histopathology 8: 641–656

Isaacson PG, Spencer J, Connolly CE et al. (1985) Malignant histiocytosis of the intestine: a T-cell lymphoma. Lancet II: 688–691

Jacobson EB, Caporale LH, Thorbecke GJ (1975) Effect of thymus cell injections on germinal center formation in lymphoid tissues of nude (thymusless) mice. Cell Immunol 13: 416–430

Jaffe ES, Shevach EM, Frank MM et al. (1974) Nodular lymphoma: evidence for origin from follicular B lymphocytes. N Engl J Med 290: 813–819

Jaffe ES, Braylan RC, Nanba K, Frank MM, Berard CW (1977) Functional markers: a new perspective on malignant lymphomas. Cancer Treat Rep 61: 953–962

Jakobiec FA, Iwamoto T, Knowles DM (1982) Ocular adnexal lymphoid tumours. Correlative ultrastructural and immunologic marker studies. Arch Ophthalmol 100:84–98

Jancelewicz Z, Takatsuki K, Sugai S, Pruzanski W (1975) IgD multiple myeloma. Arch Intern Med 135: 87–93

Jennette JC, Reddick RL, Saunders AW et al. (1982) Diffuse T-cell lymphoma preceded by nodular lymphoma. Am J Clin Pathol 78: 242–248

Johnson GJ, Oken MM, Anderson JR et al. (1984) Central nervous system relapse in unfavourable-histology non-Hodgkin's lymphomas: is prophylaxis indicated? Lancet II: 685–687

Jones SE, Fuks Z, Bull M et al. (1973) Non-Hodgkin's lymphomas. IV. Clinicopathologic correlation in 405 cases. Cancer 31: 806–823

Kadin ME (1982) Possible origin of the Reed-Sternberg cell from an interdigitating reticulum cell. Cancer Treat Rep 66: 601–608

Kadin ME, Stites DP, Levy R, Warnke R (1978) Exogenous immunoglobulin and the macrophage origin of Reed-Sternberg cells in Hodgkin's disease. N Engl J Med 299: 1208–1214

Kaiserling E (1977) Non-Hodgkin's Lymphome: Ultrastruktur and Cytogenese. Fischer, Stuttgart

Kaplan HS, Gartner S (1977) "Sternberg-Reed" giant cells of Hodgkin's disease: cultivation in vitro, heterotransplantation, and characterisation as neoplastic macrophages. Int J Cancer 19: 511–525

Kerl H, Kresbach H (1984) Germinal centre cell-derived lymphomas of the skin. J Dermatol Surg Oncol 10: 291–295

Kim H, Dorfman RF, Rappaport H (1978) Signet-ring cell lymphoma: a rare morphologic and functional expression of nodular (follicular) lymphoma. Am J Surg Pathol 2: 119–132

Kjeldsberg CR, Marty J (1981) Prolymphocytic transformation of chronic lymphocytic leukemia. Cancer 48: 2447–2457

Kjeldsberg CR, Wilson JF, Berard CW (1983) Non-Hodgkin's lymphoma in children. Hum Pathol 14: 612–627

Klein G (1971) Immunological aspects of Burkitt's lymphoma. Adv Immunol 14: 187–250

Knowles DM, Jakobiec FA, Halper JP (1979) Immunologic characterisation of ocular adnexal lymphoid neoplasms Am J Ophthalmol 87: 603–619

Knowles DM, Halper JP, Jakobiec FA (1982) The immunologic characterisation of 40 extranodal lymphoid infiltrates. Usefulness in distinguishing between benign pseudolymphoma and malignant lymphoma. Cancer 49: 2321–2335

Knowles DM, Halper JP, Azzo W et al. (1983) Reactivity of monoclonal antibodies Leu1 and OKT1 with malignant human lymphoid cells. Correlation with conventional cell markers. Cancer 52: 1369–1377

Knowles DM, Dodson L, Burke JS et al. (1985) Sig⁻ E⁻ ("null-cell") non-Hodgkin's lymphomas. Multiparametric determination of their B- or T-cell lineage. Am J Pathol 120: 356–370

Koburg E (1967) Cell production and cell migration in the tonsil. In: Cottier H, Odartchenko N, Schindler R, Congdon CC (eds) Germinal centres in the immune responses. Springer, Berlin Heidelberg New York, pp 176–182

Koss MN, Hochholzer L, Nichols PW, Wehunt PW, Lazarus AA (1983) Primary non-Hodgkin's lymphoma and pseudolymphoma of lung: a study of 161 patients. Hum Pathol 14: 1024–1038

Krishnan J, Li C, Su WPD (1983) Cutaneous lymphomas: Correlation of histochemical and immunohistochemical characteristics and clinicopathologic features. Am J Clin Pathol 79: 157–165

Kuhn C (1967) Nuclear bodies and intranuclear globulin inclusions in Waldenstrom's macroglobuline-
    mia. Lab Invest 17: 404–415
Lauder I, Bird CC, Child JA, Grigor I (1985) Surface membrane phenotypic expression and treatment
    response of malignant lymphomas. J Pathol 145: 259–268
Law IP, Dick FR, Blom J, Bergevin PR (1975) Involvement of the central nervous system in non-
    Hodgkin's lymphomas. Cancer 36: 225–231
Leech JH, Glick AD, Waldron JA, Flexner JM, Horn RG, Collins RD (1975) Malignant lymphomas
    of follicular centre cell origin in man. I. Immunologic studies. J Natl Cancer Inst 54: 11–21
Lennert K (1973) Follicular lymphoma: a tumor of the germinal centres. In: Akazaki K (ed) Malignant
    diseases of the haemopoietic system. Gann Monograph on Cancer Research No 15. University of
    Tokyo Press, Tokyo, pp 217–231
Lennert K (1978) Malignant lymphomas other than Hodgkin's disease. Springer, Berlin Heidelberg
    New York, pp 111–136
Lennert K (1981) Histopathology of non-Hodgkin's lymphomas (based on the Kiel classification).
    Springer, Berlin Heidelberg New York
Lennert K, Müller-Hermelink HK (1975) Lymphozyten und ihre Funktionsformen. Morphologie
    Organisation und immunologische Bedeutung. Verh Anat Ges 69: 19–62
Lennert K, Mohri N, Stein H et al. (1975) The histopathology of malignant lymphoma. Br J Haematol
    31 (suppl):193–203
Leong AS-Y (1983) A critique of some contemporary classifications of non-Hodgkin's lymphoma.
    Which one should we now use? Pathology 15: 437–442
Leong AS-Y, Forbes IJ, Cowled PA et al. (1979) Surface marker studies in chronic lymphocytic
    leukaemia and non-Hodgkin's lymphoma. Pathology 11: 461–471
Leong AS-Y, Sage RE, Kinnear GC, Forbes IJ (1980) Preferential epidermotrophism in adult T-cell
    leukemia-lymphoma. Am J Surg Pathol 4: 421–430
Lewin KJ, Ranchod M, Dorfman RF (1978) Lymphomas of the gastrointestinal tract: a study of 117
    cases presenting with gastrointestinal disease. Cancer 42: 693–707
Lin JJ, Farha GJ, Taylor RJ (1980) Pseuodolymphoma of the breast. In a study of 8,654 consecutive
    tylectomies and mastectomies. Cancer 45: 973–978
Linch DC, Jones HM, Berliner N et al. (1985) Hodgkin-cell leukaemia of B-cell origin. Lancet I: 78–80
Lindsay S, Dailey ME (1955) Malignant lymphoma of the thyroid gland and its relation to Hashimoto
    disease: a clinical and pathologic study of 8 patients. J Clin Endocrinol Metab 15: 1332–1353
Long JC, Aisenberg AC (1975) Richter's syndrome: a terminal complication of chronic lymphocytic
    leukemia with distinct clinico-pathologic features. Am J Clin Pathol 63: 786–795
Long JC, Mihm MC, Qazi R (1976) Malignant lymphoma of the skin. A clinicopathologic study of
    lymphoma other than mycosis fungoides diagnosed by skin biopsy. Cancer 38: 1282–1296
Lukes RJ, Collins RD (1974) Immunologic characterisation of human malignant lymphomas. Cancer
    34: 1488–1503
Lukes RJ, Taylor CR, Parker JW et al. (1978) A morphologic and immunologic surface marker study
    of 299 cases of non-Hodgkin's lymphomas and related leukemias. Am J Pathol 90: 461–485
MacLennan KA, Bennett MH, Tu A (1981) The pathology of primary gastrointestinal lymphomas.
    (Report no. 10) Clin Radiol 32: 513–528
Magrath IT, Ziegler JL (1979) Bone marrow involvement in Burkitt's lymphoma and its relationship to
    acute B-cell leukemia. Leuk Res 4: 33–59
Magrath IT, Freeman CB, Pizzo P (1980) Characterisation of lymphoma-derived cell lines: comparison
    of cell lines positive and negative for Epstein-Barr virus nuclear antigen. II. Surface Markers. JNCI
    64: 477–483
Mahoney JP, Alexander RW (1980) Primary histiocytic lymphoma of bone: a light and ultrastructural
    study of 4 cases. Am J Surg Pathol 4: 149–161
Mambo NC, Burke JS, Butler JJ (1977) Primary malignant lymphomas of the breast. Cancer 39:
    2033–2040
Mann RB, Jaffe ES, Braylan RC et al. (1976) Non-endemic Burkitt's lymphoma. A B-cell tumor
    related to germinal centres. N Engl J Med 295: 685–691
Mann RB, Jaffe ES, Berard CW (1979) Malignant lymphomas — a conceptual understanding of
    morphologic diversity. A review. Am J Pathol 94: 105–192
Mathe G, Rappaport H, O'Connor GT et al. (1976) Histological and cytological typing of neoplastic
    disease of haemopoietic and lymphoid tissues. In: World Health Organisation international
    histologic classification of tumors No 14. World Health Organisation, Geneva
Maurer R, Taylor CR, Terry R, Lukes RJ (1979) Non-Hodgkin's lymphomas of the thyroid A
    clinicopathologic review of 29 cases applying the Lukes-Collins classification and an immunoperox-
    idase method. Virchows Arch [A] 383: 293–317

McDermott MR, Bienenstock J (1979) Evidence for a common mucosal immunologic system. I. Migration of B immunoblasts into intestinal, respiratory and genital tissues. J Immunol 122: 1892–1898

McNamara JJ, Kingsley WB, Paulson DL et al. (1969) Primary lymphosarcoma of lung. Ann Surg 169: 133–140

Mellsted H, Pettersson D, Holm G (1978) Lymphocyte subpopulations in chronic lymphocytic leukemia (CLL). Acta Med Scand 204: 485–489

Moir DH (1980) Signet-ring cell lymphoma: a case report. Pathology 12: 119–122

Moore I, Wright DH (1984) Primary gastric lymphoma — a tumor of mucosa-associated lymphoid tissue. A histological and immunohistochemical study of 36 cases. Histopathology 8: 1025–1039

Morgan DR, Holgate CS, Dixon MF, Bird CC (1985) Primary small intestinal lymphoma: a study of 39 cases. J Pathol 147: 211–221

Mori Y, Lennert K (1969) Electron microscopic atlas of lymph node cytology and pathology. Springer, Berlin Heidelberg New York

Nanba K, Jaffe ES, Braylan RC et al. (1977) Alkaline phosphatase-positive malignant lymphoma: a subtype of B-cell lymphomas. Am J Clin Pathol 68: 535–542

Nathwani BN (1979) A critical analysis of the classifications of non-Hodgkin's lymphomas. Cancer 44: 347–384

Navas JJ, Battifora H (1977) Primary lymphoma of the breast. Ultrastructural study of two cases. Cancer 39: 2025–2032

Navas-Palacios JJ, Valdes MD, Laheurta-Palacios JJ (1983) Signet-ring cell lymphoma: ultrastructural and immunohistochemical features of three varieties. Cancer 52: 1613–1623

Osborne BM, Butler JJ, Mackay B (1980) Sinusoidal large cell ("histiocytic") lymphoma. Cancer 46: 2484–2491

Osborne BM, Mackay B, Butler JJ, Ordonez NG (1983) Large cell lymphoma with microvillus-like projections: an ultrastructural study. Am J Clin Pathol 79: 443–450

Otto HF, Bettmann I, Weltzien JV, Gebbers JO (1981) Primary intestinal lymphoma. Virchows Arch [A] 391: 9–31

Paladugu RR, Bearman RM, Rappaport H (1980) Malignant lymphoma with primary manifestation in the gonad A clinicopathologic study of 38 patients. Cancer 45: 561–571

Palutke M, Eisenberg L, Michandani I, Tabaczka P, Husain M (1982) Malignant lymphoma of small cleaved lymphocytes of the follicular mantle zone. Blood 59: 317–322

Pangalis GA, Nathwani BN, Rappaport H (1977) Malignant lymphoma, well differentiated lymphocytic. Its relationship with chronic lymphocytic leukemia and macroglobulinemia of Waldenström. Cancer 39: 999–1010

Papadimitriou CS, Papacharalampous NX (1979) Distribution of T lymphocytes in follicular lymphomas as revealed by acid alpha-naphthol acetate esterase. J Clin Pathol 32: 808–813

Pinkus GS, Said JW (1978) Characterization of non-Hodgkin's lymphomas using multiple cell markers. Immunologic, morphologic and cytochemical studies of 72 cases. Am J Pathol 94: 349–380

Pinkus GS, Said JW (1985) Hodgkin's disease, lymphocyte predominance type, nodular — a distinct entity? Unique staining profile for L & H variants of Reed-Sternberg cells defined by monoclonal antibodies to leukocyte common antigen, granulocyte-specific antigen, and B-cell-specific antigen. Am J Pathol 118: 1–6

Pinkus GS, Said JW, Hargreaves HK (1979) Malignant lymphoma, T-cell type: a distinct morphologic variant with large multilobated nuclei, with a report of four cases. Am J Clin Pathol 72: 540–550

Poppema S, Kaiserling E, Lennert K (1979) Hodgkin's disease with lymphocytic predominance, nodular type (nodular paragranuloma) and progressively transformed germinal centres. A cytohistological study. Histopathology 3: 295–308

Poppema S, Elema JD, Halie MR (1981a) Alkaline phosphatase positive lymphomas: a morphologic, immunologic and enzyme histochemical study. Cancer 47: 1303–1312

Poppema S, Bhan AK, Reinherz EL et al. (1981b) Distribution of T cell subsets in human lymph nodes. J Exp Med 153: 30–41

Poppema S, Bhan AK, Reinherz EL (1982) In situ immunologic characterisation of cellular constituents in lymph nodes and spleens involved by Hodgkin's disease. Blood 59: 226–232

Radaszkiewicz T, Dragosics B (1980) Primary lymphomas of the gastrointestinal tract: a clinicopathologic study of 60 cases. Pathol Res Pract 169: 353–365

Ranchod M, Lewin KJ, Dorfman RF (1978) Lymphoid hyperplasia of the gastrointestinal tract: a study of 26 cases and review of the literature. Am J Surg Pathol 2: 383–400

Rappaport H (1966) Tumors of the hemopoietic system. In: Atlas of tumor pathology, Series 3, Fascicle 8. Armed Forces Institute of Pathology, Washington, DC, p 131

Rappaport H, Winter WJ, Hicks EB (1956) Follicular lymphoma: a re-evaluation of its position in the scheme of malignant lymphoma, based on a survey of 253 cases. Cancer 9: 792–821

Richter MN (1928) Generalised reticular cell sarcoma of lymph nodes associated with lymphatic leukemia. Am J Pathol 4: 285–292

Rilke F, Pilotti S, Carbone A, Lombardi L (1978) Morphology of lymphatic cells and of their derived tumors. J Clin Pathol 31: 1009–1056

Risdall R, Hoppe RT, Warnke R (1979) Non-Hodgkin's lymphoma. A study of the evolution of the disease based upon 92 autopsied cases. Cancer 44: 529–542

Rudders RA, Ahl ET, Delellis RA et al. (1983) Surface marker identification of small cleaved follicular center cell lymphomas with a highly favourable prognosis. Cancer Res 42: 349–356

Saltzstein SL (1963) Pulmonary malignant lymphomas and pseudolymphomas: classification, therapy and prognosis.
Cancer 16: 928–955

Saraga P, Hurlimann J, Ozello L (1981) Lymphomas and pseudo-lymphomas of the alimentary tract. An immunohistochemical study with clinical pathologic correlations. Hum Pathol 12: 713–723

Schmid U, Helbron D, Lennert K (1982) Development of malignant lymphoma in myoepithelial sialadenitis (Sjogren's syndrome). Virchows Arch [A] 395: 11–43

Schneider DR, Taylor CR, Parker JW, Cramer AC, Meyer PR, Lukes RJ (1985) Immunoblastic sarcoma of T- and B-cell types: morphologic description and comparison. Hum Pathol 16: 885–900

Shustik C, Bergasgel DE, Pruzanski W (1976) Kappa and lambda light chain disease: survival rates and clinical manifestation. Blood 48: 41–51

Sibley R, Rosai J, Froelich W (1980) A case for the panel: anemone cell tumor. Ultrastruct Pathol 1: 449–453

Silberman S, Fresco R, Steinecker PH (1984) Signet-ring cell lymphoma: a report of a case and review of the literature. Am J Clin Pathol 81: 358–363

Spiro S, Galton DAG, Wiltshaw E, Lohmann RC (1975) Follicular lymphoma: a survey of 75 cases with special reference to the syndrome resembling chronic lymphocytic leukemia. Br J Cancer 31 (suppl 11): 60–72

Splinter TAW, Noorloss A, van Heerde P (1978) CLL and diffuse histiocytic lymphoma in 1 patient: clonal proliferation of two different B cells. Scand J Haematol 20: 29–36

Stein H, Bonk A, Tolksdorf G et al. (1980) Immunohistologic analysis of the organization of normal lymphoid tissue and non-Hodgkin's lymphomas. J Histochem Cytochem 28: 746–760

Stein H, Gerdes J, Mason DY (1982) The normal and malignant germinal centre. Clin Haematol 11: 531–559

Stein H, Mason DY, Gerdes J et al. (1985) The expression of the Hodgkin's disease associated antigen Ki-1 in reactive and neoplastic lymphoid tissue: evidence that Reed-Sternberg cells and histiocytic malignancies are derived from activated lymphoid cells. Blood 66: 848–858

Stein RS, Cousar J, Flexner JM et al. (1979) Malignant lymphomas of follicular centre cell origin in man. III. Prognostic features. Cancer 44: 2226–2243

Stein RS, Cousar J, Flexner JM, Collins RD (1980) Correlations between immunologic markers and histopathologic classifications: clinical implications. Semin Oncol 7: 244–254

Swerdlow SH, Murray LJ (1984) Natural killer (Leu7+) cells in reactive lymphoid tissues and malignant lymphomas. Am J Clin Pathol 81: 459–463

Swerdlow SH, Habeshaw JA, Murray LJ et al. (1983) Centrocytic lymphoma: a distinct clinicopathologic and immunologic entity. A multiparameter study of 18 cases at diagnosis and relapse. Am J Pathol 113: 181–197

Swerdlow SH, Murray LJ, Habeshaw JA, Stansfelt AG (1985) B- and T-cell subsets in follicular centroblastic/centrocytic (cleaved follicular centre cell) lymphoma: an immunohistologic analysis of 26 lymph nodes and 3 spleens. Hum Pathol 16: 339–352

Talal N, Bumin JJ (1964) The development of malignant lymphoma in the course of Sjogren's syndrome. Am J Med 36: 529–540

Tateno M, Yoshiki T, Itoh T et al. (1983) A case of primary B-cell lymphoma of the breast. Cancer 52: 671–674

Taylor CR (1983) Upon the enigma of Hodgkin's disease and the Reed-Sternberg cell. In: Bennett JM (ed) Controversies in the management of lymphomas. Martinus Nijhoff, Boston, pp 91–108

Taylor CR, Russell R, Lukes RJ, Davis RL (1978) An immunohistological study of immunoglobulin content of primary central nervous system lymphomas. Cancer 41: 2198–2205

The Non-Hodgkin's Lymphoma Classification Project (1982) National Cancer Institute sponsored study of classifications of non-Hodgkin's lymphomas. Summary and description of a Working Formulation for clinical usage. Cancer 49: 2112–2135

Thorbecke GJ, Romano TJ, Lerman SP (1974) Regulatory mechanisms and differentiation of lymphoid tissue with particular reference to germinal centre development. In: Brent L, Holborow EJ (eds) Progress in immunology II, vol 3. North Holland, Amsterdam, p 25

Tindle BH (1984) Teaching monograph. Malignant lymphomas. Am J Pathol 116: 119–174

Trump DL, Mann RB, Phelps R et al. (1980) Richter's syndrome: diffuse histiocytic lymphoma in patients with chronic lymphocytic leukemia. A report of 5 cases and review of the literature. Am J Med 68: 539–548

Tubbs RR, Sheibani K, Weiss RA et al. (1981) Immunohistochemistry of fresh-frozen lymphoid tissue with a direct immunoperoxidase technic. Am J Clin Pathol 75: 171–176

Turner RR, Colby TV, MacKintosh FR (1981) Testicular lymphoma: a clinicopathologic study of 35 cases. Cancer 48: 2095–2102

Turner RR, Egbert P, Warnke RA (1984) Lymphocytic infiltrates of the conjunctiva and orbit: immunohistochemical staining of 16 cases. Am J Clin Pathol 81: 447–452

van den Tweel JG, Taylor CR, Parker JW, Lukes RJ (1978) Immunoglobulin inclusions in non-Hodgkin's lymphomas. Am J Clin Pathol 69: 306–313

van Furth R, Cohn ZA, Hirsch JG et al. (1972) The mononuclear phagocytic system: a new classification of macrophages, monocytes and their precursor cells. Bull WHO 46: 845–852

van Heerde P, Feltkamp CA, Feltkamp-Vroom TM, Koudstal J, van Unnik JAM (1980) Non-Hodgkin's lymphoma. Immunohistochemical and electron microscopical findings in relation to lightmicroscopy. Cancer 46: 2210–2220

Venables GS, Proctor SJ, Bates D et al. (1980) Intracranial disease in non-Hodgkin's lymphoma. Q J Med 59: 111–131

Vimadalal SD, Said JW, Voyles H (1983) Gastric lymphoreticular neoplasms: an immunologic study of 36 cases. Am J Clin Pathol 80: 792–799

Warnke R, Levy R (1978) Immunopathology of follicular lymphomas. A model of B-lymphocyte homing. N Engl J Med 298: 481–486

Warnke RA, Kim H, Fuks Z, Dorfman RF (1977) The co-existence of nodular and diffuse patterns in nodular non-Hodgkin's lymphomas. Significance and clinico-pathologic correlation. Cancer 40: 1229–1233

Weisenburger DD, Nathwani BN, Diamond LW et al. (1981) Malignant lymphoma, intermediate lymphocytic type: a clinicopathologic study of 42 cases. Cancer 48: 1415–1425

Weisenburger DD, Kim H, Rappaport H (1982) Mantle-zone lymphoma: a follicular variant of intermediate lymphocytic lymphoma. Cancer 49: 1429–1438

Weiss LM, Wood GS, Dorfman RF (1985a) T-cell signet-ring cell lymphoma. A histologic, ultrastructural, and immunohistochemical study of two cases. Am J Surg Pathol 9: 273–280

Weiss LM, Yousem SA, Warnke RA (1985b) Non-Hodgkin's lymphomas of the lung. A study of 19 cases emphasising the utility of frozen section immunologic studies in differential diagnosis. Am J Surg Pathol 9: 480–490

Weissman IL, Warnke R, Butcher EC et al. (1978) The lymphoid system. Its normal architecture and the potential for understanding the system through the study of lymphoproliferative diseases. Hum Pathol 9: 25–45

Willis RA (1948) Pathology of tumours. Butterworths, London

Wiltshaw E (1976) The natural history of extramedullary plasmacytoma and its relation to solitary myeloma of bone and myelomatosis. Medicine 55: 217–238

Wolf JA, Spjut H (1981) Focal lymphoid hyperplasia of the stomach preceding gastric lymphoma: case report and review of the literature. Cancer 48: 2518–2523

Wright DH (1964) Burkitt's tumor. A postmortem study of 50 cases Br J Surg 51: 245–251

Wright DH, Isaacson P (1983) Biopsy pathology of the lymphoreticular system. Chapman and Hall, London

Yamanaka N, Ishii Y, Koshiba H et al. (1980) A study of surface markers in gastrointestinal lymphoma. Gastroenterology 79: 673–677

York JC, Glick AD, Cousar JB, Collins RE (1984) Changes in the appearance of hemopoietic and lymphoid neoplasms: clinical, pathologic, and biologic implications. Hum Pathol 15: 11–38

York JC II, Cousar JB, Glick AD et al. (1985) Morphologic and immunologic evidence of composite B- and T-cell lymphomas. A report of three cases developing in follicular centre cell lymphomas. Am J Clin Pathol 84: 35–43

Zulman J, Jaffe R, Talal N (1978) Evidence that the malignant lymphoma of Sjögren's syndrome is a monoclonal B-cell neoplasm. N Engl J Med 299: 1215–1220

18   T Cell Neoplasia

Introduction

T cell neoplasms are monoclonal populations which often produce lymphokines influencing a wide range of cell types. Lymphokines are molecules with the capacity to activate or affect the function of B cells, macrophages, bone marrow stem cells and, in the case of interleukin 1 (IL-1), connective tissue and certain neurons involved in the genesis of fever.

Lack of a marker for monoclonality in the T cell system has been a major source of frustration in the study of T cell neoplasms. In contrast to neoplasms of the B cell system, in which immunoglobulin light chain restriction has provided fairly reliable evidence of neoplasia, none of the available T cell markers can be used to distinguish reactive from neoplastic T cell populations. Subset restriction, e.g. predominance of cells of either the CD4+ or CD8+ subset, can occur in the non-neoplastic disorders, and is not an indication of monoclonality. Conversely, T cell lymphomas of one subset may contain an admixture of T cells of the other subset, and co-expression of helper and suppressor subset antigens on neoplastic T cells has also been described. Furthermore, most reactive lymphoid tissues, as well as many non-T cell lymphomas, contain numerous T cells; in some B cell lymphomas, such as follicular lymphoma, non-neoplastic T cells may even predominate. Consequently, a diagnosis of T cell neoplasia can be made with certainty only when a homogeneous population of morphologically malignant cells can be shown to have a T cell marker. This has seriously hampered our understanding of T cell neoplasia; it is likely that many of the cases of T cell lymphoma reported in the literature are in fact disorders of other cell types.

Gene technology, better techniques of chromosome analysis and gene mapping are rapidly producing fascinating information with tantalising hints that the genesis of malignancy in T cells may soon be better understood. T cell lymphomas can now be diagnosed by determining the existence of the uniform rearrangement of T receptor chain genes (Aisenberg et al. 1985; Bertness et al. 1985; O'Connor et al. 1985). In recent years, the T cell receptor for antigen has been identified, and the gene probes for the α, β and γ chains have been produced. The first probe produced was for β chain genes, which have extensive homology with the immunoglobulin heavy chain genes and undergo rearrangement during T cell maturation in a manner analogous to the rearrangement of immunoglobulin genes in B cells. Each T cell carries its gene receptor in a unique configuration; the T cell receptor gene thus becomes a unique clonal marker for the progeny of a single T cell. Detection of a rearranged T cell receptor gene (by virtue of the rearranged segment being detected by the gene probe having a different length from that of the corresponding germline segment) will simultaneously define the T cell nature of a lymphoid cell population as well as its clonal origin.

Chromosomal Abnormalities in T Cell Malignancies

The cytogenetic abnormalities which are being revealed by recent studies of T cell malignancies are frequently analogous to those found in B cell neoplasms. The locus for the α chain of the T cell receptor is frequently juxtaposed to proto-oncogenes or putative proto-oncogenes (Croce et al. 1985). The translocations are believed to cause abnormal regulation of transcription of these oncogenes and may be produced by the enzyme system involved in the normal rearrangements of genes for the T cell receptor (Croce 1986).

Some chromosomal abnormalities which have been associated with T cell neoplasms are listed in Table 18.1. In mice, T cell leukaemias bear an extra chromosome 15. No abnormality is found in other spontaneous or virus-induced leukaemias or lymphomas of mice. The chromosomal abnormalities associated with human T cell neoplasia affect particularly chromosomes 7, 11 and 14. Translocations affect the Ti_{α} genes in adult T cell leukaemia/lymphoma (ATL), T cell chronic lymphocytic leukaemia (T-CLL) and T cell lymphoma. The constant region γ chain genes which reside on the short arm of chromosome 7 are involved in chromosomal rearrangements in T cells from individuals with ataxia telangiectasia (AT). The Ti_{β} chain genes on chromosome 7 have not yet been implicated in translocations associated with T cell malignancies (Croce et al. 1985).

In AT, a dominantly transmitted disease, deficient T lymphocyte function correlates with depletion of paracortical T lymphocytes in the lymph nodes. Patients with AT show an increased frequency of T cell acute lymphoblastic leukaemia (T-ALL) and T-CLL as compared with normal subjects. Chromosomal rearrangements, involving 7p15–7p14, 7q35–7q32, 14q12–7q11 and 14q32 have been found in lymphocytes from patients with AT (Murre et al. 1985). Each of these loci include genes that rearrange during the somatic development of T cells. The 7p15–7p14 region of rearrangement contains the Ti_{γ} chain locus. Portions of the regions coding for the variable portions of the T cell receptor are subject to a high rate of spontaneous mutation during rearrangement of these genes in T cell differentiation. The same applies to the genes encoding immunoglobulin. The reason for the susceptibility to chromosomal breaks and rearrangements in AT is believed to be a defective capacity to repair DNA, perhaps after breaks occur.

Table 18.1. Chromosomal involvement in T cell neoplasia[a]

Neoplasm	Type of aberration
A. Chromosomal abnormalities in the T cell neoplasms	
ATL	Trisomy 3
	Translocations involving all or parts of
	5p15–p13, 6q14–q27, 14q32
	del (6)(q15–q21)
	inv (14)(q11;q32)
	t(14;14)(q11q12;q32)
T-ALL	t(11,14)(p13;q11)
	Rearrangements involving 7p15–7p14,
	7q32–7q35, 14q13–14q11, 14q32
T-CLL	Translocations involving
	5p15–p13, 14q11–q13
	inv (14)(q11;q32)
T-PLL	Translocations and deletions involving
	5p15–p13
B. Chromosomes involved in rearrangements in T cell neoplasia	
T-ALL	7, 11, 14
Pre-B ALL	1,19
ATL	3,5,6,14
T-CLL	5, 14
T cell malignant lymphoma	6, 14
T-PLL	5

[a]Data from Human Gene Mapping 8 (1985).

Trisomy (the occurrence of a triplicate chromosome) of chromosome 21 is the most common acquired change in ALL and is also frequent in acute myeloblastic leukaemia (AML). It has been postulated that trisomy 21 is intimately concerned with the genesis of the acute leukaemias that develop in Down's syndrome (Rowley 1981).

ALL patients with bulky disease of the lymph nodes, spleen or mediastinum, so-called lymphomatous ALL, appear to represent a distinct subgroup. In six patients with lymphomatous ALL deletions, unbalanced translocations or loss of the entire arm led to loss of bands p22-p21 on the short arm of chromosome 9. In contrast, ALL patients without lymphomatous manifestations rarely have this abnormality (Chilcote et al. 1985). Loss of chromosomal material in the region of 9p22–21 may be related to the loss of the enzyme methylthioadenosine phosphorylase, which has been reported in these patients.

The translocation t(11;14)(p13;q11), splitting the Ti$_\alpha$ locus at 14q11.2, has been described in ATL; 14q+ and non-random trisomy of chromosome 7 have also been described.

The long arm of chromosome 14 is most frequently affected in T-CLL. Abnormalities are reported to occur in 28% of cases (Pandolfi et al. 1985). Single or double breaks are found at the same bands in both HTLV-I-positive and -negative cases. It has been postulated that an oncogene (tcl-1) at 14q32 can be activated by chromosome inversion or translocation, resulting in the juxtaposition of the tcl-1 oncogene and the Ti$_\alpha$ chain locus at 14q11–14q12 (Croce et al. 1985.

Rearrangements that involve chromosome 14 are also found commonly in T cell lymphomas. The region involved is between 14q11 and 14q13.

Gene Rearrangements in T Cell Malignancies

Determination of Ti receptor gene rearrangements is the definitive and, indeed, the only way to demonstrate a monoclonal T cell population. A monoclonal population of T cells can be detected when its DNA represents only 5% of that present in a sample. This is similar to the situation for B cells when an Ig gene probe is used.

Most of the rearrangement studies to date have been made on the Ti_β chain genes, because of the availability of the genetic probe, but other probes are becoming available. Ti_α genes are also rearranged in T cell malignancies and rearrangement of Ti_γ genes has also been demonstrated in a few cases. Variable region gene fragments have been found to be deleted in some CD4 + and CD8 + T cell malignancies.

Clonal Ti receptor rearrangements have been demonstrated in leukaemia associated with mycosis fungoides, Sézary syndrome, acute non-B cell lympho-blastic leukaemias, CD4 + (T4 +) CLL, $T_{suppressor}$ lymphocytosis with granulocy-topenia and lymphoblastic lymphomas (Waldmann et al. 1985). Clonal rearrange-ment of the Ti genes can be determined in biopsies of skin and lymph nodes in mycosis fungoides (Weiss et al. 1985). These clonal rearrangements can be demonstrated when other T cell markers are absent, e.g. in ALL. It appears that all non-B, non-T cell ALL cases in children have rearranged μ heavy chains; 10% also have rearrangement of the Ti_β chain genes (Tawa et al. 1985).

Until recently, malignant lymphoma occurring in coeliac disease was con-sidered, on histological and immunohistochemical criteria, to be malignant histiocytosis. It is most probably a T cell lymphoma, as shown in four cases of so-

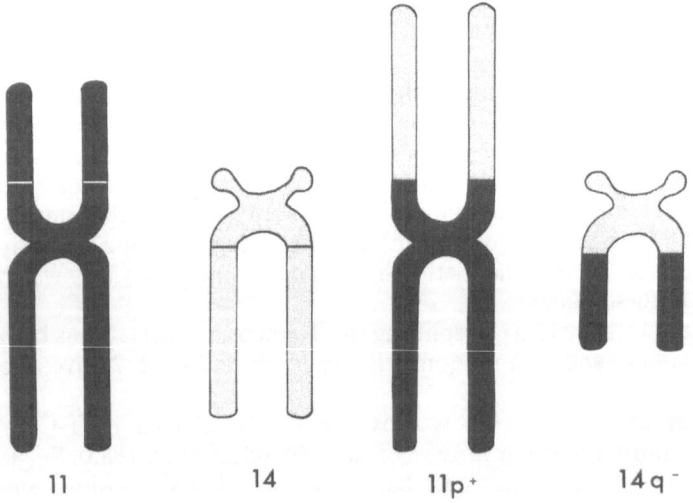

11   14   11p⁺   14q⁻

Fig. 18.1. The t(11;14) (p13;q11) translocation in ALL. The translocation breakpoint on chromosome 14 splits the gene for the α-chain of the T cell receptor, so that its variable genes remain on the truncated 14q-chromosome and its constant genes are transferred to chromosome 11 (11p+). The genes for β globulin, c-*ras* and lactic dehydrogenase A (LDHA) are also translocated to 11, and the gene for nucleoside phosphorylase remains behind.

called malignant histiocytosis of the intestine studied recently (Isaacson et al. 1985). All had T cell markers, and in the three studied by molecular hybridisation, the Ti_β chain was rearranged.

The locus for the Ti_α chain is at band q11.2 of chromosome 14. This chromosome region is involved in inversions and translocations in T cell neoplasms. The translocation t(11;14)(p13;q11) (Fig. 18.1) splits the locus for the Ti_α chain. The V_α genes remain on the 14q-chromosome and the C_α genes go to the recipient chromosome 11. This was determined by hybridising ALL cells with cultured mouse T lymphoma cells. Various hybrids contained chromosomes 14q-, 11p+ or both. Gene probe analysis showed that the V_α genes were on 14q- and the C_α genes were on 11p+ chromosomes (Erikson et al. 1985).

Although descriptions are still rather preliminary, having been made on a limited series of selected cases, it is clear that analysis of Ti gene rearrangements will have a very important impact on the classification and understanding of lymphocyte malignancies. However, clonal rearrangement of T receptor genes is not a characteristic of malignancy in itself. Pure clones of benign reactive T cells could not be distinguished from a malignant population by this technique.

Immunoglobulin Genes in T Cell Malignancies

Immunoglobulin heavy chain rearrangements have been demonstrated in about 10% of leukaemic T cell populations, but none have had Ig light chain rearrangements. For example, a case of T-ALL has been described as having immunoglobulin μ chain gene rearrangement but germline configuration of light chains (Ha et al. 1984). Ti genes are rearranged in a proportion of cases with AML.

References

Aisenberg AA, Krontiris TG, Mak TW, Wilkes BM (1985) Rearrangement of the gene for the beta chain of the T-cell receptor in T-cell chronic lymphocytic leukemia and related disorders. N Engl J Med 313: 529–533

Bertness V, Kirsch I, Hollis G, Johnson B, Bunn PA (1985) T-cell receptor gene rearrangements as clinical markers of human T-cell lymphomas. N Engl J Med 313: 534–538

Chilcote RR, Brown E, Rowley JD (1985) Lymphoblastic leukemia with lymphomatous features associated with abnormalities of the short arm of chromosome 9. N Engl J Med 313: 286–291

Croce CM (1986) Molecular mechanisms involved in human B and T cell neoplasia. In: Proceedings of the XXI congress of the International Society of Haematology, Sydney, May 1986, p 3

Croce CM, Isobe M, Palumbo M et al. (1985) Gene for α-chain of human T-cell receptor: location on chromosome 14 region involved in T-cell neoplasms. Science 227: 1044–1047

Erikson J, Williams DL, Finan J, Nowell PC, Croce CM (1985) Locus of the α-chain of the T-cell receptor is split by chromosome translocation in T-cell leukemias. Science 229: 784–786

Ha K, Minden M, Hozumi N, Gelfand EM (1984) Immunoglobulin μ-chain gene rearrangement in a patient with T cell acute lymphoblastic leukaemia. J Clin Invest 73: 1232–1236

Human Gene Mapping 8 (1985) Eighth international workshop on human gene mapping, Helsinki, Finland, 4–10 August, 1985. Cytogenet Cell Genet 40 (1–4): 1–823

Isaacson PG, O'Connor NTJ, Spencer J et al. (1985) Malignant histiocytosis of the intestine: a T-cell lymphoma. Lancet II: 688–691

Murre C, Waldmann RA, Morton CC et al. (1985) Human γ-chains are rearranged in leukaemic T cells and map to the short arm of chromosome 7. Nature 316: 549–552

O'Connor NTJ, Wainscoat JS, Weatherall DJ et al. (1985) Rearrangement of the T-cell-receptor β-chain gene in the diagnosis of lymphoproliferative disorders. Lancet I: 1295–1297

Pandolfi F, de Rossi G, Semenzato G (1985) T-helper phenotype leukaemias: role of HTLV-I. Lancet II: 1367–1368 (letter)

Rowley JD (1981) Down syndrome and acute leukaemia: increased risk may be due to trisomy 21. Lancet II: 1020–1022

Tawa A, Hozumi N, Minden M, Mak TW, Gelfand EW (1985) Rearrangement of the T-cell receptor β-chain in non-T-cell non B-cell-acute lymphoblastic leukemia of childhood. N Engl J Med 313: 1033–1037

Waldmann TA, Davis MM, Bongiovanni KF, Korsmeyer SJ (1985) Rearrangement of genes for the antigen receptor on T cells as markers of lineage and clonality in human lymphoid neoplasms. N Engl J Med 313: 776–783

Weiss LM, Hu E, Wood GS et al. (1985) Clonal rearrangements of T-cell receptor genes in mycosis fungoides and dermatopathic lymphadenopathy. N Engl J Med 313: 539–544

19 T Cell Leukaemias and Lymphomas

Introduction

Up to 30% of acute lymphoblastic leukaemias (ALLs) and 10%–20% of non-Hodgkin's lymphomas (NHLs) are of T cell lineage (Collins 1982). In many respects, much less is known of the T cell leukaemias and lymphomas then the B cell malignancies, and it is only recently that they have been studied in the detail previously accorded the B cell neoplasms. The classification of T cell malignancies is even more controversial than the classification of B cell malignancies. No more than a few authors have attempted to provide a comprehensive classification of this subject (Catovsky et al. 1982a; Collins 1982; Kadin et al. 1983; Leong 1984). As with the B cell neoplasms, it is not always possible to make a distinction between lymphoma and leukaemia. In fact, the overlap is even more pronounced in the T cell malignancies and the use of the term "lymphoma/leukaemia" is often more appropriate.

In keeping with the approach adopted for the B cell malignancies, we propose to classify the T cell neoplasms in accordance with their correspondence to the differentiation stages of normal T lymphocytes. An outline of such a classification has been proposed by Collins (1982). The maturation stages of T lymphocytes can broadly be divided into a bone marrow stage, a thymic stage and a peripheral stage. These three anatomical compartments contain T lymphocytes at different stages of maturation identified by their differentiation antigens, as discussed previously in detail (see Chap. 10, p. 115).

The bone marrow contains at least two populations of T lymphocytes: a small population of putative lymphoid precursors which are positive for terminal deoxynucleotidyl transferase (TdT) and lack T cell antigens detected by antibodies to CD1, CD2, CD3, CD4, CD5, CD8; and a larger population of T cells with a mature phenotype similar to that of peripheral T cells (Janossy et al. 1981a). Normal thymocytes originate from bone marrow precursor cells that migrate to the thymus (Stutman 1977). In the thymus, three subcompartments are identifiable, viz., the subcapsular cortex, cortex and medulla. The T cell percursors reside in the subcapsular cortex, where, postnatally, they are seen as a population of large, rapidly dividing CD2+ cells, termed "prothymocytes" (Galili et al. 1980). These prothymocytes or blast cells comprise about 10% of the total thymic cells and are reactive to two monoclonal antibodies, T10 and OKT9 (Reinherz et al.

1980). Within the thymic microenvironment, the prothymocytes undergo marked changes in surface antigens and gain some degree of functional maturity. In the thymic cortex are found the common thymocytes, comprising about 70% of the total thymocytes. They are T10+, CD1+, CD4+, CD5+ and CD8+. The thymic medulla contains the late or mature thymocytes which make up about 20% of the thymic population and segregate into T10+, CD2+, CD3+, CD4+, CD5+ helper T cells and T10+, CD2+, CD3+, CD5+, CD8+ suppressor T cells.

In the peripheral compartment, the T cells lose the T10 marker and exist as helper (CD2+, CD3+, CD4+, CD5+) and suppressor (CD2+, CD3+, CD5+ and CD8+) subsets (Reinherz et al. 1980).

A classification of T cell malignancies, based on differentiation stage in the three major compartments (Leong 1984), is shown in Table 19.1. While the neoplasms of the bone marrow compartment are all leukaemias, it will become evident that all T cell malignancies may involve the peripheral blood; thus the term "lymphoma/leukaemia" seems appropriate because of the considerable overlap between leukaemia and lymphomas. For this reason the T neoplasms will not be discussed under separate chapter headings of "Leukaemias" and "Lymphomas", as were the B cell neoplasms.

Table 19.1. T cell malignancies — a classification

Compartment	Malignancy
1. Bone marrow	*Immature T cell markers* T acute lymphoblastic leukaemia
	Mature T cell markers T prolymphocytic leukaemia T hairy cell leukaemia T chronic lymphocytic leukaemia Adult T cell leukaemia/lymphoma
2. Thymic	Lymphoblastic lymphoma
3. Peripheral	Cutaneous T cell lymphoma Node-based T cell lymphoma

T Cell Neoplasms of the Bone Marrow Compartment

There are two major populations of T lymphocytes in the bone marrow:

1. TdT+ putative lymphoid precursors, which are CD1−, CD2−, CD3−, CD4−, CD5−, CD8− and OKT10+.
2. lymphocytes of peripheral T cell phenotype, which are TdT−, CD1+, CD2+, CD3+, CD4+/CD8+, CD5+ and OKT10−.

The proportion of CD4+ inducer/helper T cells in the bone marrow is low, whereas that of CD8+ suppressor/cytotoxic T cells is high, the ratio of CD4+:CD8+ cells being between 1:6.7 and 1:2 (Janossy et al. 1981b), which contrasts with a ratio in peripheral blood of about 2: 1 (Janossy and Prentice 1982).

T cell neoplasms in the bone marrow compartment may derive from these two populations of T lymphocytes. It is possible that T acute lymphoblastic leukaemia is a neoplasm which arises from the T cells with immature phenotype, while the other forms of T cell leukaemias, viz., T prolymphocytic leukaemia, T hairy cell leukaemia, T chronic lymphocytic leukaemia and adult T cell leukaemia/lymphoma, arise from the mature T lymphocytes which are resident in the bone marrow or from peripheral T lymphocytes recirculating through the bone marrow.

T Acute Lymphoblastic Leukaemia

About 14%–30% of ALLs are identifiable as being of T cell lineage by E-rosette formation or reactivity with T cell antibodies (Brouet et al. 1976; Nadler et al. 1980; Greaves et al. 1981). Staining with an anti-T cell antibody identified 4%–5% of E– leukaemias which would otherwise be classified as common ALL (Brouet and Seligmann 1978). T-ALL occurs with equal frequency in adults and children but is four times more common in males than in females. It is characterised by high bone marrow and blood concentrations of blast cells with markedly hyperchromatic convoluted nuclei of the L1 and L2 morphology by the French-American-British (FAB) classification. The leukaemic T lymphoblasts are identified by the presence of E receptors and T surface antigens but are CD10- (CALLA-), sIg-, and do not stain for peroxidase, Sudan B or chloroacetate esterase. In about 75% of patients the blast cells will stain for acid phosphatase and acid α-naphthyl esterase and are also positive for TdT.

An anterior mediastinal mass is present in 53% of patients with T-ALL (Greaves et al. 1981), and infiltration of the central nervous system liver, spleen, lymph nodes and mediastinum is more common at diagnosis or relapse than with any other acute leukaemia. Meningeal involvement is reported to occur in 95% of children and 20% of adults with T-ALL, about five times more frequently than in patients with common ALL (Henderson 1983).

T-ALL shares many of the clinical features of T cell lymphoblastic lymphomas (LLs) in that both conditions arise predominantly in adolescent males who often present with a mediastinal mass. T-ALL differs from T-LL only in the degree of bone marrow involvement and duration of treatment-related response. By definition, LLs lack extensive involvement of bone marrow (less than 25% marrow blasts; Sen and Borella 1975; Tsukimoto et al. 1976) and blood, whereas 45% of T-ALL has been found to have a white blood count of over 10×10^9/litre and extensive bone marrow infiltration (Greaves et al. 1981). As LL progesses, however, bone marrow and peripheral blood tumour infiltration occurs and the disease then appears clinically indistinguishable from T-ALL. The many shared clinical features and the frequently observed progression of LL to T-ALL have led to the suggestion that they may represent stages of the same disease. Analysis of cell surface phenotypes of tumour cells from patients with T-ALL indicated that the majority of tumour cells had markers of early thymocytes, being T9+, T10+, without other markers. A smaller number were classed as deriving from common thymocytes, being CD1+, CD4+, CD8+ (Reinherz et al. 1980), whereas the majority of tumour cells in LL expressed the phenotypes of common or late thymocytes, lacked T9 and CD1 antigens and showed CD4 and CD8 subset segregation, i.e. expressed either CD4 or CD8 (Bernard et al. 1981; Roper et al. 1983). These results suggest that T-ALL and LL are probably not different clinical stages of a single neoplastic process but, in fact, represent separate neoplastic diseases which reflect the different stages of normal T cell differentiation. The resemblance of the phenotypic characteristics of T-ALL to those of early thymocytes or "prothymocytes" has been taken as presumptive evidence that they may be of bone marrow derivation. However, the normal marrow precursor of T-ALL has not been definitely established, as T-ALL cells are TdT+ and HuTLA+, whereas TdT+ lymphoid cells from normal juvenile bone marrow are HuTLA− (Bradstock et al. 1980).

The monoclonal antibody 3A1 (CD7), a pan-T marker present on 85% of ER+ peripheral blood lymphocytes and almost all adolescent thymocytes including prothymocytes (Haynes et al. 1979), has been shown to be the most reliable T cell marker of immature T cell leukaemias. All cases with clinically typical T-ALL, but expressing no other B, T or CALLA antigens were 3A1+ (Haynes et al. 1981; Minowada 1982).

Peanut agglutinin (PNA) has been proven useful in the study of T cell malignancies. PNA is specific for D-galactosyl-(1–3)N acetyl D-galactosamine and binds to immature cortical thymocytes that are CD1+, CD4+, CD7+, CD8+ CD1+, and CD3−. While over 80% of normal cortical thymocytes are PNA+, normal mature peripheral blood lymphocytes do not bind PNA unless treated with neuraminidase. The presence of high numbers of circulating PNA+ cells has been postulated to be of prognostic significance in T-ALL. Levin et al. (1980) reported that 8 of 13 patients in whom more than 15% of the circulating cells were PNA+ relapsed early, compared with none of 12 patients with less than 15% PNA+ cells.

In 1978, Anderson and Metzgar described several heteroantisera reactive with a T lymphocyte-associated antigen which was present on all E+ ALL as well as several cases of E− ALL. Some workers have defined T-ALL on the basis of reactivity of blasts with these antisera by using a microcytotoxicity assay (Pullen et al. 1981, 1983). A recent study suggested that CD5 or CD7 monoclonal antibodies could accurately replace the heteroantisera described by Anderson and Metzgar in the definition of T-ALL (Borowitz et al. 1985).

T Prolymphocytic Leukaemia

Prolymphocytic leukaemia (PLL), first described as a rare variant of chronic lymphocytic leukaemia (CLL), is now recognised as a separate clinicopathological entity. Only about 17% of cases of PLL have a mature T cell phenotype (Catovsky 1983). The mean age of patients with T-PLL is 64 years (range 51–74 years), with a male preponderance. They usually present with a lymphocytosis of more than 100×10^9/litre; splenomegaly, lymphadenomegaly, hepatomegaly and cutaneous deposits are the most common findings. In contrast, lymphadenomegaly and skin deposits are almost never seen in B-PLL. The white blood count tends to be higher and to rise more rapidly in T-PLL. In addition, T-PLL is a more aggressive disease, associated with a significantly shorter median survival of 7 months compared with the median survival of 24 months seen in B-PLL.

Recognition of the prolymphocyte is the most important diagnostic step. The prolymphocyte is slightly larger than the small lymphocytes in the typical case of

CLL and has a larger rim of cytoplasm. Though the chromatin is moderately clumped, there is a single prominent central nucleolus in most cells, and some condensation of peripheral nuclear chromatin is usually present. T prolymphocytes have medium to large electron-dense granules localised to one area of the cytoplasm (Costello et al. 1980), while B prolymphocytes have fewer, smaller and less electron-dense lysosomal granules. The nucleus of T-PLL cells may be quite irregular, whereas, in B-PLL, the nucleus is more often regular or, at the most, has a deep cleft. Apart from mitochondria, few cytoplasmic organelles are present in T-PLL cells.

α-napthyl acetate esterase (ANAE), β-glucuronidase and β-glucosaminidase have been found to be consistently positive in T-PLL, and acid phosphatase gives a reaction of variable intensity in about 60% of cases (Costello et al. 1980). All cases of T-PLL are E+, TdT− and none express the CD1 antigen. The majority of cases have a helper/inducer phenotype, and a cytotoxic/suppressor membrane phenotype is found in a minority (Catovsky et al. 1982a; Chan et al. 1982). Pan-T markers such as CD3 are lost in some cases, while CD4 and CD8 are co-expressed in some and absent in others. The surface marker studies suggest that the prolymphocytes are at a later stage of differentiation than cells of T-ALL and lymphoblastic lymphoma. The presence of strong ANAE activity also suggests that the cells are post-thymic lymphocytes, as this enzyme is not found in immature T cells.

Pittmann et al. (1982) reported one or more marker chromosomes and hypodiploidy in T-PLL karyotypes after stimulation with phytohaemagglutinin (PHA; Pittman et al. 1982). Catovsky reported abnormalities of chromosomes 2, 7, 8, 9, 11 and 16 in T-PLL, in comparison with 1, 3, 6, 12 and 14 in B-PLL (Catovsky et al. 1982a). The eighth Human Gene Mapping conference (Human Gene Mapping 8 1985) recorded translocations and deletions involving chromosome 5.

T Hairy Cell Leukaemia

Hairy cell leukaemia (HCL) is a distinct lymphoproliferative disorder with clearly defined diagnostic criteria of pancytopenia, splenomegaly and infiltration of bone marrow and blood by characteristic mononuclear cells with "hairy" cytoplasmic projections. While the published evidence indicates that the majority of cases of HCL are proliferations of B lymphocytes (Jansen et al. 1982; Korsmeyer et al. 1983), in rare instances HCL may express a T cell phenotype (Cawley et al. 1978; Naeim et al. 1978; Saxon et al. 1978). These cases have morphologically typical hairy HCL cells with ER+ tartrate-resistant acid phosphatase activity reacting with anti-T lymphocyte antiserum. The hairy cells from two patients switched from B to T phenotypes when stimulated with PHA in culture (Guglielmi et al. 1980).

Kalyanaraman et al. (1982) reported a case of T-HCL with leukaemic cells which showed the typical "hairy" cytoplasmic projections, contained tartrate-resistant acid phosphatase and had a CD4+, mature T cell phenotype. The patient had serum antibodies reactive with a structural protein (p24) of human T cell leukaemia/lymphoma virus (HTLV-I) and a cell line derived from the spleen cells of the patient expressed antigens cross-reactive with HTLV proteins. The viral particles found in the cultured spleen cells were not identical to HTLV-I and were considered to represent a closely related virus named HTLV-II.

T Cell Chronic Lymphocytic Leukaemia

CLL is most commonly derived from B cells. However, in less that 5% of cases the proliferating lymphocytes are malignant T cells, as defined by T cell specific heteroantisera and E-rosetting techniques. The term "T cell chronic lymphocytic leukaemia" has not yet been clearly defined so that it has even been said that "T-cell CLL has been a nosologic entity accompanied by confusion and controversy" (Simpkins et al. 1985). The term has been used loosely to encompass a wide variety of clinical and morphological entities, including T-PLL, T cell lymphoma with peripheral blood involvement, and the T cell leukaemia/lymphoma described in southwestern Japan, the Caribbean basin and the southeastern USA.

The cases originally reported from France (Brouet et al. 1975) had leukaemic cells with diverse morphology. Lymphocytes were small and mature in some, large with irregular and bizarre nuclei in others, or displayed the features of prolymphocytes. Numerous prominent azurophilic granules were present in the lymphocytes of about half the cases reported (Brouet et al. 1975). Likewise, Levine et al. (1981) recognised T-CLL with three clinicopathological expressions: a "prolymphocytic" type with round to oval nucleus, condensed chromatin, and prominent nucleolus; a "knobby" type with varied irregular, or knobby nuclear configuration, condensed chromatin, and inconspicuous nucleolus; and, lastly, a "cytoplasmic" type with round to oval nucleus, condensed chromatin, inconspicuous nucleolus and abundant cytoplasm with azurophilic granules. Costello et al. (1980), however, contended that the term "T-CLL" should be restricted to T-cell leukaemic proliferations with essentially normal mature T cell morphology which are generally indistinguishable from the B cell form of the disease.

Because of this controversy it is difficult to provide an accurate clinical picture of T-CLL. The age incidence is wide, but younger than in B-CLL, with an average age of less that 50 years at presentation. In the original French series (Brouet et al. 1975), presenting features included massive splenomegaly, anaemia, skin infiltration and moderate hepatomegaly. Lymphadenomegaly was found in only 1 of their 11 patients. In an updated series of T-CLL, Brouet and Seligmann (1981) reported lymphocyte counts below 15×10^9/litre in every one of their 21 patients. Lymphocytic infiltration in bone marrow aspirates and biopsies was moderate when compared with B-CLL but marked when the peripheral lymphocyte count was considered. Seven patients had severe neutropenia. Catovsky et al. (1982b) reported a similar experience with 16 cases of T-CLL, although high lymphocyte counts in T-CLL have occasionally been reported (Reinherz et al. 1979). Polyclonal hypergammaglobulinaemia (Brouet et al. 1975; Catovsky et al. 1982b) and pronounced hypogammaglobulinaemia associated with red cell aplasia may occur (Nagasawa et al. 1981; Thien et al. 1982).

Conspicuous azurophilic granules may be found in the malignant T cells. Electron microscopy reveals small to medium-sized membrane-bound lysosomal granules, an active Golgi apparatus and frequent parallel tubular arrays. Acid phosphatase is positive in nearly all cases with localisation in the lysosomal granules and parallel tubular arrays; β-glucuronidase and β-glucosaminidase are also strongly positive. The staining with ANAE is more variable and tends to be negative or weak and diffuse in cells with azurophilic granules, in contrast to the strong localised dot positivity seen in most other mature T cell proliferations.

Cases of T-CLL described in the literature seem to separate into two subtypes based on clinical, cytomorphological, and immunological grounds. One subtype is characterised by patients with long survival, only moderate lymphocytosis and with neoplastic lymphocytes containing prominent cytoplasmic granules (Brouet et al. 1975; Catovsky et al. 1979; Brisbane et al. 1983; Phyliky et al. 1983; Singh et al. 1984). The other subtype is characterised by patients with aggressive disease, very high lymphocyte counts, and leukaemic lymphocytes lacking azurophilic granules (Boumsell et al. 1981; Aisenberg et al. 1982; Knowles and Halper 1982; Pandolfi et al. 1982; Pizzoli et al. 1982).

In a review of the literature on T-CLL identified by the presence of ERs, Phyliky et al. (1983) found certain common characteristics among the 25 cases which expressed CD8 or cytotoxic/suppressor phenotype. Although there were some variations in the clinical picture, the symptoms came on insidiously, except when there was pure red cell aplasia or severe neutropenia. Physical findings included mild to moderate splenomegaly and, to a lesser extent, hepatomegaly. Lymphade-nomegaly and skin infiltration by neoplastic cells were uncommon. Leucocyte counts were less than 20×10^9/litre with an absolute lymphocytosis. In the moderately cellular bone marrow, 20%–70% of the cells were lymphocytes, often occurring in focal aggregates mimicking reactive nodules. There was hypergam-maglobulinaemia in one-third of cases, but the most striking feature was the indolent nature of the disease, many patients being alive at the time of review (up to 46 months without treatment; Pandolfi et al. 1982; Brisbane et al. 1983).

The CD8+ leukaemic lymphocytes were large (15–18 μm diameter), having abundant pale blue cytoplasm which contained many prominent azurophilic granules. The relatively small nuclei were round and contained clumped chroma-tin, but nucleoli were not present. Apart from being CD8+, the leukaemic cells were ER+, CD3+ (Leu-4+), CD5+ (Leu-1+), HLA-DR– and CD4–. The leukaemic cells invariably had intense activity of acid phosphatase and β-glucuronidase but showed little or no staining for ANAE and tartrate-resistant acid phosphatase.

In contrast, most reported cases of CD4+, CD8+ T-CLL have presented with relatively high white cell counts with a mean of 106×10^9/litre (range $31–270 \times 10^9$/litre) and with considerable organ involvement. The leukaemic cells were usually either small or had variable amounts of cytoplasm without azuro-philic granules. The nuclei were often irregular, either notched, indented or convoluted but were without nucleoli. Bone marrow infiltration was generally extensive and many patients died after a short duration with disease despite chemotherapy (Brisbane et al. 1983).

Although the majority of T-CLLs reported have shown mature T cell phenotype expressing either CD4 or CD8 in conjunction with other markers such as CD2, CD3, CD5, and CD6, leukaemic proliferations of lymphocytes co-expressing both CD4 and CD8 may also occur. Simpkins et al. (1985) reported a case of "knobby" type T-CLL in which the lymphocytes expressed a post-thymic phenotype except for the co-expression of CD4 and CD8 on 80%–95% of the cells. Co-expression of CD4 and CD8 in T-CLL has previously been reported (Saxon et al. 1979; Runke et al. 1982). Although post-thymic lymphocytes are identified by the absence of CD1 and TdT, and the presence of CD2 and CD3 together with one or other of the markers CD4 or CD8, there is strong evidence that these latter markers are neither mutually exclusive or reciprocal in normal or diseased states. Up to 2% of peripheral blood lymphocytes of normal subjects may be ER+, CD5+, CD3–, CD4– and CD8– (Van de Griend et al. 1982) and, conversely, a small proportion of post-thymic lymphocytes in the blood, tonsils and lymph nodes have been shown to co-express CD4 and CD8 markers (Janossy et al. 1980, 1981b; Tidman et al. 1981; Blue et al. 1985). An expanded population of CD4+, CD8+ lymphocytes has been reported in myasthenia gravis (Berrih et al. 1981) and in chronic active hepatitis (Geha and Rosen 1983). Co-expression of CD4 and CD8 has also been reported in the neoplastic lymphocytes of T-cell lymphosarcoma cell leukaemia (Ishii et al. 1982), Sézary syndrome (Habeshaw et al. 1983) and node-based T cell lymphoma (Lennert et al. 1981).

Although the occurrence of polyclonal hypergammaglobulinaemia in some cases of T-CLL with cytotoxic/suppressor phenotype is surprising, helper function has been demonstrated in a case of CD8+ T-CLL (Siegal et al. 1982), indicating that lymphocyte phenotypes as defined by monoclonal reagents may be heterogeneous with respect to functional activity. The leukaemic population may either be a clonal expansion of a minor normal subset of CD8 cells with atypical (helper) functional activity or it may function aberrantly because of the neoplastic transformation.

Neutropenia in T-CLL is evidently not caused by anti-neutrophil antibodies since such antibodies have not been found in these patients (Catovsky et al. 1982a). However, it may be the result of antibody-dependent cytotoxic activity. Removal of T cells from patients with pure red cell aplasia significantly enhanced the growth of erythrocyte precursors in vitro (BFU-E; Hoffman et al. 1978; Nagasawa et al. 1981; Linch et al. 1981), but corresponding enhancement of myeloid colony growth was not seen. In two patients with hypogammaglobulinaemia, the neoplastic T cells strongly inhibited pokeweed mitogen (PWM)-induced immunoglobulin synthesis (Nagasawa et al. 1981; Thien et al. 1982). The evidence that T cell proliferations may be directly implicated in the pathogenesis of pure red cell aplasia and hypogammaglobulinaemia is persuasive. Marrow T cells may suppress erythropoiesis in vitro (Lipton et al. 1983), but the evidence in neutropenia is less convincing.

Some authors include the HTLV-I associated adult T cell leukaemia (ATL) endemic in southwestern Japan and in people of African ancestry in the Caribbean, the southeastern USA and central Africa in discussions of T-CLL. We feel that such cases should not be classified as T-CLL as they show distinctive clinical and cytomorphological features. They are associated with HTLV-I, show lymphadenomegaly and hepatosplenomegaly, frequent skin involvement and have a rapidly progressive terminal course. ATL is largely an endemic disease and the leukaemia/lymphoma cells show marked nuclear irregularity and prominent nucleoli and are mostly of the CD4 phenotype. The cases of "T-helper phenotype chronic lymphocytic leukaemia" reported in Italian patients should also be considered to be another form of endemic ATL. Antibody to HTLV-I or integrated sequences of the virus were found in 3 of the 16 cases (Pandolfi et al. 1985).

T_γ Lymphoproliferative Disease

Cytoxic/suppressor T-CLL may be difficult to distinguish from T_γ lymphoproliferative disease. The morphologically distinct subgroup of lymphocytes known as large granular lymphocytes (LGL) have abundant cytoplasm usually containing prominent azurophilic granules which are ER+, CP03+ and bear Fc receptors for IgG. Some mediate natural killer cell (NK) activity and some have antibody-dependent cytotoxic capacity. Lymphoproliferative diseases of these T_γ cells are characterised by anaemia, hypogammaglobulinaemia, neutropenia and splenomegaly with recurrent infections. Lymphadenomegaly and skin involvement are typically absent and there are relatively low counts of circulating leucocytes with granulocytopenia (Itoh et al. 1983; Reynolds and Foon 1984; Newland et al. 1984). Cases of T_γ lymphocytosis often pursue a benign course with chronic persistent lymphocytosis that does not progress, even without therapy (Ferrarini et al. 1982). A lymphoma of LGL also occurs (Kadin et al. 1981).

The strong similarity of clinical features and the cytomorphology of the proliferating lymphocytes with their prominent azurophilic granules have led Brisbane et al. (1983) to suggest that T_γ lymphocytosis and CD8+ CLL may represent parts of a spectrum of the same disease, the former often representing an early manifestation of CD8+ CLL.

There has been debate as to whether T_γ lymphocytosis is indeed neoplastic. Rearrangement of Ti genes has now been demonstrated in a few cases, providing strong evidence of its neoplastic nature, although rearrangement of these genes has not been demonstrable in other instances (Aisenberg et al. 1985; Bertness et al. 1985). Trisomy 8 and trisomy 14 have been reported in individual cases (Loughran et al. 1985).

Adult T Cell Leukaemia/Lymphoma

Takatsuki and his co-workers in Kyoto University Hospital first described the distinct disease entity which they termed "adult T cell leukaemia" (Takatsuki et al. 1976, 1977; Uchiyama et al. 1977). This new disease showed the following characteristics:

1. Onset in adulthood
2. Subacute or chronic leukaemia with a rapidly progressive terminal course
3. Pleomorphic leukaemic cells that show markedly deformed nuclei and T cell surface markers
4. Frequent association of lymphadenopathy and hepatosplenomegaly
5. Frequent skin involvement with erythroderma and nodular infiltrates
6. Clustering of the patients' birthplaces in Kyushu and the surrounding southwestern islands of Japan.

Because of its leukaemic lymphomatous nature, this disease has also been called adult T cell leukaemia/lymphoma (ATL) (Shimoyana et al. 1979b). Its resistance to treatment with current anti-leukaemic agents and the high frequency of associated hypercalcaemia (65% of cases) and osteolysis (22% of cases) have also been more recently recognised (Kadin et al. 1983). Hypercalcaemia, the most dramatic manifestation of this disease and often the cause of death in coma, relates directly to disease activity, particularly a rising white blood count. Hypercalcaemia is rare in other malignant lymphomas, occurring in only about 1.8% of cases (Canellos 1974). Secretion of an osteoclast-activating factor has been suggested as the possible pathogenetic mechanism (Grossman et al. 1981) as hypercalcaemia does not correlate with osteolytic lesions. In Kyushu, 70%–80% of lymphoid malignancies in adults are of T cell origin (Watanabe et al. 1979), and the incidence of T cell malignancy in non-endemic areas of Japan is still higher than that of western countries. In Japan, T cell lymphoma/leukaemia accounts for about 38% of all immunologically typed cases of NHL, with B cell lymphoma accounting for 49% and "null" cell type for the remainder (Suchi and Tajima 1979).

The endemic nature of ATL led to the strong suspicion that it was caused by a virus. A new RNA virus had been isolated in 1978 from a black patient with a mature T cell malignancy and from another with Sézary-like syndrome (Poiesz et al. 1980,1981). In 1981, Hinuma et al. found a type C retrovirus-related antigen in an ATL cell line that reacted with the sera of all patients with ATL, but not with those of healthy adults in ATL non-endemic areas. This ATL-antigen (ATLA) was found in almost all patients with ATL and in up to 30% of healthy adults in disease-endemic areas. In the healthy individuals, seropositivity increased gradually with age, reaching a maximum at 40 years. Anti-ATLA antibody is found in 44% of offspring of mothers with anti-ATLA, and the highest incidence of antibody is found among wives whose husbands are antibody positive (Kadin et al. 1983), suggesting that the common routes of ATL virus transmission are from parents to children and between spouses. ATLA and HTLV-I are now believed to be identical viruses. The biology of the virus and its epidemiology are dicussed at greater length in Chapter 5 (see p. 50).

T cell malignancy in Japan is separated into four major groups: (1) T-CLL and T-PLL, (2) mycosis fungoides and Sézary syndrome, 3) lymphoblastic lymphoma, and 4) T cell lymphoma including ATL. ATL is considered to be synonymous with a histological subgroup of T cell lymphoma called malignant lymphoma, pleomorphic cell type (Watanabe et al. 1979; Suchi and Tajima 1979). Lymphadenopathy is reported to occur in 100% of cases of ATL, whereas leukocytosis (more than 10×10^9/litre) is seen in 86% and bone marrow involvement occurs in 84% of patients (Kadin et al. 1983). The 50% actuarial survival of leukaemic patients is 5.4 months, of those without manifest leukaemia 10.2 months, and the overall survival is 6 months.

The lymph node changes in ATL have been described by the Japanese Lymphoma Study Group. The diffuse pattern of infiltration which is seen in all cases can be classified according to cell type into: small cell type (2%), medium-sized cell type (38%), mixed cell type (9%), large cell type (9%) and pleomorphic cell type (42%) (Hanaoka 1981, 1982). The majority of cases (80%) were composed of tumour cells of the pleomorphic or medium-sized cell type. Cases in which the biopsy revealed the diffuse pleomorphic type of lymphoma or one of the other types in which nuclear polymorphism was a conspicuous feature had the worst prognosis (Hanaoka 1982).

Malignant lymphoma of the pleomorphic cell type is characterised by a diffuse polymorphous infiltrate of large, medium and small neoplastic cells with pleomorphic nuclei showing prominent lobation. The medium and small cells have finely stippled chromatin and variably indented or cerebriform nuclei, while the nuclei of the large cells are usually vesicular and contain large nucleoli, often resembling Reed–Sternberg cells. There is a tendency for clusters of these lymphoid cells to be compartmentalised by thin bands of fibrous tissue and by branching blood vessels. Lymph node structures such as peripheral sinuses and lymphoid follicles may occasionally be preserved. Epithelioid histiocytes are frequently present and plasma cells and eosinophils may be seen in some cases (Kikuchi et al. 1979; Watanabe et al. 1979; Kadin et al. 1983). The atypical cells in the lymph node correspond well with the atypical lobated leukaemic cells of variable size seen in the peripheral blood in patients with leukaemic change (Watanabe et al. 1979). The large Reed–Sternberg-like cells are strongly pyroninophilic and PAS-negative. Acid phosphatase and esterase activities are variable in the tumour cells.

Although cutaneous T cell lymphoma and lymphoblastic lymphoma are clearly differentiated from ATL, the separation of ATL from T-CLL is less distinct. Instances of T-CLL evolving into ATL have been well documented. Cases of T-CLL with small leukaemic lymphocytes have shown highly polymorphic lymphoid infiltrates in the lymph nodes, suggesting that the smaller cells easily become leukaemic and that smaller cells can be transformed to become larger cells in the tissues (Shimoyama et al. 1979a, b; Watanabe et al. 1979).

The spectrum of morphological changes in the lymph nodes seen in ATL is similar to that seen in T cell lymphoma in ATL non-endemic areas of Japan, the major difference being that less aggressive, non-pleomorphic types of T cell lymphomas predominate in the non-endemic areas (Kadin et al. 1983).

The cell surface antigens of the neoplastic cells of ATL are of helper/inducer T cell phenotype, being ER +, CD3 +, CD4 +, TdT−, and some display MHC class II determinants (Kadin et al. 1983). Functionally, the malignant T cells from all cases studied in different assay systems, such as B cell differentiation driven by pokeweed mitogen (PWM) (Uchiyama et al. 1978,1980; Hattori et al. 1981), lymphocyte transformation (Tatsumi et al. 1980), or allogenic mixed lymphocyte reaction (Gaeke et al. 1981) have expressed suppressor effects. ATL, therefore, has suppressor functional characteristics different from those of the bona fide CD4 + inducer-type cells of mycosis fungoides and Sézary syndrome which usually function as helper cells in vitro. The neoplastic T cells in most cases of ATL express the receptor for interleukin 2 (IL-2R; CD25 antigen), whereas those of Sézary syndrome do not (Waldmann et al. 1984). ATL leukaemic cells and HTLV-I-infected cells also often carry inappropriate or anomalous MHC class I antigens.

ATL is now recognised outside of Japan. Most of the patients with the disease have been black and predominantly of West Indian/Caribbean origin although sporadic cases in non-endemic areas have also been documented (Leong et al. 1980, 1981; Gaeke et al. 1981; Grossman et al. 1981; Catovsky et al. 1982b; Slease et al. 1984; Foucar et al. 1985). More recently, the disease has been described in southern Europe (Pandolfi et al. 1985) and in Taiwan (Su et al. 1985). The histological appearances of the lymph nodes in cases from the Caribbean were very similar to those of pleomorphic T cell lymphoma described in Japan (O'Brien et al. 1983). Of the four cases of ATL in West Indian patients which were studied with monoclonal antibodies, three were considered to be of the mature helper-inducer phenotype, being CD3 +, CD4 +, CD8−. One case was CD3 +, CD4−, CD8−, T10 + (Kadin et al. 1983). All patients were serologically positive for HTLV or had antibody to HTLV antigens. Another report of five patients with ATL born in the Caribbean revealed neoplastic cells with a CD1 +, CD4 +, CD5 +, CD7−, CD8−, M1−, phenotype. Like the cases of Japanese ATL, despite the CD4 +, CD8− phenotype, none of the patients' cells exerted helper activity on PWM-induced Ig synthesis. Instead, the neoplastic cells of three patients had suppressor activity (Miedema et al. 1984). Of 16 Italian patients with ATL, 3 patients had either HTLV-I sequences integrated into the genome of their malignant lymphocytes or anti-HTLV-I serum antibodies, or both (Pandolfi et al. 1985). It also appears that a high frequency of T cell lymphoma (42.3%) exists in Taiwan. Follicular lymphoma forms only 10.5% of malignant lymphomas and Hodgkin's disease (HD) is also uncommon (8.7%). Of 33 cases of peripheral T cell lymphomas examined, 5 were positive for HTLV antigen (Su et al. 1985).

Foucar et al. (1985) identified 15 cases of probable ATL in persons from non-endemic regions of the USA and showed that they were morphologically, clinically and immunologically similar to endemic ATL. Although antibodies to C type retrovirus were detected in three of the five patients tested, these workers concluded that the available data were not sufficient to establish a conclusive association between non-endemic forms of ATL and C type retrovirus infection.

T Cell Neoplasms of the Thymic Compartment

Lymphoblastic Lymphoma

Lymphomas may be accepted as arising in the thymus if there is an anterior mediastinal mass, if the marrow is not involved at presentation, and if tumour cells are shown to be of T lymphocyte lineage. LL occurs most commonly in adolescents and young adults. It shows a higher frequency in males than females, presenting typically with supradiaphragmatic lymphadenomegaly in association with a mediastinal mass. LL shares many clinical features with childhood T-ALL; without successful treatment, it may spread to the bone marrow and progress to a leukaemic phase and a clinical picture indistinguishable from T-ALL. The distinction of the two entities is nonetheless important because T-ALL has a poorer prognosis than LL (Weinstein et al. 1979; Pullen et al. 1982). Patients with T-ALL generally have high white blood cell counts and show bone marrow replacement by blasts at the time of presentation; this is in contrast with LL, which can be distinguished arbitrarily from T-ALL by the lack of extensive marrow involvement, i.e., less than 25% marrow blasts (Sen and Borella 1975; Tsukimoto et al. 1976).

LL has a characteristic infiltrative growth pattern. It infiltrates the lymph node and thymus diffusely by displacement of cells without destruction of the underlying architecture. Lymphoid follicles are sometimes spared, and the reticulin stain will often show preservation of the structure of the sinusoids, which become filled out and obscured by the lymphoblasts. The small to medium-sized tumour cells also infiltrate between connective tissue fibres as non-cohesive cells in a single file pattern particularly well-demonstrated in the capsule of the lymph node and around blood vessels. Numerous mitotic figures and apoptotic bodies, together with the many tingible-body macrophages in the densely cellular infiltrate impart a striking "starry sky" pattern to the section (Fig. 19.1). The nuclei of the lymphoblasts may have prominent convolutions, a characteristic which inspired Barcos and Lukes (1975) to call this neoplasm "malignant lymphoma of convoluted lymphocytes". However, subsequent studies have indicated that as many as half the cases may not show this prominent nuclear convolution (Nathwani et al. 1976; Pangalis et al. 1979; Navas-Palacios et al. 1981), having instead round to

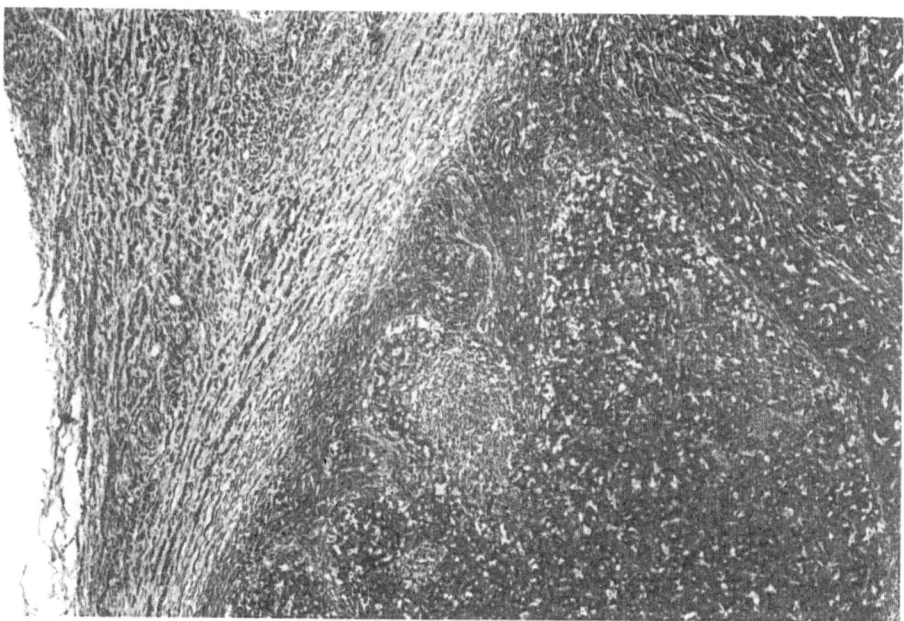

Fig. 19.1. Lymphoblastic lymphoma. The presence of scattered tingible-body macrophages in the diffuse, densely cellular infiltrate imparts a "starry sky" appearance. A preserved germinal centre is seen in the centre of the field and the neoplastic cells infiltrate in a single file in the lymph node capsule. (H & E, × 50)

oval nuclei which are slightly larger than normal lymphocytes (Figs. 19.2, 19.3). The chromatin is finely dispersed, between two and five small eosinophilic nucleoli may be present, and the nuclei contain TdT. The cytoplasm is scanty, poorly defined and moderately pyroninophilic. Cytoplasmic acid phosphatase and β-glucuronidase reactions are positive in imprints and cryostat sections.

The tumour cells from patients with T-ALL have the phenotype of early or prothymocytes (Reinherz et al. 1980). Bernard et al. (1981) using the OKT reagents found 29% of LL cells to be early thymocyte in type (ER +, T10 +); 43% were related to the common thymocyte stage, being CD1 + (T6 +), CD4 + (T4 +), CD8 + (T8 +); and 29% expressed mature thymocyte antigens, being CD3 + (T3 +) and reciprocally expressed CD4 and CD8 (Fig. 19.3). A monoclonal antibody A-50, which recognises an epitope of the CD5 antigen, was also reactive with cells from 5 of 8 patients with LL but not with cells from 12 patients with T-ALL. CD10 (CALLA) has also been reported to help distinguish T-ALL and LL, in that 40% of LL cells, but less than 10% of T-ALL cells express CD10 (Ritz et al. 1980). These and other studies suggest that the malignant cells in LL are a more mature T cell type compared with the cells of T-ALL, which are almost exclusively of the early thymocyte phenotype (Bernard et al. 1979; Reinherz et al. 1980), and that LL and T-ALL are probably not a single disease process (Nadler et al. 1980). Other workers, however, indicate that the distinction between these two diseases may be less well defined (Roper et al. 1983) and there is often heterogeneity within tumours (Cossman et al. 1983). Bernard et al. (1982) have found a shift in the

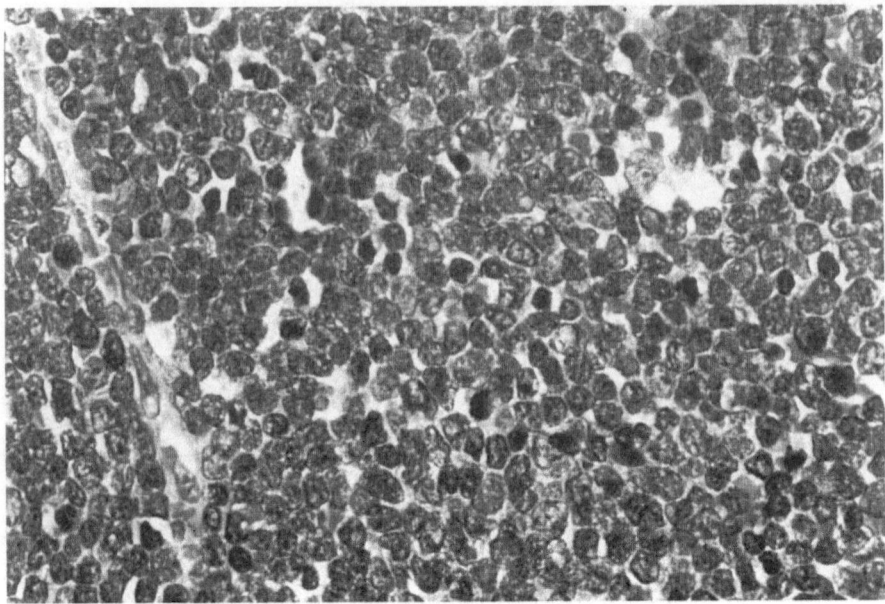

Fig. 19.2. The cells of lymphoblastic lymphoma show finely dispersed chromatin with two or three small nucleoli. Prominent folds can be seen in the nuclear membranes and the cytoplasm is scanty. Mitotic figures are frequent. (H & E, × 500)

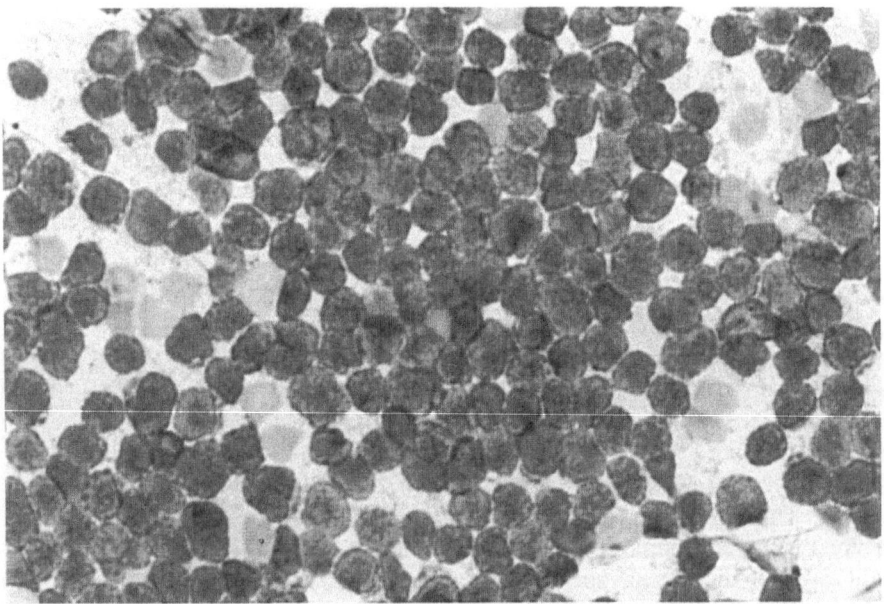

Fig. 19.3. Imprint of lymph node with lymphoblastic lymphoma stained with Leu-4 showing distinct membranous staining of the lymphoblasts. Note the presence of nuclear folds. (Modified avidin-biotin peroxidase, × 500)

surface antigen pattern during leukaemic relapse of LL towards dedifferentiation and expression of immature T cell antigens.

T Cell Neoplasms of the Peripheral Compartment

Post-thymic T lymphocytes segregate into helper/inducer and suppressor/cytotoxic subsets with CD2+, CD3+, CD4+, CD5+ and CD2+, CD3+, CD5+, CD8+ phenotypes respectively. A small percentage of T cells in the peripheral blood and lymph nodes, whose function is unknown, co-expresses CD4 and CD8 markers.

Peripheral T lymphocytes localise in specific areas within lymphoid tissues. T lymphocytes predominate in the paracortical areas of the lymph node and the periarteriolar regions of the spleen, the ratio of CD4+ to CD8+ cells being approximately 2:1, similar to that observed in the blood. CD4+ cells, however, can be observed to cluster around the interdigitating reticulum cells (IDRCs) which are strongly MHC class II+ (HLA-DR+) and S100+, while the CD8+ population surrounds these conglomerates of CD4+ cells and IDRCs (Tidman et al. 1981). T cells make up 5%–15% of lymphocyte populations in germinal centres. These, mostly of CD4+ phenotype, are distributed immediately beneath the mantle zones (Poppema et al. 1981; Stein et al. 1981). In the gut, however, intraepithelial lymphocytes are mainly CD8+ cells (Selby et al. 1981), and in the bone marrow CD8+ cells predominate (Janossy et al. 1981a).

In our classification of T cell malignancies we have chosen to separate the neoplasms of the peripheral or post-thymic compartment into cutaneous T cell lymphomas and node-based T cell lymphomas because of their very different clinicopathological features.

Cutaneous T Cell Lymphomas

Mycosis fungoides (MF) and Sézary syndrome (SS) are primary cutaneous lymphoid malignancies which are now accepted to represent different stages or manifestations of the same neoplastic process. The term "cutaneous T cell lymphoma" (CTCL) was propsed to encompass these and related disorders (Edelson 1976). CTCLs are relatively uncommon disorders, having an age-adjusted incidence of about 2 cases/10^6 individuals in the USA (Greene et al. 1979). The average age at diagnosis is 52 years. Although it has been alleged that an 8-month-old child has had MF (Serra et al. 1966), the majority of patients are 30 years or older (Epstein et al. 1972; Levi and Wiernik 1975), and the diagnosis should be made with circumspection in very young people. CTCL occurs slightly more frequently in males than in females and the incidence is similar in blacks and whites.

Although the concept of MF as a cutaneous T cell lymphoma cannot be challenged, some clinical and laboratory data, albeit controversial, point to a possible non-neoplastic aetiology for this disorder. For example, cells with large, hyperchromatic and irregularly shaped nuclei, similar in appearance to the malignant "mycosis cells" seen in MF, have been found in several non-lymphomatous conditions, including lichen planus, lupus erythematosus, psoriasis and actinic keratosis, as well as in the peripheral blood of healthy individuals (Thiers 1982). Cultured lymphocytes transformed with PHA have ultrastructural features similar to those of mycosis cells. These and other data have suggested that MF may, at least at the onset, represent a reactive rather than a neoplastic disorder.

The clinical appearance and course of MF also support the contention that the condition may begin as a reactive process. The early premycotic eruption may be indistinguishable from chronic allergic contact or psoriasiform dermatitis and often responds to conservative treatment with topical steroids or may involute spontaneously. The premycotic stage may last many years before progressing to plaque and tumour stages. This protracted clinical course, and the observation that humoral and cellular immunity are intact until the terminal stages of the illness, make this disease quite different from most other lymphomas. Three separate studies suggest a relationship between industrial exposure to potential toxins and the development of CTCL. A statistically significant link has been shown between industrial exposure and the lymphoproliferative disorder (Cohen 1977). In another study, 30% of 211 patients with MF had at least one exposure to "hazardous chemicals or materials" (Greene et al. 1979), while in the third, 91% of patients with CTCL had multiple exposures to potentially carcinogenic chemicals such as air pollutants, pesticides, solvents, vapours and detergents (Fischmann et al. 1979). However, large well-controlled prospective studies will be required to establish such an aetiological relationship.

MF is histologically diagnosable when the cutaneous involvement is at the plaque stage, which occurs in about 67% of cases, and is readily recognisable in the 17% of patients who have true cutaneous tumours and in the 15% with generalised exfoliative erythroderma (Broder and Bunn 1980). The overall frequency of lymphadenomegaly is about 45% and is related to the stage of skin involvement. Lymphadenomegaly occurs in 17% of patients with limited plaques only, compared with 56% and 79% of those with cutaneous tumours and generalised erythroderma respectively. The nature of individual types of skin lesions appears to be a reflection of the growth patterns and level of differentiation of the malignant cells. Plaques represent lateral extension; tumours, vertical extension; widespread skin disease, haematogenous spread. Disseminated nodules are associated with the worst prognosis, possibly because they indicate miliary spread of malignant cells with local aggressive growth at the sites where they settle.

There is considerable controversy over the histopathological interpretation of lymph node biopsies from patients with CTCL. The majority of such biopsies show reactive changes labelled as dermatopathic lymphadenitis. A minority of lymph node biopsies will show partial or complete effacement of the nodal architecture by neoplastic cells. What proportion of lymph node specimens currently classified as dermatopathic lymphadenitis is, in reality, infiltrated with tumour cells is not known. Bunn et al. (1980) considered that 54% of enlarged nodes were involved. Huberman et al. (1979) found evidence for neoplastic involvement in 95% of lymph node biopsies from patients with CTCL and lymphadenomegaly, suggesting that a relatively high frequency of true tumour infiltration may be found when special techniques such as electron microscopy, cytogenetics and immunohistochemistry are used to examine such specimens. Nodal involvement, as judged by histological criteria, correlated with a worse prognosis; however, it is of interest that individuals with nodal enlargement caused by so-called reactive changes have also been shown to have a shorter survival

(Fuks et al. 1973). The explanation for this finding appears to lie in the sensitivity of the techniques used to diagnose nodal involvement. Fuks et al. (1973) suggested that patients showing dermatopathic lymphadenitis should be regarded as having presumptive evidence of nodal involvement by CTCL. It is likely that phenotypic analysis of T cells in lymph nodes using monoclonal antisera will also show a higher percentage of involvement.

Some 25% of patients with classic plaque/tumour stages of MF have circulating neoplastic cells which may be referred to as Sézary cells. Using Giemsa-stained peripheral blood smears, it was possible to detect Sézary type cells in 13% of 31 patients with plaque/tumour stages and in all 18 patients with erythroderma (Schechter et al. 1979). When special techniques such as cytogenetic studies, electron microscopy and immunocytochemistry were combined, circulating neoplastic cells were found in approximately 65% of patients with plaque/tumour stages and 100% of patients in the erythrodermic stage (Guchion et al. 1979; Huberman et al. 1979; Schechter et al. 1979).

Essentially all patients with readily detectable peripheral blood involvement show lymphadenomegaly, and all patients with visceral involvement have both lymphadenomegaly and peripheral blood involvement. Patients with readily detectable peripheral blood involvement have a shorter survival than patients who do not.

The incidence of bone marrow involvement in post-mortem series ranges from 18% to 29%. Antemortem studies generally show a remarkable sparing of bone marrow. Necropsy findings show that the viscera are involved in the majority of patients, the liver, spleen and lung being the most frequently involved sites. Once extracutaneous disease has occurred, lymph nodes do not appear to impede further extension to the viscera. Dermatopathic lymphadenitis without definitive lymph node infiltration by neoplastic cells also correlates with visceral disease, suggesting underdiagnosis of lymph node involvement. Extension to lymph nodes and viscera does not indicate development of a second lymphoma since the histological findings in these sites remain representative of the original cutaneous lymphoma rather than other types of lymphoreticular neoplasm (Rappaport and Thomas 1974).

Skin biopsies from patients with MF and its leukaemic variant, SS, show a cellular infiltrate in the upper dermis, often in a band-like pattern obliterating the papillary dermis or Grenz-zone. The infiltrate tends to be polymorphous, consisting of histiocytes, eosinophils, small lymphocytes as well as larger cells with multiple or polylobated nuclei, prominent nucleoli and darkly staining cytoplasm. These mycosis cells infiltrate the epidermis singly or in clusters within acantholytic spaces forming the so-called Pautrier's microabscesses (Fig. 19.4). Histologically, the dermal infiltrates in MF are similar to those seen in SS.

Although the histological pattern described above has been reported as being pathognomonic of MF and SS (Lever and Schaumberg-Lever 1975; Van Scott and Haynes 1977), it is now recognised that preferential epidermotropism as single cell exocytosis or as Pautrier's microabscesses may be manifested by neoplastic cells in T cell leukaemia/lymphoma (Leong et al. 1980), as well as in Japanese ATL (Watanabe et al. 1981).

The diagnosis of CTCL still requires close interaction between the experienced dermatologist and the pathologist. More often than not, the clinician makes the diagnosis before the pathologist. Relatively rarely will the pathological diagnosis antedate clinical suspicion, indeed, the latter situation is fraught with hazard

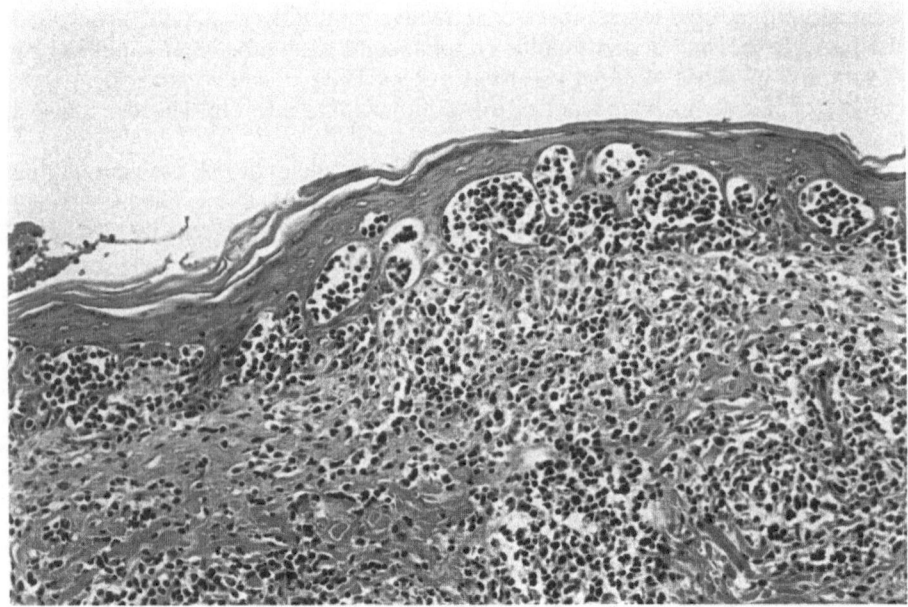

Fig. 19.4. Mycosis fungoides showing band-like infiltrate in the superficial dermis which obliterates the papillary dermis. Clusters of tumour cells lie within acantholytic spaces in the epidermis. (H & E, × 125)

because many non-neoplastic conditions can histologically simulate CTCL (Ackerman et al. 1974).

The microscopic findings in the lymph nodes from patients with CTCL encompass a spectrum of changes which range from dermatopathic lymphadenitis only, through various combinations of dermatopathic lymphadenitis and partial replacement by CTCL, to total replacement by CTCL. Distinction between dermatopathic lymphadenitis and malignant lymphoma is not possible on macroscopic grounds. In dermatopathic lymphadenitis the enlarged lymph nodes show prominent germinal centres as well as expansion of the paracortical regions which contain numerous interdigitating reticulum cells. Macrophages with phagocytosed lipid and melanin are seen in the subcapsular sinus and the sinusoids. A positive diagnosis of CTCL can only be made when focal clusters of mycosis cells are recognised. The earliest of these clusters are localised in the paracortex of the lymph node and a focus of increased mitotic figures may be the first clue to the recognition of involvement by CTCL (Fig. 19.5). The mycosis cells have hyperconvoluted, cerebriform nuclei (Figs. 19.6, 19.7) and should be distinguished from the IDRCs, which may also have irregular but vesicular nuclei and display abundant faintly eosinophilic or pale cytoplasm with prominent cytoplasmic processes. The mycosis cells may progressively replace the T cell zones of the lymph node in a diffuse manner, although occasional germinal centres may be preserved.

The spleen, like the lymph nodes, shows selective involvement of the periarteriolar sheath or T cell zone without involvement of the germinal centres and follicles, although with progression of the disease, the lymphoma cells spill over into the red

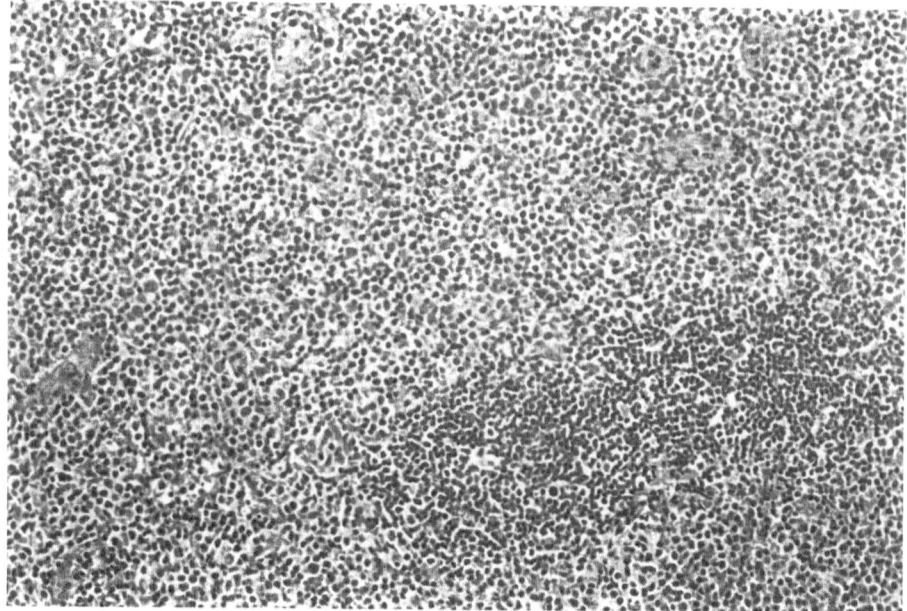

Fig. 19.5. Focal replacement of lymph node by mycosis cells. A cluster of small lymphocytes is present, possibly representing remnants of a lymphoid follicle. (H & E, × 125)

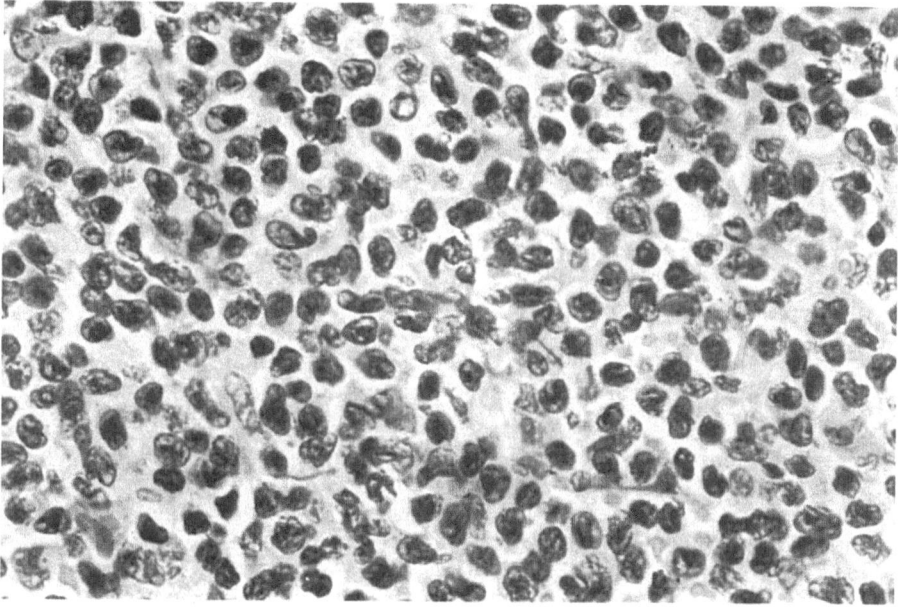

Fig. 19.6. Lymph node in a case of Sézary syndrome, showing diffuse infiltration by cells with marked nuclear convolution. (H & E, × 500)

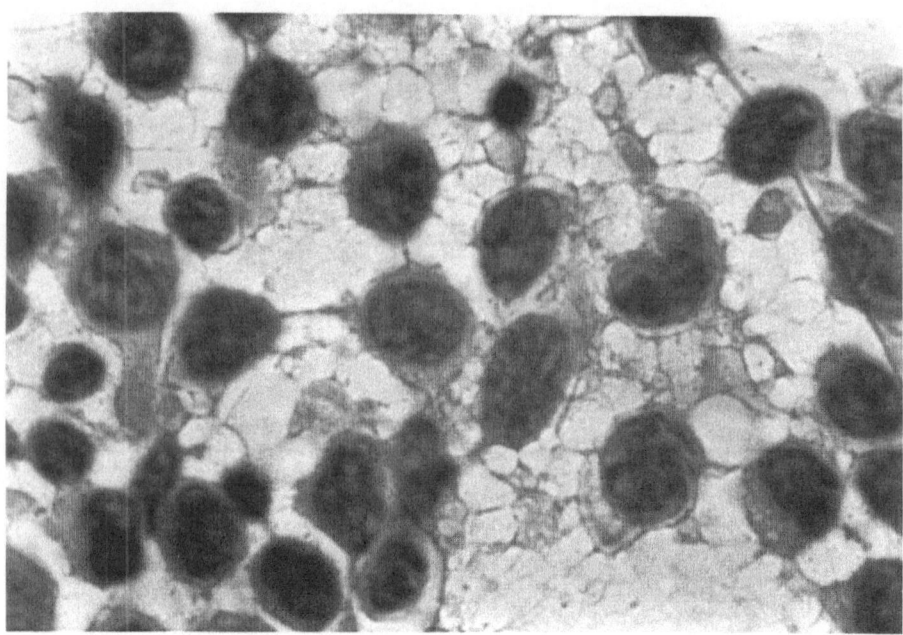

Fig. 19.7. Imprint of lymph node infiltrated by Sézary cells. The cerebriform nuclei are well demonstrated. (H & E, × 1250)

pulp. About 60% of patients with extracutaneous involvement show splenic infiltration.

Thomas and Rappaport (1975) showed a strong positive correlation between lymph node involvement and the spread of mycosis fungoides to visceral organs. Infiltration of viscera is diffuse, more akin to a leukaemic infiltration, often with preservation of architecture. In the liver, lungs, heart and kidneys, gross nodules may be visible, but the neoplastic cells are seen to infiltrate diffusely through the parenchymal tissues.

The difficulties in diagnosing CTCL in its early stages have led to the use of more advanced techniques of investigation. One of these is the determination of the nuclear contour index (NCI = perimeter/area$^{1/2}$). The measurement of the NCI of lymphocytes in electron micrographs proved to be a reliable method of separating CTCL from the benign dermatoses (Meijer et al. 1980; McNutt and Crain 1981). DNA cytophotometry may be a useful technique to identify CTCL. Benign inflammatory diseases sometimes show tetraploid as well as diploid DNA values but neoplastic lesions are hypertetraploid. The techniques correlate well but the morphometry appeared to be more sensitive than DNA cytophotometry in detection of CTCL (Meijer et al. 1980; van der Loo et al. 1981). Light microscopic analysis of sectioned Epon-embedded lymphocyte fractions is also an accurate alternative to electron microscopy for counting circulating Sézary cells (Myrie et al. 1980). Recently, Payne et al. (1984) showed that the most sensitive ultrastructural method for confirming the diagnosis of CTCL was a simple scoring of the number of sharply angled nuclear invaginations in 100 lymphocytes (Fig. 19.8). Control biopsy specimens had many more lymphocytes with no sharply angled

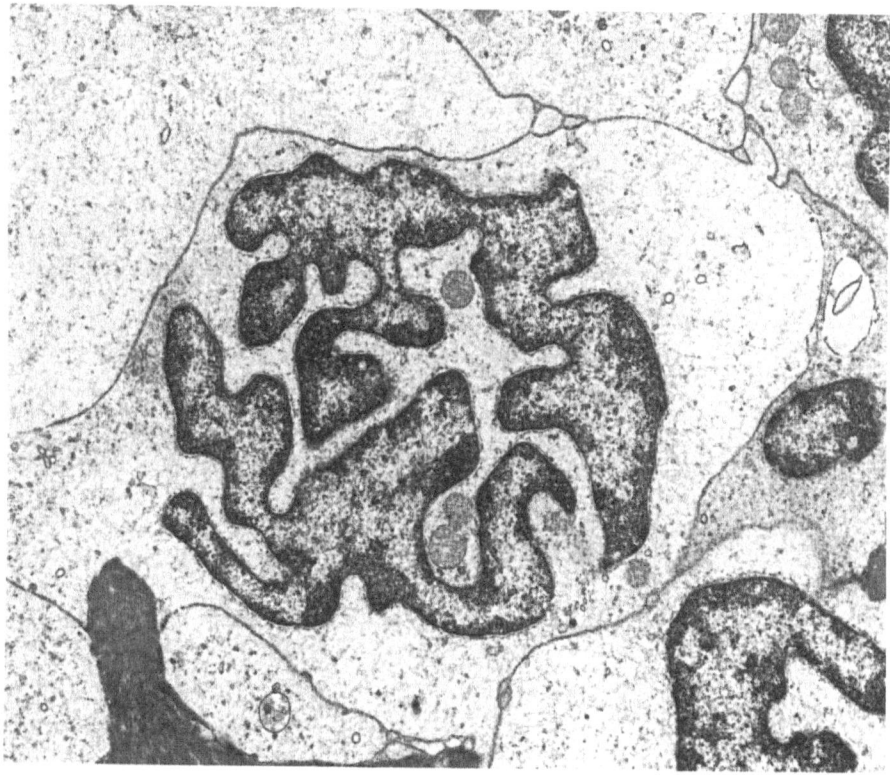

Fig. 19.8. Ultrastructure of mycosis cell showing the marked nuclear convolution and the large number of sharply angled nuclear invaginations. (Uranyl acetate, lead citrate, × 9000)

nuclear invaginations (19%–55%) compared with those from patients with CTCL (3%–15%). Using this method of assessment, these authors confirmed the diagnosis of CTCL in 100% of patients, whereas measurement of the NCI identified only 67% of the patients with CTCL.

In as much as the initial clinical manifestations of CTCL are cutaneous, it was generally assumed that the proliferating lymphocytes originate in the skin. Current evidence, however, suggests the contrary. Miller et al. (1980) provided kinetic evidence to show that Sézary cells accumulate in the blood and migrate preferentially to the skin. Shackney et al. (1979) and Schwarzmeier et al. (1981) postulated a common extravascular site for the production of Sézary cells, probably the lymphoid tissues.

The demonstration that the neoplastic cells of most cases of CTCL are of CD4 phenotype (Broder et al. 1976; Haynes et al. 1981; Kung et al. 1981) has provided some insights into the pathogenesis of CTCL (Fig. 19.9). A normal population of CD4+ cells which ordinarily "homes" in the skin may be the origin of the clonally-derived malignant T cells (Fig. 19.10). These neoplastic cells initially closely resemble their normal ancestor and retain the functional and phenotypic features of helper T cells as well as the tendency for epidermotropism. As progressively more poorly differentiated subclones of malignant T cell develop, the

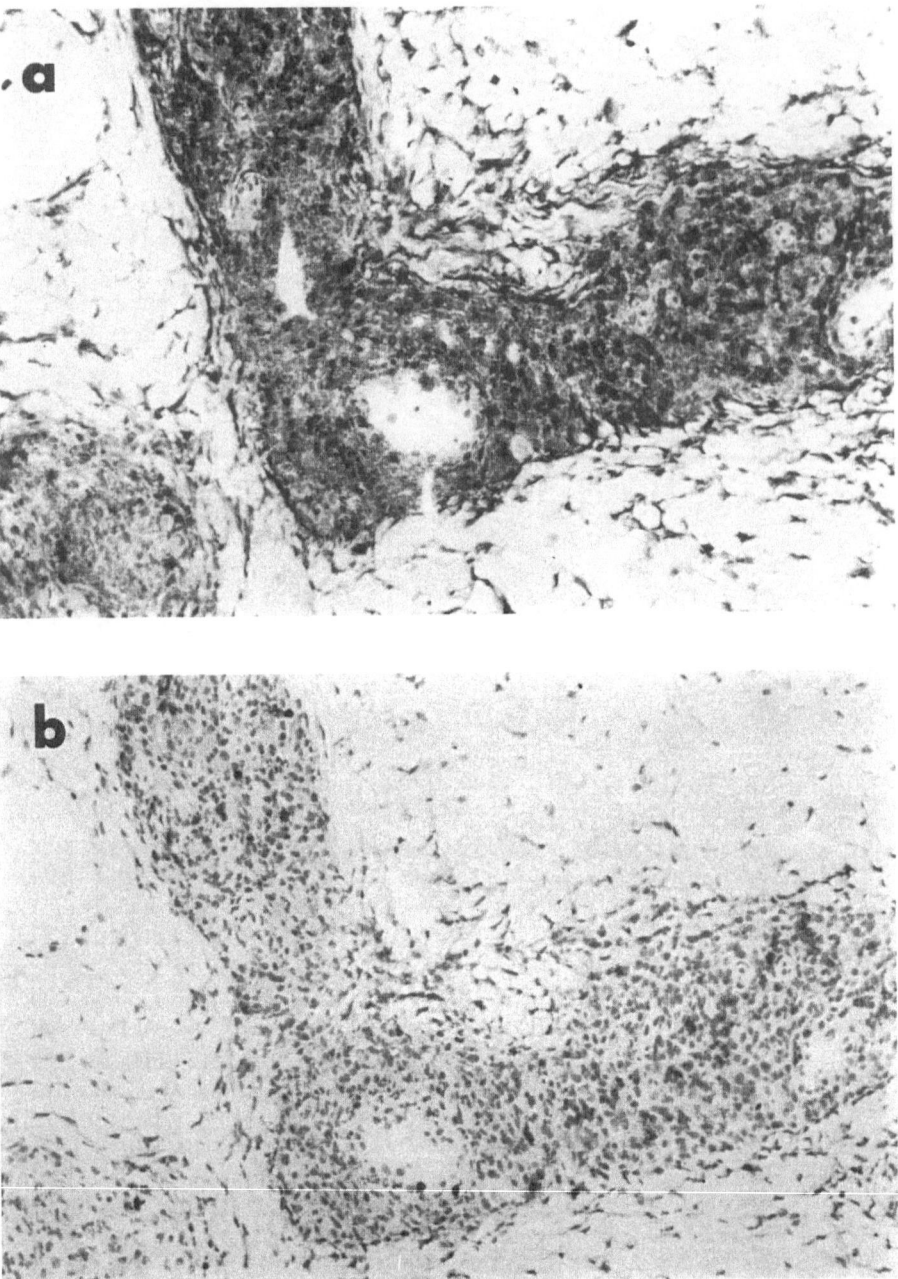

Fig. 19.9a, b. Consecutive frozen sections of skin with mycosis fungoides. The majority of lymphoid cells in the periappendageal dermal infiltrates stain with Leu-3a (CD4) (**a**), whereas only scattered cells stain with Leu-2a (CD8) (**b**). (Modified avidin-biotin peroxidase, × 125)

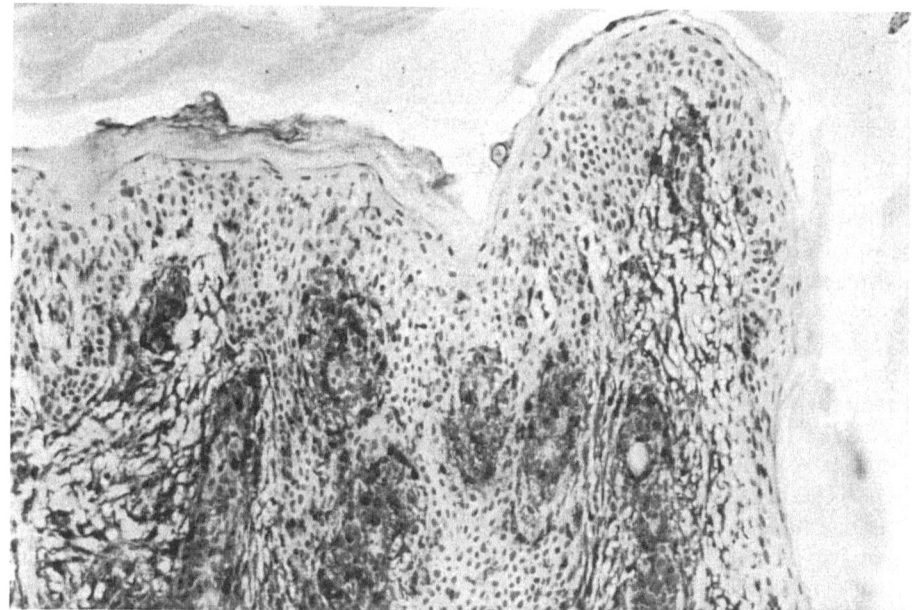

Fig. 19.10. The neoplastic cells in Pautrier's abscesses stain with Leu-3a (CD4). (Modified avidin-biotin peroxidase, × 125)

abnormal cells will exhibit a parallel decrease in their affinity for epidermotropism as well as a tendency to disseminate widely to visceral organs. Edelson (1980) considers CTCL in terms of an epidermotropic and a non-epidermotropic form. He suggests that a natural progression generally occurs from epidermotropic to non-epidermotropic CTCL, a trend sometimes reversed by therapy.

The tissue distribution of extracutaneous spread of CTCL has been explained in terms of T cell biology. The often absent or limited bone marrow infiltration, even in the presence of circulating neoplastic cells, probably reflects the extramedullary proliferation of the neoplastic post-thymic cells and their tendency to spare the marrow in their circulatory pathway. Bone marrow function is thus preserved until late in the course of CTCL, when a generalised blast crisis may supervene. The neoplastic T cells may also resemble their normal counterparts in their propensity to recirculate rapidly through the soft tissues, explaining, at least partly, why the lymph nodes do not appear to be barriers to the spread of the disease once the neoplastic cells escape the confines of the skin.

There are several suggestions for the demonstrated affinity for the epidermis. That the epidermis might mediate effects parallel to those of the thymus has been suspected for many years. Safai et al. (1979, 1980) have found high levels of a small, biologically active peptide called Facteur Thymique Sérique as well as thymopoietin-like activity in the serum of patients with MF. They also showed that the epidermal cells of patients with MF can produce Facteur Thymique Sérique-like activity in tissue cultures. Facteur Thymique Sérique induces differentiation of T cell precursors. Chu et al. (1982) have reported that basal keratinocytes synthesise a thymopoietin-like substance, and Rubenfeld et al. (1980)

supported the role of the skin as an inducer of T cell differentiation. They showed that epidermal cells can induce Thyl (a marker of cortical thymic T cells in mice) and TdT in lymphocytes. The role of the Langerhans cell in CTCL has also been the subject of much discussion. Immunochemical analysis has demonstrated receptors for Fc and C3b as well as MHC class II antigens on the surface of Langerhans cells. The number of Langerhans cells in the epidermis of MF lesions has been shown to increase with advancing disease (Tjernlund 1978). It is interesting that in cases of ATL, neoplastic T cell infiltration in the skin is accompanied by an increase in Langerhans cells (Shamoto 1983). These findings are in keeping with the view that Langerhans cells may induce antigen-specific and allogenic T cell activation. In contrast, the observation that Langerhans cells are significantly decreased in older adults with chronic actinically damaged skin (Thiers et al. 1984) may be related to the reportedly low incidence of CTCL in people living in sunny climates such as Australia. Ultraviolet light is known to render Langerhans cells incapable of acting as antigen-presenting cells (APCs) (Stingl and Wolff 1982), and ultraviolet light (PUVA) treatment has been shown to reduce the number of Langerhans cells in the skin (MacKie and Turbitt 1982).

Langerhans cells, in their role as antigen-trapping cells of the monocyte-histiocyte-macrophage system, can transport antigens from the epidermis to the local lymph nodes where a primary immune response is initiated (Silberberg et al. 1975). Their rich expression of MHC class II determinants is related to cellular collaboration in initiation of immune responses. The sensitised lymphocytes produced in the lymph nodes may "home" to the epidermis as a result of attraction to intraepidermal Langerhans cells (Rowden and Lewis 1976) or as a result of thymic hormone-like substances synthesised by the keratinocytes (Safai et al. 1979,1980; Rubenfeld et al. 1980; Chu et al. 1982). The observation that increased numbers of Langerhans cells are present even in the early stages of CTCL has led to the suggestion that the disease may be the result of antigen persistence, such as may occur with recurrent exposure to industrial chemicals (Edelson 1980). The discovery of HTLV-I in neoplastic T cells maintained in vitro from patients with CTCL (Poiesz et al. 1980) has led MacKie (1981) to hypothesise that infection of Langerhans cells by retrovirus may be the initiating event. Prolonged antigenic stimulation within the skin and lymph node could result in T helper/inducer cells homing to the epidermis, with modulation by T suppressor/cytotoxic cells. This may eventually result in the development of a malignant clone of T helper/inducer cells. CTCL may thus represent a neoplastic amplification of the normal protective biological function of the skin (Edelson 1980).

The neoplastic cells of CTCL rosette with sheep red blood cells and have Fc_μ receptors. In virtually all cases studied, a mature T-helper/inducer phenotype (CD4+, CD8−) has been demonstrated (Haynes et al. 1981; Kung et al. 1981), although an increased proportion of suppressor T cells has been shown rarely (Wassermann et al. 1980). In the skin and lymph nodes, the CD4+ cells form clusters with abundant MHC class II+ "indeterminate" macrophage-like cells (MacKie 1981; Thomas et al. 1982), closely mimicking the relationship of CD4+ cells and IDRCs in normal lymph nodes. In accordance with the helper/inducer phenotype of CTCL cells, lymphocytes from many cases provide helper activity in pokeweed-driven polyclonal B cell differentiation (Broder et al. 1976; Kung et al. 1981). Some cases of CTCL have raised immunoglobulin levels (Broder et al. 1976), suggesting that the tumour cells also have some helper activity in vivo. T cell responses to mitogen and delayed cutaneous hypersensitivity reactions are reduced and overwhelming infection in the absence of neutropenia is the commonest cause of death in these patients.

Cytogenetic studies of 36 patients with CTCL showed extensive aneuploidy, with both numerical and structural aberrations, a wide range of heteroploidy, and a lack of clone formation until the terminal phases of the disease as a characteristic feature (Whang-Peng et al. 1979). Therefore, broken, reduplicated, lost, or rearranged chromosomes can be readily found in the cells of CTCL and can be considered strong evidence to indicate neoplastic involvement of the tissue studied. It must be emphasised that although karyotype analysis is one of the most sensitive diagnostic indicators presently available, gross structural chromosomal changes are probably secondary phenomena in malignant lymphocytes.

CTCL is associated with HTLV-I infection. In fact, one of the first HTLV isolates was obtained from a T cell line derived from the lymph node of a patient with a malignant variant of cutaneous T lymphoma and several additional isolates were also obtained from separate blood samples from the patient (Poiesz et al. 1980; Gallo et al. 1982). Van der Loo et al. (1979) have found C type virus particles in the Langerhans cells of skin biopsies and lymph nodes from patients with MF and SS.

The different staging systems used for CTCL make it difficult to compare treatment results from various centres. Epstein et al. (1972) showed a mean survival of less than 5 years from the time of diagnosis for MF; the mean interval between onset of skin lesions and histological diagnosis was 3.8 years. Additional findings indicative of a poor prognosis were the presence of tumours or palpable lymphadenomegaly, each associated with a mean survival of 2.5 years. Definitive histological evidence of lymph node involvement was also associated with decreased longevity (18 months) as compared with those without such evidence (34 months). Clinically recognised splenomegaly or hepatomegaly was indicative of a median survival of only 3 months. Median survival between 8 and 9 years has been reported more recently, the difference probably being due to earlier diagnosis without much improvement in the overall course of the disease (Broder and Bunn 1980).

Node-based T Cell Lymphoma

When Lukes and Collins (1974) first proposed their immunologically based classification of NHL, they included the category of a "yet to be identified immunoblastic sarcoma of T cells". In a subsequent paper describing their findings in 790 cases of NHL studied with immunological surface marker techniques, Lukes et al. (1982) reported that 20% of the cases were of T cell lineage. Node-based T cell lymphomas made up 8% of the cases, while the remainder were cases of LL and cutaneous T cell lymphoma. By applying immunoperoxidase techniques to frozen sections, Tubbs et al. (1983) showed that of 257 cases of NHL classified by the International Working Formulation, T cell lymphomas comprised 10 out of 49 (20%) cases of low-grade lymphomas, 6 out of 82 (7.3%) cases of diffuse large cell lymphomas, and 9 out of 21 (43%) cases of diffuse mixed cell lymphomas in the intermediate-grade category and 50% of the lymphomas in the high-grade category. Thus, although initially conceived to be uncommon, immunological techniques have shown that T cell lymphomas form a significant percentage of all NHLs, particularly among the diffuse mixed cell type and the diffuse immunoblastic sarcomas. The high proportion of T cell lymphomas in Japan has already been mentioned. In endemic areas such as the southwestern islands of Japan, the proportion of T cell lymphomas is over 70% of all NHLs (Tajima et al. 1979), and even in the non-endemic areas of Japan, T cell lymphomas account for 40% (35% peripheral T cell phenotype, 5% thymic T cell phenotype) of all NHLs (presented by Suchi T. in Kadin et al. 1983).

Despite the obvious importance of this group of neoplasms, there is currently no satisfactory classification of T cell lymphoma, and the terminology used to describe this entity is confusing and controversial. The terminologies used in the Working Formulation are not appropriate to the T cell lymphomas. The main prognostic factors in the Working Formulation such as a nodular or diffuse pattern of infiltration and cell size, are probably not applicable to the T cell lymphomas. Furthermore, many of the characteristics of the T cell lesions, including polymorphism of cellular infiltrate and bizarre nuclear morphology of the neoplastic cells are not catered for in the Working Formulation.

Following their proposal of the term "immunoblastic sarcoma of T cells", Lukes and associates have expanded its use to include all malignant lymphomas of T cell type except for T-CLL, LL and the CTCL. Waldron et al. (1977) used the term "peripheral T cell lymphoma" in their description of six patients with lymphomas which they postulated to be of peripheral T cell origin in contrast with those of central or thymic origin. From the many terms used for this group of T cell malignancies (Table 19.2) we chose "node-based T cell lymphoma" (NBTCL; Leong et al. 1981), as it reflected not only the mature peripheral phenotype of the malignant cells but also their initial presentation in the lymph node as opposed to the skin, thus distinguishing this neoplasm from CTCL, the other neoplasm of mature T lymphocytes in the peripheral T cell compartment.

Table 19.2. Node-based T cell lymphoma: some other terms and subtypes described in the literature

---

T-immunoblastic sarcoma (Lukes and Collins 1974).
Peripheral T cell lymphoma (Waldron et al. 1977).
T zone lymphoma (Helbron et al. 1979).
Malignant lymphoma with high content of epithelioid histiocytes (so-called Lennert's lymphoma; Lukes et al. 1978).
Hyperlobated T cell lymphoma (Pinkus et al. 1979).
Pleomorphic lymphoma (Watanabe et al. 1979).
Immunoblastic lymphadenopathy (IBL)-like T cell lymphoma (Shimoyama et al. 1979a).
Erythrophagocytic T $_\gamma$ lymphoma (Kadin et al. 1981).
Plasmacytoid T cell lymphoma (Müller-Hermelink et al. 1983).
Signet-ring lymphoma, T cell type (Weiss et al. 1985a).

Several authors have attempted histological subtyping of the T cell lymphomas, and the many different names which have been used probably reflect the great variability of these tumours and the frustration in attempting to identify a dominant and characteristic clinicopathological feature. Lennert presented a classification of T cell lymphomas and leukaemias in Europe at a seminar on lymphoproliferative diseases in Japan and western countries in 1982 (Kadin et al. 1983). This classification is shown in Table 19.3. The Japanese classification of 101

Table 19.3. Classification of T cell lymphomas and leukaemias in Europe[a]

I. Thymic T cell lymphomas/leukaemias
  1. T lymphoblastic lymphoma, including T-type acute lymphoblastic leukaemia (T-ALL; thymic and prethymic types)

II. Peripheral T cell lymphomas/leukaemias
  1. T lymphoblastic lymphoma/T-ALL, peripheral type
  2. T type chronic lymphocytic leukaemia (T-CLL) ·
  3. T prolymphocytic leukaemia
  4. Cutaneous T cell lymphomas: mycosis fungoides, Sézary's syndrome and others
  5. Multilobated T cell lymphoma (Pinkus)
  6. Plasmacytoid T cell lymphoma
  7. Pleomorphic (polymorphic) T cell lymphomas: special variant, lymphoepithelioid lymphoma
  8. T immunoblastic lymphoma

---

[a] Presented by Lennert K. in Kadin et al. (1983).

cases of adult T cell leukaemia/lymphoma (ATL) is shown in Table 19.4. It appears from the Japanese reports that although cases of HTLV-I adult T cell lymphomas are most commonly classified as the "pleomorphic type" (Suchi and Tajima 1979), there is a large overlap in the histological appearances of the lymph nodes in ATL (presented by Hanaoka M. in Kadin et al. 1983) and in the cases labelled as T cell lymphoma (Watanabe et al. 1979; Kikuchi et al. 1979). Some of the latter came from non-endemic areas of Japan and did not appear to be associated with HTLV infection. Jaffe (1984) classified post-thymic T cell malignancies into: (1) T-CLL, (2) mycosis fungoides/Sézary syndrome, (3) peripheral T cell lymphomas, (4) adult T cell leukaemia/lymphoma and (5) angiocentric immunoproliferative lesions. We believe the separation of ATL from NBTCL on histological grounds is extremely difficult. Matsumoto et al. (1979) have shown the close similarities in clinicopathological features of ATL and T cell type NHL and have suggested a close relationship between the two entities. These workers use the term "adult T cell leukaemia/lymphoma" for both these entities. Indeed, the lymph node morphology in cases of T cell lymphoma associated with HTLV can be quite varied. Jaffe and associates (Blayney et al. 1983; Jaffe et al. 1983) identified 4 patients with antibodies to HTLV in a series of 34 cases of "peripheral T cell lymphoma". Three of these cases were histologically classified as malignant

Table 19.4. Distribution of 101 cases of adult T cell leukaemia/lymphoma (ATL) classified histologically from lymph nodal biopsy specimens[a]

	No. of Cases
Diffuse lymphoma	
Small cell type	2
Medium-sized cell type	38
Mixed cell type	9
Large cell type	9
Pleomorphic type	43
Total	101

---

[a] Presented by Hanaoka M. in Kadin et al (1983).

lymphoma, diffuse mixed cell type and one as malignant lymphoma, diffuse large cell type. It appears that although the pleomorphic type is most commonly associated with Japanese ATL, the lymph node changes in cases of T cell lymphoma associated with HTLV-I can be quite varied, without absolute correlation between any one histological subtype and HTLV infection.

Lennert has been reported to use the term "pleomorphic T cell lymphoma" interchangeably with "peripheral T cell lymphoma", as well as for the main part of the T cell immunoblastic sarcoma of the Lukes classification, and for the T-zone lymphoma of the Kiel classification (Kadin et al. 1983). Additional confusion is imparted by the term "pleomorphic T cell lymphoma" proposed by the Japanese workers, as the majority of cases of NBTCLs of various histological subtypes also show a marked degree of nuclear pleomorphism, which has been described variously as squiggly, Reed–Sternberg-like, multilobated, hyperlobated, deeply clefted, sinuate, mulberry, corrugated, cerebriform, etc.

We propose to classify NBTCL into two major groups: (1) a polymorphous type and (2) a monomorphous type (Table 19.5), believing that such a classification will encompass all the histological subtypes of NBTCL which have been described and will also allow a logical approach to the subject as many of the different histological appearances may represent different parts of the same morphological spectrum. We have seen progression from the polymorphous type to a monomorphous picture in rare cases of NBTCL (Leong et al. 1981).

Table 19.5. Classification of node-based T cell lymphoma

1. *Polymorphous type*
   a) Pleomorphic type, peripheral T cell lymphoma, T zone lymphoma
   b) Immunoblastic lymphadenopathy-like T cell lymphoma
   c) Lymphoepithelioid T cell lymphoma

2. *Monomorphous type*
   a) T-immunoblastic sarcoma
   b) Multilobated T cell lymphoma
   c) Monomorphous medium-sized T cell lymphoma
   d) Plasmacytoid T cell lymphoma
   e) Erythrophagocytic T lymphoma
   f) Signet-ring lymphoma, T cell type

NBTCL, Polymorphous Type

The polymorphous subtype of NBTCL is characterised by a polymorphous infiltrate within which are found the malignant T cells with their atypical and often characteristic nuclear morphology. The cellular infiltrate contains a mixture of small and large lymphoid cells, the smaller cells having dark but finely stippled chromatin and irregular sinuous nuclei, while the scattered larger cells are T-immunoblasts with round open vesicular nuclei which are often multilobated and contain two or three prominent nucleoli. Their cytoplasm is abundant, varying from amphophilic to pale staining. Some of these polylobated cells may resemble Reed–Sternberg cells, and all gradations between the large and small cells may be present. There is a background infiltrate of plasma cells, macrophages, epithelioid histiocytes and eosinophils in varying numbers. Blood vessels lined by plump endothelial cells are usually abundantly distributed throughout the lymph node. There may be a diffuse proliferation of collagenous twigs, apparently related to the blood vessels, which compartmentalise the tumour into small nests of cells (Figs. 19.11, 19.12, 19.13).

In the lymph nodes, NBTCL characteristically involves the paracortical T cell zones and infiltrates the sinusoids, and in the spleen, the periarteriolar areas are involved (Fig. 19.14). With progression of the disease, however, this typical zonal distribution is obscured.

The presence of these morphological features, which are common to the polymorphous subtypes of NBTCL, particularly the polymorphous nature of the infiltrate and the neoplastic cells with their characteristic nuclear morphology, should alert the pathologist to the diagnosis. A study by Jaffe et al. (1982) has revealed that in only 61% of aggressive diffuse NHL could immunological phenotype be correctly predicted on the basis of the histological examination of tissue sections. For this reason it is recommended that suspected cases of polymorphous NBTCL be confirmed with immunological studies.

Several subtypes of pleomorphic NBTCL have been described and are discussed below. However, we believe that there may be considerable overlap between these subtypes making a clear-cut histological distinction very difficult.

Pleomorphic Type, Peripheral T Cell Lymphoma and T-zone Lymphoma. We are of the opinion that there are strong morphological similarities among the NBTCLs which have been named pleomorphic type (Kikuchi et al. 1979;

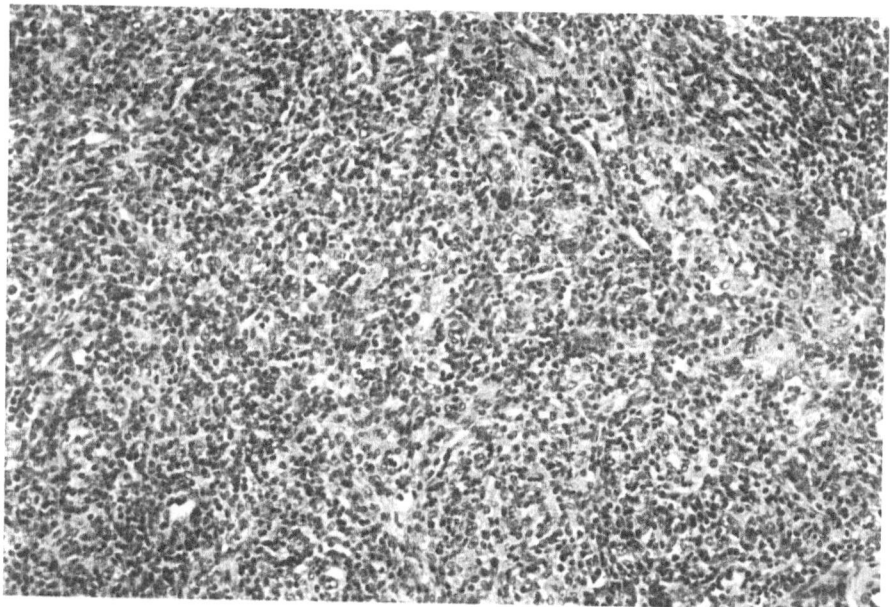

Fig. 19.11. Node-based T cell lymphoma, pleomorphic type. Note the polymorphous infiltrate of large and small lymphoid cells, epithelioid cells, and the prominent vessels in the background. (H & E, ×125)

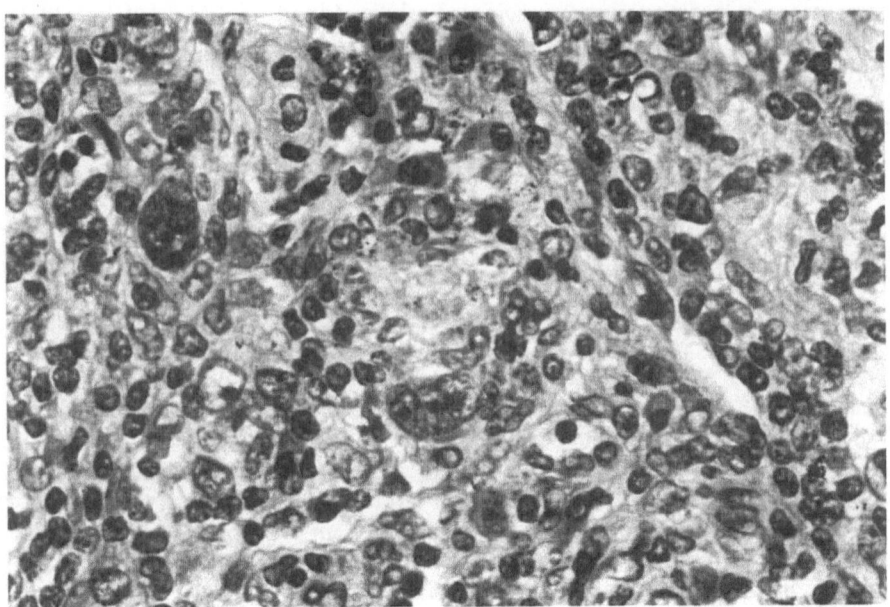

Fig. 19.12. Node-based T cell lymphoma, polymorphous type. The neoplastic cells have large multilobated nuclei and often large nucleoli. The range of smaller lymphocytes in the background display marked nuclear irregularities and occasional plasma cells are present. (H & E, × 500)

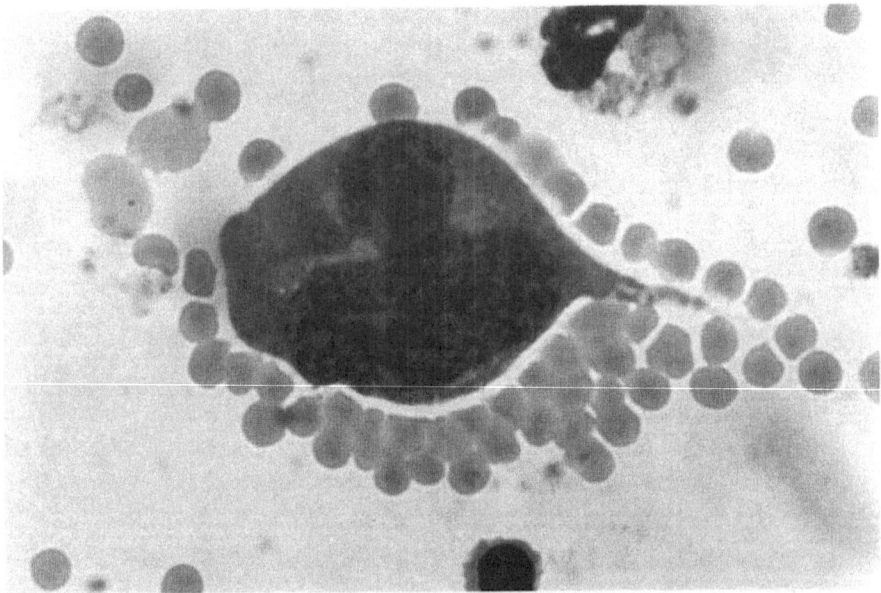

Fig. 19.13. E-rosette preparation stained with ANAE. E-rosetting and fine red granules of ANAE positivity (the red staining not visible in this photograph) identify the large polylobated neoplastic cell as a T cell. (ANAE stain, × 1250)

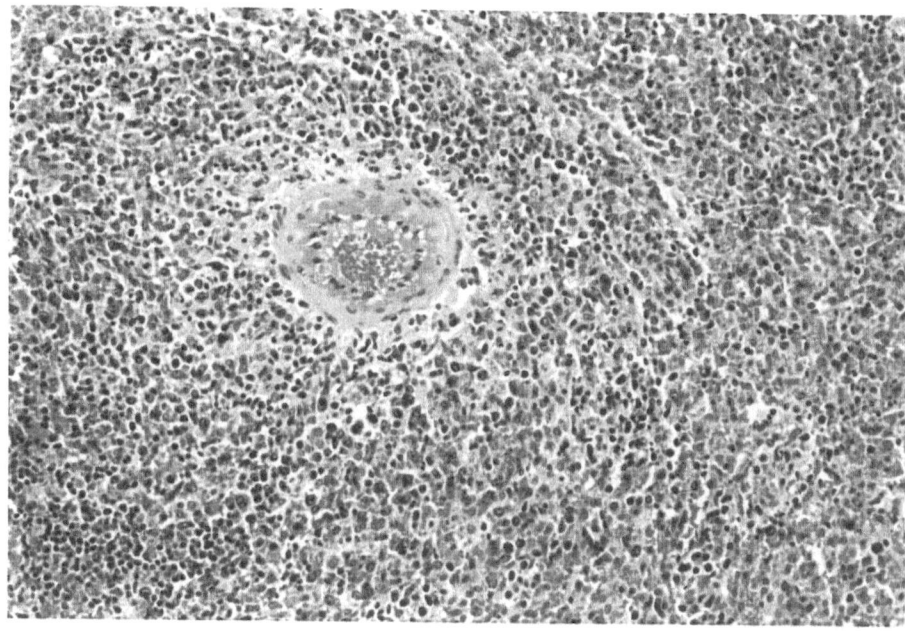

Fig. 19.14. T cell lymphomas of polymorphous type involving the periarteriolar sheath of the spleen. (H & E, × 125)

Watanabe et al. 1979; Watanabe et al. 1981), peripheral T cell lymphoma (Waldron et al. 1977) and T-zone lymphoma (Helbron et al. 1979). Although ATL has distinctive clinicopathological features, pleomorphic T cell lymphoma, albeit the most common (43% of cases), is only one of the five histological subtypes which have been described in association with ATL (see Table 19.4) and the same pleomorphic subtype can be seen in patients with NBTCL from non-endemic areas of Japan.

The pleomorphic type of NBTCL has been described as showing "intermingled lymphoid cells of widely varying size and degree of nuclear transformation. Nuclear folding was appreciable throughout the lymphoid population. A considerable number of giant cells with nuclear hyperlobation and multinucleation were distributed among the cells. The lymphoid infiltrate was generally compartmentalised into microscopic clusters of cells partially demarcated by delicate collagenous or reticulum bands in 43.2% of the cases. A histiocytic reaction was conspicuous in 10 cases and eosinophils were seen in 4" of a total of 44 cases studied (Kikuchi et al. 1979). A polymorphous infiltrate of lymphocytes of varying sizes with pronounced nuclear irregularities, mixed with hyperlobated giant cells, histiocytes and occasionally eosinophils, and compartmentalisation into clusters by fine bands of collagen fibres, would fit the description of peripheral T cell lymphoma of Waldron et al. (1977) as well as the T zone lymphoma of Lennert (Helbron et al. 1979). Additional features which have been described in the latter two conditions include bands of collagen fibres which seem to arise from prominent high endothelial vessels, and the epithelioid nature of many of the histiocytes in the infiltrate.

The vast majority of patients having this type of NBTCL are adults, only rare cases being reported under the age of 20 years. Most patients present with generalised lymphadenopathy. Other frequent sites of involvement include skin, liver, peripheral blood, lungs and pleura. Skin involvement, when present, is usually dermal in location and spares the epidermis, a feature which allows the distinction from CTCL. However, in some cases epidermotropism is marked and the cutaneous infiltrate may mimic that of CTCL (Leong et al. 1980). The bone marrow is rarely involved at presentation but, in as many as one-third of cases, atypical lymphocytes may be seen in the peripheral blood and lymphopenia may be present in another third (Catovsky et al. 1982a). Other unusual sites of involvement include Waldeyer's ring (Leong et al. 1981).

This group of T cell lymphomas pursues an aggressive clinical course. In the Japanese series, about 80% of the patients died within 1 year despite intensive chemotherapy (Kikuchi et al. 1979), and in Lennert's series the median survival was 9.4 months with poor response to therapy (Helbron et al. 1979). At variance with the Japanese experience, Jaffe et al. (1984) suggest that the histological subtype in ATL seen in the USA does not appear to influence prognosis. Unlike other forms of NHL in which an increasing proportion of large neoplastic cells is correlated with a more aggressive natural history, in ATL neither complete remission nor survival has been correlated with histological subtype. These authors suggested that ATL should be considered a single clinicopathological entity and should be diagnosed as such.

Immunoblastic Lymphadenopathy (IBL)-like T Cell Lymphomas. In 1979, Shimoyama and associates (1979a) described the disease they named "IBL-like T cell lymphoma". They felt that this disease was distinctly different from ATL, although it bore some resemblance to immunoblastic lymphadenopathy or angioimmunoblastic lymphadenopathy. The clinical characteristics of IBL-like T cell lymphoma include:

1. Generalised lymphadenopathy that may respond initially to steroids
2. High fever, cutaneous rash, and weakness
3. Fequent hepatosplenomegaly without a mediastinal mass
4. Polyclonal hypergammaglobulinaemia
5. Autoimmune haemolytic anaemia
6. Elevation of various antiviral titres such as rubella, rubeola, varicella, EBV and/or antitoxoplasma
7. Leukocytosis with neutrophilia, lymphocytopenia and atypical plasmacytoid cells
8. Marked male predominance
9. Progressive course with fatal outcome
10. No endemic distribution of patients' birthplaces.

The histological features of lymph nodes in IBL-like T cell lymphoma include a diffuse or multifocal neoplastic infiltrate consisting of immunoblasts and large lymphoid cells with abundant water-clear cytoplasm or pale cells, which are frequently associated with angioimmunoblastic and granulomatous lesions. There is zonal proliferation of plasma cells, disappearance of germinal centres, depletion of small lymphocytes, and deposition of amorphous and eosinophilic interstitial material. The patients are often initially considered to have immunoblastic lymphadenopathy or angioimmunoblastic lymphadenopathy with dysproteinae-mia, until subsequent studies reveal the neoplastic nature of the disease. To date, although only rare cases of this subtype of T cell lymphoma have been described outside of Japan, the prominent post-capillary venules seen in NBTCL, polymor-phous type can cause a resemblance to immunoblastic lymphadenopathy. The distinction between the two entities can be difficult and NBTCL is identified by cytological atypia in the setting of the polymorphous infiltrate of peripheral T cell lymphoma. It is likely that some cases previously diagnosed as immunoblastic lymphadenopathy represent a form of NBTCL. Up to 35% of patients with immunoblastic lymphadenopathy develop a large cell immunoblastic lymphoma, and even in patients without overt histological progression, the median survival is only about 2 years (Nathwani et al. 1978). The exact relationship between NBTCL and immunoblastic lymphadenopathy needs to be defined further.

Lymphoepithelioid T Cell Lymphoma. In 1968, Lennert and Mestdagh de-scribed a malignant lymphoma with a high content of epithelioid cells. Since then there has been considerable debate as to the nature of this tumour which was originally thought to be a form of HD. Because of the frequent absence of Reed–Sternberg cells and the progression of some of these cases, Lennert et al. (1975) subsequently recommended the term "lymphoepithelioid lymphoma". Intense epithelioid cell infiltration may occur in a number of lymphomas of differing histogenic type (Kim et al. 1980). Of 12 cases of lymphoepithelioid lymphoma, 3 were shown to be NBTCL, 6 had markers of HD, being positive for Ki-1 and 3C4 antigens, and the remaining 3 cases were of an "undefined type" (Kadin et al. 1983). In a study of 33 cases of NBTCL in Taiwan, Su et al. (1985) found 2 cases of lymphoepithelioid lymphoma, both of which revealed T helper phenotype. Other cases of lymphoepithelioid lymphoma with T cell phenotype have been rarely described (Bogomoletz et al. 1983). It is important to attempt to identify the malignant lymphoid cells intervening between the large and prominent clusters of epithelioid cells seen in lymphoepithelioid lymphoma. In the cases of lymphoepithelioid T cell lymphoma (Fig. 19.15), the characteristic neoplastic T cells may be found. These show a range of appearances between small, irregular, sinuous T cells and T-immunoblasts (Fig. 19.16). Other characteristics of NBTCL such as prominent blood vessels with plump endothelial cells, eosinophils and plasma cells may also be present.

NBTCL, Monomorphous Type

In contrast to the polymorphous type, this type of NBTCL shows a more homogeneous infiltrate. The various histological subtypes which have been described are discussed below.

T-immunoblastic Sarcoma. Lukes and associates have used the term "immu-noblastic sarcoma of T cells" to encompass almost all malignant lymphomas of peripheral T cell type with the exception of T-CLL, LL and CTCL, thereby emphasising that these tumours are derived from effector lymphocytes. We feel that the use of this term for all such cases is misleading. The term "B-immunoblastic sarcoma" defines a certain large cell lymphoma of B cell type. T-

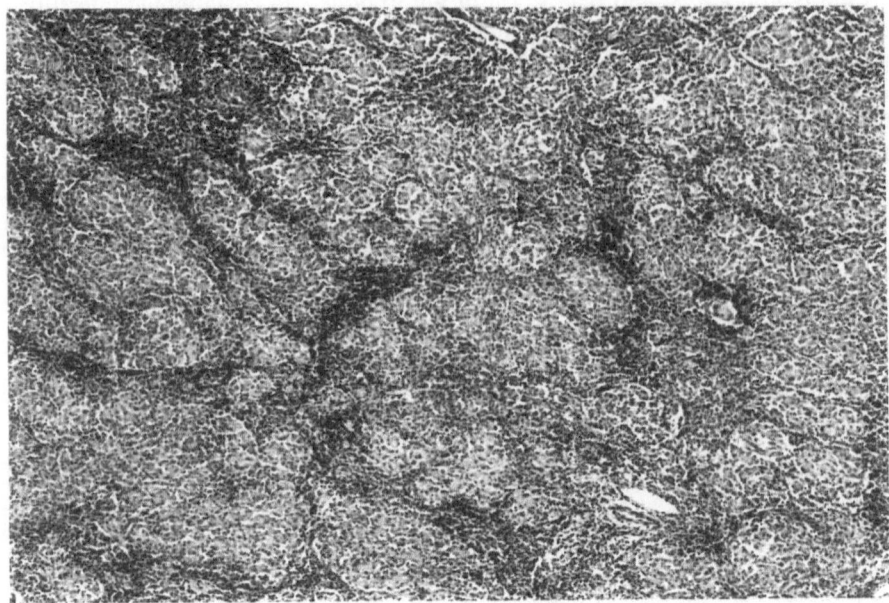

Fig. 19.15. So-called Lennert's lymphoma or lymphoepithelioid T cell lymphoma showing prominent clusters of epithelioid histiocytes with the small darker areas in between representing the neoplastic infiltrate. (H & E, ×125)

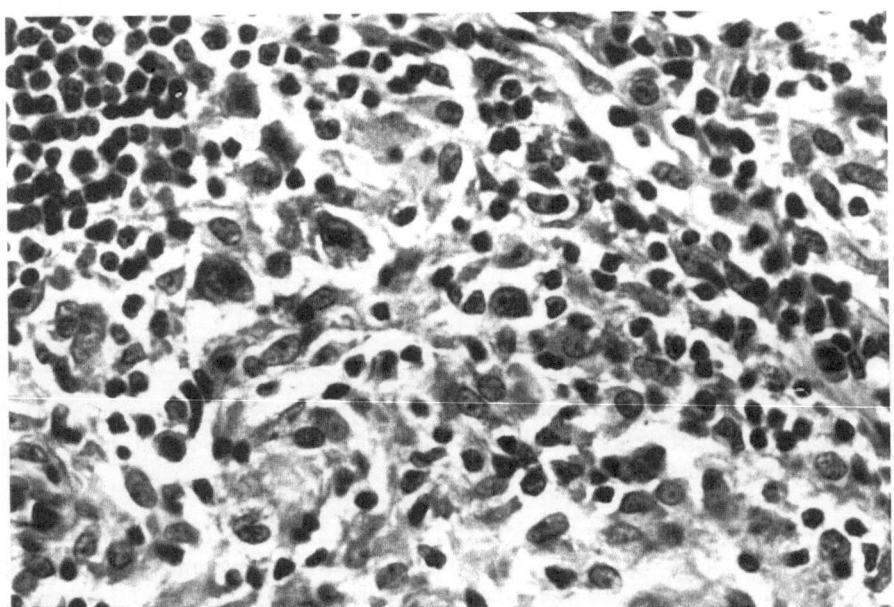

Fig. 19.16. Lymphoepithelioid T cell lymphoma showing the neoplastic cells, which range in appearance from large T-immunoblasts to small lymphocytes with irregular nuclear outlines. (H & E, ×500)

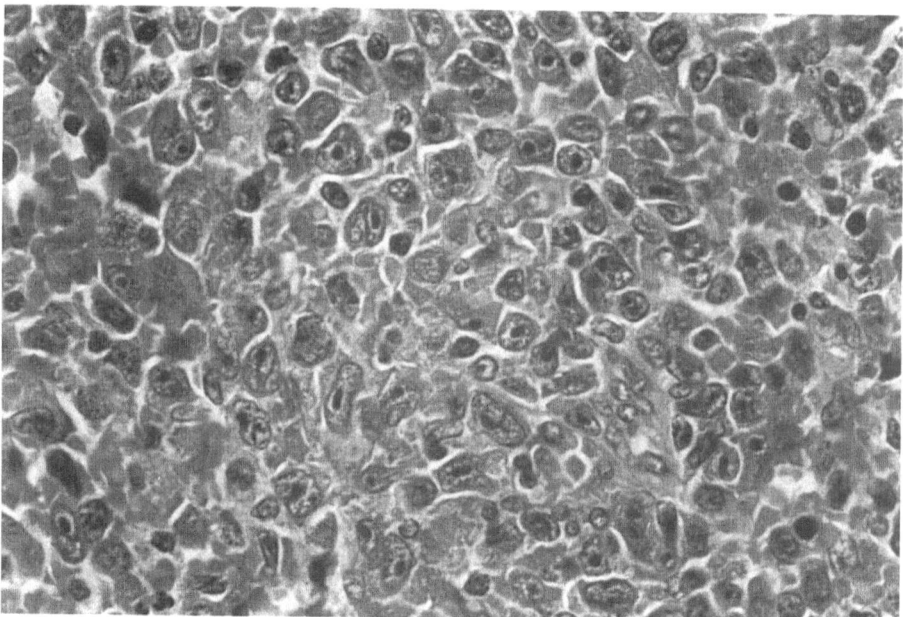

Fig. 19.17. T-IBS composed of a diffuse homogeneous infiltrate of immunoblasts with abundant dense cytoplasm and large nuclei with one to three prominent nucleoli. There is fine speckling of the chromatin. (H & E, × 500)

immunoblastic sarcoma therefore, by implication, defines its T cell counterpart, i.e. a large cell lymphoma of T cell type. We prefer to use the term "T-immunoblastic sarcoma" (T-IBS) for a specific histological type of NBTCL which is composed of a relatively homogeneous infiltrate of T-immunoblasts. The latter are characterised by large round to oval vesicular nuclei, which are frequently polylobated, two to four prominent nucleoli and abundant cytoplasm. The cytoplasm of varying density may be amphophilic or pale staining, and cytoplasmic membranes are often fine and distinct (Fig. 19.17). It is not unusual for this lesion to contain a small population of admixed transformed lymphocytes. These have scanty cytoplasm and show varying degrees of nuclear folding and irregularity. The nuclear membranes are distinct and the chromatin is finely dispersed; the nucleoli are small. T-IBS may be associated with varying degrees of sclerosis, but the prominent vascular pattern seen in polymorphous NBTCL is not observed. Mitotic figures are frequent.

In our experience, T-IBS may be preceded by polymorphous NBTCL and, in some lesions, areas of polymorphous infiltrate merge with more homogeneous areas of T-immunoblasts, suggesting a morphological continuum (Fig. 19.18).

Multilobated T Cell Lymphoma. Pinkus and associates (Pinkus et al. 1979; Weinberg and Pinkus 1981) described a distinct morphological variant of NBTCL with large multilobated nuclei. Their 14 patients, aged from 25 to 69 years, presented with features which included fever, night sweats and weight loss. There was a predilection for extranodal involvement, and the skin and subcutaneous tissue, bone and central nervous system were frequent sites of infiltration by the

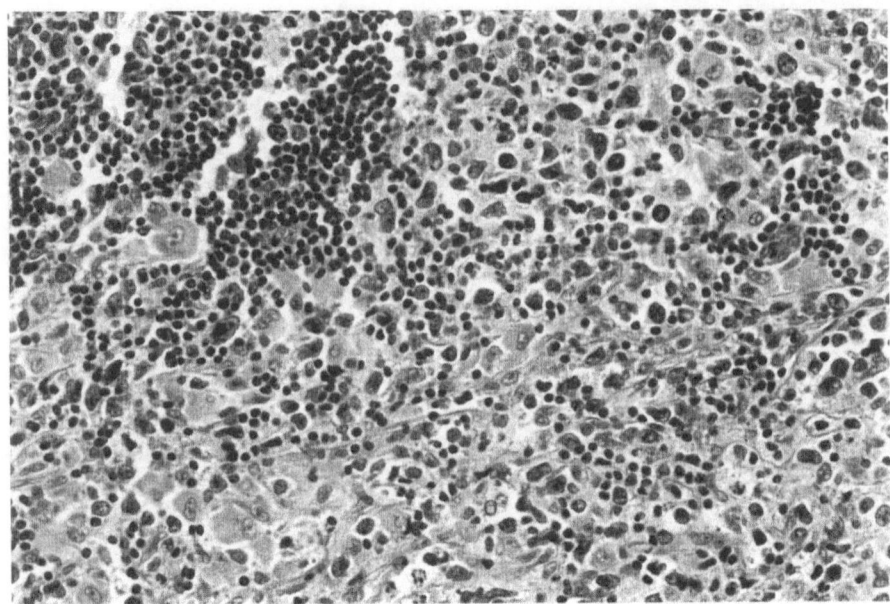

Fig. 19.18. Another area of the node with T-IBS shown in Fig. 19.17, where a polymorphous infiltrate of small and large atypical lymphoid cells and epithelioid cells is seen. This polymorphous infiltrate merged with homogeneous areas of T-immunoblasts. (H & E, × 300)

lymphoma. Lymphadenopathy was present in all cases but splenomegaly was not observed. The striking feature of all but one of nine patients in whom the course was followed for a long period was the excellent clinical response to therapy. This has yet to be confirmed.

The diffuse relatively monomorphic lymphomatous infiltrate was characterised by large lymphoid cells with markedly irregular, multilobated or hypersegmented nuclei which imparted a clover leaf or mulberry appearance in histological sections (Fig. 19.19). The nuclei had relatively fine chromatin and small to inconspicuous nucleoli and were surrounded by a broad rim of water-clear cytoplasm. Occasionally, the tumour cells had elongated nuclei. The tumour cells were relatively monomorphous and were not accompanied by the same proliferation of blood vessels, eosinophils and epithelioid cells seen in polymorphous NBTCL. The tumour cells in the cases initially reported by Pinkus et al. (1979) were identified as being of T-cell lineage by E-rosette formation. They also demonstrated strong punctate cytoplasmic acid phosphatase activity, and α-naphthyl butyrate esterase activity. We have also observed transition from the polymorphous type to this form of monomorphous multilobated NBTCL.

Monomorphous Medium-sized T Cell Lymphoma. Next to the pleomorphic type, the monomorphous medium-sized cell type is the most common form of NBTCL seen in Japan (presented by Hanaoka M. in Kadin et al. 1983). This lesion is characterised by a diffuse infiltrate which consists of medium-sized lymphoid cells with round to oval nuclei which show marked nuclear membrane irregularities (Figures 19.20, 19.21). The chromatin is finely dispersed and the

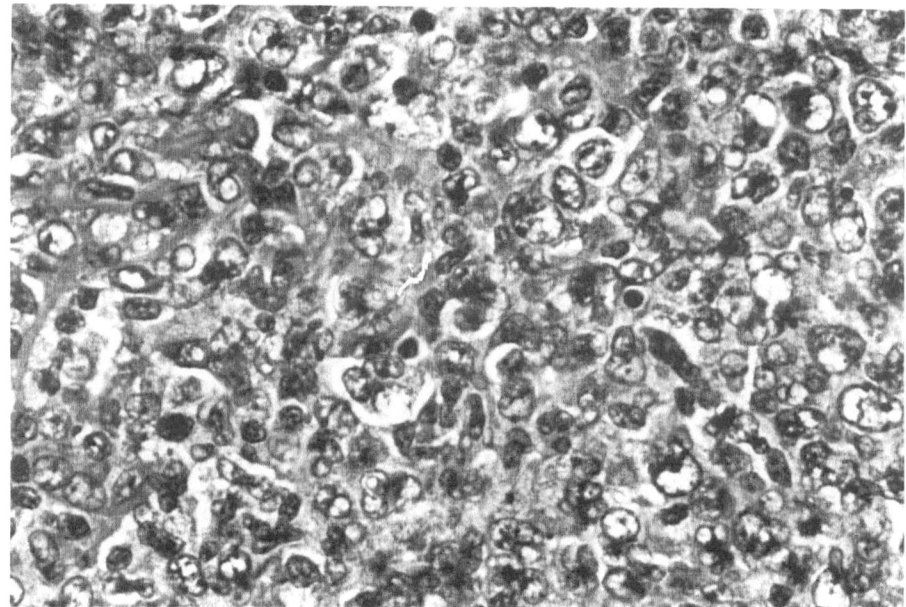

Fig. 19.19. Multilobated T cell lymphoma. The monomorphous infiltrate is composed of large cells with moderate amounts of cytoplasm and characteristic multilobated nuclei which display fine chromatin and small nucleoli. (H & E, × 500)

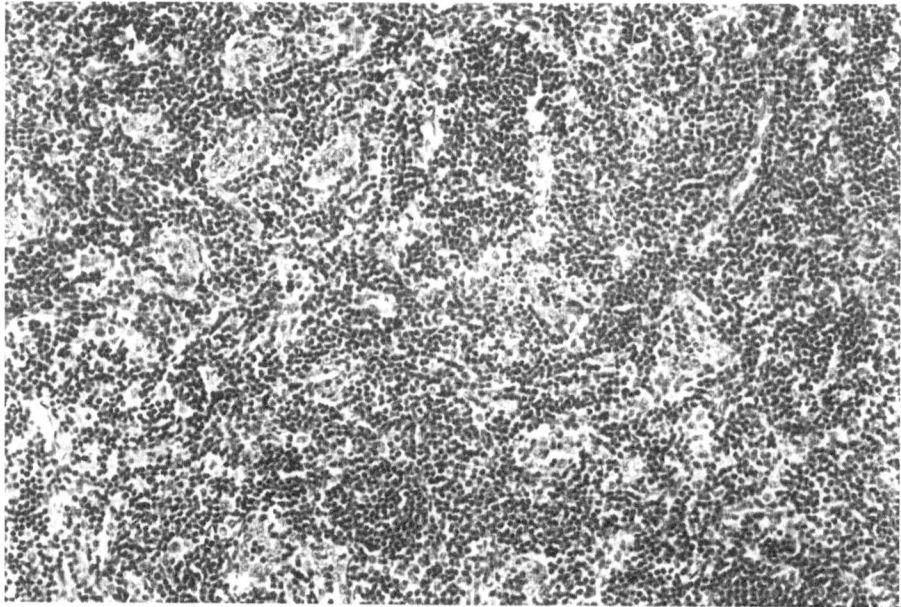

Fig. 19.20. Monomorphous medium-sized T cell lymphoma. A diffuse monomorphous infiltrate is seen with a prominent vascular background. (H & E, × 125)

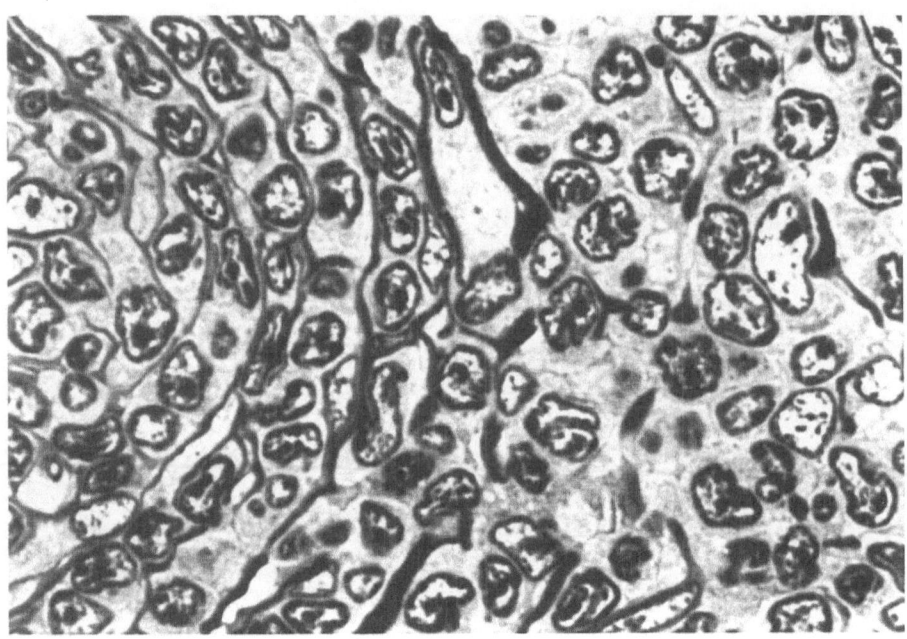

Fig. 19.21. Monomorphous medium-sized T cell lymphoma. Note the marked nuclear irregularities of the neoplastic lymphocytes which are seen infiltrating the wall of a blood vessel on the *left*. (Epon-embedded, toluidine blue, × 1250)

nuclei have a twisted or cerebriform appearance. The cytoplasm is scanty to moderate in amount and the cytoplasmic outlines are distinct. Elongated nuclei are also common. Mitotic activity is brisk. Survival of patients with this subtype has been short, the 50% survival being only 2.5 months (Kikuchi et al. 1979).

Plasmacytoid T Cell Lymphoma. Plasmacytoid T cell lymphoma is a variant of low-grade NBTCL recently described by Müller-Hermelink et al. (1983). We are aware of only one other case report of this very rare entity (Prasthofer et al. 1985). Lennert and Remmelle (1958) reported the presence of plasmacyte-like cells in the paracortex of reactive lymph nodes, i.e. in non-specific lymphadenitis. These cells were arranged in clusters that showed a topographic relationship with IDRCs and with the high endothelium-lined vessels of the T cell zones. Ultrastructural examination has shown that T-associated plasma cells are indistinguishable from plasmablasts and plasma cells detected in the B-dependent areas of lymphoid tissues, as they display eccentric nuclei with marginal chromatin and prominent nucleoli, abundant rough endoplasmic reticulum cisternae arranged in parallel arrays, expanded Golgi apparatus, numerous Golgi-related smooth and coated vesicles, and some lysosomal granules. The T-associated plasmacytoid cells have been shown to lack surface or cytoplasmic immunoglobulin and to express T helper markers, but do not bear surface receptors for sheep erythrocytes.

The monomorphous infiltrate of plasmacytoid T cells described by Müller-Hermelink et al. (1983) was CD5+ (Leu-1+), CD4+ (Leu-3+) and MHC class II+, but other T cell markers such as CD2, CD3 and CD8 were not detected. Cells were also negative for B and myelomonocytic lineage markers, C3b receptors and TdT but reacted weakly with a CD10 monoclonal antibody. Shortly after the diagnosis of plasmacytoid T cell lymphoma was made, the patient developed a myelomonocytic leukaemia and died 7 months later. In the case reported by Prasthofer et al. (1985) lymph node architecture was completely effaced by an infiltrate predominantly of medium-sized cells with round central nuclei and slightly basophilic cytoplasm. The peripheral distribution of heterochromatin and the presence of nucleoli, often located centrally, suggested plasmablastic morphology. Numerous tingible-body macrophages were present with a "starry sky" appearance. The plasmacytoid cells were consistently negative for surface or cytoplasmic immunoglobulin, myelomonocytic surface markers and peroxidase. They expressed T cell markers CD4 (OKT4, Leu-3), T9 and T10, and a proportion was also positive for sheep erythrocyte receptors. The association between plasmacytoid T cell lymphoma and a myeloproliferative disorder in both the reported cases has suggested that plasmacytoid T cells might exert a regulatory role on proliferation of myeloid cells.

Erythrophagocytic T_γ Lymphoma. Kadin et al. (1981) reported two patients, aged 30 and 33 years, with a variant of NBTCL which mimicked malignant histiocytosis in that the neoplastic T cells displayed erythrophagocytosis and had a tissue distribution similar to that of cells of the monocyte-macrophage system. Both patients had hepatosplenomegaly and minimal lymphadenopathy, and lymph node biopsies showed infiltration of medullary cords and medullary and subcapsular sinuses. The neoplastic cells were medium-sized, had peripherally condensed chromatin and one or two small nucleoli, but prominent nuclear convolutions and hypersegmentation or multinucleated cells were not a feature of this lymphoma. Erythrophagocytosis by tumour cells was the most remarkable finding in the lymph node biopsies. In the enlarged spleens, the tumour cells infiltrated the red pulp cords, the sinuses, and the area immediately outside the white pulp sheaths that surrounded central arterioles. The periarteriolar white pulp contained mostly small lymphocytes and infrequent mitoses so that its involvement by tumour was unclear. Tumour erythrophagocytosis was found only infrequently in the spleen. Tumour cells also infiltrated sinusoids in the liver.

Most tumour cells had receptors for both sheep erythrocytes and IgG-coated sheep or ox erythrocytes. When tumour cells were incubated with IgG-coated erythrocytes at 37° C, there was a twofold to fivefold increase in the number of phagocytic tumour cells. The tumour cells lacked non-specific esterase and TdT but stained with acid phosphatase in a focal pattern typical of T lymphocytes. Kadin et al. (1981) suggested that erythrophagocytosis by these T_γ cells was mediated by the Fc receptor, since phagocytosis by tumour and normal T_γ cells occurred in vitro only with IgG-coated erythrocytes and was usually limited to just one or two erythrocytes.

Erythrophagocytosis by tumour cells has also been observed in SS (Schechter et al. 1981). A pronounced benign erythrophagocytic reaction may also be observed in patients with NBTCL. Jaffe and associates (Costa et al. 1980; Jaffe et al. 1981) have reported a variable degree of erythrophagocytic activity in benign histiocytes in the splenic red pulp, hepatic sinusoids, lymph node sinuses and bone marrow infiltrated by NBTCL. At times, the erythrophagocytosis can be so conspicuous as to overshadow the noteworthy but less conspicuous malignant lymphoid infiltrate.

These authors have suggested that activated T cells can produce a lymphokine that induces Fc receptors and phagocytosis in mononuclear phagocytes.

Signet-ring Lymphoma, T Cell Type.   The term "signet-ring cell lymphoma" was proposed for a rare morphological variant of follicular centre cell and immunoblastic lymphomas in which signet-ring-like cells were a prominent feature. The morphological appearance of the signet-ring-like cells was thought to be due to the presence of a clear vacuolated or eosinophilic cytoplasmic inclusion, resembling a Russell body, which displaces the nucleus to one side of the cell. It was speculated that the cytoplasmic inclusions represent the morphological expression of immunoglobulin production and that signet-ring cell lymphoma is a morphological feature specific to lymphomas of B cell derivation. Recently, however, two reports have described the occurrence of the signet-ring morphology in three cases of lymphoma of T cell origin (Grogan et al. 1985a; Weiss et al. 1985a). Histologically, all three cases were diffuse large cell lymphomas with many neoplastic cells containing cytoplasmic vacuoles imparting a signet-ring configuration. Ultrastructural examination revealed the vacuoles to consist of electron-lucent spaces containing variable numbers of microspherules. The neoplastic cells expressed T cell phenotypes, lacking reactivity with antibodies to B cell antigens.

The electron-lucent cytoplasmic spaces and microspherules in cases of signet-ring lymphoma have been thought to represent immunoglobulin. However, these recently reported cases of signet-ring lymphoma of T cell type support the arguments of Harris et al. (1981), who questioned this concept and hypothesised that the microspherules found in this type of lymphoma may be derived from multivesicular bodies. Multivesicular bodies are membrane-bound vacuoles containing small vesicles seen in many cell types. Because they stain for acid phosphatase, they are regarded as a category of lysosomes. Grogan et al. (1985a) suggest that aberrant membrane recycling may be the common denominator of signet-ring formation in both B and T cell signet-ring lymphomas. They hypothesise that the large vacuoles containing microvesicules are most probably giant multivesicular bodies resulting from endocytosis or internalisation of surface T-antigens or the sequestration of Golgi-derived vesicles containing T cell antigens.

Immunological Phenotypes

The cell surface antigens of neoplastic cells in 29 cases of ATL were reported by Kikuchi (in Kadin et al. 1983). A helper/inducer T cell phenotype (CD3+, CD4+), with or without MHC class II antigens, was the most common. Of 12 cases of medium-sized type, 8 were CD3+, CD4+ and CD8-, and 4 were CD3-, CD4+ and CD8-. Of 9 cases of pleomorphic type, 4 were CD3+, CD4+ and CD8-, 1 was CD3+, CD4+ and CD8+, and 4 were CD3-, CD4+, CD8-. Of 8 cases of large cell type, 3 were CD3+, CD4+ and CD8-, 1 was CD3+, CD4+ and CD8+, and 4 were CD3-, CD4+ and CD8-. A recent study by Weiss et al. (1985b) of 50 cases of NBTCL revealed no correlation between immunophenotype and classification by the Working Formulation: 64% of the lymphomas were of helper/inducer phenotype (Figs. 19.22, 19.23), 12% were of suppressor/cytotoxic phenotype, 8% co-expressed both helper/inducer and suppressor/cytotoxic antigenic markers, and 16% lacked detectable markers for either helper/inducer or suppressor/cytotoxic cells. A common finding was the loss of one or more of the pan-T antigens CD2, CD3, CD5 and CD7 in 32 cases. The expression of CD5 and

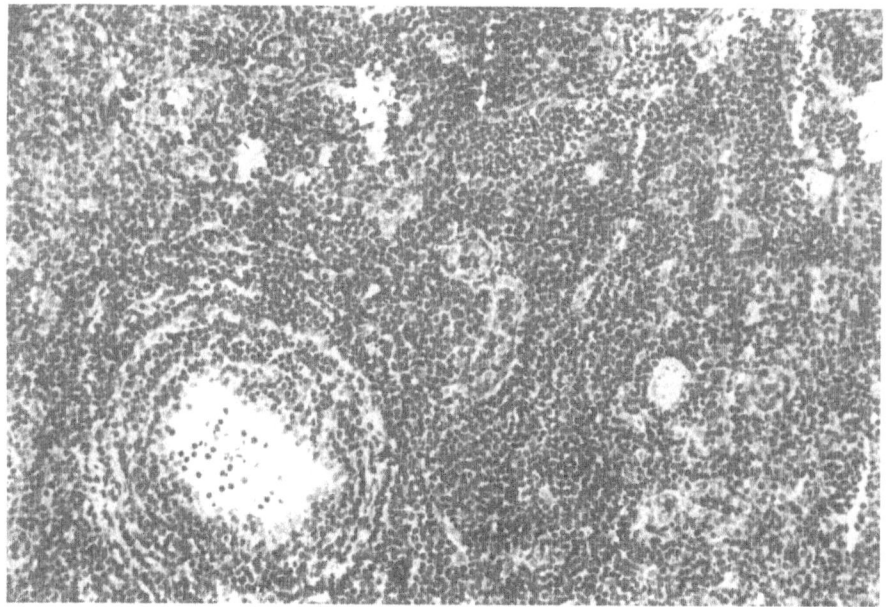

Fig. 19.22. Node-based T cell lymphoma, monomorphous medium-sized type, showing T-helper/inducer phenotype. There is staining with Leu-3a (CD4) of most of the neoplastic cells, which are seen infiltrating a blood vessel. (Leu-3a, modified avidin-biotin peroxidase, haematoxylin counterstain, × 125)

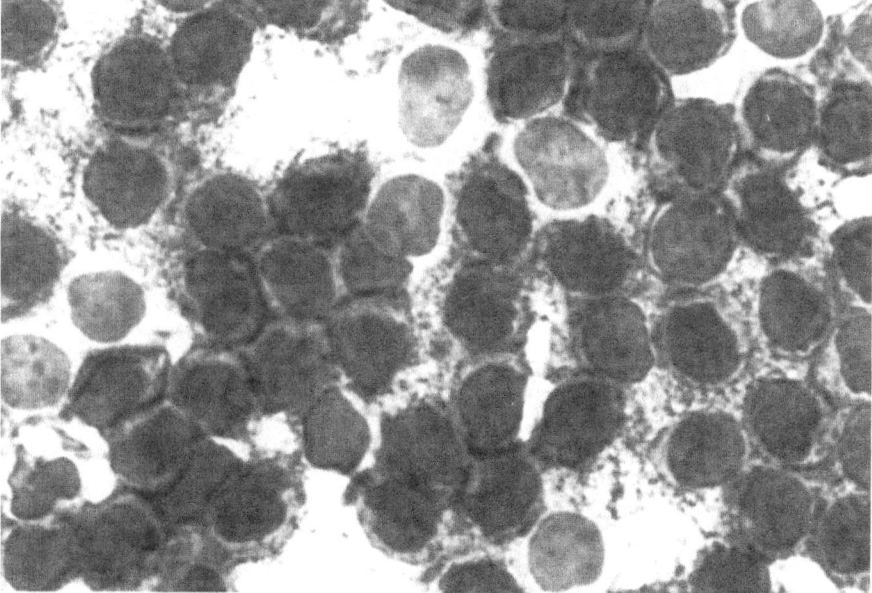

Fig. 19.23. Cytospin preparation of lymph node tissue from case of NBTCL, monomorphous medium-sized type stained with Leu-3a (CD4). The atypical lymphocytes with marked nuclear irregularity show positive staining. (Modified avidin-biotin peroxidase, haematoxylin counterstain, × 1250)

CD7 was lost in 46% of cases, expression of CD3 was lost in 26%, and expression of CD2 was lost in 24%. About three-quarters of the lymphomas expressed MHC class II antigens. This immunotype heterogeneity of NBTCL has also been demonstrated in other similar studies (Wood et al. 1983). Unusual or "novel" phenotypes, i.e. phenotypes of patterns of antigen expression not usually identified with normal T cell ontogeny, were found in 7 out of 11 cases (Grogan et al. 1985b). These included cases with E-rosette formation without E-rosette receptor, cases with subset antigens without universal antigens, and cases with some universal antigens and not others.

The Leu-M1 antigen has recently been proposed as a valuable immunodiagnostic marker of the Reed–Sternberg cells of HD and as being particularly helpful in distinguishing HD from other lymphoproliferative disorders such as peripheral T cell lymphomas. Wieczorek et al. (1985), however, showed that of 38 cases of well-characterised NBTCL, the neoplastic cells in 19 (50%) expressed the Leu-M1 antigen, suggesting that Leu-M1 is not a specific immunodiagnostic marker and has limited value in distinguishing between HD and NBTCL, which simulates HD morphologically.

Conclusions

The classification of NBTCL is currently confusing and controversial and a wide variety of histological and eponymic designations identify the morphological variants. We propose that this group of neoplasms can be divided into two groups, a polymorphous and a monomorphous type. The polymorphous group encompasses several variants which include T zone lymphoma, peripheral T cell lymphoma, pleomorphic lymphoma, lymphoepithelioid lymphoma, T-IBS of Lukes and IBL-like T cell lymphoma. Histologically, these cases are characterised by a polymorphous infiltrate of a spectrum of transformed T lymphocytes admixed with epithelioid histiocytes, plasma cells and eosinophils. The neoplastic T cells range from small cells with scanty cytoplasm and dark nuclei with finely dispersed chromatin and strikingly irregular nuclear membranes to large cells with abundant pale or amphophilic cytoplasm and large vesicular round to oval nuclei which are polylobated and contain two to four large nucleoli. The sections containing the diffuse infiltrate display prominent blood vessels which are lined by plump endothelial cells. The infiltrate may, in its earlier stages, be confined to the T cell zones of the lymph node and spleen. There appears to be sufficient overlap in the descriptions of these various subtypes to make their separation difficult and we suggest that they are best grouped together as a polymorphous type. The differential diagnosis of this type of NBTCL includes immunoblastic lymphadenopathy and HD.

We suggest that one explanation for this admixture of cell types in NBTCL is the secretion of lymphokines by the neoplastic T cells. The current list of such soluble factors includes IL-1, IL-2, colony-stimulating factors, macrophage activating factor, macrophage inhibition factor, B cell growth factor and interferon. The monomorphous type, in contrast, is relatively homogeneous, perhaps because the neoplastic cells do not secrete lymphokines to induce an admixture of benign cells. We have observed transformation or progression of the polymorphous to the monomorphous type and in some lesions we have observed the merging of areas of lymphomatous infiltrate of the two types, suggesting a morphological continuum. This observation is not without precedent. Schneider et al. (1985) separated T-IBS of Lukes into tumours composed of varying mixtures of small, medium-sized, and large transformed cells and tumours with more homogeneous populations of medium-sized or large transformed cells. However, they made the observation that "the groups tended to merge with one another such that a morphologic continuum appeared to exist".

It is not clear at present if the histological variants can be correlated with specific clinical features or if they have any bearing on prognosis and clinical response. However, it is clear that the T cell malignancies, in particular NBTCL, will be the focus of future attention and interest.

References

Ackerman AB, Breza TS, Caplan DL (1974) Spongiotic simulants of mycosis fungoides. Arch Dermatol 109: 218–220

Aisenberg AC, Wilkes BM, Harris NL, Koh HK (1982) T-cell chronic lymphocytic leukemia. Report of a case studied with monoclonal antibody. Am J Med 72: 695–699

Aisenberg AC, Krontiris TG, Mak TW et al. (1985) Rearrangement of the gene for the β chain of the T-cell receptor in T-cell chronic lymphocytic leukemia and related disorders. N Engl J Med 313: 529–533

Anderson JK, Metzgar RS (1978) Detection and partial characterization of human T and B lymphocyte membrane antigens with antisera to HSB and SB cell lines. J Immunol 120: 262–271

Barcos MP, Lukes RJ (1975) Malignant lymphoma of convoluted lymphocytes: a new entity of possible T-cell type. In: Sinks LF, Godden JO (eds) Conflicts in childhood cancer. An evaluation of current management. Alan R Liss, New York, pp 147–178

Bernard A, Boumsell L, Bayle C et al. (1979) Subsets of malignant lymphomas in children related to the cell phenotype. Blood 54: 1058–1068

Bernard A, Boumsell L, Reinherz EL et al. (1981) Cell surface characterization of malignant T cells from lymphoblastic lymphoma using monoclonal antibodies: evidence for phenotypic differences between malignant T cells from patients with acute lymphoblastic leukemia and lymphoblastic lymphoma. Blood 57: 1105–1110

Bernard A, Raynal B, Lemerle J, Boumsell L (1982) Changes in surface antigens on malignant T cells from lymphoblastic lymphomas at relapse: an appraisal with monoclonal antibodies and microfluorometry. Blood 59: 809–815

Berrih S, Gaud C, Bach AM et al. (1981) Evaluation of T cell subsets in myasthenia gravis using anti-T cell monoclonal antibodies. Clin Exp Immunol 45: 1–8

Bertness V, Kirsch I, Hollis G et al. (1985) T-cell receptor gene rearrangements as clinical markers of human T-cell lymphomas. N Engl J Med 313: 534–538

Blayney DW, Jaffe ES, Fisher RI et al. (1983) The human T-cell leukemia/lymphoma virus, lymphoma, lytic bone lesions and hypercalcemia. Ann Intern Med 98: 144–151

Blue ML, Daley JF, Levine H, Schlossman SF (1985) Coexpression of T4 and T8 on peripheral blood T cells demonstrated by two-color fluorescence flow cytometry. J Immunol 134: 2281–2286

Bogomoletz WV, Bernard J, Capron F, Diebold J (1983) T-cell origin of Lennert's lymphoma — immunohistochemical and immunologic study of one case. Arch Pathol Lab Med 107: 586–588

Borowitz MJ, Dowell BL, Boyett JM et al. (1985) Monoclonal antibody definition of T-cell acute leukemia: a Paediatric Oncology Group study. Blood 65: 785–788

Boumsell L, Bernard A, Reinherz EL et al. (1981) Surface antigens on malignant Sézary and T-CLL cells correspond to those of mature T cells. Blood 57: 526–530

Bradstock KF, Janossy G, Pizzolo G et al. (1980) Subpopulations of normal and leukemic human thymocytes: an analysis with the use of monoclonal antibodies. JNCI 65: 33–42

Brisbane JU, Berman LD, Osband ME, Neiman RS (1983) T8 chronic lymphocytic leukemia. A distinctive disorder related to T8 lymphocytosis. Am J Clin Pathol 80: 391–396

Broder S, Bunn PA Jr (1980) Cutaneous T-cell lymphomas. Semin Oncol 7: 310–331

Broder S, Edelson R, Lutzner M (1976) The Sézary syndrome. A malignant proliferation of helper T cells. J Clin Invest 58: 1297–1306

Brouet JC, Seligmann M (1978) The immunological classification of acute lymphoblastic leukemias. Cancer 42: 817–821

Brouet JC, Seligmann M (1981) T-derived chronic lymphocytic leukemia. Main clinical and immunological features Pathol Res Pract 171: 262–267

Brouet JC, Flandrin G, Sasportes M et al. (1975) Chronic lymphocytic leukaemia of T-cell origin. Lancet II: 890–893

Brouet JC, Valensi F, Daniel MT et al. (1976) Immunological classification of acute lymphoblastic leukaemias: evaluation of its clinical significance in 100 patients. Br J Haematol 33: 319–328

Bunn P Jr, Huberman M, Whang-Peng J et al. (1980) Prospective staging evaluation of patients with cutaneous T-cell lymphomas. Demonstration of a high frequency of extracutaneous dissemination. Ann Intern Med 93: 223–230

Canellos GP (1974) Hypercalcemia in malignant lymphoma and leukemia. Ann NY Acad Sci 230: 240–246

Catovsky D (1983) Prolymphocytic and hairy cell leukemias. In: Gunz FW, Henderson ES (eds) Leukemia, 4th edn. Grune and Stratton, New York, pp 759–781

Catovsky D, Pittmann S, O'Brien M et al. (1979) Multiparameter studies in lymphoid leukemias. Am J Clin Pathol 72: 736–745

Catovsky D, Linch DC, Beverley PCL (1982a) T cell disorders in haematological diseases. Clin Haematol 11: 661–695

Catovsky D, Rose M, Goolden AWG et al. (1982b) Adult T-cell lymphoma-leukaemia in blacks from the West Indies. Lancet I: 639–643

Cawley JC, Burns GF, Nash TA, Higgy KE, Child JA, Roberts BE (1978) Hairy cell leukemia with T cell features. Blood 51: 61–69

Chan WC, Check IJ, Heffner LT et al. (1982) Prolymphocytic leukemia of helper cell phenotype: report of a case and review of the scientific literature. Am J Clin Pathol 77: 643–647

Chu A, Eisinger M, Lee JS, Takezaki S, Kung PC, Edelson RL (1982) Immunoelectron microscopic identification of Langerhans cells using a new antigen marker. J Invest Dermatol 78: 177–180

Cohen SR (1977) Mycosis fungoides — Clinicopathologic relationships, survival and therapy in 59 patients. Master of Public Health Thesis, Yale University

Collins RD (1982) T-neoplasms. Their significance in relation to the classification system of lymphoid neoplasms. Am J Surg Pathol 6: 745–754

Cossman J, Chused TM, Fisher RI, Magrath I, Bollum F, Jaffe ES (1983) Diversity of immunological phenotypes of lymphoblastic lymphoma. Cancer Res 43: 4486–4490

Costa JC, Jaffe ES, Tsokos M et al. (1980) Peripheral T-cell lymphoma with pulmonary involvement and erythrophagocytosis mimicking malignant histiocytosis. Lab Invest 42: 108

Costello C, Catovsky D, O'Brien M, Morilla R, Varadi S (1980) Chronic T-cell leukemias. I. Morphology, cytochemistry and ultrastructure. Leuk Res 4: 463–476

Edelson RL (1976) Cutaneous T-cell lymphomas: clues of a skin-thymus interaction. J Invest Dermatol 67: 419–424

Edelson RL (1980) Cutaneous T-cell lymphoma: mycosis fungoides, Sèzary syndrome and other variants. J Am Acad Dermatol 2: 89–106

Epstein EH Jr, Levin DL, Croft JD et al. (1972) Mycosis fungoides. Survival, prognostic features, response to therapy and autopsy findings. Medicine (Baltimore) 15: 61–72

Ferrarini M, Romagnani S, Montesoro E et al. (1982) A lymphoproliferative disorder of the large granular lymphocytes with natural killer activity. J Clin Immunol 3: 30–36

Fischmann AB, Bunn PA Jr, Guccion JG, Matthews MJ, Minna JD (1979) Exposure to chemicals, physical agents, and biologic agents in mycosis fungoides and the Sézary syndrome. Cancer Treat Rep 63: 591–596

Foucar K, Carroll TJ, Tannous R et al. (1985) Non-endemic adult T-cell leukemia/lymphoma in the United States: report of two cases and review of the literature. Am J Clin Pathol 83: 18–26

Fuks ZY, Bagshaw MA, Farber EM (1973) Prognostic signs and the management of the mycosis fungoides. Cancer 32: 1385–1395

Gaeke ME, Vardiman JW, Miller W, Medenica M, Hopper JE, Rowley JD (1981) Human T-cell lymphoma with suppressor effects on the mixed lymphocyte reaction (MLR). I. Morphological and cytogenetic analysis. Blood 57: 634–641

Galili U, Polliack A, Okon E et al. (1980) Human prothymocytes. Membrane properties, differentiation patterns, glucocorticoid sensitivity, and ultrastructural features. J Exp Med 152: 796–807

Gallo RC, Mann D, Broder S et al. (1982) Human T-cell leukemia-lymphoma virus (HTLV) is in T but not B lymphocytes from a patient with cutaneous T-cell lymphoma. Proc Natl Acad Sci USA 79: 5680–5683

Geha RS, Rosen FS (1983) Immunoregulatory T-cell defects. Immunol Today 4: 233–236

Greaves MF, Janossy G, Peto J, Kay H (1981) Immunologically defined subclasses of acute lymphoblastic leukemia in children: their relationship to presentation features and prognosis. Br J Haematol 48: 179–197

Greene MH, Dalarger NA, Lamberg SI et al. (1979) Mycosis fungoides: epidemiologic observations. Cancer Treat Rep 63: 597–606

Grogan TM, Richter LC, Payne CM, Rangel CS (1985a) Signet-ring cell lymphoma of T-cell origin. An immunocytochemical and ultrastructural study relating giant vacuole formation to cytoplasmic sequestration of surface membrane. Am J Surg Pathol 9: 684–692

Grogan TM, Fielder K, Rangel C et al. (1985b) Peripheral T-cell lymphoma: aggressive disease with heterogenous immunotypes. Am J Clin Pathol 83: 279–288

Grossman B, Schechter GP, Horton JH et al. (1981) Hypercalcemia associated with T-cell lymphoma-leukemia. Am J Clin Pathol 75: 149–155

Guccion JG, Fischmann AB, Bunn PA Jr, Schechter GP, Patterson RH, Matthews MJ (1979) Ultrastructural appearance of cutaneous T cell lymphomas in skin, lymph nodes and peripheral blood. Cancer Treat Rep 63: 565–570

Guglielmi P, Preud'homme J, Flandrin G (1980) Phenotypic changes of phytohemoglutinin-stimulated hairy cells. Nature 286: 166–168

Habeshaw JA, Bailey D, Stansfeld AG, Greaves MF (1983) The cellular content of non Hodgkin lymphomas: a comprehensive analysis using monoclonal antibodies and other surface marker techniques. Br J Cancer 47: 327–351

Hanaoka M (1981) Clinical pathology of adult T-cell leukemia. Nippon Ketsueki Gakkai Zasshi 44: 1420–1430

Hanaoka M (1982) Progress in adult T-cell leukemia research. Acta Pathol Jpn 32(suppl 1): 171–185

Harris M, Eyden B, Read G (1981) Signet ring cell lymphoma: a rare variant of follicular lymphoma. J Clin Pathol 34: 884–891

Hattori T, Uchiyama T, Toibana T et al. (1981) Surface phenotype of Japanese adult T-cell leukemia cells characterised by monoclonal antibodies. Blood 58: 645–647

Haynes BF, Eisenbarth GS, Fauci AS (1979) Human lymphocyte antigens: production of a monoclonal antibody that defines functional thymus-derived lymphocyte subsets. Proc Natl Acad Sci USA 76: 5829–5833

Haynes BF, Metzgar R, Minna J et al. (1981) Phenotypic characterization of cutaneous T-cell lymphoma. Use of monoclonal antibodies to compare to other malignant T cells. N Engl J Med 304: 1319–1323

Helbron D, Brittinger G, Lennert K (1979) T-zone lymphoma. Clinical features, therapy and prognosis (in German). Blut 39: 117–131

Henderson ES (1983) Clinical diagnosis. In: Gunz FW, Henderson ES (eds) Leukemia, 4th edn. Grune and Stratton, New York, pp 393–462

Hinuma Y, Nagata K, Hanaoka M et al. (1981) Adult T-cell leukemia: antigen in an ATL cell line and detection of antibodies to the antigen in human sera. Proc Natl Acad Sci USA 78: 6476–6480

Hoffman R, Kopel S, Hsu SD, Dainiak N, Zanjani ED (1978) T-cell chronic lymphocytic leukemia: presence in bone marrow and peripheral blood of cells that suppress erythropoiesis in vitro. Blood 52: 255–260

Huberman M, Bunn PA Jr, Matthews MJ et al. (1979) Extracutaneous involvement in patients with cutaneous T-cell lymphomas (mycosis fungoides and Sézary syndrome). Proc AACR and ASCO 20: 410–418

Human Gene Mapping 8 (1985) Eighth international workshop on human gene mapping, Helsinki, Finland, 4–10 August, 1985 Cytogenet Cell Genet 40(1–4): 1–823

Ishii Y, Fujimoto J, Kon S et al. (1982) Surface antigenic phenotypes of human T-cell leukemia corresponding to those of post-thymic T cells. Am J Hematol 12: 251–260

Itoh K, Tsuchikawa AK, Awataguchi T et al. (1983) A case of chronic lymphocytic leukemia with properties characteristic of natural killer cells. Blood 61: 940–948

Jaffe ES (1984) Pathologic and clinical spectrum of post-thymic T-cell malignancies. Cancer Invest 2: 413–426

Jaffe ES, Costa JC, Fauci AS (1981) Erythrophagocytic T γ lymphoma. N Engl J Med 305: 103–104

Jaffe ES, Strauchen JA, Berard CW (1982) Predictability of immunologic phenotype by morphologic criteria in diffuse aggressive non-Hodgkin's lymphomas. Am J Clin Pathol 77: 46–49

Jaffe ES, Blayney DW, Blattner W et al. (1983) The human T-cell leukemia/lymphoma virus: its association with disease in the United States. Lab Invest 48: 40A

Jaffe ES, Blattner WA, Blayney DW et al. (1984) The pathologic spectrum of adult T-cell leukemia/lymphoma in the United States. Am J Surg Pathol 8: 263–275

Janossy G, Prentice HG (1982) T cell subpopulations monoclonal antibodies and their therapeutic applications. Clin Haematol 11: 631–660

Janossy G, Tidman N, Selby WS et al. (1980) Human T lymphocytes of inducer and suppressor type occupy different microenvironments. Nature 288: 81–86

Janossy G, Tidman N, Papageorgiou ES, Kung PC, Goldstein G (1981a) Distribution of T lymphocyte subsets in the human bone marrow and thymus: an analysis with monoclonal antibodies. J Immunol 126: 1608–1613

Janossy G, Panayi G, Duke O et al. (1981b) Rheumatoid arthritis: a disease of T-lymphocyte/macrophage immunoregulation. Lancet II: 839–842

Jansen J, LeBien TW, Kersey JH (1982) The phenotype of the neoplastic cells of hairy cell leukemia: studies with monoclonal antibodies. Blood 59: 609–614

Kadin MD, Kamoun M, Lamberg J (1981) Erythrophagocytic T γ lymphoma. A clinicopathologic entity resembling malignant histiocytosis. N Engl J Med 304: 648–653

Kadin ME, Berard CW, Nanba K, Wakasa H (1983) Lymphoproliferative diseases in Japan and Western countries: proceedings of the United States-Japan Seminar, September 6th and 7th 1982 in Seattle, Washington. Hum Pathol 14: 745–772

Kalyanaraman V, Sarngadharan M, Robert-Guroff M et al. (1982) A new subtype of human T-cell leukemia virus (HTLV-II) associated with a T-cell variant of hairy cell leukemia. Science 218: 571–573

Kikuchi M, Mitsui T, Matsui N et al. (1979) T-cell malignancies in adults: histopathological studies of lymph nodes in 110 patients. Jpn J Clin Oncol 9 (suppl): 407–422

Kim H, Nathwani BN, Rappaport H (1980) So-called "Lennert's lymphoma". Is it a clinicopathologic entity? Cancer 45: 1379–1399

Knowles DM II, Halper JP (1982) Human T-cell malignancies. Correlative clinical, histopathologic, immunologic and cytochemical analysis of 23 cases. Am J Pathol 106: 187–203

Korsmeyer SJ, Greene WC, Crossman J et al. (1983) Rearrangement and expression of immunoglobulin genes and expression of Tac antigen in hairy cell leukemia. Proc Natl Acad Sci USA 80: 4522–4526

Kung P, Berger C, Goldstein G et al. (1981) Cutaneous T-cell lymphoma: characterisation by monoclonal antibodies. Blood 57: 261–266

Lennert K, Mestdagh J (1968) Lymphogranulomatosen mit konstant hohen Epithelioidzellgehalt. (Hodgkin's disease with constantly high content of epithelioid cells.) Virchows Arch [Pathol Anat] 344: 1–20

Lennert K, Remmelle W (1958) Karyometrische Untersuchungen an Lymphknotenzellen des Menschen. I Germinoblasten Lymphoblasten und Lymphozyten. Acta Hematol (Basel) 19: 99–113

Lennert K, Stein H, Kaiserling E (1975) Cytological and functional criteria for the classification of malignant lymphoma. Br J Cancer 31(suppl II): 29–43

Lennert K, Stein H, Feller AC, Gerdes J (1981) Morphology cytochemistry and immunohistology of T-cell lymphomas. In: Vitetta ES (ed) B and T-cell tumours. Academic, Orlando, Florida, pp 9–26

Leong AS-Y (1984) An evolving classification of malignancies of the T lymphocyte series. Pathology 16: 482–483

Leong AS-Y, Sage RE, Kinnear GC, Forbes IJ (1980) Preferential epidermotrophism in adult T-cell leukaemia-lymphoma. Am J Surg Pathol 4: 421–430

Leong AS-Y, Dale BM, Liew SH et al. (1981) Node-based T cell lymphoma The clinical, immunological and morphological spectrum. Pathology 13: 79–95

Lever WF, Shaumberger-Lever G (1975) Histopathology of the skin, 5th edn. Lippincott, Philadelphia, p 698

Levi JA, Wiernik PH (1975) Management of mycosis fungoides: current status and future prospects. Medicine (Baltimore) 54: 73–88

Levin S, Russell E, McWilliams N et al. (1980) Receptors for peanut agglutinin (*Arachus hypogea*) in childhood acute lymphoblastic leukemia. Possible clinical significance. Blood 55: 37–41

Levine AM, Meyer PR, Lukes RJ, Feinstein DI (1981) Clinical and morphologic heterogeneity of T-cell chronic lymphocytic leukemia. Blood 58 (suppl 1): 144a (abstract)

Linch DC, Cawley JC, MacDonald SM et al. (1981) Acquired pure red cell aplasia associated with an increase of T cells bearing receptors for the Fc of IgG. Acta Haematol 65: 270–274

Lipton JM, Nadler LM, Canellos GP (1983) Evidence for genetic restriction in the suppression of erythropoiesis by a unique subset of T lymphocytes in man. J Clin Invest 72: 694–706

Loughran TP, Kadin ME, Starkebaum G et al. (1985) Leukemia of large granular lymphocytes: association with clonal chromosomal abnormalities and autoimmune neutropenia, thrombocytopenia, and hemolytic anemia. Ann Intern Med 102: 169–175

Lukes RJ, Collins RD (1974) Immunologic characterization of human malignant lymphomas. Cancer 34: 1488–1503

Lukes RJ, Taylor CR, Parker JW (1982) Immunological surface marker studies in the histopathological diagnosis of non-Hodgkin's lymphomas based on multiparameter studies of 790 cases. In: Rosenberg SA, Kaplan HS (eds) Malignant lymphoma aetiology, immunology, pathology and treatment. Academic, New York, pp 310–349

MacKie RM (1981) Initial event in mycosis fungoides of the skin is viral infection of epidermal Langerhans cells. Lancet II: 283–284

MacKie RM, Turbitt ML (1982) The use of a double-label immunoperoxidase monoclonal antibody technique in the investigation of patients with mycosis fungoides. Br J Dermatol 106: 379–384

Matsumoto M, Nomura K, Matsumoto T (1979) Adult T-cell leukemia/lymphoma in Kagoshima district South-western Japan: clinical and haematological characteristics. Jpn J Clin Oncol 9 (suppl):325–336

McNutt N, Crain W (1981) Quantitative electron microscopic comparison of lymphocyte nuclear contours in mycosis fungoides and in benign infiltrate in skin. Cancer 47: 698–709

Meijer C, van der Loo E, van Vloten W et al. (1980) Early diagnosis of mycosis fungoides and Sézary's syndrome by morphometric analysis of lymphoid cells in the skin. Cancer 45: 2864–2871

Miedema F, Terpstra FG, Smit JW et al. (1984) Functional properties of neoplastic T-cells in adult T-cell lymphoma/leukemia patients from the Caribbean. Blood 63: 477–481

Miller RA, Coleman CN, Fawcett HD et al. (1980) Sézary syndrome: a model for migration of T lymphocytes to skin. N Engl J Med 303: 89–92

Minowada J (1982) Membrane and other phenotypes of leukemia cells. In: Mirand EA, Hutchinson EB, Mihich E (eds) Proceedings of the 13th international cancer congress. Alan R Liss, New York, pp 213–217

Müller-Hermelink HK, Steinmann G, Stein H, Lennert K (1983) Malignant lymphoma of plasmacytoid T-cells. Morphologic and immunologic studies characterising a special type of T-cell. Am J Surg Pathol 7: 849–862

Myrie C, Zucker-Franklin D, Ramsey D (1980) Light-microscopic analysis of sectioned Sézary cells. Am J Pathol 99: 243–252

Nadler LM, Reinherz EL, Weinstein HJ, D'Orsi CJ, Schlossman SF (1980) Heterogeneity of T-cell lymphoblastic malignancies. Blood 55: 806–810

Naeim F, Gatti RA, Johnson CE Jr et al. (1978) "Hairy cell" leukemia. A heterogenous chronic lymphoproliferative disorder. Am J Med 65: 479–487

Nagasawa T, Abe T, Nakagawa T (1981) Pure red cell aplasia and hypogammaglobulinemia associated with T-cell chronic lymphocytic leukemia. Blood 57: 1025–1031

Nathwani BN, Kim H, Rappaport H (1976) Malignant lymphoma, lymphoblastic. Cancer 38: 964–983

Nathwani BN, Rappaport H, Moran EM, Pangalis GA, Kim H (1978) Malignant lymphoma arising in angioimmunoblastic lymphadenopathy. Cancer 41: 578–606

Navas-Palacios JJ, Valdes MD, Montalban Pallares MA et al. (1981) Lymphoblastic lymphoma/leukemia of T cell origin: ultrastructural, cytochemical, and immunologic features of ten cases. Cancer 48: 1982–1991

Newland AC, Catovsky D, Linch D et al. (1984) Chronic T-cell lymphocytosis: a review of 21 cases. Br J Haematol 58: 433–436

O'Brien C, Lampert IA, Catovsky D (1983) The histopathology of adult T-cell lymphoma/leukemia in blacks from the Caribbean. Histopathology 7: 349–364

Pandolfi F, De Rossi G, Semenzato G et al. (1982) Immunologic evaluation of T chronic lymphocytic leukemia cells: correlations among phenotype, functional activities and morphology. Blood 59: 688–695

Pandolfi F, DeRossi G, Lauria F et al. (1985) T-helper phenotype chronic lymphocytic leukaemia and "adult T-cell leukaemia" in Italy. Endemic HTLV-I-related T-cell leukaemias in Southern Europe. Lancet II: 633–636

Pangalis GA, Nathwani BN, Rappaport H, Rosen RB (1979) Acute lymphoblastic leukemia. The significance of nuclear convolutions. Cancer 43: 551–557

Payne CM, Nagle RB, Lynch PJ (1984) Quantitative electron microscopy in the diagnosis of mycosis fungoides. A simple analysis of lymphocytic nuclear convolutions. Arch Dermatol 120: 63–75

Phyliky RL, Li C-Y, Yam LT (1983) T-cell chronic lymphocytic leukemia with morphologic and immunologic characteristics of cytotoxic/suppressor phenotype. Mayo Clin Proc 58: 709–720

Pinkus GS, Said JW, Hargreaves H (1979) Malignant lymphoma T-cell type. A distinct morphologic variant with large multilobated nuclei, with a report of four cases. Am J Clin Pathol 72: 540–550

Pittman S, Morilla R, Catovsky D (1982) Chronic T-cell leukemias. II. Cytogenetic studies. Leuk Res 6: 33–42

Pizzoli G, Chilosi M, Cetto GL et al. (1982) Immunohistological analysis of bone marrow involvement in lymphoproliferative disorders. Br J Haematol 50: 95–100

Poiesz BJ, Ruscetti FW, Gazdar AF, Bunn PA, Minna JD, Gallo RC (1980) Detection and isolation of type C retrovirus particles from fresh and cultured lymphocytes of a patient with cutaneous T-cell lymphoma. Proc Natl Acad Sci USA 77: 7415–7419

Poiesz BJ Ruscetti FW, Reitz MS, Kalyanaraman VS, Gallo RC (1981) Isolation of a new type C retrovirus (HTLV) in primary uncultured cells of a patient with Sézary T cell leukaemia. Nature 294: 268–271

Poppema S, Bhan AK, Reinherz EL et al. (1981) Distribution of T cell subsets in human lymph nodes. J Exp Med 153: 30–41

Prasthofer EF, Grizzle WE, Prchal JT, Grossi CE (1985) Plasmacytoid T-cell lymphoma associated with chronic myeloproliferative disorder. Am J Surg Pathol 9: 380–387

Pullen DJ, Falletta JM, Christ WM et al. (1981) Southwest Oncology Group experience with immunological phenotyping in acute lymphoblastic leukemia of childhood. Cancer Res 41: 4802–4809

Pullen DJ, Sullivan MP, Falletta JM et al. (1982) Modified LSA-2L2 treatment in 53 children with E-rosette positive T-cell leukemia: results and prognostic factors. Blood 60: 1159–1168

Pullen DJ, Christ WM, Falletta JM et al. (1983) A Paediatric Oncology Group classification protocol for acute lymphocytic leukemia: immunologic phenotypes and correlation with treatment results. In: Murphy SB, Gilbert JF (eds) Leukemia research: advances in cell biology and treatment. Elsevier, Amsterdam, p 221

Rappaport H, Thomas LB (1974) Mycosis fungoides: the pathology of extracutaneous involvement. Cancer 34: 1198–1229

Reinherz EL, Nadler LM, Rosenthal TS, Moloney WC, Schlossman SF (1979) T-cell subset characterisation of human T-CLL. Blood 53: 1066–1075

Reinherz EL, Kung PC, Goldstein G, Levey RH, Schlossman SF (1980) Discrete stages of human intrathymic differentiation: analysis of normal thymocytes and leukemic lymphoblasts of T-cell lineage. Proc Natl Acad Sci 77: 1588–1592

Reynolds CW, Foon KA (1984) T_γ lymphoproliferative disease and related disorders in humans and experimental animals: a review of the clinical, cellular and functional characteristics. Blood 64: 1146–1158

Ritz J, Pesando JM, Notis-McConarty J et al. (1980) A monoclonal antibody to human acute lymphoblastic leukemia antigen. Nature 283: 583–585

Roper M, Christ WM, Metzgar R et al. (1983) Monoclonal antibody characterization of surface antigens in childhood T-cell lymphoid malignancies. Blood 61: 830–837

Rowden G, Lewis MG (1976) Langerhans cells: involvement in the pathogenesis of mycosis fungoides. Br J Dermatol 95: 665–672

Rubenfeld M, Silverstone A, Knowles D et al. (1980) Induction of T-cell differentiation by human epidermal cells. Clin Res 28: 581a (abstract)

Rümke HC, Miedema F, tenBerge IJM et al. (1982) Functional properties of T cells in patients with chronic T_γ lymphocytosis and chronic T cell neoplasia. J Immunol 129: 419–426

Safai B, Good RA, Towmey JJ, Lewis V, Goldstein G (1979) A novel lymphocyte differentiating factor in serum of patients with mycosis fungoides and Sézary syndrome. Blood 54: 837–841

Safai B, Incefy GS, Good RA (1980) T-cell differentiating activity in tissue cultures containing mycosis fungoides epidermal cells. N Engl J Med 303: 113

Saxon A, Stevens RH, Golde DW (1978) T-lymphocyte variant of hairy-cell leukaemia. Ann Intern Med 88: 323–326

Saxon A, Stevens RH, Golde DW (1979) Helper and suppressor T-lymphocyte leukemia in ataxia telangiectasia. N Engl J Med 300:700-704

Schechter GP, Bunn PA Jr, Fischmann AB et al. (1979) Blood and lymph node T lymphocytes in cutaneous T-cell lymphoma: evaluation by light microscopy. Cancer Treat Rep 63: 571–574

Schechter GP, Guccion J, Matthews M et al. (1981) Erythrophagocytic T_γ lymphoma. N Engl J Med 305: 103

Schneider DR, Taylor CR, Parker JW, Cramer AC, Meyer PR, Lukes RL (1985) Immunoblastic sarcoma of T- and B-cell types: morphologic description and comparison. Hum Pathol 16: 885–900

Schwarzmeier J, Paitta E, Radaszkiewicz T et al. (1981) Proliferation kinetics of Sézary cells. Blood 57: 1049–1054

Selby SWS, Janossy G, Goldstein G, Jewell DP (1981) T lymphocyte subsets in human intestinal mucosa: the distribution and relationship to MHC-derived antigens. Clin Exp Immunol 44: 453–458

Sen L, Borella L (1975) Clinical importance of lymphoblasts with T markers in childhood acute leukemia. N Engl J Med 292: 828–832

Serra JM, Venuti A, Castane DM (1966) Mycosis fungoides en un lactante. Rev Argent Dermatol 30: 161–164

Shackney S, Edelson R, Bunn P Jr (1979) The kinetics of Sèzary cell production. Cancer Treat Rep 63: 659–661

Shamoto M (1983) Langerhans cells increase in the dermal lesions of adult T cell leukemia in Japan. J Clin Pathol 36: 307–311

Shimoyama M, Minato K, Saito H et al. (1979a) Immunoblastic lymphadenopathy (IBL)-like T-cell lymphoma. Jpn J Clin Oncol 9(suppl): 347–356

Shimoyama M, Minato K, Saito H et al. (1979b) Comparison of clinical morphologic and immunologic characteristics of adult T-cell leukemia-lymphoma and cutaneous T-cell lymphoma. Jpn J Clin Oncol 9(suppl): 357–372

Siegal FP, Rambotti P, Siegal M et al. (1982) Helper cell function of leukemic Leu-2a + histamine receptor, and T$_\gamma$ lymphocytes. J Immunol 129: 1775–1781

Silberberg I, Thorbecke GJ, Baer RL et al. (1975) Antigen-bearing Langerhans cells in skin dermal lymphatics and in lymph nodes. Cell Immunol 25: 137–151

Simpkins H, Kiprof DD, Davis JL et al. (1985) T cell chronic lymphocytic leukemia with lymphocytes of unusual immunologic phenotype and function. Blood 65: 127–133

Singh AK, Lewis P, Wetherley-Mein G (1984) Heterogeneity of T-lymphocytic chronic lymphatic leukemia. Scand J Haematol 32: 195–206

Slease RB, Pitha JV, Eichner ER (1984) Adult T-cell leukemia: clinical and immunologic characterization of a nonendemic case. Am J Clin Pathol 82: 495–501

Stein H, Mason DY, Gerdes J et al. (1981) Immunohistology of B-cell lymphomas. In: Knapp W (ed) Leukemia markers. Academic, London, pp 99–108

Stingl G, Wolff K (1982) Origin and function of Langerhans cells and their role in disease. In: Goos M, Christophers E (eds) Lymphoproliferative diseases of the skin. Springer, Berlin Heidelberg New York, pp 34–40

Stutman O (1977) Two main features of T cell development: thymus traffic and postthymic maturation. Contemp Top Immunobiol 7: 1–46

Su I-J, Shih L-Y, Kadin ME et al. (1985) Pathologic and immunologic characterization of malignant lymphoma in Taiwan with special reference to retrovirus-associated adult T-cell lymphoma/leukemia. Am J Clin Pathol 84: 715–723

Suchi T, Tajima K (1979) Peripheral T-cell malignancy as a problem in lymphoma classification. Jpn J Clin Oncol 9(suppl): 443–450

Tajima K, Tominagas S, Kuroishi T et al. (1979) Geographical features and epidemiological approach to endemic T-cell leukemia/lymphoma in Japan. Jpn J Clin Oncol 9(suppl):495–504

Takatsuki K, Uchiyama T, Sagawa K, Yodoi J (1976) Adult T-cell leukemia (in Japanese). Jpn J Clin Hematol 17: 416–427

Takatsuki K, Uchiyama T, Sagawa K, Yodoi J (1977) Adult T-cell leukemia in Japan. In: Seno S, Tkaku F, Irino S (eds) Topics in haematology. Excerpta Medica, Amsterdam, pp 73–77

Tatsumi E, Takiguchi Y, Domae N et al. (1980) Suppressive activity of some leukemic T cells from adult patients in Japan. Clin Immunol Immunopathol 15: 190–199

Thien SL, Catovsky D, Oscier D et al. (1982) T-chronic lymphocytic leukaemia presenting as primary hypogammaglobulinemia — evidence of a proliferation of T suppressor cells. Clin Exp Immunol 47: 670–676

Thiers BH (1982) Controversies in mycosis fungoides. J Am Acad Dermatol 7: 1–16

Thiers BH, Maize JC, Spicer SS, Cantor AB (1984) The effect of ageing and chronic sun exposure on human Langerhans cell populations. J Invest Dermatol 82: 223–226

Thomas JA, Janossy G, Graham-Brown RAC, Kung PC, Goldstein G (1982) The relationship of T lymphocyte subsets and Ia-like antigen positive non-lymphoid elements in early stages of cutaneous T-cell lymphoma J Invest Dermatol 78: 169–176

Thomas LB, Rappaport H (1975) Mycosis fungoides and its relationship to other malignant lymphomas. In: Rebuck JW, Berard CW, Abell MR (eds) International Academy of Pathology monograph. The reticulo-endothelial system. Williams and Wilkins, Baltimore, pp 243–261

Tidman N, Janossy G, Broder M et al. (1981) Delineation of human thymocyte differentiaton pathways utilizing double-staining techniques with monoclonal antibodies. Clin Exp Immunol 45: 457–467

Tjernlund U (1978) Epidermal expression of Langerhans cells in mycosis fungoides. Arch Dermatol Res 261: 81–86

Tsukimoto I, Wong KY, Lampkin BC (1976) Surface markers and prognostic factors in acute lymphoblastic leukemia. N Engl J Med 294: 245–248

Tubbs RR, Fishleder A, Weiss RA et al. (1983) Immunohistologic cellular phenotypes of lymphoproliferative disorders. Comprehensive evaluation of 564 cases including 257 non-Hodgkin's lymphomas classified by the International Working Formulation. Am J Pathol 113: 207–221

Uchiyama T, Yodoi J, Sagawa K et al. (1977) Adult T-cell leukemia: clinical and hematologic features of 16 cases. Blood 50: 481–492

Uchiyama T, Sagawa K, Takatsuki K, Uchino H (1978) Effect of adult T-cell leukemia cells on pokeweed mitogen-induced normal B-cell differentiation. Clin Immunol Immunopathol 10: 24–34

Uchiyama T, Broder S, Bonnard GD, Waldmann T (1980) Immunoregulatory functions of cultured human T lymphocytes. Trans Assoc Am Physicians 93: 251–262

Van de Griend RJ, DeBruin HG, Rümke HC et al. (1982) Isolation and partial characterisation of a novel subset of human T lymphocytes defined by monoclonal antibodies. Immunology 47: 317–320

van der Loo EM, van Muijen GNP, van Vloten WA, Beens W, Scheffer E, Meijer CJ (1979) C-type virus like particles specifically localised in Langerhans cells and related cells of skin and lymph nodes of patients with mucosis fungoides and Sézary's syndrome. A morphological and biochemical study. Virchows Arch [Cell Pathol] 31: 193–203

van der Loo EM, van Vloten W, Cornelisse CJ, Scheffer E, Meijer CJ (1981) The relevance of morphometry in the differential diagnosis of cutaneous T cell lymphomas. Br J Dermatol 104: 257–269

Van Scott EJ, Haynes HA (1971) Cutaneous lymphomas. In: Fitzpatrick TB, Arndt KA, Clark WH et al. (eds) McGraw-Hill, New York, pp 556–559

Waldmann TA, Greene WC, Sarin PS et al. (1984) Functional and phenotypic comparison of human T cell leukemia/lymphoma virus positive adult T cell leukemia with human T cell leukemia/lymphoma virus negative Sézary leukemia and their distinction using anti-Tac. Monoclonal antibody identifying the human receptor for T cell growth factor. J Clin Invest 73: 1711–1718

Waldron JA, Leech JH, Glick AD, Flexner JM, Collins RD (1977) Malignant lymphoma of peripheral T lymphocyte origin: immunologic pathologic and clinical features in 6 patients. Cancer 40: 1604–1617

Wassermann J, Bieberfeld G, Baral E, Blomgren H, Thyresson N, Brehmer-Andersson E (1980) Suppressor T cells in mycosis fungoides and socalled pre-mycotic eruptions. Acta Derm Venereol (Stockh) 60: 139–143

Watanabe S, Nakajima T, Shimosato Y et al. (1979) T-cell malignancies: subclassification and interrelationships. Jpn J Clin Oncol 9(suppl): 423–442

Watanabe S, Shimosato Y, Shimoyama M (1981) Lymphoma and leukemia of T lymphocytes. In: Sommers SC, Rosen PP (eds) Pathology Annual Monograph. Appleton Century Crofts, New York, pp 155–203

Weinberg DS, Pinkus GS (1981) Non-Hodgkin's lymphoma of large multilobated cell type. A clinicopathologic study of ten cases. Am J Clin Pathol 76: 190–196

Weinstein HJ, Vance ZB, Jaffe N, Buell D, Cassady JR, Nathan DG (1979) Improved prognosis for patients with mediastinal lymphoblastic lymphoma. Blood 53: 687–694

Weiss LM, Wood GS, Dorfman RF (1985a) T-cell signet-ring cell lymphoma. A histologic, ultrastructural and immunohistochemical study of 2 cases. Am J Surg Pathol 9: 273–280

Weiss LM, Crabtree GS, Rouse RV, Warnke RA (1985b) Morphologic and immunologic characterization of 50 peripheral T-cell lymphomas. Am J Pathol 118: 316–324

Whang-Peng J, Bunn P Jr, Knutsen T et al. (1979) Cytogenetic abnormalities in patients with cutaneous T-cell lymphomas. Cancer Treat Rep 63: 575–580

Wieczorek R, Burke JS, Knowles DM II (1985) Leu-M1 antigen expression in T-cell neoplasia. Am J Pathol 121: 374–380

Wood GS, Burke JS, Horning S, Doggett RS, Levey R, Warnke RA (1983) The immunologic and clinicopathologic heterogeneity of cutaneous lymphomas other than mycosis fungoides. Blood 62: 464–472

20 Treatment, Treatment Failure and Future Possibilities

Introduction

It is probably not an incorrect generalisation to state that current methods of treatment of the lymphomas and lymphocytic leukaemias have met with limited success. In this chapter we will not discuss the details of treatments but will consider why treatment may be unsuccessful and will also discuss the potential of contemporary therapeutic approaches.

Treatment of Hodgkin's disease (HD), a tumour of the lymphoid system of unknown lineage, by radiotherapy and/or chemotherapy, is now capable of curing as many as 70% of all patients with this disease (DeVita et al. 1985, p. 1691). This has aroused hopes of similar success in the treatment of other lymphomas that have not been fulfilled. In general, cancers are curable if they can be removed *in toto* or completely destroyed by radiotherapy, less commonly by chemotherapy and rarely by other means. The first cures of HD were obtained by giving the tumour an adequate dose of radiotherapy. Standard radiotherapeutic practice is to treat lymph nodes contiguous to the site of the primary tumour. The curability of HD may be due to the late migration or dissemination of malignant cells from the primary site. Spread, when it occurs, is orderly, with extension to contiguous lymphoid tissue. Irradiation of lymphoid tissue along the line of spread may therefore eradicate all malignant cells. It is doubtful, however, whether this is really the explanation of the curability of HD. It is curious that even when HD is so widely disseminated that it cannot be excised or destroyed by radiotherapy, the patients still have a chance of cure by chemotherapy. Perhaps tumours can also be cured if the initial chemotherapeutic onslaught leaves relatively few cells to be dealt with by the host. Such destruction of remaining tumour cells by the poorly understood defence mechanisms of the host may also explain cure of some cases of non-Hodgkin's lymphoma (NHL) by chemotherapy.

NHLs are classified into two groups for treatment purposes: lymphomas of low grade, and lymphomas of intermediate and high grades. Overall, the low-grade lymphomas respond to treatment better, but the cure rate is low. This is not surprising in view of the fact that more than 50% of cases of follicular small cleaved B cell lymphoma are disseminated by the time of diagnosis, and in such cases more than 75% have circulating malignant cells, as shown by the use of a DNA probe on peripheral blood (Hu et al. 1985). About 50% cure rates have been obtained in the diffuse "histiocytic" lymphomas by the use of aggressive chemotherapy, and it appears increasingly possible to produce long-term disease-free survivals in the nodular and lymphoblastic lymphomas, which have a high proportion of large cells in involved nodes.

We have previously discussed the assumption that the cell of origin of the lymphomas corresponds to a normal lymphocyte at the same stage of differentiation residing in a particular location in the lymphoid tissues. It is commonly assumed that this cell is the target of treatment. A reason for treatment failure may be the incorrectness of this assumption. The cells acting as stem cells for the tumour should be the therapeutic targets, but we do not know what they are, because the techniques for their detection are not yet fully developed. There is therefore a great need to develop techniques for identification of stem cells of the various types of lymphoma. With this knowledge of the stem cells it may be possible to employ their characteristics and properties as targets for selective chemotherapy. This is a particularly important consideration in purging of the bone marrow with monoclonal antibodies.

The clinician's first choice of treatment is often very important. If the disease is considered potentially curable, treatment must be chosen accordingly. Failure of initial therapy often portends a bad outcome. The reasons why this should be so can only be guessed; the treatment may kill susceptible cells and allow a resistant population of malignant cells to emerge. Also the tolerance of the patient for another round of aggressive treatment may be reduced, particularly through the vulnerability of the haematopoietic stem cells in his bone marrow, which may have suffered a serious reduction in numbers during the first treatment. Treatment should be commenced only after proper histological and immunological assessment and clinical staging, and the choice of treatment should be based on accumulated wisdom and the latest reliable data from clinical trials.

A wide range of drugs is available for the attempt to destroy malignant lymphocytes. The biochemical action of most of these chemotherapeutic agents is known, more or less precisely, but the reason for their selective action on malignant cells or for the relatively better resistance of normal cells to them is poorly understood. If these drugs are given inadvisedly or recklessly the malignant lymphocytes may survive the onslaught, but the innocent cells of the host may not.

Treatment Failure Exemplified by Lymphocytic Leukaemias

Although patients with chronic lymphocytic leukaemia (CLL) usually survive for many years, the disease is incurable. Treatment of CLL has never been assessed satisfactorily, and very few studies have included adequate controls. In the 1960s, it was thought that chlorambucil, administered daily, was better than the other alkylating agents and that the prognosis was not improved by the addition of corticosteroids. Unfortunately, chlorambucil caused the development of acute leukaemias in some patients. Treatment with this drug is now conventionally reserved for patients with "active" disease (Rai stage II), with splenomegaly, progressing lymphadenopathy, unexplained fever, weight loss, recurrent infections and thrombocytopenia. Patients in stage II have a median survival of 6 years. Patients with stages III and IV, also included in the "active" category, have a mean survival of 1.5 years. Intermittent, higher doses of chlorambucil are now used and adrenal corticosteroids are added to enhance the effect. This treatment may confer good symptomatic benefit and usually reduces the counts of circulating malignant cells, but has not been shown to improve survival (Gale and Foon 1985). Until recently, multiple intermittent chemotherapy has not been shown to improve the prognosis in CLL. The tumour masses resolve and the circulating lymphocyte count falls, but the manifestations relapse quite quickly. A French cooperative trial has provided evidence of improved survival in patients with poor prognosis with the use of a regimen containing doxorubicin (French Cooperative Group on Chronic Lymphocytic Leukaemia 1986). Alkylating agents usually fail to produce a significant response in prolymphocytic leukaemia (PLL), and combination therapy also fails. Splenic irradiation may be beneficial, particularly if the differentiation is not so advanced, as indicated by a relatively high percentage of prolymphocytes forming rosettes with mouse erythrocytes, i.e. relatively immature B cells (Oscier et al. 1984). The response to chemotherapy in hairy cell leukaemia (HCL) is usually suboptimal. Splenectomy does not benefit patients with asymptomatic disease but is beneficial in the treatment of deficiencies of circulating erythrocytes, granulocytes and platelets. Chemotherapy before operation increases unduly the risks of surgery.

Removal of the circulating leukaemia cells by leukapheresis or extracorporeal irradiation is of limited benefit in the chronic B cell leukaemias. Besides bringing relatively little relief of symptoms to the patient, removal of vast numbers of cells has a small effect on the numbers of circulating leukaemic cells, because there is rapid replacement and rapid influx from sites of sequestration. It is clearly necessary to influence the production of malignant cells by treatment of the malignant stem cells. It is possible that bone marrow purging of all immunologically recognisable tumour cells could produce a cure.

Dramatic improvement may be obtained with interferon (IFN_α) in HCL, indicating that cytokines may have a profound influence on malignant cells, but the mode of action of interferon in HCL is unknown. The disease could conceivably be sustained by a virus, or the effect of IFN could be on the differentiation block. Differentiation arrest, an attribute of all neoplasms, causes an accumulation of malignant cells at particular stages of differentiation. Treatment causes a striking reduction in the numbers of specific receptors for IFN on circulating hairy cells, which is possibly a manifestation of a shift in the state of differentiation (Billard et al. 1986). A third possibility is that IFN is acting as a so-called biological response modifier, enhancing the host's immune response to the tumour.

These questions can be approached systematically when the stem cells of lymphoid neoplasms can be grown in culture. The requirement for successful culture of the stem cells may be simply the requirement for the appropriate growth factors, of which virtually nothing is known at present. Culture of T cells appeared to be equally difficult until interleukin 2 (IL-2) became available. Conventional treatment and advances in the treatment of CLL have been reviewed recently by Gale and Foon (1985).

Immunotherapy

There is no doubt that cells of an individual's immune system may kill other types of cell in his own body, as occurs in autoimmune disease, yet the emergence of a tumour evidently indicates that the immunological surveillance of tumours developing in his own body has failed. It has been said that immune surveillance is only effective against those tumours which do not develop to a detectable size (Weiss 1984). Immunological defences may not be effective against spontaneous tumours, because these tumours may not have the capacity to express unique antigens, in contrast to the tumours induced by chemical and viral agents. However, new genes that arise by translocation and fusion of chromosomes may result in expression of unique antigens.

Despite the unconvincing arguments supporting the concept of immune surveillance, attempts have been made in the past three or four decades to eliminate tumours by immunological means, through a great variety of approaches. Vaccines have been injected, antibodies from immunised animals have been administered and drugs have been given to stimulate the allegedly flagging immune response. Conceptually, immune responsiveness against tumour antigens may be enhanced by increasing the immunogenicity of a tumour-associated antigen, by, for example, attaching a hapten or by other chemical or physical modification of the tumour antigen used for immunisation. Alternatively, the efficiency of the immune system could be enhanced by biological response modifiers (reviewed by Chirigos and Talmadge 1985). Biological response modifiers are substances that enhance immunological function. They include micro-organisms and compounds isolated from micro-oganisms, synthetic compounds and cytokines. Immunological adjuvants, such as Bacille Calmette-Guérin (BCG), *Corynebacterium parvum* and levamisole have been given to humans as non-specific immune stimulators. The use of these agents has been controversial and definitive proof of benefit is still lacking. Studies in the 1960s of the use of BCG indicated improvement in the duration of the response and the survival of children with acute lymphoblastic leukaemia (ALL).

Monoclonal Antibodies

An alternative to the stimulation of active immune responses against tumours is the administration of antibodies or immunologically competent cells. Early attempts to exploit immunoglobulin as a target for passive immunotherapy were performed with murine plasmacytomas. Anti-idiotypic alloantiserum specific for the immunoglobulin synthesised by the plasmacytoma prolonged survival time in inbred mice, if the antiserum was administered before the mice received the tumour transplant. An ever-present concern of immunotherapy by passive immunisation is enhancement of tumour growth, which can be produced regularly under certain experimental conditions.

There are advantages in using monoclonal antibodies for passive immunotherapy of tumours, the most important being purity. Once a clone has been generated there is no limitation on the supply of the same antibody, which can then be used in multicentre trials throughout the world. Potential obstacles to effective treatment with monoclonal antibodies (Ritz and Schlossman 1982; Kirch 1984b) include:

1. Presence of circulating antigen
2. Antigenic modulation of the target antigen, i.e. change of its expression, without death of the cells
3. Reactivity of antibody with normal cells
4. Immune response to murine immunoglobulin
5. Inefficiency of natural immune effector mechanisms
6. Sparseness of antigen.

If the antigen, e.g. an idiotype, is modulated, it may aggregate on the cell surface, whereupon the cell may be refractory to lysis by anti-idiotypic antibody plus complement. The greatest problem in treating tumours with antibody may be the immunity of the stem cells from which the malignant cells arise, particularly if these stem cells are too immature to express the target antigen. Another problem may be the exhaustion of effector cells, e.g. macrophages, that destroy the malignant cells to which the administered antibody has bound.

T cell neoplasms have been treated with Leu-1 and T101 antibodies of CD5 specificity. The antibody binds to leukaemic T cells, which may disappear from circulation within 2 h of treatment, but malignant cells in the bone marrow are not affected and the circulating T cell count rises to pretreatment levels within 3–4 days (Miller and Levy 1981). Anti-CD5 antibodies do not lyse the target cells in vitro, and better results may be obtained with lytic antibody. Partial responses have been reported in cutaneous and lymph node T cell lymphoma, especially in cutaneous T cell lymphoma (mycosis fungoides) where regressions may occur. Some patients develop an immunological response against mouse antigens after 3 weeks, which neutralises further benefit. Side effects include urticaria, diarrhoea, dyspnoea, cough and hypotension.

For treatment of B cell neoplasms, target antigens can be the B cell-specific antigens of the CD19–22 clusters, or the idiotype expressed by the individual B cell tumour. Remission of chemotherapy-resistant, diffuse, poorly differentiated B cell lymphoma has been achieved with anti-idiotype antibody (Miller et al. 1982). In another study, 1 of 11 patients who received anti-idiotypic antibody has remained in remission for 42 months and 5 others have had remissions of shorter duration (Meeker et al. 1985). High doses of anti-idiotypic antibodies are necessary to achieve remission in B cell tumours which secrete antibody, because the administered antibody is diverted from its target idiotype on the malignant cell by forming complexes with secreted antibody. Plasmapheresis may achieve some reduction of this secreted immunoglobulin in the circulation.

Complement-fixing antibodies reacting with peripheral B cells can be used to eliminate residual lymphoma cells from a patient's bone marrow in vitro ("bone marrow purging") before retransplantation, a procedure which does not damage the haematopoietic stem cells. Before the marrow is harvested, patients are treated with chemotherapy, radiotherapy or both, to induce a minimal disease state with less than 5% involvement of the bone marrow with tumour (Nadler et al. 1984). The marrow is then harvested, treated with the monoclonal antibodies and stored at low temperatures. After the patient has received high-dose cyclophosphamide and whole body radiation, the marrow is reinfused. Haematopoietic regeneration after purging autologous marrow with Y29/55 or CD20 has been rapid (Nadler et al. 1980; Baumgartner et al. 1984). Six of eight patients with relapsed NHL treated by this regimen remained free of disease for 1–18 months (Nadler et al. 1984).

Bone marrow transplantation with heterologous marrow has potential advantages as an alternative to retransplantation of purged autologous marrow, but the problems of heterologous marrow transplantation are considerable. Only 40% of patients have a relative who shares identity at the major histocompatibility complex (MHC). Removal of T cells with soybean agglutinin or by other means reduces markedly the incidence of graft versus host disease, but graft rejection may occur. A monoclonal rat anti-human lymphocyte antibody which triggers human complement to lyse T cells has been used with good effect to deplete bone marrow allografts of donor T cells before transplantation, thereby avoiding graft versus host disease (Waldmann et al. 1984).

Immunotoxins

Diphtheria toxin, abrin, ricin, pokeweed antiviral protein, photoactive dyes and radioisotopes are cell toxins which may be coupled to monoclonal antibodies (reviewed by Uhr 1984; Reisfeld and Cheresh 1985). The most studied of these, ricin, is a protein derived from the castor bean, having two polypeptide chains. The A chain of ricin is a potent toxin which inhibits protein synthesis by inactivating ribosomes after it enters cells. The B chain is a lectin, i.e. a plant protein which binds specifically to sugar residues, in this case galactose residues present on most mammalian cells. Conjugates of monoclonal antibody with the intact ricin molecule appear to be more effective than immunotoxins of antibody-A chain conjugates, which have proved to be unstable and ineffective. The activity of the B chain in whole ricin conjugates can be inhibited by lactose when the immunotoxin is used in vitro, for example in the purging of bone marrow of malignant cells. Studies in mice and rats have shown that such immunotoxins can destroy 99.9% of leukaemic cells in bone marrow with little or no harm to haematopoietic stem cells (Mason et al. 1982), and ricin-antibody conjugates have been considered for purging neoplastic B cells from human bone marrow (Muirhead et al. 1983). Clinical trials of the use of ricin immunotoxin for the purging of bone marrow in acute lymphoblastic leukaemia (ALL) are in progress.

The localisation of a cytotoxic drug may be enhanced by conjugating it with a monoclonal antibody, increasing the anti-tumour effect and reducing the toxicity of the cytotoxic agents to normal tissues (Baldwin and Byers 1986). Since most tumours are heterogeneous in their expression of antigen, a cocktail of antibodies of different specificities may be required for effective treatment. The optimal target antigen is one located primarily on the surface of the tumour cells. The antibody-drug conjugate is internalised and the drug is cleaved from the antibody. Preliminary studies indicate that methotrexate can be coupled to mouse monoclonal antibodies with preservation of their capacity to localise to human tumours such as colorectal cancer and osteogenic sarcoma. Conjugates of antibody with vindesin and Adriamycin have been shown to be effective against human tumour xenografts in immunodeficient mice (Baldwin and Byers 1986). If the drug is linked to a carrier such as human serum albumin and the albumin-drug complex is then linked to the antibody, at least ten times more drug can be linked to the antibody than by direct conjugation. Drugs that are likely to be effective, but are too toxic in the free state, may be used in this way.

Radioisotope-labelled monoclonal antibodies have been investigated extensively as agents for the detection of tumours. Most clinical studies on the localisation of radiolabelled monoclonal antibodies have been carried out in patients with colorectal cancer. One antibody used for this purpose is an antibody to carcinoembryonic antigen. Radioimmunodetection of cancer with radiolabelled monoclonal antibodies has been reviewed by Primus et al. (1984).

Antibodies Against Growth Factor Receptors

The first example of this kind to be used clinically is antibody to CD25, the IL-2 receptor. Anti-CD25 treatment (anti-Tac) has resulted in temporary remission in some patients with adult T cell leukaemia/lymphoma (ATL) (Waldmann et al. 1985).

Adoptive Immunity with Cytotoxic T Cells

Cellular immunity has been manipulated with increasing success in animal models. It is now possible to grow sensitised T cells in vitro and to select out individual clones which react against target cells. Established subcutaneous Moloney virus-induced sarcomas in rats (Fernandez-Cruz et al. 1979, 1980) and Friend virus-induced lymphoma leukaemia in mice (Eberlein et al. 1982) can be eliminated completely by infusion of immune lymphocytes primed in vitro, but a very high ratio of cytotoxic T lymphocytes to tumour cells is necessary for a successful outcome. The lymphocyte populations may be expanded in vitro by culturing in the presence of IL-2. The procedure for obtaining adequate numbers of specifically reactive cytotoxic lymphocytes is arduous (Hirshaut and Slovin 1985). It involves primary sensitisation of T lymphocytes in vitro by exposure to irradiated tumour cells in an environment containing IL-2. Over a thousandfold increase can be achieved in 3 or 4 weeks and it is possible to stimulate the patient's own tumour cells to form clones of cytotoxic lymphocytes which can be infused back into the patient. The biggest problem with this approach has been to obtain enough specifically active cells. Extrapolation from animal models suggests that 10^{10} immune cells are necessary to treat human cancers.

The recent accent in the adoptive immunity approach has been to use the naturally occurring tumour-killing lymphokine-activated killer (LAK) cells, avoiding the need to select specifically sensitised classic cytotoxic T cells (Rayner et al. 1985; Rosenberg 1985; Rosenberg et al. 1985). LAK cells are distinct both from natural killer (NK) cells and classic cytotoxic T cells, requiring the collaboration of macrophages in vivo. Interruption of the function of host macrophages abrogates the anti-tumour effect of LAK cells in experimental models. Infusion of LAK cells has few side effects, mainly fever and chills, but IL-2, which is given to the patients after they have received the infusion of cells, can cause severe fluid retention. Preliminary reports record good remissions (Rosenberg et al. 1985). Of 25 patients, in whom standard therapy had failed, reduction of tumour volume by more than 50% was achieved in 11, and complete regression, lasting at least 10 months, was seen in 1 patient with metastatic melanoma. The latter patient received 4.2×10^{10} LAK cells as well as 47 doses of IL-2.

Recombinant IL-2 has a short half-life in the body — about 4 min after intravenous injection in the mouse and 6 min in humans, as determined in two patients with advanced melanoma (Bindon et al. 1983). IL-2 can reconstitute some functions in T cells from patients with the acquired immunodeficiency syndrome (AIDS) in vitro (Lifson et al. 1984) and is necessary for the action of LAK cells. Commercial development of IL-2 production from human cell lines is proceeding, but published details are few.

Activated Macrophages

Macrophages kill tumour cells in experimental situations (Chirigos and Talmadge 1985). They can be activated to become tumoricidal by immunomodulators, for example by interaction with phospholipid vesicles containing macrophage activating factor (MAF), which is probably IFN_γ. Natural activation of macrophages by micro-organisms can be simulated by muramyl-L-alanyl-D-isoglutamine peptide (MDP), the smallest structure that can replace mycobacteria in Freund's complete adjuvant. Unfortunately, 90% of MDP injected intravenously is excreted in the urine within 1 h. When given encapsulated in liposomes to mice it produces a tumoricidal effect.

Cytokines and Other Biological Agents

Interferon

Interferons are a group of proteins which, as well as possessing antiviral activity, have antiproliferative, differentiation-inducing and immunoregulatory activity. Interferons inhibit the development and growth of virus-induced, transplantable and spontaneous tumours by direct action on malignant cells. There are at least 15 α forms, differing subtly in their amino acid composition. Purified leucocyte IFN_α (Helsinki Red Cross), purified lymphoblastoid IFN_α (Wellcome) and recombinant leucocyte IFN_α from Hoffman-La Roche and Schering Plough have been used in clinical trials. The Wellcome product, named Wellferon, is a mixture of interferons made by cultures of the Namalva malignant B cell line.

The interferons from biological sources are very impure. IFN_α employed in the American Cancer Society Trial (Horning et al. 1985) was 1% pure. Recombinant IFN_α preparations of approximately 95% purity have recently become available for clinical investigation (Gutterman et al. 1982). It is too early to compare the doses required for recombinant material with those required for material from cellular sources.

The side effects of even the highly purified recombinant interferons are profound. These side effects are due to the interferon, not the impurities. They include fever, malaise, an influenza-like syndrome, myalgia and weight loss. There may also be mild haematological toxicity with cytopenias. Severe effects on brain function have been seen, such as mental confusion and loss of speech. Profound neurotoxicity can lead to coma if the administration of the drug is continued. The malaise, fever and other constitutional symptoms may reverse with reduction of dose and may not recur with re-introduction of higher doses of interferons. Acute myelocytic leukaemia has been reported 30 months after treatment in one patient with nodular poorly differentiated lymphoma. Myeloid leukaemia, not being a recognised complication of lymphoma, may have been related to the treatment received.

In a multi-institutional trial of IFN$_\alpha$ in 49 patients with NHL and HD, partial responses were seen in 3 of 18 patients with nodular lymphoma at the highest dose used, 9×10^6 units (Horning et al. 1985). IFN$_\alpha$ was not useful in other subtypes of NHL or HD. The best results appear to have been obtained with recombinant IFN$_\alpha$ at doses five to ten times higher than this, but all reports are preliminary. Treatment was considered particularly effective in advanced refractory cutaneous T cell lymphomas (Bunn et al. 1984). Objective partial remissions lasting from 3 months to more than 25 months were seen in 9 of 20 patients with advanced cutaneous T cell lymphomas treated with recombinant leucocyte interferon (50×10^6 units/m^2 three times weekly).

HCL is the condition in which treatment with IFN has been most uniformly successful (Porzsolt et al. 1985; Quesada et al. 1984; Worman et al. 1985; Billard et al. 1986), with more than 90% of cases responding (Gale and Foon 1985). Partial or complete remissions are induced by doses of IFN too low to give detectable serum levels. After treatment, bone marrow aspirates may show an absence of leukaemic cells or very substantial reduction. Subnormal peripheral blood values may return to normal in patients with anaemia, granulocytopenia, and thrombocytopenia. Relapses occur and continuous substitution may be required to maintain remissions. Both natural IFN$_\alpha$ or recombinant IFN$_{\alpha 2}$ are effective. A small proportion of patients with HCL does not respond to treatment with IFN. So far, no clinical, morphological or phenotypic features have been recognised to distinguish the non-responders.

Reports suggest that IFN provides effective treatment of renal cell carcinoma, chronic myelogenous leukaemia (CML), juvenile laryngeal papillomatosis, bladder papillomas, myeloma, breast cancer, malignant melanoma and Kaposi's sarcoma. Most patients receiving IFN have already had chemotherapy and/or radiotherapy. IFN is not effective in relapsed acute myeloblastic leukaemia (AML). It will be logical to extend the trials to include treatment in combination with cytotoxic agents.

Tumour Necrosis Factor

In 1975, Carswell et al. reported that serum of endotoxin-treated mice, rats and rabbits, previously infected with BCG, caused haemorrhagic necrosis of various tumours in mice with no apparent effect on the host (Carswell et al. 1975). Tumour necrosis factor (TNF) is produced by macrophages in vivo, and induced by bacterial lipopolysaccharide (LPS). The naturally occurring TNFs are glycoproteins (Aggarwal et al. 1985). T cells may also produce TNF or be involved in its production in a helper capacity. A human cell line has been established from peripheral blood lymphocytes which produces TNF. From its product the amino acid sequence was partially determined and with this knowledge a 42 base-long deoxynucleotide was synthesised. This DNA sequence was used as a probe to identify the gene (Pennica et al. 1984). The gene was cloned and a recombinant TNF lacking sugar side chains was produced.

Recombinant TNF lyses some tumour cell lines in vitro and augments the growth of normal fibroblasts. TNF is synergistic with IFN_γ in inhibiting the proliferation of some cell lines (Sugarman et al. 1985). TNF binds to receptors on the plasma membrane and is internalised and degraded, probably within lysosomes (Tsujimoto et al. 1985). Growth of tumour cell lines that have few surface receptors to TNF is not inhibited (Baglione et al. 1985), but some cell types that do have receptors are not affected by TNF (Tsujimoto et al. 1985). No clinical trials have been reported.

Thymic Cytokines

The thymosins (see Table 10.2, p. 117) are a group of polypeptides produced by epithelial cells of the thymus. Their main function is apparently to induce differentiation in thymocytes. They are potentially useful in restoring immunological competence in a variety of situations, including lymphomas and leukaemias of the lymphoid system, although their use in this capacity has hardly been explored.

Thymosin V (thymosin fraction 5) from fetal thymus contains several polypeptides. One of these, $thymosin_{\alpha 1}$, is also available as a synthetic preparation. Thymosin V has been used in immunodeficient children and both thymosin V and $thymosin_{\alpha 1}$ have been tried in cancer patients. Thymosin V treatment has been reported to prolong the survival of patients with oat cell carcinoma of the lung who had achieved a remission with chemotherapy (Cohen et al. 1979). It was considered to cause its effect through restoration of immune deficiency. In patients with autoimmune diseases such as systemic lupus erythematosus and rheumatoid arthritis treated with thymosin V there is a significant increase of circulating T cells and a decrease in null cells. Thymosin V treatment also decreases the level of a cytotoxic factor in the serum of many of these patients that lyses murine thymocytes in the presence of complement. Thymosin V is suspected to induce a subpopulation of suppressor T cells.

Thymopoietin and Facteur Thymique Sérique are under clinical investigation. A biologically active pentapeptide synthesised from thymopoietin has been used with benefit in children suffering from primary T cell defects (Aiuti et al. 1983). A thymic extract designated thymopoietin 1 was reported to increase the proportion of CD4+ cells, nearly normalising the CD4+:CD8+ ratio in B-CLL (Lauria et al. 1984).

New Drugs and Other Treatments

Cyclosporin

Cyclosporin, a metabolite of two soil fungi (reviewed by Cohen et al. 1984), is a cyclic peptide with a molecular weight of 1203. Cyclosporin stops the production of IL-1 by monocytes and IL-2 by helper T cells (reviewed in a Lancet editorial; Editorial 1985). Its effect on T cells is thought to depend on binding to the MHC class II-CD3 molecular complex on T cells. This may interfere with signal transduction, causing complete inhibition of transcription of the gene encoding IL-2 (Krönke et al. 1984). The result is that the expansion of helper T cell population is inhibited, B cells are not activated, cytotoxic T cells are not generated and IFN$_\gamma$ is not produced. Another action is thought to be the expansion of antigen-specific suppressor T cells, despite the fact that this effect normally requires IL-2. Cyclosporin is now known also to block other early events in B cell activation. Cyclosporin seems to enable antigen-specific tolerance to be achieved in vivo. It may not act in vivo in entirely the same way as has been deduced from experiments in vitro (Klaus and Chisholm 1986). T cells can apparently proliferate in vivo in the presence of concentrations of cyclosporin which inhibit production of IL-2 in vitro.

Cyclosporin is selectively cytotoxic to several types of human leukaemic T cells in vitro but not to other types of malignant T cells, including those in T-CLL. Cyclosporin has toxic side effects on the liver, peripheral nerves and central nervous system, causing tremor, and may cause inappropriate growth of hair and enlargement of the gums. It is implicated in causing lymphomas, presumably through severe immunodeficiency (see Chap. 5, p. 56).

Purine and Pyrimidine Analogues

Acyclovir, a purine nucleoside analogue, is a representative of a class of drugs of established therapeutic value which act as false building blocks in DNA and RNA metabolism. Acyclovir establishes the principle that drugs of this class may have a selective action against viruses. 3'-azido-3'-deoxythymidine (AZT) is a new thymidine analogue with potent antiviral activity against HTLV-III (now renamed the human immunodeficiency virus; HIV). In the first clinical study AZT increased the numbers of circulating helper T lymphocytes in 15 of 19 patients with AIDS or the AIDS-related complex. The drug may be taken by mouth and appears to be tolerated well (Yarchoan et al. 1986). The development of drugs of this kind seems therefore to have potential for the treatment of T cell malignancies associated with HTLV-I.

Deoxycoformycin (dCF) is a potent and irreversible inhibitor of adenosine deaminase (ADA), an essential enzyme for purine nucleoside metabolism. An inherited deficiency of this enzyme is related to severe combined immunodeficiency in children affecting both humoral and cellular immunity. Responses to dCF have been reported in both T- and B-CLL (Yu et al. 1981; Grever et al. 1981, 1985).

Hyperthermia

Malignant cells are more sensitive than normal cells to hyperthermia, and tumour cells can be killed selectively by exposure to a raised temperature for a limited time. Hyperthermia should be applicable to the treatment of lymphomas and, via extracorporeal circulation, to the treatment of CLL (Robbins et al. 1984).

Preclinical studies have been made, but no clinical trials have been undertaken. Whole-body hyperthermia is synergistic with whole-body irradiation in the treatment of leukaemia in mice.

Vaccines Against HTLV

As a final note in this catalogue of potentially effective strategies against lymphoid neoplasms, the possibility must be mentioned of developing effective vaccines against those viruses closely associated with the genesis of human cancers. Gene technology may already offer the necessary tools; non-pathogenic genes encoding antigens of the serious microbial pathogens can be inserted into harmless organisms for immunisation. The approach has received a great impetus from the pressing need to combat HIV. Strategies for developing vaccines to HTLV are discussed by Fischinger et al. (1985).

Conclusions

This brief discussion of the current situation in the treatment of malignant diseases of lymphocytes illustrates a number of new approaches that offer hope of substantial improvement of therapy. However, the ultimate victory will be prevention. It is to be hoped that the implementation of effective measures, once the causative factors are known, will not be so difficult as the control of tobacco-related cancers has proved. It may be easier to immunise against a virus such as HTLV-I than to alter lifestyles. The only conceivable way to treat established cancer is to use agents which strike at the fundamental abnormalities of the malignant cells; the abnormalities may well be somewhat different for each kind of cell. While this goal is still not within our grasp, the picture we have of the malignant process is far more comprehensive and credible than it was a few years ago.

   If the emerging concepts of the nature of malignant transformation as a derangement of the genome conferring freedom from normal controls on growth prove to be generally correct, we may be permitted some excitement in the anticipation of possessing agents with greater specificity for their neoplastic targets. Neoplastic lymphocytes are particularly promising in this respect, having idiotypic targets and requiring specific growth factors and cellular interactions for their growth. Agents directed at idiotypes and growth factor receptors are aimed at the products of genes expressed by malignant cells. Another set of agents affecting the function of enzymes is beginning to emerge in step with the better understanding of the enzymes involved in gene expression, in viral replication and nucleic acid synthesis, and in the mechanisms of gene amplification. These agents also have their effect on products of the genes active in malignant cells. Since the principle underlying the specific targetting of genes, DNA hybridisation, is widely used in vitro, it will surely not be long before the genes involved in the disordered growth of malignant cells can themselves be the specific targets in therapy.

References

Aggarwal BB, Kohr WJ, Hass PE et al. (1985) Human tumor necrosis factor. Production purification and characterization. J Biol Chem 260: 2345–2354

Aiuti F, Businco L, Fiorilli M et al. (1983) Thymopoietin pentapeptide treatment of primary immunodeficiencies. Lancet I: 551–555

Baglioni C, McCandless S, Tavernier J, Fiers W (1985) Binding of human tumor necrosis factor to high affinity receptors on HeLa and lymphoid cells sensitive to growth inhibition. J Biol Chem 260: 13395–13397

Baldwin RW, Byers VS (1986) Monclonal antibodies in cancer treatment. Lancet I: 603–605

Baumgartner C, Bleher EA, Brum del Re G et al. (1984) Autologous bone marrow transplantation in the treatment of children and adolescents with advanced malignant tumors. Med Paediatr Oncol 12: 104–111

Billard C, Sigaux F, Castaigne S et al. (1986) Treatment of hairy cell leukemia with recombinant alpha interferon. II. In vivo down-regulation of alpha interferon receptors on tumor cells. Blood 67: 821–826

Bindon C, Czernecki M, Ruell P et al. (1983) Clearance rates and systemic effects of intravenously administered interleukin 2 (IL-2) containing preparations in human subjects. Br J Cancer 47: 123–133

Bunn PA Jr, Foon KA, Ihde DC et al. (1984) Recombinant leukocyte A interferon: an active agent in advanced cutaneous T-cell lymphomas. Ann Intern Med 101: 484–487

Carswell EA, Old LJ, Kassel RI, Green S, Fiore N, Williamson B (1975) An endotoxin-induced serum factor that causes necrosis of tumours. Proc Natl Acad Sci USA 72: 3666–3670

Chirigos MA, Talmadge JE (1985) Immunotherapeutic agents; their role in cellular immunity and their therapeutic potential. Semin Immunopathol 8: 327–346

Cohen DJ, Loertscher R, Rubin MF et al. (1984) Cyclosporine: a new immunosuppressive agent for organ transplantation. Ann Intern Med 101: 667–682

Cohen MH, Chretien PB, Ihde DC et al. (1979) Thymosin fraction V and intensive combination therapy. Prolonging the survival of patients with small cell lung cancer. J Am Med Assoc 241: 1813–1815

De Vita VT, Jaffe ES, Hellman S (1985) Hodgkin's disease and the non-Hodgkin's lymphomas. In: DeVita VT, Hellman S, Rosenberg SA (eds) Cancer. Principles and practice of oncology, 2nd edn. Lippincott, Philadelphia, pp 1623–1709

Eberlein TJ, Rosenstein M, Rosenberg SA (1982) Regression of a disseminated syngeneic solid tumor by systemic transfer of lymphoid cells expanded in interleukin 2. J Exp Med 156: 385–397

Editorial (1985) Cyclosporin in autoimmune disease. Lancet I: 909–911

Fernandez-Cruz E, Halliburton B, Feldman JD (1979) In vivo elimination by specific effector cells of an established syngeneic rat Moloney virus-induced sarcoma. J Immunol 123: 1772–1777

Fernandez-Cruz E, Woda BA, Feldman JD (1980) Elimination of syngeneic sarcomas in rats by a subset of T lymphocytes. J Exp Med 152: 823–841

Fischinger PJ, Robey WG, Koprowski H, Gallo RC, Bolognesi DP (1985) Current status and strategies for vaccines against diseases induced by human T-cell lymphotropic retroviruses (HTLV-I, -II, -III). Cancer Res (Suppl 9) 45: 4694s-4699s

French Cooperative Group on Chronic Lymphocytic Leukaemia (1986) Effectiveness of "CHOP" regimen in advanced untreated chronic lymphocytic leukaemia. Lancet I: 1346–1349

Gale RP, Foon K (1985) Chronic lymphocytic leukemia. Recent advances in biology and treatment. Ann Intern Med 103: 101–120

Grever MR, Wilson HE, Kraut EH et al. (1981) Deoxycoformycin in the treatment of refractory chronic lymphocytic leukemia. Proc Am Assoc Cancer Res 22: 487

Grever MR, Leiby EH, Kraut EH et al. (1985) Low-dose deoxycoformycin in lymphoid malignancy. J Clin Oncol 3: 1196–1201

Gutterman JU, Fine S, Quesada J et al. (1982) Recombinant leukocyte A interferon: pharmacokinetics, single-dose tolerance, and biologic effects in cancer patients. Ann Intern Med 96: 549–556

Hirshaut Y, Slovin SF (1985) Harnessing T-lymphocytes for human cancer immunotherapy. Cancer 56: 1366–1373

Horning SJ, Merigan TC, Krown S et al. (1985) Human interferon α in malignant lymphoma and Hodgkin's disease. Results of the American Cancer Society Trial. Cancer 56: 1305–1310

Hu E, Trela M, Thompson J et al. (1985) Detection of B-cell lymphoma in peripheral blood by DNA hybridization. Lancet II: 1092–1095

Kirch ME (1984) Approaches to cancer therapy using monoclonal antibodies. In: Wright GL (ed) Monoclonal antibodies and cancer. (Immunology Series 23.) Marcel Dekker, New York, pp 325–360

Klaus GGB, Chisholm PM (1986) Does cyclosporine act *in vivo* as it does *in vitro*? Immunol Today 7: 100-103

Krönke M, Leonard WJ, Depper JM et al. (1984) Cyclosporin A inhibits T-cell growth factor gene expression at the level of mRNA transcription. Proc Natl Acad Sci (USA) 81: 5214–5218

Lauria F, Raspadori D, Tura S (1984) Effect of a thymic factor on T lymphocytes in B cell chronic lymphocytic leukemia: in vitro and in vivo studies. Blood 64: 667–671

Lifson JD, Benike CJ, Mark DF, Koths K, Engelman EG (1984) Human recombinant interleukin-2 partly reconstitutes deficient in-vitro immune responses of lymphocytes from patients with AIDS. Lancet I: 698–702

Mason DW, Thorpe PE, Ross WCJ (1982) Elimination of leukemic cells from rodent bone marrow *in vitro* with antibody ricin conjugates: implications for autologous bone marrow transplantation in man. Cancer Surv 1: 389

Meeker TC, Loweder J, Maloney DG et al. (1985) A clinical trial of anti-idiotype therapy for B cell malignancy. Blood 65: 1349–1363

Miller RA, Levy R (1981) Response of cutaneous T cell lymphoma to therapy with hybridoma monoclonal antibody. Lancet II: 226–230

Miller RA, Maloney DG, Warnke R, Levy R (1982) Treatment of B-cell lymphoma with monoclonal anti-idiotype antibody. N Engl J Med 306: 517–522

Muirhead M, Martin PJ, Torok-Storb B, Uhr JW, Vitetta ES (1983) Use of antibody-ricin A-chain conjugate to delete neoplastic B cells from bone marrow. Blood 62: 327–332

Nadler LM, Stashenko P, Hardy R et al. (1980) Serotherapy of a patient with a monoclonal antibody directed against a human lymphoma-associated antigen. Cancer Res 40: 3147–3154

Nadler LM, Takvorian T, Botnick L et al. (1984) Anti-B1 monoclonal antibody and complement treatment in autologous bone-marrow transplantation for relapsed B-cell non-Hodgkin's lymphoma. Lancet II: 427–431

Oscier DG, Catovsky D, Errington RD et al. (1984) Splenic irradiation in B-prolymphocytic leukaemia. Br J Haematol 48: 577–584

Pennica D, Nedwin GE, Hayflick JS et al. (1984) Human tumour necrosis factor; precursor structure, expression and homology to lymphotoxin. Nature 312: 724–729

Porzsolt F, Thomä J, Unsöld M et al. (1985) Platelet-adjusted IFN dosage in the treatment of advanced hairy cell leukemia. Blut 51: 73–82

Primus FJ, DeLand FH, Goldenberg DM (1984) Monoclonal antibodies for the detection of cancer. In: Wright GL (ed) Monoclonal antibodies and cancer. (Immunology Series 23.). Marcel Dekker, New York, pp 305–323

Quesada JR, Reuben J, Manning JT, Hersh EM, Gutterman JU (1984) Alpha interferon for induction of remission in hairy cell leukemia. N Engl J Med 310: 15–18

Rayner AA, Grimm EA, Lotze MT, Chu EW, Rosenberg SA (1985) Lymphokine-activated killer (LAK) cells. Analysis of factors relevant to the immunotherapy of human cancer. Cancer 55: 1327–1333

Reisfeld RA, Cheresh DA (1985) Human tumour-associated antigens: targets for monoclonal antibody-mediated cancer therapy. Cancer Surv 4: 271–299

Ritz J, Schlossman SF (1982) Utilisation of monoclonal antibodies in the treatment of leukemia and lymphoma. Blood 59: 1–11

Robbins IH, Dennis WH, Steeves RA, Sondel PM (1984) A proposal for the addition of hyperthermia to treatment regimens for acute and chronic leukemia. J Clin Oncol 2: 1050–1056

Rosenberg SA (1985) Lymphokine-activated killer cells: a new approach to immunotherapy of cancer. J Natl Cancer Inst 75: 595–603

Rosenberg SA, Lotze MT, Muul LM et al. (1985) Observations on the systemic administration of autologous lymphokine-activated killer cells and recombinant interleukin-2 to patients with metastatic cancer. N Engl J Med 313: 1485–1492

Sugarman BJ, Aggarwal BB, Hass PE et al. (1985) Recombinant human tumour necrosis factor-alpha: effects on proliferation of normal and transformed cells in vitro. Science 230: 943–945

Tsujimoto M, Yip YK, Vilcek J (1985) Tumor necrosis factor: specific binding and internalisation in sensitive and resistant cells. Proc Natl Acad Sci USA 82: 7626–7630

Uhr JW (1984) Immunotoxins: harnessing nature's poisons. J Immunol 133: i–x

Waldmann H, Polliak A, Hale G et al. (1984) Elimination of graft-versus-host disease by in-vitro depletion of alloreactive lymphocytes with a monclonal rat anti-human lymphocyte antibody (CAMPATH-1). Lancet II: 483–486

Waldmann TA, Davis MM, Bongiovanni KF, Korsmeyer SJ, (1985) Rearrangements of genes for the antigen receptor on T cells as markers of lineage and clonality in human lymphoid neoplasms. N Engl J Med 313: 776–783

Weiss DW (1984) Reflections on tumour origin, immunogenicity and immunotherapy. Cancer Immunol Immunother 18: 1–4

Worman CP, Catovsky D, Bevan PC et al. (1985) Interferon is effective in hairy cell leukaemia. Br J Haematol 60: 759–763

Yarchoan R, Klecker RW, Weinhold KJ et al. (1986) Administration of 3'-azido-3'-deoxythymidine, an inhibitor of HIV/LAV replication, to patients with AIDS or AIDS-related complex. Lancet I: 575–580

Yu A, Bakay B, Matsumoto S et al. (1981) The effects of deoxycoformycin (dCF) on T-cell chronic lymphocytic leukemia (CLL). Proc Am Assoc Cancer Res 22: 226

Glossary

ADCC Cytotoxicity mediated by a subclass of lymphocytes which recognise target cells via specific antibody

Adenine Organic base, building block of DNA and RNA

Allele Alternative version of a gene, occupying the same locus

Alloantigen Foreign cell surface antigenic determinant

Allosteric Refers to proteins with the capacity to undergo reversible change in conformation determined by occupation of binding sites by ligand or the formation of other chemical bonds

Allotype Product of an allele. Inherited variant of a particular molecule

Amino acid Building block of peptides and proteins. Twenty different amino acids are found in proteins in nature. The genetic information for the sequence of amino acids in proteins is encoded in DNA base triplets

Autologous Belonging to the organism in question

Autosomes Chromosomes other than the X or Y sex chromosomes

Avidity The power with which an antibody combines with its antigen

Banding Use of special techniques to demonstrate banded structure of chromosomes, and identify the individual bands. Banding usually involves fluorescent staining with quinacrine and/or treatment with trypsin before Giemsa staining (trypsin-Giemsa banding)

Bases Building blocks of nucleic acid: adenine (A), cytosine (C), guanine (G) and thymine (T) in DNA; A, G, C and uracil (U) in RNA

Bence Jones protein Immunoglobulin light chains in blood and urine of patients with multiple myeloma and other lymphoproliferative diseases

Bursa of Fabricius Lymphoepithelioid organ of birds at the junction of the hindgut and cloaca in which B cells are generated

Capping Redistribution of molecules of the same type to one part of the surface of a lymphocyte

Capsid The protein coat or shell of a virus

Carcinogenesis The process of development of cancer

Cell cycle The process cell division. This is divided into four major stages: G_1 (first growth phase); S (DNA synthesis); M (mitosis); and G_2 (second growth phase)

Clone   A family of genetically identical cells, derived from the same cell

Cold agglutinin   Antibody which agglutinates erythrocytes bearing target antigen at temperatures below 37° C only

Congenic inbred strain   Strains bred to differ by a small part of the genome, preferably at one genetic locus

Cyclophosphamide   Cytotoxic drug

Cyclosporin   Drug used for immunosuppression

Cytokine   Generic name for lymphokines, monokines or other cell products influencing the behaviour of other cells involved in immunological mechanisms (excluding hormones and other metabolites)

Cytosine   Organic base, building block of DNA

Cytotoxic   Having the capacity to kill cells

Deletion   Consistent loss of the same portion of a specific chromosome

Deoxyribose   Sugar molecule, building block of DNA, not RNA

DNA   Genetic material of all living creatures. Consists of two strands, coupled by base pairing and wound into a double helix. The sequence of the four building blocks (nucleotides) determines the sequences of amino acids. The code is read in triplets. The bases are adenine, thymine, guanine and cytosine

Domain   A segment of a protein possessing a distinct, compact shape

Down regulation   Reduction in number of receptors resulting from binding of specific ligand

Enhancer   DNA segment which, when activated, influences the transcription of DNA at a distance

env   A viral gene encoding the envelope glycoproteins

Envelope   Viral outer membrane containing lipid and protein. The lipids are the same as in the plasma membrane of mammalian cell and the proteins are specific for the virus

Epitope   A single antigenic determinant on a molecule, which will combine with a particular site on antibody or T cell receptor

Exon   Segment of a gene coding for protein, interrupted by introns

Fc   Segment of immunoglobulin molecule by which it binds to cell receptors specific for it, and to the C1q component of complement

Freund's adjuvant   Mixture containing oil and *Mycobacterium tuberculosis* into which antigen is emulsified for enhancement of the immune response

gag   A viral gene coding for the group-specific antigens which are the internal structural proteins of the virus

Gene   Set of adjacent nucleotides specifying the amino acid sequence of a polypeptide chain

Genome   The total complement of genes of a cell

Genotype   The characteristics encoded in the genome. These are not necessarily expressed (i.e. not necessarily observable) in the phenotype

Germline   Genotype in the undifferentiated cell

Haplotype   Set of genes on a single chromosome, as inherited from one parent

Hapten   A small molecule capable of combining with antibody but not capable of evoking an antibody response when injected alone. If chemically bonded to a large unrelated protein molecule, "carrier", a hapten will evoke an immune response

Heterologous   Of another species

Homologous   Of the same species

Hybridisation   When used in molecular biology, refers to the binding of two single complementary strands of DNA by base pairing, similarly DNA to RNA

Hybridoma   A cell line arising by fusion of a B lymphocyte with a malignant plasma cell line, producing a single protein, e.g. monoclonal antibody or lymphokine

Idiotope   A single antigenic determinant on the variable region of a specific antibody molecule

Idiotype   Set of idiotopes on an antibody molecule

Inbred strain   A strain in which members of the same sex are genetically identical

Initiation   Initial step in carcinogenesis involving a subtle permanent alteration of the genome

Intron   A sequence of DNA containing information not encoded into protein, interrupting protein-encoding sequences (exons). Introns and exons are transcribed, and then the intron regions are cut out of the RNA

Isoantibody   An antibody that reacts with antigen in another member of the same species, e.g. blood group antibody

Isologous   Of identical genetic constitution

Karyotype   Chromosome complement of an individual cell. This is obtained by spreading cells at metaphase, staining and photography. The karyotype is obtained by arrangement of the chromosomes in pairs according to the Paris convention

Kupffer cell   Phagocytic cells lining sinusoids of the liver

Leukotrienes   Locally acting metabolites of arachidonic acid having powerful metabolic effects

Ligand   A molecule with the capacity to bind to another (usually designated the receptor)

Linkage   Close proximity of two genes on a chromosome. Individual chromosomes are inherited after breakage and rejoining of parental chromosomes. Linked genes are close together and are highly likely to be inherited together

Lipopolysaccharide   Constituent of cell walls of many Gram negative bacteria

Locus   Position of a gene on a chromosome

Lymphokine   Molecule produced by lymphocytes affecting the metabolism of other cells involved in immunological responses

Monoclonal   Derived from a single cell

Monokine   Product of mononuclear phagocytes (monocytes and macrophages) which influences the behaviour of other cells involved in immunological responses

Monosomy   Consistent loss of the same whole chromosome

Mutation   Alteration of the genome (damage to DNA bases, DNA strands, or addition, deletion, translocation or transposition of chromosome structure) usually affecting its coding or expression of a gene product

Nucleotide   Building block of the nucleic acids, consisting of a sugar (deoxyribose for DNA, ribose for RNA), phosphoric acid residue and an organic base (adenine, thymine, guanine, cytosine, uracil)

Nude mouse   Species genetically lacking a thymus, as well as carrying a gene which produces a defect in production of hair

Phenotype   Detectable products of the genotype. Characteristics of a cell or individual

Phytohaemagglutinin   T cell mitogen derived from red kidney beans

Plasmid   Ring form of DNA in bacteria carrying information, amongst other, for antibiotic resistance. Plasmids can be replicated in bacteria independently from the other DNA. In gene technology foreign DNA can be built into plasmids for replication

pol   A viral gene coding for reverse transcriptase (RNA polymerase), the viral polymerase

Polyclonal   Applying to cells deriving from (genetically) different ancestors

Polyclonal B cell activator (PBA)   Agent which can induce partial or complete activation of B cells polyclonally, i.e. irrespective of the antibody specificity of the B cell

Promoter   A starting signal on DNA for the beginning of RNA synthesis. To begin RNA synthesis, RNA polymerase binds to the promoter

Provirus   Virus integrated into host chromosome

Rearrangement   When applied to T and B lymphocytes, the translocation, insertion and excision of genetic material involved in expression of the T cell receptor or Ig during development of T and B cells. It is detected by alteration of the size of the restriction fragment which is detected by a specific probe by the Southern blotting technique

Recombination   The process of rearrangement of the genetic material which occurs during meiosis

Restriction enzyme   Enzyme cutting a DNA strand at a specific point, e.g. EcoR1 cuts at the sequence GAATC. Bacterial restriction enzymes normally function to defend micro-organisms against foreign DNA

Restriction fragment length polymorphism (RFLP)   Difference in length of DNA fragments bearing a gene excised by a restriction enzyme. This indicates that the genes bear a different relationship to the genome, e.g. may be in different sites

Ribosomes   Bodies in the cytoplasm on which a protein chain is formed by joining amino acids according to the sequence dictated by messenger RNA

RNA   Ribonucleic acid. Nucleic acid complementary to DNA acting as code for synthesis of proteins. Bases are adenine, guanine, cytosine and uracil. (*See* Transcription)

RNA polymerase   Also known as reverse transcriptase. An enzyme initiating the transcription process after binding to a specificic DNA sequence called a promoter (q.v.), that signals where RNA synthesis should begin

Somatic   Pertaining to the cells of the body other than the germ cells

Syngeneic   Of (virtually) identical genetic constitution, as in member of an inbred strain produced by continuous brother-sister mating

Tolerance   State of immunological unresponsiveness to a specific antigen

Transcription   Transfer of genetic information of DNA into messenger RNA. The DNA strands part, and then particular enzymes synthesise a complementary RNA strand according to the rules of base pairing

Transfection   DNA-mediated gene transfer into cells. Insertion of genes from one cell or group of cells into another population of cells

Translation   Production of protein on ribosomes according to the sequence encoded in messenger RNA

Translocation   Transfer of material from one chromosome to another. This is often reciprocal

Trisomy   Presence of three instead of two chromosomes of any given chromosome number

Xenogeneic   Referring to a different species, particularly with respect to antigenic differences

Subject Index

Terms with abbreviations are indexed under the full name and not the abbreviation.
For entries that extend over more than one page, only the first page number is given.